Pediatric Oncology

Each volume of the series "Pediatric Oncology" covers the whole spectrum of the disease concerned, from research issues to clinical management, and is edited by internationally highly respected experts in a comprehensive and clearly structured way. The user-friendly layout allows quick reference to in-depth information. The series is designed for all health-care personnel interested in high-level education in pediatric oncology.

James H. Feusner • Caroline A. Hastings
Anurag K. Agrawal

Editors

Supportive Care in Pediatric Oncology

A Practical Evidence-Based Approach

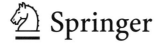 Springer

Editors
James H. Feusner
Hematology/Oncology
Children's Hospital and Research
Center Oakland
Oakland, CA
USA

Anurag K. Agrawal
Hematology/Oncology
Children's Hospital and Research
Center Oakland
Oakland, CA
USA

Caroline A. Hastings
Hematology/Oncology
Children's Hospital and Research
Center Oakland
Oakland, CA
USA

ISSN 1613-5318   ISSN 2191-0812   (electronic)
ISBN 978-3-662-44316-3   ISBN 978-3-662-44317-0   (eBook)
DOI 10.1007/978-3-662-44317-0
Springer Heidelberg New York Dordrecht London

Library of Congress Control Number: 2014959419

Springer is part of Springer Science+Business Media (www.springer.com)

Preface

Many of the gains in overall survival in pediatric oncology over the past 50 years have come about through the utilization of combination chemotherapy, pioneered by the work done at the National Institutes of Health by Freireich and Frei and St. Jude Children's Hospital by Pinkel in children with acute lymphoblastic leukemia (ALL) (Pearson 2002). The ALL model was subsequently expanded to the management of other pediatric malignancies through the utilization of a multimodal approach including chemotherapy, radiation therapy and surgery (Pearson 2002). Due to smaller numbers as compared to the adult cohort, advances in therapy required the utilization of cooperative group studies to develop common therapeutic protocols and secondarily assess therapy effectiveness and toxicities. The modern advancement of these early initiatives has been the utilization of hematopoietic stem cell transplantation (HSCT) in certain pediatric malignancies which are refractory or recurrent where HSCT has been shown beneficial.

Underlying the gains in survival through the progression of therapy intensiveness has been the supportive care of pediatric patients with malignancies. Many of the early pioneers found that children were able to handle intensive therapies but needed the appropriate environment as well as supportive care measures to prevent infection and treat complications of therapy such as thrombocytopenia (with subsequent bleeding), tumor lysis syndrome (with metabolic complications) and infection. Again taking the ALL model, the newest drugs to be commonly utilized were developed in the mid-1980s, stressing that the improvement in cure has come about through changing the timing and intensity of known drugs as well as through improvements in supportive care. For ALL, decrease in both relapse/disease progression and treatment-related death prior to relapse/disease progression have significantly contributed to the gains in overall survival (Gaynon et al. 2010; Hunger et al. 2012).

Supportive care refers to the standard of care to support a child or adolescent during the active treatment process. The art and science of anticipating, preventing and managing treatment-related complications and toxicities vary considerably by individual experience and institutional practice. The editors have chosen the topics in this book to represent some of the most common and significant challenges impacting the success of treatment for our patients, recognizing many more areas are in need of future consideration. We have asked the authors to provide an evidence-based approach utilizing a standard grading system (Table 1) in management of common complications and toxicities as well as reporting practice based on consensus guidelines and institutional experience when validated data are lacking (Guyatt et al. 2006). The chapters

Table 1 Grading recommendations

Grade of recommendation/description	Benefit versus risk and burdens	Methodological quality of supporting evidence	Implications
1A/strong recommendation, high-quality evidence	Benefits clearly outweigh risk and burdens, or vice versa	RCTs without important limitations or overwhelming evidence from observational studies	Strong recommendation, can apply to most patients in most circumstances without reservation
1B/strong recommendation, moderate-quality evidence	Benefits clearly outweigh risk and burdens, or vice versa	RCTs with important limitations (inconsistent results, methodological flaws, indirect, or imprecise) or exceptionally strong evidence from observational studies	Strong recommendation, can apply to most patients in most circumstances without reservation
1C/strong recommendation, low-quality or very low-quality evidence	Benefits clearly outweigh risk and burdens, or vice versa	Observational studies or case series	Strong recommendation but may change when higher quality evidence becomes available
2A/weak recommendation, high-quality evidence	Benefits closely balanced with risks and burdens	RCTs without important limitations or overwhelming evidence from observational studies	Weak recommendation, best action may differ depending on circumstances or patients' or societal values
2B/weak recommendation, moderate-quality evidence	Benefits closely balanced with risks and burdens	RCTs with important limitations (inconsistent results, methodological flaws, indirect, or imprecise) or exceptionally strong evidence from observational studies	Weak recommendation, best action may differ depending on circumstances or patients' or societal values
2C/weak recommendation, low-quality or very low-quality evidence	Uncertainty in the estimates of benefits, risks, and burdens; benefits, risks, and burdens may be closely balanced	Observational studies or case series	Very weak recommendations; other alternatives may be equally reasonable

RCT randomized controlled trial
With permission from Guyatt et al. (2006)

herein provide tools for recognition, assessment, and effective management of commonly encountered emergencies and treatment complications for pediatric oncology patients.

The editors would like to acknowledge the contribution of the authors, our colleagues at Children's Hospital and Research Center Oakland and the editorial staff at Springer-Verlag in preparation of this book as well as the numerous patients and families that we have had the privilege of joining on their unique cancer journeys. We have invited leading experts in the field and encouraged them to mentor young investigators to contribute to this book.

Oakland, CA, USA   James H. Feusner
                                                                          Caroline A. Hastings
                                                                          Anurag K. Agrawal

References

Gaynon PS, Angiolillo AL, Carroll WL et al (2010) Long-term results of the children's cancer group studies for childhood acute lymphoblastic leukemia 1983–2002: a Children's Oncology Group report. Leukemia 24:286–297

Guyatt G, Gutterman D, Baumann MH et al (2006) Grading strength of recommendations and quality of evidence in clinical guidelines: report from an American College of Chest Physicians task force. Chest 129:174–181

Hunger SP, Lu X, Devidas M et al (2012) Improved survival for children and adolescents with acute lymphoblastic leukemia between 1990 and 2005: a report from the Children's Oncology Group. J Clin Oncol 30:1663–1669

Pearson HA (2002) History of pediatric hematology oncology. Pediatr Res 52:979–992

Contents

Febrile Neutropenia

1

Blanca E. Gonzalez, Linda S. Cabral,
and Jeffery J. Auletta

Contents

B.E. Gonzalez, MD
Center for Pediatric Infectious Diseases,
Cleveland Clinic,
Cleveland, OH, USA

L.S. Cabral, PAC
Pediatric Blood and Marrow Transplant Program,
Rainbow Babies and Children's Hospital,
Cleveland, OH, USA

J.J. Auletta, MD (✉)
Host Defense Program,
Hematology/Oncology/BMT and Infectious Diseases,
Nationwide Children's Hospital,
700 Children's Drive, ED557,
Columbus, OH 43205, USA
e-mail: jeffery.auletta@nationwidechildrens.org

Abstract

Febrile neutropenia (FN) is a common, potentially life-threatening complication in pediatric oncology patients due to deficiencies in both innate and adaptive immunity usually secondary to treatment of the underlying malignancy. Although a majority of oncology patients experience FN, large randomized controlled trials to determine appropriate management strategies in pediatric FN are lacking and much of the decision-making process is based on extrapolation of adult guidelines, consensus pediatric guidelines, and institutional protocols. Here we review the relevant literature focusing on available models for risk stratification, appropriate diagnostic evaluations, applicable empiric therapies as well as proper location, timing, and duration of such therapies.

J. Feusner et al. (eds.), *Supportive Care in Pediatric Oncology:
A Practical Evidence-Based Approach*, Pediatric Oncology,
DOI 10.1007/978-3-662-44317-0_1, © Springer Berlin Heidelberg 2015

1.1   Introduction

Febrile neutropenia (FN) is a life-threatening complication of cancer therapy. FN is a medical emergency that requires thorough patient evaluation and prompt initiation of broad-spectrum empiric antibiotics. Fever is defined as a single oral temperature $\geq$38.3 °C (101.0 °F) or an oral temperature $\geq$38.0 °C (100.4 °F) that is sustained for >1 h (Freifeld et al. 2011). Recent consumption of hot or cold beverages should not be a factor if these thresholds are met. Temperatures taken via alternate routes including axillary, otic, and temporal should be discouraged but all are considered real if fever is documented by these modes. Families should be advised against rectal temperatures due to the potential underlying neutropenia. Clinically significant neutropenia in the context of FN is an absolute neutrophil count (ANC) <0.5×10^9/L or ANC <1.0×10^9/L that is expected to decrease to <0.5×10^9/L over the subsequent 48 h. Profound neutropenia is defined as ANC $\leq$$0.1 \times 10^9$/L, while prolonged neutropenia is defined as neutropenia lasting >7 days (Freifeld et al. 2011). Neutropenia decreases the patient's ability to resolve infection in the background of anticancer treatment, which may alter both innate (natural protection barriers such as the skin and mucous membranes) and adaptive (pathogen specific B and T cell) immunity, predisposing the child to common pathogens as well as opportunistic infections (Lehrnbecher et al. 1997).

Despite thorough investigation, pathogens are identified in only approximately 15–30 % of FN episodes (Rackoff et al. 1996; Baorto et al. 2001; Duncan et al. 2007; Bakhshi et al. 2008; Stabell et al. 2008; Wicki et al. 2008; Meckler and Lindemulder 2009). Bacteremia is the most common cause of microbiologically documented infection in pediatric oncology patients with FN, particularly in patients who have received intensive therapy for hematologic malignancies (Castagnola et al. 2007). Gram-positive bacteria like coagulase-negative *Staphylococci* are the most common isolates (Zinner 1999; Duncan et al. 2007). However, Gram-negative bacteria are also common, particularly in patients with significant mucositis, and are associated with higher mortality (Aledo et al. 1998). Fungi are isolated less frequently and occur most often in patients with prolonged and profound neutropenia (Freifeld et al. 2011). Although a majority of oncology patients experience FN, large randomized controlled trials to determine appropriate management strategies in pediatric FN are lacking and much of the decision-making process is based on extrapolation of adult guidelines, consensus pediatric guidelines, and institutional protocols. Here we review the relevant literature focusing on available models for risk stratification, appropriate diagnostic evaluations, applicable empiric therapies as well as proper location, timing, and duration of such therapies. A grading of evidence-based recommendations is presented in Table 1.1.

1.2   History and Physical Examination

Critical assessment of the child with FN begins by obtaining a complete medical history and performing a thorough physical examination. This initial assessment will direct initial risk stratification and subsequent diagnostic evaluations (Table 1.2). It is important to inquire about the characteristics and height of the fever as temperature >39.0 °C has been noted as an independent risk factor for serious bacterial infection, and children (mainly inpatient) with a median fever of 39.4 °C have been reported to be at significantly increased risk of viridans streptococcal shock syndrome with underlying viridans strep bacteremia (Klaassen et al. 2000; Gassas et al. 2004). Fever may be the only sign of infection given the blunted inflammatory response associated with neutropenia. One must inquire about the presence of rigors or chills with central line flushing, recent therapy (potential for prolonged neutropenia), current medications (including antibiotic

Table 1.1 Graded recommendations for management of pediatric febrile neutropenia

Clinical scenario	Recommendation	Level of evidence[a]
Risk stratification	Must be individualized at local institutions due to lack of evidence to support the needs of each individual treatment area	2C
Baseline laboratory recommendations	CBC/diff to assess level of neutropenia and monocytopenia in addition to other cytopenias; CMP for potential drug interactions; CVC culture or peripheral culture if no CVC; viral studies if symptomatic and appropriate season	1B
Utilization of DTP at FN presentation	Peripheral blood cultures in addition to CVC cultures can be done at the discretion of individual institutions but may not impact management	2C
Baseline imaging	Not recommended except CXR if with respiratory symptoms	1B
Antibiotic management at FN presentation in the clinically stable patient	Monotherapy with piperacillin/tazobactam, cefepime, or carbapenem; based on institutional preference, initial dual therapy with an antipseudomonal cephalosporin plus aminoglycoside (e.g., ceftazidime + tobramycin) can also be considered; aminoglycosides may be preferably administered once daily; initial antibiotic therapy should not include vancomycin unless there is concern for a Gram-positive infection due to such findings as sepsis, severe mucositis, skin infection, pneumonia or recent high-dose cytarabine administration	1A
Location of FN management	All patients should initially be managed as inpatients; if early discharge is considered, a multidisciplinary approach to determine appropriate risk stratification and outpatient therapy is required with IRB approval of such a prospective study to ensure safety and efficacy; patients identified as low risk may be discharged after 48 h per protocol if stable and without microbiologic-documented infection	1B
Management of low-risk patients	Empiric antibiotic therapy may be discontinued after 48 h if the patient is afebrile ≥24 h with signs of bone marrow recovery; patients may also be discharged after 72 h if afebrile ≥24 h even without signs of bone marrow recovery if close follow-up is ensured based on institutional preference	1B
Management of high-risk patients	Antibiotic therapy should be continued until resolution of FN episode	1A
FN ≥5 days	Empiric CT of the chest ± sinuses can be considered to rule out occult fungal infection; serial galactomannan can be considered	1C
FN ≥5 days in high-risk patients	Empiric antifungal therapy can be considered; appropriate empiric antifungal agent is unclear and must be chosen based on institutional preference; preemptive management may also be considered on a local basis as there is unclear evidence that prophylaxis prevents IFI	1C

CBC complete blood count, *CMP* complete metabolic panel, *CVC* central venous catheter, *DTP* differential time to positivity, *FN* febrile neutropenia, *CXR* chest radiography, *IRB* institutional review board, *CT* computed tomography, *IFI* invasive fungal infection
[a]Per Guyatt et al. (2006); see Preface

prophylaxis), and possible infectious exposures at home and school as well as recent travel (Orudjev and Lange 2002). Additional history should focus on community outbreaks of specific pathogens (i.e., respiratory viruses), prior history of fevers and documented infections, and pathogen colonization (e.g., methicillin-resistant *Staphylococcus aureus* [MRSA],

Table 1.2 Diagnostic evaluation based upon organ system involvement and physical findings

Organ system	Physical findings	Diagnostic evaluation based upon physical finding(s)
Head, ears, nose, and throat	Mucositis Thrush Oral lesions Pre-septal/orbital cellulitis Facial pain Rhinorrhea Otorrhea	HSV, VZV, *Enterovirus/Parechovirus* PCR/DFA/viral culture (PCR preferred) Biopsy unusual oral lesions (histology and microbiology) CT scan of the sinuses, orbits, temporal bones (obtain sample) Sinus drainage sample if able to perform and send for bacterial, fungal, and viral culture Nasopharyngeal secretions for respiratory viral culture/antigen panel and PCR
Respiratory	Cough/respiratory distress Hypoxemia Chest radiograph infiltrates	CT chest *Legionella* urine antigen PCP evaluation: BAL, (1,3)-β-D-glucan, LDH Sputum culture if able to perform *Aspergillus* galactomannan, (1,3)-β-D-glucan *Histoplasma* urine and serum antigen
Vascular access sites	Exit site/tunnel erythema or discharge	Blood culture from all ports (consider bacteria, fungus, mycobacteria) Gram stain and culture (bacteria, fungal) exit site discharge
Gastrointestinal	Diarrhea Perirectal pain Abdominal pain	*C. difficile* PCR Viral stool culture/PCR (adenovirus, norovirus, etc.) SSYC and/or O&P if exposure by history Ultrasound or CT abdomen/pelvis Liver function test, amylase, lipase
Skin	Rash Cellulitis	DFA/PCR/viral culture of vesicular lesion Dermatology evaluation and biopsy of cellulitis or undiagnosed rash/lesion and send for culture (bacterial, fungal, and atypical mycobacteria)
Musculoskeletal	Arthritis Limp/point tenderness Lower back pain	Arthrocentesis: fluid for cell count and differential, cultures for bacteria, fungus, and mycobacteria CT/MRI extremity or site Urine culture (bacteria, fungal, consider adenovirus, BK, CMV PCR)
Central nervous system	Change in mental status Headache	CT/MRI brain (consider MRA/V) Lumbar puncture: cell count, bacterial and fungal stain and culture, viral PCR (consider CMV, EBV, *Enterovirus*, HHV-6, HSV, VZV)

HSV herpes simplex virus, *VZV* varicella zoster virus, *DFA* direct fluorescence antibody, *CT* computed tomography, *PCR* polymerase chain reaction, *PCP Pneumocystis jiroveci (carinii)* pneumonia, *BAL* bronchoalveolar lavage, *LDH* lactate dehydrogenase, *SSYC Salmonella, Shigella, Yersinia, Campylobacter, O&P* ova and parasites, *MRI* magnetic resonance imaging, *CMV* cytomegalovirus, *MRA/V* magnetic resonance arterio/venogram, *EBV* Epstein-Barr virus, *HHV-6* human herpesvirus-6

vancomycin-resistant *Enterococcus* [VRE]). A comprehensive review of each organ system is important to determine possible etiologies of the fever. The physical exam should be thorough and not focus only on common sites of infection unique to the febrile neutropenic child (i.e., oral and perirectal mucosa, central venous access sites), but rather on all sites of common childhood infection such as the ears, throat, and skin (Auletta et al. 1999). Information obtained from the review of systems and physical findings will direct laboratory and ancillary evaluations and influence the choice of antimicrobial therapy.

1.3 Defining the Risk for Serious Infection

Risk stratification for serious infection incorporates the following variables: presenting clinical signs and symptoms, underlying cancer diagnosis and remission status, type of antitumor therapy received, and medical comorbidities (Orudjev and Lange 2002; Paganini et al. 2007; Freifeld et al. 2011). Sepsis signs and symptoms, presence of a central venous access device (CVAD), mucositis, infant acute lymphoblastic leukemia (ALL), acute myelogenous leukemia (AML), induction or intensification chemotherapy, and leukemia in relapse have all been shown to increase infection-related morbidity and mortality in pediatric patients and should be regarded as high-risk features at initial FN presentation (Orudjev and Lange 2002; Wicki et al. 2008; Badiei et al. 2011). Social factors including history of noncompliance and distance >1 h from clinical facility must be considered high-risk conditions (Orudjev and Lange 2002; Paganini et al. 2007). Paganini et al. (2007) showed that advanced disease stage, bacteremia, and associated comorbities including persistent bleeding, refractory hypoglycemia, hypotension, altered mental status, renal insufficiency and hepatic dysfunction were independent risk factors for mortality.

The Multinational Association for Supportive Care in Cancer (MASCC) risk index has been prospectively validated in adults allowing for potential outpatient management of low-risk patients (Klastersky et al. 2000; Uys et al. 2004). Multiple risk prediction models for pediatric oncology patients have been presented in the literature and are reviewed by Orudjev and Lange (2002), Härtel et al. (2007), Phillips et al. (2010), and Lehrnbecher et al. (2012). No one system has been found superior, none have undergone rigorous prospective validation to ensure patient safety across populations, and no prospectively validated stratification for high-risk patients has been identified (Härtel et al. 2007; te Poele et al. 2009; Phillips et al. 2010; Lehrnbecher et al. 2012). With the lack of significant randomized prospective data, Härtel et al. (2007) strongly recommend against outpatient management of FN in pediatric patients outside of clinical trials. In the recent pediatric FN expert consensus guidelines, Lehrnbecher et al. (2012) recommend the use of local population-based stratification systems with careful prospective and continuous evaluation to ensure safety and efficacy.

In particular risk stratification schemata, initial laboratory values such as platelet count $<50 \times 10^9$/L and C-reactive protein (CRP) ≥ 90 mg/L have been noted to increase risk, while absolute monocytosis ≥ 0.1–0.155×10^9/L (depending on study) has tempered risk (Rackoff et al. 1996; Baorto et al. 2001; Santolaya et al. 2002; Ammann et al. 2010). Multiple laboratory assessments including CRP, procalcitonin, IL-6, and IL-8 have all been studied in pediatric and adult oncology patients to potentially define high-risk patients but none has been uniformly shown as an effective marker (Santolaya et al. 1994; Lehrnbecher et al. 1999; Uys et al. 2007; Semeraro et al. 2010; Phillips et al. 2012). These studies have been recently reviewed by Phillips et al. (2012).

1.4 Diagnostic Evaluation

1.4.1 Initial Laboratory Evaluation

The diagnostic evaluation for the pediatric patient with FN should be guided by clinical history and physical findings to optimize detecting an etiology for the fever. Initial work-up includes a complete blood cell count (CBC), a comprehensive metabolic panel, and blood cultures from each port of a central catheter. The CBC will demonstrate the degree of neutropenia and monocytopenia, and the metabolic panel will evaluate renal and hepatic function, which could be affected by previous chemotherapeutic agents and may influence antimicrobial selection and dosing. For example, if the patient's creatinine is elevated, antimicrobials like aminoglycosides, vancomycin or amphotericin B should be used with caution and appropriate trough levels followed (Fisher et al. 2010; Lahoti et al. 2010).

Peripheral blood cultures should be obtained if cultures are not or are unable to be obtained from the patient's central venous access device. Peripheral blood cultures in addition to central line cultures are recommended in infection guidelines but remains controversial as the yield for detection from peripheral cultures is <15 % and the utility of differential time to positivity (DTP) between central and peripheral cultures in treatment decision-making is unclear in FN (Gaur et al. 2003; Raad et al. 2004; Gaur et al. 2005; Mermel et al. 2009; Scheinemann et al. 2010; Lehrnbecher et al. 2012; Rodriguez et al. 2012; Carraro et al. 2013). To increase the blood culture yield, ≥ 1 mL of blood should be added to the culture bottles for children ≥ 1 month of age (Connell et al. 2007). Repeating blood cultures in patients who are persistently febrile has been shown useful in identifying bacteremia in a subset with initial negative cultures (Rosenblum et al. 2013). Most contemporary blood culture vials support the growth of *Candida* spp; however, other fungal species may not grow, so sending fungal blood cultures from all ports should be considered with persistent fever (i.e., ≥ 5 days) (Hennequin et al. 2002; Kosmin and Fekete 2008). If clinically suspected, acid-fast bacteria (AFB) cultures from the blood should also be sent to best isolate mycobacterial species.

Urinary tract infection (UTI) in the neutropenic patient may be subclinical given that patients may have minimal symptoms and pyuria may not be present in urinalysis (Klaassen et al. 2011). A recent study utilizing midstream urine samples reported UTI frequency of 8.6 % in 45 children with 58 episodes of FN, with all patients being asymptomatic and the majority having normal urinalyses, supporting the recommendation to obtain clean-catch bacterial urine cultures at the time of initial FN presentation (Lehrnbecher et al. 2012; Sandoval et al. 2012).

1.4.2 Radiographic Imaging

1.4.2.1 Chest Radiography (CXR)
A supine CXR may identify pleural effusions, allow for assessment of central line catheter position and detect pulmonary congestion. However CXR is less useful in identifying early pneumonia (Heussel 2011). CXR has not been found beneficial without the presence of respiratory symptoms and therefore should only be obtained in the symptomatic patient (Feusner et al. 1988; Roberts et al. 2012).

1.4.2.2 Computed Tomography (CT)
Institutional practice may recommend CT of the chest, abdomen and pelvis in neutropenic patients with ≥ 5 days of persistent fever although a recent pediatric study challenges this practice (Agrawal et al. 2011). Specifically, for 52 children with 68 episodes of FN for whom CT (sinuses, chest, abdomen and pelvis) was performed at day five of fever, minimal changes in clinical management occurred based upon results from imaging. The authors conclude that patients with prolonged FN (defined as >4 consecutive days of fever), in which occult fungal infections are being sought, should have CT imaging limited to the chest (Agrawal et al. 2011). Other pediatric studies have similarly found CT chest as well as sinuses to be most useful in prolonged FN (Archibald et al. 2001). CT of the sinuses can be performed in the context of pulmonary symptoms to rule out invasive fungal infections, as some patients with fungal sinusitis can present with minimal symptoms. Of note, patients with fungal sinusitis usually have positive findings on chest CT, and endoscopic biopsy of the sinuses has the highest yield for determining the microbiologic cause (Ho et al. 2011).

High-resolution chest CT with thin sections (1 cm slices) is the preferred imaging modality in patients with neutropenia and pulmonary symptoms, given its ability to characterize lesions and discriminate between infectious and noninfectious etiologies (Heussel 2011). In addition, CT imaging can be used for diagnostic purposes such as CT-guided biopsy of lung lesions for histologic and microbiologic assessment. Importantly, radiologic findings of common molds in children may differ from those in adults. For example, pulmonary nodules are common findings in pediatric patients with *Aspergillus*, while the halo and crescent signs occur less frequently than in adult patients (Thomas et al. 2003; Burgos et al. 2008). Therefore, consultation with pediatric radiologists is critical when interpreting these studies. Providing the radiologist with information about the patient's clinical presentation, level of neutropenia, and current supportive therapy including specific antimicrobial and growth factor use increases the diagnostic utility of CT (Heussel 2011).

1.4.2.3 Magnetic Resonance Imaging (MRI)

MRI is advantageous over CT due to a lack of radiation exposure although at a much higher cost. MRI is also more affected by motion related to cardiorespiratory function increasing artifact incidence especially in the chest. Furthermore, given its increased imaging time, MRI usually requires sedation for pediatric patients, decreasing its convenience as a diagnostic tool. However, MRI remains the imaging of choice for assessing lesions in the liver, spleen, and central nervous system (CNS) (brain and spine) (Sahani and Kalva 2004; Luna et al. 2006).

1.4.2.4 Positron Emission Tomography (PET)

PET is now used frequently alongside CT for the diagnosis of cancer, but experience using PET/CT for FN is limited. A recent study from Australia compared diagnostic yields of PET/CT and conventional imaging in 20 adult patients with FN of >5 days duration (Guy et al. 2012). By using conventional imaging, the authors found 14 infections sites, 13 of which were also confirmed by PET/CT; in addition, PET/CT identified 9 more sites of infection (8 of which were subsequently confirmed as true infection), suggesting that PET/CT may be useful in the study of prolonged FN. However, more data are needed

to support the use of this modality as first-line imaging in pediatrics given its inherent expense and associated radiation exposure (Xu et al. 2010; Haroon et al. 2012).

1.4.3 Biomarkers for Invasive Fungal Infection (IFI)

Early identification of infection in FN, especially IFI, critically affects patient survival. Biomarkers for IFI have proven useful in the adult population as adjuncts to clinical findings and imaging. Limited pediatric data suggest these biomarkers may also be used in children with similar sensitivities and specificities as defined in adults.

1.4.3.1 *Aspergillus* Galactomannan (GMN)

GMN is a cell-wall component of growing hyphae and can be detected by assay from the serum, urine and bronchoalveolar (BAL) fluid (Klont et al. 2004; Pfeiffer et al. 2006). The GMN assay has been shown effective in adult populations with hematologic malignancies and limited data in children suggest utility in pediatric oncology patients as well (Sulahian et al. 2001; Pfeiffer et al. 2006; Steinbach et al. 2007; Castagnola et al. 2010). A recent observational, prospective, multicenter study found the specificity of urine and serum GMN assays were 80 % and 95 %, respectively. This study found that the false-positive rate was lower than previously described (Fisher et al. 2012).

The GMN assay must be interpreted with caution, particularly in the context of a single positive value, and should be utilized in conjunction with corroborative clinical and radiologic findings. Serial repetition of the assay can be used as a surveillance marker either for potential IFI or disease response to antifungal therapy (Groll et al. 2014). The GMN assay may have false-positive results in patients receiving beta-lactam antimicrobials (especially piperacillin/tazobactam), although recent studies suggest the false-positive rate may not be as high as previously published (Zandijk et al. 2008; Metan et al. 2010; Mikulska et al. 2012).

1.4.3.2 (1,3)-β-ᴅ-glucan (BDG)

Serum BDG, an important cell-wall component of most fungi including *Pneumocystis jiroveci* (former *carinii*), has been measured in adult patients with IFI and hematologic malignancies (Marty and Koo 2009). Like GMN, studies using serum BDG in the pediatric population are limited. In fact, few studies performed to date even establish a normal value for children, which may be higher than the 60 pg/mL cutoff used in adult patients (Smith et al. 2007; Mularoni et al. 2010). In immunocompromised adult patients, serum BDG levels exceeding 500 pg/mL have been used to diagnose *P. jiroveci* (Del Bono et al. 2009; Koo et al. 2009; te Poele et al. 2009). One pediatric study found serum BDG potentially useful for *P. jiroveci* diagnosis in three patients with hematologic malignancies, one with BAL fluid confirmation (Gonzalez et al. 2011). The sensitivity of BAL for diagnosing *P. jiroveci* pneumonia is lower in non-HIV patients and in patients receiving aerosolized pentamidine. Therefore, serum BDG may be a useful adjunctive, noninvasive diagnostic tool (Levine et al. 1992; Azoulay and Schlemmer 2006; Jiancheng et al. 2009). More pediatric studies are needed to define serum BDG as a reliable indicator of IFI such as *P. jiroveci*.

Serum BDG does not detect *Cryptococcus* or *Zygomycetes* spp. (e.g., *Mucor*, *Rhizopus*, *Absidia*), which do not produce BDG. False positives also occur in patients receiving antimicrobial agents such as piperacillin/tazobactam in addition to hemodialysis with cellulose membranes, intravenous albumin and immunoglobulin (Marty and Koo 2009; Karageorgopoulos et al. 2011). Finally, the test may serve as a prognostic marker for invasive candidiasis when serial levels are measured, but data supporting this indication are limited (Ginocchio et al. 2012; Glotzbecker et al. 2012; Jaijakul et al. 2012).

1.4.3.3 Polymerase Chain Reaction (PCR)

Molecular methodology such as PCR testing may improve the detection of IFI as well as bacterial or viral organisms in children with FN (Santolaya et al. 2011; Kourkoumpetis et al. 2012). However, lack of standardization has limited its current use and more data are required to make firm recommendations.

1.4.4 Viral Studies

Viral infections may cause prolonged fevers in neutropenic patients. Seasonal viral infections such as influenza A/B and respiratory syncytial virus (RSV) in the winter and enterovirus in the summer must be considered (Lindblom et al. 2010; Ozdemir et al. 2011). In patients with mucositis, herpes simplex virus (HSV) should be considered. Viral PCR (whole blood and plasma, cerebrospinal fluid, stool) is commercially available and enables faster identification of viral etiologies at higher sensitivity and specificity compared to viral culture. In addition, direct fluorescent antibody (DFA) testing of cutaneous lesions may expedite diagnosis of herpetic skin infections (i.e., HSV, varicella).

1.4.5 Invasive Procedures: Bronchoalveolar Lavage (BAL) and Tissue Biopsy

Tissue is necessary for diagnosis when physical examination or radiographic imaging is concerning for abscess formation or lesions of the skin, sinuses, or organ parenchyma but without corroborative microbiologic confirmation. Microbiologic evaluations should include proper sample collection for assessing AFB and other bacterial and fungal pathogens. For IFI such as chronic disseminated candidiasis or invasive *Aspergillus* spp., hepatic or splenic biopsy may be required (Masood and Sallah 2005).

In children with pulmonary lesions, BAL should be attempted first as it has a low complication rate and may yield an etiologic agent (Pattishall et al. 1988; Jain et al. 2004; Efrati et al. 2007). CT-guided lung biopsy or wedge resection may be necessary if BAL sampling is nondiagnostic in the patient with persistent fever and pulmonary nodules (Wingard et al. 2012). In addition to routine cultures, BAL samples should be analyzed by GMN assay (Wingard et al. 2012).

In patients with neutropenia, skin lesions may be a manifestation of localized or systemic infection (Mays et al. 2006). Ecthyma gangrenosum, a black eschar with surrounding erythema originally attributed to *Pseudomonas* spp., can be caused by many other bacterial as well as fungal and viral pathogens (Moyer et al. 1977; Reich et al. 2004; Son et al. 2009). Many invasive systemic fungal infections with high potential for dissemination like *Zygomycetes* spp., *Aspergillus* spp. and *Candida* spp. may present as nonspecific lesions that require prompt evaluation (Mays et al. 2006). Contaminated medical equipment such as adhesive tape has been associated with nosocomial outbreaks of *Zygomycetes* spp., so it is imperative to consider such infections in skin lesions found under dressings near tape (Everett et al. 1979; Lalayanni et al. 2012). Prompt punch biopsy and consideration for consultation with a dermatology specialist is advisable.

1.5 Empiric Management of Febrile Neutropenia (FN)

Management of FN in pediatric oncology is often based on institutional and consensus guidelines. To inform decision-making we review the appropriate literature regarding specific topics including the use of monotherapy versus combination antibiotic therapy, use of vancomycin, empiric utilization of antifungals, emergence of resistant pathogens, duration and location of therapy, and criteria for central venous catheter removal. Pediatric FN guidelines from one institution are provided as an example of how these concepts can be practically implemented.

1.5.1 Adult FN Guidelines for Empiric Therapy: Do They Apply to Children?

Infectious Diseases Society of America (IDSA) guidelines for empiric antimicrobial therapy for FN patients serve as the foundation for institutional protocols treating pediatric cancer patients (Freifeld et al. 2011). Notably, the International Pediatric Fever and Neutropenia Guideline Panel has also published guidelines for FN in pediatric oncology patients (Lehrnbecher et al. 2012). Recommendations from such practice guidelines are mostly based upon level III evidence (expert opinion) versus level I and II evidence (results from randomized clinical trials) (Lee and Vielemeyer 2011). Furthermore, no formal guidelines for FN have been published by the American Society of Pediatric Hematology/Oncology (ASPHO) or the Pediatric Infectious Diseases Society (PIDS) despite notable disparity among adult and pediatric cancer patients, including differences in underlying malignant diseases and associated therapies, immunity and susceptibility to pathogens, and antimicrobial pharmacodynamics (PD) and pharmacokinetics (PK) (Sung et al. 2011; Watt et al. 2011). Defining such PD/PK differences are critical, particularly in the cancer patient as cancer therapy can affect antimicrobial efficacy, promoting pathogen resistance (Theuretzbacher 2012). Whether such differences significantly impact infection-related morbidity and mortality in pediatric cancer patients remains largely unstudied.

The International Antimicrobial Therapy Cooperative Group (IATCG) published the largest series comparing FN episodes in adult ($n = 2,321$) and pediatric ($n = 759$) patients receiving standardized disease assessment and empiric therapy and noted significant differences in patient demographics and outcomes by age: (1) malignant diagnoses associated with FN episodes differed across patient age with ALL being most frequent in children and AML most frequent in adults; (2) adult patients more frequently received antibacterial and antifungal prophylaxes; (3) children tended to have lower ANCs at presentation but shorter durations of granulocytopenia; (4) children had less defined sites of infection and more fever of unknown origin; (5) children and adults had similar rates of Gram-positive and Gram-negative bacteremia, but children had more streptococcal bacteremia; and (6) children had lower infection-related mortality and overall mortality (3 % vs. 10 %) than adult FN patients (Hann et al. 1997). Together, these data suggest that children and adults with FN are indeed distinct both in presentation and outcome.

Additional studies are needed to investigate further these suggestive data. However, such clinical investigation is practically limited by the large numbers of patients required for accurate statistical analysis as well as by the inherent expense associated with large randomized clinical trials (RCTs) (Mullen 2012). Likewise, reproducible and accurate biomarkers of response to infection and clinical end points are needed to ensure sound clinical trials addressing antimicrobial efficacy and safety (Powers 2012). Given their limitations in study design and expense, RCTs comparing FN episodes and response to therapy among adult and pediatric cancer patients will likely not be performed. Yet, extensive pediatric literature incorporating antimicrobial agents used in adult FN demonstrates that empiric antibacterial and antifungal therapies are comparable in their efficacy. For these reasons, extrapolation of adult FN guidelines to the pediatric population is unavoidable.

1.5.2 Choice of Empiric Antimicrobial Therapy

As discussed, determination of initial risk stratification can help guide utilization of appropriate antimicrobial agents and specifically the route (oral vs. intravenous), setting (inpatient vs. outpatient), and duration of use. In general, antimicrobial choices for empiric pediatric FN are comparable in their efficacy in either high-risk or low-risk scenarios as serious medical complications remain low with use of contemporary treatments (Baorto et al. 2001; Luthi et al. 2012; Manji et al. 2012b, c). Therefore, institutional guidelines for empiric antimicrobial therapy should consider the following: (1) published experience with using the antimicrobial agent in the context of FN; (2) physician experience with using the proposed antimicrobial agent; (3) pathogen epidemiology and resistance patterns to the antimicrobial agent inherent to the institution and its surrounding community; and (4) the antimicrobial agent's toxicity profile, cost and availability. In essence, choice of empiric antimicrobial therapy should integrate the patient's clinical history and presentation with institutional experience of local

microbial patterns and specific antimicrobial therapies.

1.5.2.1 Monotherapy Versus Combination Therapy

Pizzo et al. (1986) first showed that cephalosporin monotherapy is as effective as combination therapy in adult oncology patients. Since that time, institutional guidelines are slowly adopting the recommendation for monotherapy that is supported in both the IDSA as well as the recent pediatric guidelines (Freifeld et al. 2011; Lehrnbecher et al. 2012). In a Cochrane review of 71 published trials, monotherapy with broad-spectrum, antipseudomonal beta-lactams was found to be non-inferior to combination therapy with a trend toward improved survival and a significantly decreased risk of adverse events, specifically fungal infection and nephrotoxicity secondary to aminoglycosides as part of combination therapy (Paul et al. 2013). The observations of Paul et al. (2013) have been corroborated by a previous systematic meta-analysis by Furno et al. (2002). Specifically for pediatric oncology patients, Manji et al. (2012b) conducted a meta-analysis and found no significant difference between antipseudomonal penicillins and antipseudomonal cephalosporins either as monotherapy or when combined with an aminoglycoside. The authors therefore recommend choosing a regimen based on cost, availability and local factors such as institutional resistance patterns. Whether the increased utilization of a more broad-spectrum agent as monotherapy over a more narrow-spectrum antipseudomonal cephalosporin plus an aminoglycoside will lead to increased resistance for these agents is unknown.

In an additional Cochrane review of anti-Gram-positive antibiotics (often vancomycin) in FN, Paul et al. (2005) showed that the addition of such therapy does not improve outcomes without a documented Gram-positive infection. Use of vancomycin as initial empiric FN therapy is not recommended in consensus guidelines as it does not significantly affect survival or length of stay (Freifeld et al. 2011; Lehrnbecher et al. 2012). Furthermore, imprudent use of vancomycin has been associated with emergence of resistant pathogens (e.g., VRE) and nephrotoxicity. Clinical indications for empiric vancomycin include skin/soft-tissue and catheter-related infection, hemodynamic instability, severe mucositis, and pneumonia. In these situations, targeted vancomycin trough levels and renal function surveillance are recommended (Rybak et al. 2009). If susceptible bacteria are not recovered or if concern for Gram-positive infection abates, vancomycin should be discontinued within 72 h (Lehrnbecher et al. 2012).

Consensus guidelines recommend combination therapy be reserved for specific clinical indications including patient instability, concern for resistant pathogens (e.g., extended spectrum β-lactamase [ESBL]-producing *Serratia*, *Pseudomonas*, *Acinetobacter*, *Citrobacter*, *Enterobacter* and *Klebsiella* spp.), and need for synergism to treat specific pathogens (e.g., *Enterococcus*, *Mycobacterium* spp., MRSA) or infections (e.g., endocarditis, cryptococcal meningitis) (Freifeld et al. 2011; Lehrnbecher et al. 2012). Of note, if combination therapy is required, meta-analyses in pediatrics recommend utilization of once rather than multiple daily doses of aminoglycosides due to trends toward improved efficacy and decreased nephrotoxicity (Sung et al. 2003; Contopoulos-Ioannidis et al. 2004).

1.5.2.2 Which Monotherapy to Choose

A Cochrane review of antipseudomonal beta-lactams for initial management of FN compared studies with ceftazidime, cefepime, piperacillin/tazobactam, meropenem and imipenem (Paul et al. 2010). Cefepime monotherapy was shown to have a significantly higher all-cause mortality which had been previously reported (Yahav et al. 2007). The Cochrane meta-analysis reported a nonsignificant higher rate of bacterial superinfection with cefepime which has been a reported concern due to its limited anaerobic profile and poor coverage for skin infections (Yahav et al. 2007; Paul et al. 2010; Kalil 2011). A follow-up meta-analysis did not find a statistically significant increased mortality with cefepime and current pediatric consensus guidelines consider cefepime a reasonable choice for monotherapy (Kim et al. 2010; Lehrnbecher

et al. 2012). Ceftazidime is not a good first-line choice for monotherapy due to reduced Gram-positive coverage as well as induction of β-lactamase production leading to subsequent emergence of resistant pathogens and inferior clinical outcomes in pediatric patients (Mebis et al. 1998; Ariffin et al. 2000; Greenberg et al. 2005). Paul et al. (2010) additionally noted that carbapenem monotherapy had similar all-cause mortality as other monotherapy regimens but was associated with higher rates of antibiotic- and *Clostridium difficile*-associated diarrhea. Pediatric meta-analyses have shown similar effectiveness between antipseudomonal cephalosporins, antipseudomonal penicillins and carbapenems as monotherapy but without the noted increase in *Clostridium difficile*-associated diarrhea (Manji et al. 2012b, c).

1.5.2.3 Alterations in Initial Empiric FN Antibiotic Management

Once empiric therapy has been initiated, alterations in FN antibiotic management may be required to optimize treatment; these changes occur at the discretion of the practitioner or institution without significant evidence basis. For instance, Lehrnbecher et al. (2012) recommend discontinuing combination therapy (if initiated at presentation) after 24–72 h in the stable patient without microbiologic evidence to continue both agents. Similarly, patients who are stable but with persistent fever should not have their initial regimen escalated. Those who become unstable should have additional coverage for potential resistant Gram-negative, Gram-positive and anaerobic causes initiated with consideration for fungal and viral etiologies.

1.5.2.4 Outpatient Management of FN

Although there remains a lack of one uniform pediatric oncology risk stratification system, many institutions have begun to utilize outpatient management of low-risk FN which can include outpatient oral or parenteral therapy as either initial management or as step-down to outpatient treatment after initial inpatient management; such options and the evidence surrounding them are reviewed by Chisholm and Dommett (2006). This differs from previous studies in which low-risk patients were discharged early (ANC $<0.5 \times 10^9$/L) but only after defervescence (Mullen and Buchanan 1990; Aquino et al. 1997; Wacker et al. 1997). Meta-analyses of efficacy and safety from adult and pediatric studies found no significant difference in treatment failure in the inpatient versus outpatient setting and no significant difference in the efficacy of outpatient oral versus parenteral therapy in low-risk FN (Teuffel et al. 2011b). Studies were extremely heterogenous in terms of choice of antibiotics (both oral and parenteral) as well as timing of step-down making generalizations difficult. A recent Cochrane review of randomized controlled trials comparing oral versus intravenous antibiotic therapy for FN found no significant difference in treatment failure or mortality (Vidal et al. 2013).

The utilization of outpatient oral therapy specifically for pediatric patients either at FN presentation or as step-down after initial inpatient management was most recently reviewed by Manji et al. (2012a). Sixteen prospective trials were reviewed in the meta-analysis with no significant difference between oral and parenteral regimens and no outpatient infection-related mortality. None of the trials were randomized controlled trials specifically comparing inpatient versus outpatient management and outcomes of low-risk FN (Manji et al. 2012a). The types of oral agents utilized in pediatric studies are quite heterogenous and include amoxicillin/clavulanate, cefixime, fluoroquinolones (ciprofloxacin, gatifloxacin) and combination therapy (ciprofloxacin plus amoxicillin) (Mullen et al. 1999; Aquino et al. 2000; Paganini et al. 2000, 2001; Shenep et al. 2001; Park et al. 2003; Petrilli et al. 2007; Dommett et al. 2009; Brack et al. 2012). Ciprofloxacin plus amoxicillin/clavulanate is recommended as the oral regimen of choice in adult patients (Freifeld et al. 2011). Brack et al. (2012) recently reported on an RCT comparing continued inpatient treatment versus oral outpatient management and found non-inferiority for

efficacy but lack of power to prove non-inferiority for safety.

Many centers are continuing to initially admit all pediatric oncology FN patients with the potential for early discharge with or without continued antibiotic support depending on the clinical context (Gibson et al. 2013). The United Kingdom recommends such a management strategy after 48 inpatient hours in patients >1 year of age, without medical or social comorbidities, not receiving extremely intensive therapy, appearing clinically well without a source of infection, with some marrow recovery (i.e., ANC $>0.1 \times 10^9$/L), and with fever improvement (but not full defervescence necessary), for outpatient oral antibiotics to complete a 5-day course (Gibson et al. 2013). A recent survey of Canadian pediatric oncology centers found heterogenous treatment strategies from full inpatient care, to step-down care, to full outpatient care exemplifying the perceived lack of sufficient data to uniformly modify practice (Boragina et al. 2007). Sung et al. (2004) reported in a survey of parents that only 53 % supported initial FN outpatient management (as compared to 71 % of practitioners) due to perceived increased fear and anxiety balanced with increased comfort, while early discharge and outpatient intravenous management are reportedly associated with improved health-related quality of life (Cheng et al. 2011). Finally, Teuffel et al. (2011a) calculated that the most cost-effective model is one in which low-risk FN patients are treated entirely at home but through a parenteral rather than oral route. The risk of nosocomial infection (NI) with inpatient management must also be considered and was reported to be 5.2 NI per 100 admissions by one group (Simon et al. 2000). The recent pediatric FN expert consensus guidelines allow for consideration of initial or step-down outpatient management for the low-risk patient in the appropriate setting although as a weak recommendation (Lehrnbecher et al. 2012).

1.5.2.5 Choice of Empiric Antifungal Therapy

The use of empiric antifungal therapy in neutropenic children is also based upon limited data (Pizzo et al. 1982). Despite the low incidence of

IFI in pediatric FN, cost of associated antifungal therapy and supportive care and IFI-related mortality are high (Zaoutis et al. 2006; Kim et al. 2011; Mor et al. 2011; Steinbach 2011). Therefore, recent emphasis has been placed on defining risk factors for IFI and providing empiric antifungal therapy only to high-risk FN patients (Cordonnier et al. 2009; Caselli et al. 2012; Lehrnbecher et al. 2012). Notable risk factors for IFI include hematologic malignancy, especially AML and relapsed disease, prolonged and profound neutropenia and lymphopenia, and adolescent age (Groll et al. 1999; Rosen et al. 2005; Castagnola et al. 2006; Mor et al. 2011).

The number of antifungals has increased dramatically over the last decade but efficacy data in prevention of IFI in pediatric oncology are very limited (Blyth 2011; Steinbach 2011). Meta-analyses on the utilization of empiric antifungal therapy has shown mixed benefit in decreasing all-cause mortality (Gøtzsche and Johansen 2002; Goldberg et al. 2008). Similarly, one small prospective pediatric study showed no benefit with antimycotic prophylaxis as compared to early therapeutic treatment (Uhlenbrock et al. 2001). Additional meta-analyses of limited trial data mainly from adult oncology patients have shown that intravenous liposomal amphotericin B and potentially caspofungin (2 trials) are the most effective empiric agents (Johansen and Gøtzsche 2000; Jørgensen et al. 2006; Goldberg et al. 2008). Voriconazole was reported to be non-inferior to liposomal amphotericin B as empiric antifungal therapy by Walsh et al. (2002), but this was refuted by a subsequent Cochrane review and not approved by the US Food and Drug Administration (FDA) for this indication (Jørgensen et al. 2006). Clinical trials incorporating empiric antifungal therapy in pediatric FN are extremely limited. Maertens et al. (2010) report that liposomal amphotericin B and caspofungin are comparable in their efficacy and safety although patient numbers were small and it is unclear if the study was powered to make this conclusion (Sekine et al. 2010). Generalizability in regard to the efficacy of other echinocandins is unknown. Consensus guidelines recommend initiation of empiric antifungal therapy in high-risk patients with persistent FN without a source while receiving broad-spectrum antibiotics for ≥4 days (Freifeld et al. 2011; Lehrnbecher et al. 2012). Pediatric guidelines recommend either liposomal amphotericin B or caspofungin while the adult IDSA guidelines admit there is insufficient evidence to recommend any one particular agent beyond ensuring for anti-mold coverage (Freifeld et al. 2011; Lehrnbecher et al. 2012; Groll et al. 2014). Due to unclear efficacy of empiric antifungal prophylaxis in the prevention of IFI, the IDSA guidelines also suggest consideration for "preemptive antifungal management" (i.e., withholding empiric therapy) as an alternative strategy in patients who remain febrile >4 days but are clinically stable and have no clinical, radiographic (CT sinus and chest), laboratory (negative fungal serology screens), or microbiologic (positive culture from sterile site) evidence of fungal infection (Freifeld et al. 2011).

1.5.3 Duration of Antimicrobial Therapy: Empiric Versus Therapeutic Intent

In the absence of documented or clinical concern for infection, empiric antimicrobial therapy is often continued until resolution of FN in both low- and high-risk patients. As mentioned, in low-risk pediatric patients, discontinuing antibiotics prior to attaining an ANC $>0.5 \times 10^9$/L has been shown safe if afebrile ≥24 h and with negative cultures ≥48 h (Mullen and Buchanan 1990; Aquino et al. 1997; Wacker et al. 1997; Lehrnbecher et al. 2002; Hodgson-Viden et al. 2005; Lehrnbecher et al. 2012). Risk stratification in these studies was heterogenous with no set ANC threshold for early discharge; therefore, consensus pediatric guidelines recommend evidence of bone marrow recovery (i.e., post nadir ANC $≥0.1 \times 10^9$/L) prior to antimicrobial discontinuation (Lehrnbecher et al. 2012). Santolaya et al. (1997) have also shown in a small low-risk carefully selected pediatric cohort that antimicrobials can be discontinued on day 3 of hospital admission prior to defervescence or neutrophil recovery; thus, consensus guidelines suggest discontinuation of antimicrobials after 72 h of intravenous antibiotic therapy in the patient who is afebrile ≥24 h even without evidence of bone marrow recovery as long as close follow-up is ensured (Lehrnbecher et al. 2012). Again, the data to support this practice comes from small prospective trials with no uniform risk stratification system. In high-risk patients, empiric antifungal therapy is usually discontinued once fever has resolved for ≥48 h with an ANC >0.5 × 10^9/L. If the patient remains afebrile and clinically stable, antibiotic therapies are discontinued. Although definitive evidence is lacking, the usual clinical practice is to remove one antimicrobial agent per 24 h time interval to observe for fever recrudescence if the patient is on combination antimicrobial therapy. No pediatric studies address the appropriate management strategy in high-risk pediatric FN patients and specific management of these patients is not addressed in the pediatric consensus guidelines (Lehrnbecher et al. 2012).

For documented infection, duration of therapy is determined by the site, pathogen and clinical response to therapy. Most bacterial infections (with notable exceptions including CNS infection, abscess formation and endovascular focus) require 10–14 days of appropriate therapy, assuming complete clinical and microbiologic response. In general, duration of antimicrobial therapy should be continued through a time of neutrophil recovery (i.e., at least 5 days beyond ANC >0.5 × 10^9/L), although there is little evidence to support the efficacy of this practice. For established IFI, prolonged therapy (4–6 weeks) is necessary and concomitant immune recovery is critical for favorable outcomes (Nucci et al. 2003). The role for combination antifungal therapy, particularly in the context of mold infection, requires further investigation; potential utilization of combination therapy must balance the significant drug interactions and potential side effects with questionable benefit (Vazquez 2008; Spellberg et al.

2012). The interested reader is directed to recently published IDSA guidelines for a more extensive discussion of infections due to *Aspergillus*, *Candida* and *Cryptococcus* (Walsh et al. 2008; Pappas et al. 2009; Perfect et al. 2010).

1.5.4 Endovascular Sources of Infection: Catheter Removal

Any central venous access device (CVAD) can cause central line-associated bloodstream infection (CLABSI), including a peripherally inserted central catheter (PICC) (Advani et al. 2011). As mentioned, although DTP between peripheral and central cultures can allow for determination of line infection versus bacteremia, such information rarely changes management. Rather, CVAD removal is necessary in the following clinical contexts: any bloodstream infection in which the CVAD is no longer required, tunneled catheter site infection, hemodynamic instability/sepsis, endocarditis or other endovascular infection (e.g., thrombophlebitis), persistent positive blood culture despite appropriate antimicrobial therapy for >72 h, and CLABSI due to highly resistant pathogens (e.g., MRSA, ESBL Gram-negative bacilli, VRE) or pathogens that are difficult to eradicate, particularly due to adhesive biofilm production (e.g., fungi, *Propionibacterium* spp., *Bacillus* spp. *Mycobacterium* spp.) (Mermel et al. 2009). Delay in catheter removal for less virulent pathogens increases the risk for recurrent CLABSI (Raad et al. 2009). Antibiotic lock therapy, instilling high concentrations of susceptible antibiotic or ethanol into the CVAD lumen, has been successfully used in combination with systemic antimicrobial therapy to both eradicate and prevent CLABSI and should be considered when the CVAD cannot be removed (e.g., limited access sites in the patient) (Fortun et al. 2006; Flynn 2009).

1.5.5 Adjunctive Treatment Modalities

Additional treatment modalities such as granulocyte transfusion and hematopoietic growth factors are of unclear benefit in pediatric FN and are discussed in detail in Chaps. 2 and 15 respectively.

1.5.6 Emergence of Resistant Pathogens: Dwindling Antimicrobial Options and Focus on Prevention

Judicious use of antimicrobial therapy is imperative to curb emergence of resistant pathogens which have been shown to negatively affect clinical outcomes in pediatric FN patients (El-Mahallawy et al. 2011). In particular, prevalence of highly resistant ESBL- and carbapenemase-producing organisms is increasing while development of novel effective antimicrobial therapy is both limited and associated with significant side effects (Prasad et al. 2012). Institutional prevention through implementation of surveillance and antimicrobial stewardship programs is vital, particularly for heavily exposed patient populations like cancer patients (Rolston 2005). Similarly, establishing guidelines for resistant pathogens and their associated therapies is also imperative (Rybak et al. 2009; Liu et al. 2011).

1.6 Summary: Building Institutional FN Guidelines

It is clear that without sufficient data guiding uniform treatment strategies, institutional guidelines addressing FN in pediatric oncology are critical in effective clinical management for this life-threatening complication and in monitoring institutional trends in resistance and infectious sequelae. A multidisciplinary team approach is required to create comprehensive and critically reviewed guidelines that are supported at all levels of the hospital, from primary patient managers including hematology/oncology physicians to consultants such as infectious disease specialists and pediatric surgeons to additional caregivers such as emergency medicine physicians and pediatric intensivists. Cooperation between all care providers will ensure uniformity and successful treatment of this patient population. In a recent survey of time to antibiotic delivery for presenting FN in the emergency department, Burry et al. (2012) note many factors to improve care including administrative barriers, communication between oncology and emergency department staff, and patient education. As noted, implementing potential practices such as early discharge will require multidisciplinary discussion, institutional review board (IRB) approval, and prospective study and ongoing analysis to ensure patient safety as well as efficacy of the treatment strategy.

Here we provide examples of institutional guidelines incorporating the various diagnostic and management concepts throughout this chapter and compiled into a practical algorithm to illustrate a standard supportive care approach for FN in pediatric oncology patients (Figs. 1.1, 1.2, and 1.3). These guidelines should be regarded as quality of evidence level III recommendations as they are based mainly on expert opinion and published reports from expert committees due to the lack of randomized clinical trials in pediatrics; additionally, the reader should refer back to the text for full details as many reasonable treatment options are equally valid. As discussed, institutional guidelines must incorporate local microbial prevalence and incidence and local clinical expertise which may not necessarily be equal across institutions. Lastly, available guidelines assist with decision-making but an individualized approach must be taken when evaluating and treating each episode of FN in pediatric oncology patients.

Fever and Neutropenia in Children Receiving Cancer Treatment Emergency Department/Outpatient Algorithm[a]

- Access central venous access device (CVAD); If unable or none present, place peripheral IV & obtain culture
- Obtain T&S, CBC with differential, renal and hepatic function, blood cultures from all lumens
- Obtain urinalysis and urine culture (but do not delay antibiotic admininstration)
- CXR, stool cultures, respiratory viral PCR panel if symptoms exist
- Order appropriate antibiotics (see below)
  ANTIBIOTICS GIVEN WITHIN 1 HOUR OF ARRIVAL TO EMERGENCY ROOM
- Contact oncology service after assessment

* Signs and Symptoms (S/Sx) Sepsis
- Chills
- Age-specific vital signs:

Age	Heart Rate	Systolic BP
1 wk – 1 m	>180 or <100	<80
1 m – 1 y	>180 or <90	<75
1 y – 5 y	>140	<75
5 y – 12 y	>130	<80
12 y – 18 y	>110	<90

Definition of fever:
- HSCT patient: Any oral T ≥ 38°C
- Oncology patient:
  -- Single oral T ≥ 38.3°C (101°F)
  -- Oral T ≥ 38°C (100.4°F) for ≥ 1h

S/Sx Sepsis *∇   No / Yes

Yes → Admit on combination therapy:
- Piperacillin/tazobactam
- Tobramycin
- Vancomycin
Consider infectious disease consult

ANC < 0.5 x 10⁹/L   No / Yes

Antimicrobial allergies:
Penicillin allergy:
- Cefepime + Metronidazole OR
- Meropenem
Cephalosporin allergy:
- Meropenem
β-lactam allergy:
- Fluoroquinolone
Vancomycin allergy:
- Daptomycin (if no pulmonary infection) OR
- Linezolid

No →
- Assess risk‡
- Observe 1h post-ceftriaxone
- Discharge if clinically well
- Return to clinic next day if remains febrile, sooner if new symptoms

Admit Assess Risk‡

Low Risk

High Risk

Admit on monotherapy:
- Piperacillin/tazobactam (Zosyn)

Admit on combination therapy:
- Piperacillin/tazobactam
- Tobramycin
Add vancomycin if meets criteria†

‡Risk assessment criteria
Patient is considered High Risk if ANY
of the following is present:
- Signs/symptoms of sepsis
- ANC < 0.1 x 10⁹/L
- Focal infection (e.g. mucositis, abdominal pain, perianal tenderness)
- Patient receiving therapeutic dexamethasone or prednisone
- Infant ALL, ALL (Induction, Delayed Intensification), AML
- HSCT patient < 100 days from transplant

†Vancomycin criteria
- Skin infection/cellulitis
- CVAD site infection
- Mucositis
- AML or recent high-dose cytarabine administration
- Isolation of vancomycin-sensitive organism
- Previous MRSA or *Streptococcus viridans*
- Note: Discontinue vancomycin after 72 h if none of the above

∇Consider stress-dose steroids
- If patient receiving systemic steroids ≥ 7 days
- If presentation within 4 weeks of ALL induction

Fig. 1.1 Emergency room algorithm for fever and neutropenia in pediatric oncology patients
[a]see text for full detail as other treatment algorithms are equally justifiable
T&S type and screen, *CBC* complete blood count, *PCR* polymerase chain reaction, *HSCT* hematopoietic stem cell transplant, *ANC* absolute neutrophil count, *ALL* acute lymphoblastic leukemia, *AML* acute myelogenous leukemia, *MRSA* methicillin resistant *S. aureus*

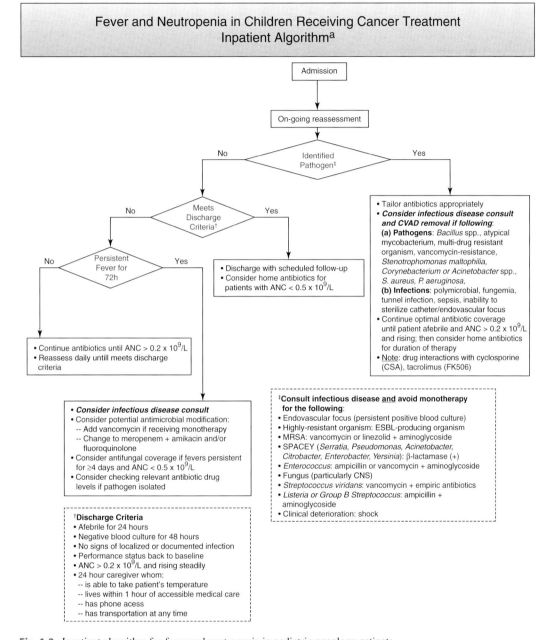

Fig. 1.2 Inpatient algorithm for fever and neutropenia in pediatric oncology patients
[a]see text for full detail as other treatment algorithms are equally justifiable
CVAD central venous access device, *ANC* absolute neutrophil count, *MRSA* methicillin resistant *S. aureus*

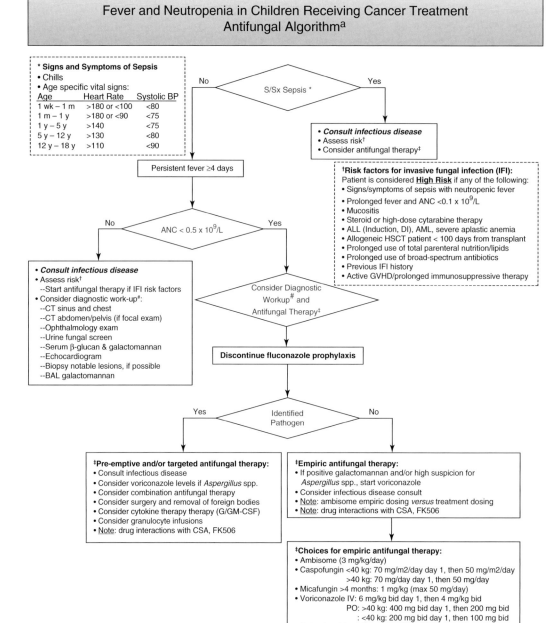

Fig. 1.3 Antifungal algorithm for fever and neutropenia in pediatric oncology patients
[a]see text for full detail as other treatment algorithms are equally justifiable
ANC absolute neutrophil count, *ALL* acute lymphoblastic leukemia, *DI* delayed intensification, *AML* acute myelogenous leukemia, *HSCT* hematopoieic stem cell transplant, *GVHD* graft-versus-host disease, *CT* computed tomography, *BAL* bronchoalveolar lavage, *CSA* cyclosporine, *FK506* tacrolimus, *bid* twice daily

References

Advani S, Reich NG, Sengupta A et al (2011) Central line-associated bloodstream infection in hospitalized children with peripherally inserted central venous catheters: extending risk analyses outside the intensive care unit. Clin Infect Dis 52:1108–1115

Agrawal AK, Saini N, Gildengorin G et al (2011) Is routine computed tomographic scanning justified in the first week of persistent febrile neutropenia in children with malignancies? Pediatr Blood Cancer 57:620–624

Aledo A, Heller G, Ren L et al (1998) Septicemia and septic shock in pediatric patients: 140 consecutive cases on a pediatric hematology-oncology service. J Pediatr Hematol Oncol 20:215–221

Ammann RA, Bodner N, Hirt A et al (2010) Predicting adverse events in children with fever and chemotherapy-induced neutropenia: the prospective multicenter SPOG 2003 FN study. J Clin Oncol 28:2008–2014

Aquino VM, Tkaczewski I, Buchanan GR (1997) Early discharge of low-risk febrile neutropenic children and adolescents with cancer. Clin Infect Dis 25:74–78

Aquino VM, Herrera L, Sandler ES et al (2000) Feasibility of oral ciprofloxacin for the outpatient management of febrile neutropenia in selected children with cancer. Cancer 88:1710–1714

Archibald S, Park J, Geyer JR et al (2001) Computed tomography in the evaluation of febrile neutropenic pediatric oncology patients. Pediatr Infect Dis J 20:5–10

Ariffin H, Navaratnam P, Mohamed M et al (2000) Ceftazidime-resistant Klebsiella pneumoniae bloodstream infection in children with febrile neutropenia. Int J Infect Dis 4:21–25

Auletta JJ, O'Riordan MA, Nieder ML (1999) Infections in children with cancer: a continued need for the comprehensive physical examination. J Pediatr Hematol Oncol 21:501–508

Azoulay E, Schlemmer B (2006) Diagnostic strategy in cancer patients with acute respiratory failure. Intensive Care Med 32:808–822

Badiei Z, Khalesi M, Alami MH et al (2011) Risk factors associated with life-threatening infections in children with febrile neutropenia: a data mining approach. J Pediatr Hematol Oncol 33:e9–e12

Bakhshi S, Padmanjali KS, Arya LS (2008) Infections in childhood acute lymphoblastic leukemia: an analysis of 222 febrile neutropenic episodes. Pediatr Hematol Oncol 25:385–392

Baorto EP, Aquino VM, Mullen CA et al (2001) Clinical parameters associated with low bacteremia risk in 1100 pediatric oncology patients with fever and neutropenia. Cancer 92:909–913

Blyth CC (2011) Antifungal azoles: old and new. Pediatr Infect Dis J 30:506–507

Boragina M, Patel H, Reiter S et al (2007) Management of febrile neutropenia in pediatric oncology patients: a Canadian survey. Pediatr Blood Cancer 48:521–526

Brack E, Bodmer N, Simon A et al (2012) First-day step-down to oral outpatient treatment versus continued standard treatment in children with cancer and low-risk fever in neutropenia. A randomized controlled trial within the multicenter SPOG 2003 FN study. Pediatr Blood Cancer 59:423–430

Burgos A, Zaoutis TE, Dvorak CC et al (2008) Pediatric invasive aspergillosis: a multicenter retrospective analysis of 139 contemporary cases. Pediatrics 121:e1286–e1294

Burry E, Punnett A, Mehta A et al (2012) Identification of educational and infrastructural barriers to prompt antibiotic delivery in febrile neutropenia: a quality improvement initiative. Pediatr Blood Cancer 59:431–435

Carraro F, Cicalese MP, Cesaro S et al (2013) Guidelines for the use of long-term central venous catheter in children with hemato-oncological disorders. On behalf of supportive therapy working group of Italian Association of Pediatric Hematology and Oncology (AIEOP). Ann Hematol 92:1405–1412

Caselli D, Cesaro S, Ziino O et al (2012) A prospective, randomized study of empirical antifungal therapy for the treatment of chemotherapy-induced febrile neutropenia in children. Br J Haematol 148:249–255

Castagnola E, Cesaro S, Giacchino M et al (2006) Fungal infections in children with cancer: a prospective, multicenter surveillance study. Pediatr Infect Dis J 25:634–639

Castagnola E, Fontana V, Caviglia I et al (2007) A prospective study on the epidemiology of febrile episodes during chemotherapy-induced neutropenia in children with cancer or after hemopoietic stem cell transplantation. Clin Infect Dis 45:1296–1304

Castagnola E, Furfaro E, Caviglia I et al (2010) Performance of the galactomannan antigen detection test in the diagnosis of invasive aspergillosis in children with cancer or undergoing haemopoietic stem cell transplantation. Clin Microbiol Infect 16:1197–1203

Cheng S, Teuffel O, Ethier MC et al (2011) Health-related quality of life anticipated with different management strategies for paediatric febrile neutropaenia. Br J Cancer 105:606–611

Chisholm JC, Dommett R (2006) The evolution towards ambulatory and day-case management of febrile neutropenia. Br J Haematol 135:3–16

Connell TG, Rele M, Cowley D et al (2007) How reliable is a negative blood culture result? Volume of blood submitted for culture in routine practice in a children's hospital. Pediatrics 119:891–896

Contopoulos-Ioannidis DG, Giotis ND, Baliatsa DV et al (2004) Extended-interval aminoglycoside administration for children: a meta-analysis. Pediatrics 114:e111–e118

Cordonnier C, Pautas C, Maury S et al (2009) Empirical versus preemptive antifungal therapy for high-risk, febrile, neutropenic patients: a randomized, controlled trial. Clin Infect Dis 48:1042–1051

Del Bono V, Mularoni A, Furfaro E et al (2009) Clinical evaluation of a (1,3)-beta-D-glucan assay for presumptive diagnosis of Pneumocystis jiroveci pneumonia in immunocompromised patients. Clin Vaccine Immunol 16:1524–1526

Dommett R, Geary J, Freeman S et al (2009) Successful introduction and audit of a step-down oral antibiotic strategy for low risk paediatric febrile neutropaenia in a UK, multicentre, shared care setting. Eur J Cancer 45:2843–2849

Duncan C, Chisholm JC, Freeman S et al (2007) A prospective study of admissions for febrile neutropenia in secondary paediatric units in South East England. Pediatr Blood Cancer 49:678–681

Efrati O, Gonik U, Bielorai B et al (2007) Fiberoptic bronchoscopy and bronchoalveolar lavage for the evaluation of pulmonary disease in children with primary immunodeficiency and cancer. Pediatr Blood Cancer 48:324–329

El-Mahallawy HA, El-Wakil M, Moneer MM et al (2011) Antibiotic resistance is associated with longer bacteremic episodes and worse outcome in febrile neutropenic children with cancer. Pediatr Blood Cancer 57:283–288

Everett ED, Pearson S, Rogers W (1979) Rhizopus surgical wound infection with elasticized adhesive tape dressings. Arch Surg 114:738–739

Feusner J, Cohen R, O'Leary M et al (1988) Use of routine chest radiography in the evaluation of fever in neutropenic pediatric oncology patients. J Clin Oncol 6:1699–1702

Fisher BT, Zaoutis TE, Leckerman KH et al (2010) Risk factors for renal failure in pediatric patients with acute myeloid leukemia: a retrospective cohort study. Pediatr Blood Cancer 55:655–661

Fisher BT, Zaoutis TE, Park JR et al (2012) Galactomannan antigen testing for diagnosis of invasive Aspergillosis in pediatric hematology patients. J Pediatr Infect Dis 1:116–124

Flynn PM (2009) Diagnosis and management of central venous catheter-related bloodstream infections in pediatric patients. Pediatr Infect Dis J 28:1016–1017

Fortun J, Grill F, Martin-Davila P et al (2006) Treatment of long-term intravascular catheter-related bacteremia with antibiotic-lock therapy. J Antimicrob Chemother 58:816–821

Freifeld AG, Bow EJ, Sepkowitz KA et al (2011) Clinical practice guideline for the use of antimicrobial agents in neutropenic patients with cancer: 2010 update by the Infectious Diseases Society of America. Clin Infect Dis 52:e56–e93

Furno P, Bucaneve G, Del Favero A (2002) Monotherapy or aminoglycoside-containing combinations for empirical antibiotic treatment of febrile neutropenic patients: a meta-analysis. Lancet Infect Dis 2:231–242

Gassas A, Grant R, Richardson S et al (2004) Predictors of viridans streptococcal shock syndrome in bacteremic children with cancer and stem-cell transplant recipients. J Clin Oncol 22:1222–1227

Gaur AH, Flynn PM, Giannini MA et al (2003) Difference in time to detection: a simple method to differentiate catheter-related from non-catheter-related bloodstream infection in immunocompromised pediatric patients. Clin Infect Dis 37:469–475

Gaur AH, Flynn PM, Heine DJ (2005) Diagnosis of catheter-related bloodstream infections among pediatric oncology patients lacking a peripheral culture, using differential time to detection. Pediatr Infect Dis J 24:445–449

Gibson F, Chisholm J, Blandford E et al (2013) Developing a national 'low-risk' febrile neutropenia framework for use in children and young people's cancer care. Support Care Cancer 21:1241–1251

Ginocchio F, Verrina E, Furfaro E et al (2012) Case report of the reliability 1,3-beta-D-glucan monitoring during treatment of peritoneal candidiasis in a child receiving continuous peritoneal dialysis. Clin Vaccine Immunol 19:626–627

Glotzbecker B, Duncan C, Alyea E 3rd et al (2012) Important drug interactions in hematopoietic stem cell transplantation: what every physician should know. Biol Blood Marrow Transplant 18:989–1006

Goldberg E, Gafter-Gvili A, Robenshtok E et al (2008) Empirical antifungal therapy for patients with neutropenia and persistent fever: systematic review and meta-analysis. Eur J Cancer 44:2192–2203

Gonzalez BE, Faverio LA, Marty FM et al (2011) Elevated serum beta-D-glucan levels in immunocompromised children with clinical suspicion for Pneumocystis jirovecii pneumonia. Clin Vaccine Immunol 18:1202–1203

Gøtzsche PC, Johansen HK (2002) Routine versus selective antifungal administration for control of fungal infections in patients with cancer. Cochrane Database Syst Rev (2):CD000026

Greenberg D, Moser A, Yagupsky P et al (2005) Microbiological spectrum and susceptibility patterns of pathogens causing bacteraemia in paediatric febrile neutropenic oncology patients: comparison between two consecutive time periods with use of different antibiotic treatment protocols. Int J Antimicrob Agents 25:469–473

Groll AH, Kurz M, Schneider W et al (1999) Five-year-survey of invasive aspergillosis in a paediatric cancer centre. Epidemiology, management and long-term survival. Mycoses 42:431–442

Groll AH, Castagnola E, Cesaro S et al (2014) Fourth European Conference on Infections in Leukaemia (ECIL-4): guidelines for diagnosis, prevention, and treatment of invasive fungal diseases in paediatric patients with cancer or allogeneic haemopoietic stem-cell transplantation. Lancet Oncol 15:e327–e340

Guy SD, Tramontana AR, Worth LJ et al (2012) Use of FDG PET/CT for investigation of febrile neutropenia: evaluation in high-risk cancer patients. Eur J Nucl Med Mol Imaging 39:1348–1355

Guyatt G, Gutterman D, Baumann MH et al (2006) Grading strength of recommendations and quality of evidence in clinical guidelines: report from an American College of Chest Physicians task force. Chest 129:174–181

Hann I, Viscoli C, Paesmans M et al (1997) A comparison of outcome from febrile neutropenic episodes in children compared with adults: results from four EORTC studies. International Antimicrobial Therapy Cooperative Group

(IATCG) of the European Organization for Research and Treatment of Cancer (EORTC). Br J Haematol 99: 580–588

Haroon A, Zumla A, Bomanji J (2012) Role of fluorine 18 fluorodeoxyglucose positron emission tomography-computed tomography in focal and generalized infectious and inflammatory disorders. Clin Infect Dis 54:1333–1341

Härtel C, Deuster M, Lehrnbecher T et al (2007) Current approaches for risk stratification of infectious complications in pediatric oncology. Pediatr Blood Cancer 49:767–773

Hennequin C, Ranaivoarimalala C, Chouaki T et al (2002) Comparison of aerobic standard medium with specific fungal medium for detecting fusarium spp in blood cultures. Eur J Clin Microbiol Infect Dis 21: 748–750

Heussel CP (2011) Importance of pulmonary imaging diagnostics in the management of febrile neutropenic patients. Mycoses 54(Suppl 1):17–26

Ho DY, Lin M, Schaenman J et al (2011) Yield of diagnostic procedures for invasive fungal infections in neutropenic febrile patients with chest computed tomography abnormalities. Mycoses 54:59–70

Hodgson-Viden H, Grundy PE, Robinson JL (2005) Early discontinuation of intravenous antimicrobial therapy in pediatric oncology patients with febrile neutropenia. BMC Pediatr 5:10

Jaijakul S, Vazquez JA, Swanson RN et al (2012) (1,3)-beta-D-Glucan as a prognostic marker of treatment response in invasive candidiasis. Clin Infect Dis 55:521–526

Jain P, Sandur S, Meli Y et al (2004) Role of flexible bronchoscopy in immunocompromised patients with lung infiltrates. Chest 125:712–722

Jiancheng W, Minjun H, Yi-jun A et al (2009) Screening Pneumocystis carinii pneumonia in non-HIV-infected immunocompromised patients using polymerase chain reaction. Diagn Microbiol Infect Dis 64: 396–401

Johansen HK, Gøtzsche PC (2000) Amphotericin B lipid soluble formulations versus amphotericin B in cancer patients with neutropenia. Cochrane Database Syst Rev (3):CD000969

Jørgensen KJ, Gøtzsche PC, Johansen HK (2006) Voriconazole versus amphotericin B in cancer patients with neutropenia. Cochrane Database Syst Rev (1):CD004704

Kalil AC (2011) Is cefepime safe for clinical use? A Bayesian viewpoint. J Antimicrob Chemother 66: 1207–1209

Karageorgopoulos DE, Vouloumanou EK, Ntziora F et al (2011) Beta-D-glucan assay for the diagnosis of invasive fungal infections: a meta-analysis. Clin Infect Dis 52:750–770

Kim PW, Wu YT, Cooper C et al (2010) Meta-analysis of a possible signal of increased mortality associated with cefepime use. Clin Infect Dis 51:381–389

Kim A, Nicolau DP, Kuti JL (2011) Hospital costs and outcomes among intravenous antifungal therapies for patients with invasive aspergillosis in the United States. Mycoses 54:e301–e312

Klaassen RJ, Goodman TR, Pham B et al (2000) "Low-risk" prediction rule for pediatric oncology patients presenting with fever and neutropenia. J Clin Oncol 18:1012–1019

Klaassen IL, de Haas V, van Wijk JA et al (2011) Pyuria is absent during urinary tract infections in neutropenic patients. Pediatr Blood Cancer 56:868–870

Klastersky J, Paesmans M, Rubenstein EB et al (2000) The Multinational Association for Supportive Care in Cancer risk index: a multinational scoring system for identifying low-risk febrile neutropenic cancer patients. J Clin Oncol 18:3038–3051

Klont RR, Mennink-Kersten MA, Verweij PE (2004) Utility of Aspergillus antigen detection in specimens other than serum specimens. Clin Infect Dis 39:1467–1474

Koo S, Bryar JM, Page JH et al (2009) Diagnostic performance of the (1 >3)-beta-D-glucan assay for invasive fungal disease. Clin Infect Dis 49:1650–1659

Kosmin AR, Fekete T (2008) Use of fungal blood cultures in an academic medical center. J Clin Microbiol 46:3800–3801

Kourkoumpetis TK, Fuchs BB, Coleman JJ et al (2012) Polymerase chain reaction-based assays for the diagnosis of invasive fungal infections. Clin Infect Dis 54:1322–1331

Lahoti A, Kantarjian H, Salahudeen AK et al (2010) Predictors and outcome of acute kidney injury in patients with acute myelogenous leukemia or high-risk myelodysplastic syndrome. Cancer 116:4063–4068

Lalayanni C, Baliakas P, Xochelli A et al (2012) Outbreak of cutaneous zygomycosis associated with the use of adhesive tape in haematology patients. J Hosp Infect 81:213–215

Lee DH, Vielemeyer O (2011) Analysis of overall level of evidence behind Infectious Diseases Society of America practice guidelines. Arch Intern Med 171:18–22

Lehrnbecher T, Foster C, Vazquez N et al (1997) Therapy-induced alterations in host defense in children receiving therapy for cancer. J Pediatr Hematol Oncol 19:399–417

Lehrnbecher T, Venzon D, de Haas M et al (1999) Assessment of measuring circulating levels of interleukin-6, interleukin-8, C-reactive protein, soluble Fcγ receptor type III, and mannose-binding protein in febrile children with cancer and neutropenia. Clin Infect Dis 29:414–419

Lehrnbecher T, Stanescu A, Kuhl J (2002) Short courses of intravenous empirical antibiotic treatment in selected febrile neutropenic children with cancer. Infection 30:17–21

Lehrnbecher T, Phillips R, Alexander S et al (2012) Guideline for the management of fever and neutropenia in children with cancer and/or undergoing hematopoietic stem-cell transplantation. J Clin Oncol 30: 4427–4438

Levine SJ, Kennedy D, Shelhamer JH et al (1992) Diagnosis of Pneumocystis carinii pneumonia by multiple lobe, site-directed bronchoalveolar lavage with immunofluorescent monoclonal antibody staining in human immunodeficiency virus-infected patients receiving aerosolized pentamidine chemoprophylaxis. Am Rev Respir Dis 146:838–843

Lindblom A, Bhadri V, Soderhall S et al (2010) Respiratory viruses, a common microbiological finding in neutropenic children with fever. J Clin Virol 47:234–237

Liu C, Bayer A, Cosgrove SE et al (2011) Clinical practice guidelines by the infectious diseases society of america for the treatment of methicillin-resistant Staphylococcus aureus infections in adults and children: executive summary. Clin Infect Dis 52:285–292

Luna A, Ribes R, Caro P et al (2006) MRI of focal splenic lesions without and with dynamic gadolinium enhancement. AJR Am J Roentgenol 186:1533–1547

Luthi F, Leibundgut K, Niggli FK et al (2012) Serious medical complications in children with cancer and fever in chemotherapy-induced neutropenia: results of the prospective multicenter SPOG 2003 FN study. Pediatr Blood Cancer 59:90–95

Maertens JA, Madero L, Reilly AF et al (2010) A randomized, double-blind, multicenter study of caspofungin versus liposomal amphotericin B for empiric antifungal therapy in pediatric patients with persistent fever and neutropenia. Pediatr Infect Dis J 29:415–420

Manji A, Beyene J, Dupuis LL et al (2012a) Outpatient and oral antibiotic management of low-risk febrile neutropenia are effective in children – a systematic review of prospective trials. Support Care Cancer 20:1135–1145

Manji A, Lehrnbecher T, Dupuis LL et al (2012b) A meta-analysis of antipseudomonal penicillins and cephalosporins in pediatric patients with fever and neutropenia. Pediatr Infect Dis J 31:353–358

Manji A, Lehrnbecher T, Dupuis LL et al (2012c) A systematic review and meta-analysis of anti-pseudomonal penicillins and carbapenems in pediatric febrile neutropenia. Support Care Cancer 20:2295–2304

Marty FM, Koo S (2009) Role of (1→3)-beta-D-glucan in the diagnosis of invasive aspergillosis. Med Mycol 47:S233–S240

Masood A, Sallah S (2005) Chronic disseminated candidiasis in patients with acute leukemia: emphasis on diagnostic definition and treatment. Leuk Res 29:493–501

Mays SR, Bogle MA, Bodey GP (2006) Cutaneous fungal infections in the oncology patient: recognition and management. Am J Clin Dermatol 7:31–43

Mebis J, Goossens H, Bruyneel P et al (1998) Decreasing antibiotic resistance of Enterobacteriaceae by introducing a new antibiotic combination therapy for neutropenic fever patients. Leukemia 12:1627–1629

Meckler G, Lindemulder S (2009) Fever and neutropenia in pediatric patients with cancer. Emerg Med Clin North Am 27:525–544

Mermel LA, Allon M, Bouza E et al (2009) Clinical practice guidelines for the diagnosis and management of intravascular catheter-related infection: 2009 Update by the Infectious Diseases Society of America. Clin Infect Dis 49:1–45

Metan G, Agkus C, Buldu H et al (2010) The interaction between piperacillin/tazobactam and assays for

Aspergillus galactomannan and 1,3-beta-D-glucan in patients without risk factors for invasive fungal infections. Infection 38:217–221

Mikulska M, Furfaro E, Del Bono V et al (2012) Piperacillin/tazobactam (TazocinTM) seems to be no longer responsible for false-positive results of the galactomannan assay. J Antimicrob Chemother 67:1746–1748

Mor M, Gilad G, Kornreich L et al (2011) Invasive fungal infections in pediatric oncology. Pediatr Blood Cancer 56:1092–1097

Moyer CD, Sykes PA, Rayner JM (1977) Aeromonas hydrophila septicaemia producing ecthyma gangrenosum in a child with leukaemia. Scand J Infect Dis 9:151–153

Mularoni A, Furfaro E, Faraci M et al (2010) High Levels of beta-D-glucan in immunocompromised children with proven invasive fungal disease. Clin Vaccine Immunol 17:882–883

Mullen CA (2012) "Good Enough" medicine: noninferiority clinical trials and the management of fever and neutropenia. Pediatr Blood Cancer 59:415–416

Mullen CA, Buchanan GR (1990) Early hospital discharge of children with cancer treated for fever and neutropenia: identification and management of the low-risk patient. J Clin Oncol 8:1998–2004

Mullen CA, Petropoulos D, Roberts WM et al (1999) Outpatient treatment of fever and neutropenia for low risk pediatric cancer patients. Cancer 86:126–134

Nucci M, Anaissie EJ, Queiroz-Telles F et al (2003) Outcome predictors of 84 patients with hematologic malignancies and Fusarium infection. Cancer 98:315–319

Orudjev E, Lange BJ (2002) Evolving concepts of management of febrile neutropenia in children with cancer. Med Pediatr Oncol 39:77–85

Ozdemir N, Celkan T, Midilli K et al (2011) Novel influenza A (H1N1) infection in a pediatric hematology oncology clinic during the 2009–2010 pandemia. Pediatr Hematol Oncol 28:288–293

Paganini HR, Sarkis CM, De Martino MG et al (2000) Oral administration of cefixime to lower risk febrile neutropenic children with cancer. Cancer 88:2848–2852

Paganini H, Rodriguez-Brieschcke T, Zubizarreta P et al (2001) Oral ciprofloxacin in the management of children with cancer with lower risk febrile neutropenia. Cancer 91:1563–1567

Paganini HR, Aguirre C, Puppa G et al (2007) A prospective, multicentric scoring system to predict mortality in febrile neutropenic children with cancer. Cancer 109:2572–2579

Pappas PG, Kauffman CA, Andes D et al (2009) Clinical practice guidelines for the management of candidiasis: 2009 update by the Infectious Diseases Society of America. Clin Infect Dis 48:503–535

Park JR, Coughlin J, Hawkins D et al (2003) Ciprofloxacin and amoxicillin as continuation treatment of febrile neutropenia in pediatric cancer patients. Med Pediatr Oncol 40:93–98

Pattishall EN, Noyes BE, Orenstein DM (1988) Use of bronchoalveolar lavage in immunocompromised children with pneumonia. Pediatr Pulmonol 5:1–5

Paul M, Borok S, Fraser A et al (2005) Additional anti-Gram-positive antibiotic treatment for febrile neutropenic cancer patients. Cochrane Database Syst Rev (3):CD003914

Paul M, Yahav D, Bivas A et al (2010) Anti-pseudomonal beta-lactams for the initial, empirical, treatment of febrile neutropenia: comparison of beta-lactams. Cochrane Database Syst Rev (11):CD005197

Paul M, Dickstein Y, Schlesinger A et al (2013) Beta-lactam versus beta-lactam-aminoglycoside combination therapy in cancer patients with neutropenia. Cochrane Database Syst Rev (6):CD003038

Perfect JR, Dismukes WE, Dromer F et al (2010) Clinical practice guidelines for the management of cryptococcal disease: 2010 Update by the Infectious Diseases Society of America. Clin Infect Dis 50:291–322

Petrilli AS, Carlesse FA, Pereira CA (2007) Oral gatifloxacin in the outpatient treatment of children with cancer fever and neutropenia. Pediatr Blood Cancer 49:682–686

Pfeiffer CD, Fine JP, Safdar N (2006) Diagnosis of invasive aspergillosis using a galactomannan assay: a meta-analysis. Clin Infect Dis 42:1417–1427

Phillips B, Wade R, Stewart LA et al (2010) Systematic review and meta-analysis of the discriminatory performance of risk prediction rules in febrile neutropaenic episodes in children and young people. Eur J Cancer 46:2950–2964

Phillips RS, Wade R, Lehrnbecher T et al (2012) Systematic review and meta-analysis of the value of initial biomarkers in predicting adverse outcome in febrile neutropenic episodes in children and young people with cancer. BMC Med 10:6

Pizzo PA, Robichaud KJ, Gill FA et al (1982) Empiric antibiotic and antifungal therapy for cancer patients with prolonged fever and granulocytopenia. Am J Med 72:101–111

Pizzo PA, Hathorn JW, Hiemenz J et al (1986) A randomized trial comparing ceftazidime alone with combination antibiotic therapy in cancer patients with fever and neutropenia. N Engl J Med 315:552–558

Powers JH (2012) Editorial commentary: asking the right questions: morbidity, mortality, and measuring what's important in unbiased evaluations of antimicrobials. Clin Infect Dis 54:1710–1713

Prasad P, Sun J, Danner RL et al (2012) Excess deaths associated with tigecycline after approval based on noninferiority trials. Clin Infect Dis 54:1699–1709

Raad I, Hanna HA, Alakech B et al (2004) Differential time to positivity: a useful method for diagnosing catheter-related bloodstream infections. Ann Intern Med 140:18–25

Raad I, Kassar R, Ghannam D et al (2009) Management of the catheter in documented catheter-related coagulase-negative staphylococcal bacteremia: remove or retain? Clin Infect Dis 49:1187–1194

Rackoff WR, Gonin R, Robinson C et al (1996) Predicting the risk of bacteremia in children with fever and neutropenia. J Clin Oncol 14:919–924

Reich HL, Williams Fadeyi D et al (2004) Nonpseudomonal ecthyma gangrenosum. J Am Acad Dermatol 50:S114–S117

Roberts SD, Wells GM, Gandhi NM et al (2012) Diagnostic value of routine chest radiography in febrile, neutropenic children for early detection of pneumonia and mould infections. Support Care Cancer 20:2589–2594

Rodriguez L, Ethier MC, Phillips B et al (2012) Utility of peripheral blood cultures in patients with cancer and suspected blood stream infections: a systematic review. Support Care Cancer 20:3261–3267

Rolston KV (2005) Challenges in the treatment of infections caused by gram-positive and gram-negative bacteria in patients with cancer and neutropenia. Clin Infect Dis 40:S246–S252

Rosen GP, Nielsen K, Glenn S et al (2005) Invasive fungal infections in pediatric oncology patients: 11-year experience at a single institution. J Pediatr Hematol Oncol 27:135–140

Rosenblum J, Lin J, Kim M et al (2013) Repeating blood cultures in neutropenic children with persistent fevers when the initial blood culture is negative. Pediatr Blood Cancer 60:923–927

Rybak MJ, Lomaestro BM, Rotschafer JC et al (2009) Vancomycin therapeutic guidelines: a summary of consensus recommendations from the Infectious Diseases Society of America, the American Society of Health-System Pharmacists, and the Society of Infectious Diseases Pharmacists. Clin Infect Dis 49:325–327

Sahani DV, Kalva SP (2004) Imaging the liver. Oncologist 9:385–397

Sandoval C, Sinaki B, Weiss R et al (2012) Urinary tract infections in pediatric oncology patients with fever and neutropenia. Pediatr Hematol Oncol 29:68–72

Santolaya ME, Cofre J, Beresi V (1994) C-reactive protein: a valuable aid for the management of febrile children with cancer and neutropenia. Clin Infect Dis 18:589–595

Santolaya ME, Villarroel M, Avendaño LF (1997) Discontinuation of antimicrobial therapy for febrile, neutropenic children with cancer: a prospective study. Clin Infect Dis 25:92–97

Santolaya ME, Alvarez AM, Avilés CL et al (2002) Prospective evaluation of a model of prediction of invasive bacterial infection risk among children with cancer, fever, and neutropenia. Clin Infect Dis 35:678–683

Santolaya ME, Farfan MJ, De La Maza V et al (2011) Diagnosis of bacteremia in febrile neutropenic episodes in children with cancer: microbiologic and molecular approach. Pediatr Infect Dis J 30:957–961

Scheinemann K, Ethier MC, Dupuis LL et al (2010) Utility of peripheral blood cultures in bacteremic pediatric cancer patients with a central line. Support Care Cancer 18:913–919

Sekine L, Humbwavali J, Wolff FH et al (2010) Caspofungin versus liposomal amphotericin B: are they really comparable? Pediatr Infect Dis J 29:985–986

Semeraro M, Thomée C, Rolland E et al (2010) A predictor of unfavourable outcome in neutropenic paediatric patients presenting with fever of unknown origin. Pediatr Blood Cancer 54:284–290

Shenep JL, Flynn PM, Baker DK et al (2001) Oral cefixime is similar to continued intravenous antibiotics in the empirical treatment of febrile neutropenic children with cancer. Clin Infect Dis 32:36–43

Simon A, Fleischhack G, Hasan C et al (2000) Surveillance for nosocomial and central line related infections among pediatric hematology-oncology patients. Infect Control Hosp Epidemiol 21:592–596

Smith PB, Benjamin DK Jr, Alexander BD et al (2007) Quantification of 1,3-beta-D-glucan levels in children: preliminary data for diagnostic use of the beta-glucan assay in a pediatric setting. Clin Vaccine Immunol 14:924–925

Son YM, Na SY, Lee HY et al (2009) Ecthyma gangrenosum: a rare cutaneous manifestation caused by Stenotrophomonas maltophilia in a leukemic patient. Ann Dermatol 21:389–392

Spellberg B, Ibrahim A, Roilides E et al (2012) Combination therapy for mucormycosis: why, what, and how? Clin Infect Dis 54:S73–S78

Stabell N, Nordal E, Stensvold E et al (2008) Febrile neutropenia in children with cancer: a retrospective Norwegian multicentre study of clinical and microbiological outcome. Scand J Infect Dis 40:301–307

Steinbach WJ (2011) Rational approach to pediatric antifungal therapy. Adv Exp Med Biol 697:231–242

Steinbach WJ, Addison RM, McLaughlin L et al (2007) Prospective Aspergillus galactomannan antigen testing in pediatric hematopoietic stem cell transplant recipients. Pediatr Infect Dis J 26:558–564

Sulahian A, Boutboul F, Ribaud P et al (2001) Value of antigen detection using an enzyme immunoassay in the diagnosis and prediction of invasive aspergillosis in two adult and pediatric hematology units during a 4-year prospective study. Cancer 91:311–318

Sung L, Dupuis LL, Bliss B et al (2003) Randomized controlled trial of once- versus thrice-daily tobramycin in febrile neutropenic children undergoing stem cell transplantation. J Natl Cancer Inst 95:1869–1877

Sung L, Feldman BM, Schwamborn G et al (2004) Inpatient versus outpatient management of low-risk pediatric febrile neutropenia: measuring parents' and healthcare professionals' preferences. J Clin Oncol 22:3922–3929

Sung L, Phillips R, Lehrnbecher T (2011) Time for paediatric febrile neutropenia guidelines – children are not little adults. Eur J Cancer 47:811–813

Sung L, Manji A, Beyene J et al (2012) Fluoroquinolones in children With fever and neutropenia: a systematic review of prospective trials. Pediatr Infect Dis J 31:431–435

te Poele EM, Tissing WJ, Kamps WA et al (2009) Risk assessment in fever and neutropenia in children with cancer: what did we learn? Crit Rev Oncol Hematol 72:45–55

Teuffel O, Amir E, Alibhai SM et al (2011a) Cost-effectiveness of outpatient management for febrile neutropenia in children with cancer. Pediatrics 127:e279–e286

Teuffel O, Ethier MC, Alibhai SM et al (2011b) Outpatient management of cancer patients with febrile neutropenia: a systematic review and meta-analysis. Ann Oncol 22:2358–2365

Theuretzbacher U (2012) Pharmacokinetic and pharmacodynamic issues for antimicrobial therapy in patients with cancer. Clin Infect Dis 54:1785–1792

Thomas KE, Owens CM, Veys PA et al (2003) The radiological spectrum of invasive aspergillosis in children: a 10-year review. Pediatr Radiol 33:453–460

Uhlenbrock S, Zimmermann M, Fegeler W et al (2001) Liposomal amphotericin B for prophylaxis of invasive fungal infections in high-risk paediatric patients with chemotherapy-related neutropenia: interim analysis of a prospective study. Mycoses 44:455–463

Uys A, Rapoport BL, Anderson R (2004) Febrile neutropenia: a prospective study to validate the Multinational Association of Supportive Care of Cancer (MASCC) risk-index score. Support Care Cancer 12:555–560

Uys A, Rapoport BL, Fickl H et al (2007) Prediction of outcome in cancer patients with febrile neutropenia: comparison of the Multinational Association of Supportive Care in Cancer risk-index score with procalcitonin, C-reactive protein, serum amyloid A, and interleukins-1β, -6, -8 and -10. Eur J Cancer Care 16:475–483

Vazquez JA (2008) Clinical practice: combination antifungal therapy for mold infections: much ado about nothing? Clin Infect Dis 46:1889–1901

Vidal L, Ben dor I, Paul M et al (2013) Oral versus intravenous antibiotic treatment for febrile neutropenia in cancer patients. Cochrane Database Syst Rev (10):CD003992

Wacker P, Halperin DS, Wyss M et al (1997) Early hospital discharge of children with fever and neutropenia: a prospective study. J Pediatr Hematol Oncol 19:208–211

Walsh TJ, Pappas P, Winston DJ et al (2002) Voriconazole compared with liposomal amphotericin B for empirical antifungal therapy in patients with neutropenia and persistent fever. N Engl J Med 346:225–234

Walsh TJ, Anaissie EJ, Denning DW et al (2008) Treatment of aspergillosis: clinical practice guidelines of the Infectious Diseases Society of America. Clin Infect Dis 46:327–360

Watt K, Benjamin DK Jr, Cohen-Wolkowiez M (2011) Pharmacokinetics of antifungal agents in children. Early Hum Dev 87:S61–S65

Wicki S, Keisker A, Aebi C et al (2008) Risk prediction of fever in neutropenia in children with cancer: a step towards individually tailored supportive therapy? Pediatr Blood Cancer 51:778–783

Wingard JR, Hiemenz JW, Jantz MA (2012) How I manage pulmonary nodular lesions and nodular infiltrates in patients with hematologic malignancies or undergoing hematopoietic cell transplantation. Blood 120:1791–1800

Xu B, Shi P, Wu H et al (2010) Utility of FDG PET/CT in guiding antifungal therapy in acute leukemia patients with chronic disseminated candidiasis. Clin Nucl Med 35:567–570

Yahav D, Paul M, Fraser A et al (2007) Efficacy and safety of cefepime: a systematic review and meta-analysis. Lancet Infect Dis 7:338–348

Zandijk E, Mewis A, Magerman K et al (2008) False-positive results by the platelia Aspergillus galactomannan antigen test for patients treated with amoxicillin-clavulanate. Clin Vaccine Immunol 15:1132–1133

Zaoutis TE, Heydon K, Chu JH et al (2006) Epidemiology, outcomes, and costs of invasive aspergillosis in immunocompromised children in the United States, 2000. Pediatrics 117:e711–e716

Zinner SH (1999) Changing epidemiology of infections in patients with neutropenia and cancer: emphasis on gram-positive and resistant bacteria. Clin Infect Dis 29:490–494

Transfusion Support

2

Esteban Gomez, Anurag K. Agrawal,
and Caroline A. Hastings

Contents

E. Gomez, MD • A.K. Agrawal, MD (✉)
C.A. Hastings, MD
Department of Hematology/Oncology,
Children's Hospital and Research Center Oakland,
747 52nd Street, Oakland, CA 94609, USA
e-mail: aagrawal@mail.cho.org

Abstract

The utilization of appropriate transfusion therapy is a vital aspect in the prevention of morbidity in pediatric oncology patients. Practitioners must be cognizant of the risks and benefits of transfusion as well as the appropriate transfusion practices in immunocompromised patients. Here we review the evidence regarding transfusion management practices in pediatric cancer patients with anemia, thrombocytopenia and neutropenia as well as practice in managing potential transfusion reactions. Where an evidence basis is lacking, we review consensus guidelines in both the pediatric and adult cohorts.

2.1 Introduction

The utilization of appropriate transfusion therapy is a vital aspect in the prevention of morbidity in pediatric oncology patients. Practitioners must be cognizant of the risks and benefits of transfusion as well as the appropriate transfusion practices in immunocompromised patients. Here we review the evidence regarding transfusion management practices in pediatric cancer patients with anemia, thrombocytopenia and neutropenia as well as practice in managing potential transfusion reactions. Where an evidence basis is lacking, we review consensus guidelines in both the pediatric and adult cohorts.

J. Feusner et al. (eds.), *Supportive Care in Pediatric Oncology:
A Practical Evidence-Based Approach*, Pediatric Oncology,
DOI 10.1007/978-3-662-44317-0_2, © Springer Berlin Heidelberg 2015

2.2   Anemia

Anemia is a deficiency of red blood cells (RBCs) and secondarily hemoglobin (hgb) concentration leading to a reduced oxygen-carrying capacity. Anemia is widely prevalent in pediatric oncology patients at presentation and during the course of their treatment. Studies document an overall incidence of anemia in >50 % of children with malignancy at diagnosis and during the course of treatment; as many as 97 % of those with pediatric leukemia have been reported to be affected (Green et al. 1998; Nachman et al. 1998; Hockenberry et al. 2002; Michon 2002). The specific hemoglobin concentration at which anemia becomes symptomatic is dependent on several variables including age, time over which anemia develops, and the clinical status of the patient and is usually unique to each individual patient. Understanding the etiology of anemia, its signs and symptoms and how it can be appropriately managed is essential to providing effective supportive care in the pediatric oncology patient.

Anemia develops due to suppressed erythropoiesis secondary to marrow infiltration with malignant cells, suppression related to chemotherapy, radiation therapy, or infection, impaired use of iron stores, and decreased endogenous erythropoietin (EPO) and blood loss secondary to hemorrhage, infection, repetitive blood sampling, and hemolysis (Groopman and Itri 1999; Cazzola 2000; Sobrero et al. 2001; Hockenberry et al. 2002; Stasi et al. 2003). Parvovirus B19, cytomegalovirus (CMV) and Epstein-Barr virus (EBV) have specifically been reported to suppress erythropoiesis (Alpert and Fleisher 1984; Almeida-Porada and Ascensao 1996; El-Mahallawy et al. 2004; Eid et al. 2006). Recognition of the major contributors toward anemia can provide insight into the expected course and potential optimal interventions.

Clinical symptoms of anemia include fatigue, weakness, loss of appetite, headache, dizziness, irritability, fainting and poor concentration while signs of anemia include tachycardia, tachypnea, dyspnea, flow murmurs and, in severe cases, congestive heart failure (Cunningham 2003; Mock and Olsen 2003). The severity of signs and symptoms depends both on the degree of anemia and the rapidity of decline. With a gradual onset, patient physiology has time to undergo compensatory changes that minimize symptoms. For example, the newly diagnosed leukemia patient often presents with severe anemia yet minimal symptoms. The gradual onset of anemia allows for physiologic compensation through plasma expansion and increased cardiac output allowing the patient to maintain near-normal activity despite profound decrement in hemoglobin concentration.

2.2.1   Red Blood Cell Transfusion Guidelines

The transfusion of packed red blood cells (PRBCs) is the primary treatment modality for anemia in pediatric oncology patients and provides rapid and relatively safe correction of anemia and its concurrent symptoms. Utilization of hematopoietic growth factors (i.e., recombinant erythropoietin, rhEPO) remains controversial and is discussed in Chap. 15; specific populations such as Jehovah's Witnesses, whose religious practice forbids the transfusion of blood products, may be able to avoid transfusion in certain cases with the utilization of rhEPO. The potential risk-benefit ratio of PRBC transfusion must be considered in each individual case and discussed with the patient and family; transfusion should therefore be avoided in the clinically stable child who is recovering from chemotherapy-induced aplasia. Evidence-based guidelines on appropriate thresholds for PRBC transfusion are lacking in the pediatric oncology literature since the decision to transfuse should be individualized (Buchanan 2005; Wong et al. 2005). Factors to consider include the effect of anemia on quality of life (i.e., fatigue, patient preference), cardiovascular stability, safety of procedures and sedation, the clinical condition of the patient, the presence or risk of bleeding, comorbidities such as infection and the anticipated length of suppressed erythropoiesis (Rossetto and McMahon 2000). Studies have demonstrated that adolescent and adult patients with higher hgb levels have improved quality of life measures (Hockenberry-Eaton and Hinds

Table 2.1 Red blood cell transfusion guidelines and level of evidence

Clinical status	Description	Hemoglobin level for transfusion (g/dL)	Level of evidence[a]
Stable	Asymptomatic, imminent marrow recovery	<7	1C
Vital sign changes	Tachycardia, tachypnea, hypotension	<8	1C
Thrombocytopenia	Recent or active hemorrhage	8–10	1C
Procedure	Potential blood loss	8–10	1C
	Anesthesia requirement	<7	1C
Oxygen requirement	Pulmonary or cardiac comorbidities	8–10	1C
Fatigue	Decreased quality of life, especially in adolescents	8–10	1B
Chronic anemia, infancy	Impact on growth or development	8–10	1C
Radiation therapy	Radiosensitizer	See text	2C

With permission from Agrawal et al. (2011)
[a]Per Guyatt et al. (2006); see Preface

2000; Mock and Olsen 2003; Knight et al. 2004). Generally young children compensate for anemia better than adolescents and thus it is not uncommon for adolescents to have a higher hgb threshold at which they become symptomatic and at which transfusion should be considered (Davies and Kinsey 1994; Ruggiero and Riccardi 2002).

Generally, severe anemia (i.e., hgb <7 g/dL) is the threshold utilized for PRBC transfusion in pediatric oncology patients although may not be required for the well-compensated patient recovering from chemotherapy-induced aplasia (Table 2.1) (Ruggiero and Riccardi 2002; Marec-Berard et al. 2003). As expected, the need for PRBC transfusion is directly related to the intensity of therapy (Tas et al. 2002; Marec-Berard et al. 2003; Ruccione et al. 2012). Management of moderate anemia (i.e., hgb >7 g/dL) should be individualized based on physical findings, symptoms and patient preference; usually close monitoring is sufficient. Particular clinical situations may alter the threshold for PRBC transfusion: (1) the patient with planned surgery may require PRBC transfusion to minimize risks of induction anesthesia or blood loss; (2) the critically ill patient; (3) the patient with bleeding; (4) the patient with recent severe hemorrhage; and (5) the febrile patient with risk of sepsis and increased RBC and coagulation factor consumption (Table 2.1). Evidence is lacking to guide specific transfusion thresholds for each of these clinical situations and therefore provider and

institutional preference must be considered. Infants generally can be managed with the same hgb thresholds although underlying cardiopulmonary status, ability to feed, and effect on growth and development should be specifically considered (Roseff et al. 2002; Gibson et al. 2004). Utilization of PRBC transfusion for increased hgb thresholds in pediatric oncology patients with solid tumors receiving radiotherapy as a means to increase radiosensitivity remains controversial; see Chap. 13 for a summary of the evidence and recommendations which should occur in discussion with radiation oncology. Patients with leukemia and hyperleukocytosis (white blood cell [WBC] count $>100 \times 10^9$/L) are at risk for leukostasis secondary to the increase in the cytocrit. Often a compensatory decrease in the hgb (erythrocrit) is seen and may aid in the prevention of symptom development. Therefore, PRBC transfusion must be avoided in the asymptomatic patient with hyperleukocytosis; see Chap. 6 for a full discussion of PRBC transfusion with hyperleukocytosis.

2.2.2 Red Blood Cell Administration

Informed consent must be obtained prior to PRBC transfusion with a discussion of the risks, benefits and treatment alternatives to transfusion therapy. PRBCs are often stored in adsol (adenine saline, AS) secondary to a longer storage life (42 days) with a resultant hematocrit of 55–60 % due to the addition of 100 mL of AS per unit blood. All pediatric oncology patients should receive leukoreduced, irradiated PRBCs. Leukocytes are implicated as contributory to the majority of transfusion reactions; leukoreduction has been shown to significantly reduce febrile nonhemolytic transfusion reactions (FNHTRs) as well as infection with viral, bacterial, and protozoal pathogens, and specifically CMV transmission (van Marwijk Kooy et al. 1991; Chu 1999; Vamvakas and Blajchman 2001; Dzik 2002; Heddle 2004; King et al. 2004; Paglino et al. 2004; Yazer et al. 2004; Blumberg et al. 2005). Although leukoreduction decreases CMV transmission, CMV-seronegative units are thought safer in at-risk populations; specifically for pediatric oncology, consensus guidelines recommend CMV-seronegative units in patients receiving hematopoietic stem cell transplantation (HSCT) although this recommendation is controversial (Hillyer et al. 1994; Blajchman et al. 2001; Nichols et al. 2003; Gibson et al. 2004; Ljungman 2004; Vamvakas 2005). Additional studies have shown no difference in CMV transmission rates in HSCT patients receiving leukoreduced versus CMV-seronegative PRBCs (Bowden et al. 1995; Thiele et al. 2011; Nash et al. 2012). PRBC irradiation is recommended in all immunocompromised patients to prevent transfusion-associated graft-versus-host disease (TA-GVHD) by inactivating donor T-cell replication and engraftment in the host (Anderson et al. 1991; Moroff and Luban 1992; Dwyre and Holland 2008; Rühl et al. 2009). Similar to HSCT-related GVHD, TA-GVHD can present with fever, anorexia, vomiting, diarrhea, skin rash, as well as pancytopenia and hepatic dysfunction. Directed donation of PRBCs from family members is generally not recommended due to the cost and time required in addition to not being shown more safe in the prevention of transfusion-associated infection (Strauss et al. 1990).

Determination of the goal hgb should direct the volume of PRBCs transfused and is dependent on the patient's clinical status, potential for ongoing blood loss and time to recovery from myelosuppressive chemotherapy. Generally 10–20 mL/kg of PRBCs are transfused, rounding to the nearest unit to avoid blood product wastage and historically given over 4 h although this practice is not well studied in hemodynamically stable children. In the patient without ongoing blood loss or alloimmunization, the expected rise in hgb is dependent on the hematocrit concentration of the PRBC product; for an AS preserved unit, the hgb is expected to increase by approximately 2 g/dL for each 10 mL/kg of PRBCs transfused (Davies et al. 2007). Anecdotal teaching that repeat hgb measurement must wait a certain period of time for reequilibration is poorly studied and likely unnecessary (Glatstein et al. 2005; Davies et al. 2007). Patients with severe chronic anemia (i.e., hgb <5 g/dL) are potentially at risk for transfusion-associated circulatory overload (TACO) due to the theoretical concern for cardiogenic pulmonary edema with transfusion in the patient with existing compensatory increase in plasma blood volume to near-normal levels. Variable practice exists, including slow transfusion of 5 mL/kg over 4 h, sometimes with the addition of a diuretic agent such as furosemide. Limited evidence suggests more liberal transfusion rates such as 2 mL/kg/h can be safely used in those patients without underlying evidence of hemodynamic instability or cardiopulmonary compromise (Jayabose et al. 1993; Agrawal et al. 2012).

2.3   Thrombocytopenia

Thrombocytopenia is a common side effect of intensive pediatric oncology therapy with potential risks for morbidity, dependent on the rate of platelet drop and seen more commonly when the platelet count is $<20 \times 10^9$/L (Belt et al. 1978; Rintels et al. 1994). Petechiae, spontaneous hemorrhage and mucosal bleeding are common with platelet count $<20 \times 10^9$/L while the risk for severe spontaneous or life-threatening hemorrhage is rare (Slichter and Harker 1978; Consensus Conference 1987; Gmür et al. 1991; Contreras 1998; Norfolk et al. 1998; Schiffer et al. 2001; Athale and Chan 2007). Thrombocytopenia occurs most commonly secondary to suppressed thrombopoiesis from chemotherapy,

Table 2.2 Platelet transfusion guidelines and level of evidence

Clinical scenario	Description	Platelet count for transfusion (×10⁹/L)	Level of evidence[a]
Stable	Asymptomatic, imminent marrow recovery	<10	1B
Procedures	Diagnostic LP	50–100 (see text)	1B
	Subsequent LP	<20	1C
	Bone marrow aspiration	Not indicated	1C
	Minor surgery: central line placement, bronchoscopy with lavage, sinus aspiration, endoscopy with biopsy	<50	1C
	Major surgery: CNS or solid tumor resection or biopsy	<100	1C
Signs/symptoms or underlying diagnosis	Minor bleeding: epistaxis, mild mucosal bleeding	<20	1C
	Major bleeding: hemoptysis, hemorrhagic cystitis, GI, CNS, tumor necrosis	<100	1C
	Fever	<20	2C
	APL induction	<50	1C
	Newborns	<20–50	1C
	Radiation	<20–50	2C
	DIC	<50	1C
	Coagulopathy	<50	1C

LP lumbar puncture, *CNS* central nervous system, *GI* gastrointestinal, *APL* acute promyelocytic leukemia, *DIC* disseminated intravascular coagulation
With permission from Agrawal et al. (2011)
[a]Per Guyatt et al. (2006); see Preface

radiation therapy or infection. Thrombocytopenia at diagnosis in leukemia patients can be secondary to marrow infiltration as well as splenic sequestration in those with splenomegaly. Increased platelet consumption can occur due to hemorrhage and sepsis with secondary disseminated intravascular coagulation (DIC). Frequent platelet transfusion increases the risk of developing platelet antibodies and subsequent refractoriness to further transfusion; therefore, as with PRBC transfusion, the risks and benefits of platelet transfusion must be considered in each individual case prior to the decision to transfuse.

2.3.1 Platelet Transfusion Guidelines

Platelet transfusion guidelines generally recommend prophylactic transfusion at threshold levels depending on the underlying risks of bleeding (Table 2.2). Although no specific pediatric oncology guidelines have been published, the American

Society of Clinical Oncology (ASCO) practice guidelines incorporate clinical trials in pediatric oncology (Schiffer et al. 2001). Factors that must be considered when deciding to transfuse platelets include: (1) cause of thrombocytopenia; (2) time to expected resolution; (3) rapidity of platelet count drop; (4) clinical condition of the patient including fever, infection, mucositis, coagulopathy or bleeding; (5) history of severe hemorrhage; (6) recent surgical procedure or planned surgery; and (7) concomitant medications such as amphotericin, enoxaparin and tyrosine kinase inhibitors.

Prospective, randomized trials in adolescents and adults with acute leukemia have reported that prophylactic transfusion can be safely given for a platelet threshold of 10×10^9/L in clinically stable patients (Gmür et al. 1991; Heckman et al. 1997; Rebulla et al. 1997; Wandt et al. 1998).

What platelet threshold is appropriate for patients undergoing procedures, for those with a history of hemorrhage and in those with potential concurrent bleeding risk factors such as fever, infection, and coagulopathy has not been well studied. Similarly, social factors such as distance to clinic and ease of accessing care must also be considered when determining the need for platelet transfusion (Benjamin and Anderson 2002). Although definitive evidence is lacking, consensus panels have concluded that platelets $>50 \times 10^9$/L and $>20 \times 10^9$/L are sufficient for major and minor surgical procedures, respectively (Norfolk et al. 1998; Rebulla 2001; Schiffer et al. 2001; BCSH 2003). Risk of bleeding has been found to correlate most with a history of severe hemorrhage rather than platelet count (Friedmann et al. 2002).

What platelet threshold should be utilized for lumbar puncture in pediatric oncology patients is poorly studied. One large retrospective study concluded that a platelet threshold of $>10 \times 10^9$/L was sufficient for lumbar puncture (LP) although only 3.8 % of patients had platelet count $<20 \times 10^9$/L at the time of LP (Howard et al. 2000). A follow-up study analyzing risk factors for traumatic LP concluded that African American race, age <1 year, prior traumatic tap within 2 weeks, prior LP with platelets $<50 \times 10^9$/L, lack of general anesthesia, platelet count $<100 \times 10^9$/L, interval of <15 days between LPs and a less experienced practitioner were all significant (Howard et al. 2002). What effect this analysis has on practice is unclear. The study was also confounded by a high rate of traumatic (29.3 %; ≥ 10 RBC/µL) and bloody (10.4 %; ≥ 500 RBC/µL) LPs (Howard et al. 2002). Based on this analysis the authors conclude that a platelet count $>100 \times 10^9$/L should be the threshold for diagnostic LP and the procedure be performed by the most experienced practitioner (Howard et al. 2002). Data on the prognostic significance of traumatic LP and theoretical potential of introduction of leukemic blasts into the cerebrospinal fluid are controversial although multiple studies have shown it to be a risk factor for poor outcome (Gajjar et al. 2000; Bürger et al. 2003; te Loo et al. 2006). Whether a lower platelet count in the hands of an experienced practitioner remains a risk factor for traumatic LP is unknown.

Unlike LP procedures, bone marrow aspiration and biopsy can be performed without regard to platelet count as long as pressure is applied to the area after the procedure (BCSH 2003). For patients undergoing central line placement, adult studies have shown that platelet counts >30–50×10^9/L are safe (Stellato et al. 1985; Coit and Turnbull 1988; Lowell and Bothe 1991; Barrera et al. 1996; Doerfler et al. 1996; Ray and Shenoy 1997; Loh and Chui 2007). No similar studies have been reported in pediatric patients. Additionally, the need for a particular platelet count for some post-procedure time period to prevent development of bleeding has not been reported.

2.3.2 Platelet Administration

Platelets for transfusion come as either pooled platelet concentrates (PPCs) or as an apheresis unit. PPCs are aggregated from red blood cell donations and contain $\geq 5.5 \times 10^{10}$ platelets. Four to six platelet units are combined to make a PPC. On the other hand, an apheresis platelet unit is obtained from a single donor and is the equivalent of 6–10 PC units (i.e., $\geq 3 \times 10^{11}$ platelets). Transfusion with apheresis platelets minimizes exposure to multiple blood donors although whether this decreases the risk of alloimmunization and therefore is of benefit in patient populations requiring frequent transfusion such as pediatric oncology is controversial (NEJM 1997). Apheresis platelet units undergo leukodepletion during the collection procedure, whereas PPCs must be subsequently filtered. Leukodepletion has been shown to decrease the risk of alloimmunization in both PPCs and apheresis units (NEJM 1997). Risk of bacterial contamination is low with both PPCs and apheresis units and has not been found to be significantly different (Schrezenmeier et al. 2007). Storage of platelet units at 20–24 °C with gentle horizontal agitation has been found safe up to 5 days after collection; longer storage times increase the risk for bacterial proliferation and cytokine-mediated reactions (Schiffer et al. 1986; Klein et al. 1997).

As with PRBCs, platelets should be dosed by weight with 10 mL/kg of either PPCs or an apheresis product resulting in an increase of

$50–100 \times 10^9/L$ (Roseff et al. 2002; Fasano and Luban 2008). Determination of response as well as clinical status of the patient can guide future transfusions; generally patients are not given more than one apheresis unit although those with a poor response to transfusion or active bleeding may require higher doses. Platelets are transfused over 30–60 min although more rapid infusion rates have been found safe and effective (Norville et al. 1997). Although considered a risk factor, a direct relationship between number of transfused platelet units and incidence of platelet refractoriness has not been consistently shown in the literature (Howard and Perkins 1978; Dutcher et al. 1981; Schiffer et al. 2001). Platelet refractoriness is defined as an insufficient platelet increment after transfusion on at least two occasions and is the most significant long-term complication of platelet transfusion (Schiffer 1991). ABO incompatibility has been shown to be a risk factor in development of platelet refractoriness (Carr et al. 1990). HLA-matched platelets and crossmatching have been shown effective in improving platelet increment in patients found refractory (Duquesnoy et al. 1977; Heal et al. 1987; Kickler et al. 1988; Welch et al. 1989; O'Connell et al. 1992; Friedberg et al. 1993, 1994; Gelb and Leavitt 1997). As with PRBCs, platelets should be irradiated to prevent TA-GVHD in immunocompromised patients, while CMV seronegativity may be unnecessary in the apheresis product for the CMV-seronegative patient (Luban et al. 2000; Nichols et al. 2003; Dwyre and Holland 2008).

2.4 Granulocyte Transfusion

Patients with prolonged neutropenia are at increasing risk of infection and secondarily lack neutrophils to eradicate infection. Therefore it has been theorized that frequent granulocyte transfusion may be an effective method to fight serious infection in the severely neutropenic patient without imminent count recovery. Although theoretically promising and potentially shown beneficial in small observational studies, consistent data are lacking and some meta-analyses have failed to show a significant benefit

(Vamvakas and Pineda 1997; Bishton and Chopra 2004; Robinson and Marks 2004; Grigull et al. 2006; Sachs et al. 2006; van de Wetering et al. 2007; Seidel et al. 2008; Massey et al. 2009; Peters 2009).

In the patient with severe, refractory or progressive bacterial or fungal infection and severe neutropenia likely to continue >1 week, granulocyte transfusion can be considered (Bishton and Chopra 2004). Donors should be mobilized with G-CSF and dexamethasone with a goal transfusion dose of $>1.0 \times 10^9$ cells/kg in the pediatric patient transfused daily for a minimum of 4–7 days (Chanock and Gorlin 1996; Klein et al. 1996; Massey et al. 2009). Granulocyte transfusion should be ABO compatible and crossmatched as well as irradiated to prevent TA-GVHD (Bishton and Chopra 2004). CMV-seronegative products should be used in CMV-seronegative patients to prevent CMV transmission (Bishton and Chopra 2004).

2.5 Risks of Blood Product Therapy and Their Management

In the past, clerical error leading to ABO-incompatible blood transfusion and secondary acute hemolysis, as well as infectious complications, were the most common transfusion reactions (Williamson et al. 1999; Linden et al. 2000; Myhre and McRuer 2000; Stainsby et al. 2006). Now, due to improved blood safety, transfusion-related acute lung injury (TRALI) has become most common in the adult literature due to increased recognition, and generally noninfectious causes are much more common (Bolton-Maggs and Murphy 2004; Stainsby et al. 2006). Reactions to transfusion may range from mild to life-threatening and the clinician must be able to promptly recognize the potential severe reaction in the face of common transfusion-related symptoms such as fever. Acute reactions are defined as occurring within 24 h while delayed reactions occur beyond the acute period. Potential reactions include acute and delayed hemolysis, FNHTR, allergic reactions, TRALI, TACO, TA-GVHD and infectious complications. In the chronically transfused, alloimmunization to PRBC transfusion must be considered in addition to iron overload. Management of transfusion reactions is generally based on best practice and consensus guidelines rather than an evidence basis (Table 2.3).

2.5.1 Hemolytic Transfusion Reactions

Acute hemolytic transfusion reactions (AHTRs) present with fever, chills, nausea and vomiting as well as anxiety and discomfort. Additional signs and symptoms include dyspnea, hypotension or shock, oliguria, hemoglobinuria, hemoglobinemia and disseminated intravascular coagulation (DIC). AHTRs generally occur secondary to IgM antibodies to anti-A and anti-B isohemagglutinins but may additionally develop due to other IgM and IgG antibodies. Bystander hemolysis can secondarily lyse recipient red blood cells. AHTR is generally due to ABO incompatibility but may also occur with other immune and nonimmune causes including RBCs damaged by blood warmers, incorrectly prepared frozen PRBCs, bacterial contamination, as well as autoimmune and drug-induced causes of hemolysis. Delayed hemolytic transfusion reactions (DHTRs) present with milder symptoms including low-grade fever, jaundice, and a lower than expected posttransfusion hgb increment and are due to previously sensitized patients without detectable antibody at the time of crossmatch. DHTR occurs with IgG antibody-mediated complement fixation, manifesting as extravascular hemolysis.

Evaluation of a potential AHTR should include each blood unit transfused. Laboratory evaluation involves repeat crossmatch, performance of a direct antibody test (DAT; direct Coombs), as well as measurement of hgb, urinalysis, and plasma-free hgb or haptoglobin. With a more insidious DHTR leading to extravascular hemolysis, laboratory assessment should include hgb, reticulocyte count, DAT, indirect bilirubin and lactate dehydrogenase. Management of an AHTR is based on best practice and includes immediately stopping the transfusion, providing fluid support, and monitoring perfusion and urine output. Vasopressor support may be required as well as management of DIC with platelets and fresh frozen plasma (FFP). Transfusion of additional PRBCs should be avoided due to the potential for continued bystander hemolysis but can be given in the symptomatic patient or if with continued active bleeding.

2.5.2 Infection and Sepsis

Transfusion-transmitted viral infections have markedly decreased with improved donor screening and viral testing measures; current estimated rates of transmission include approximately <1 in 1.5 million for HIV, 1 in 300,000 for hepatitis B virus, and <1 in 2 million for hepatitis C virus (Busch et al. 2005; Dodd 2007; Dwyre et al. 2011). Advanced serologic screening measures have decreased the window period in which viral transmission has recently transpired but without positive testing measures, although, false-negative tests can still occur (Dwyre et al. 2011). Posttransfusion hepatitis is generally caused by viruses including hepatitis A, B, C and E in addition to CMV and EBV. CMV transmission can lead to primary infection in the previously CMV-seronegative recipient or reactivation in the previously infected recipient. CMV can lead to a mononucleosis-type syndrome and immunocompromised patients are at risk for more severe manifestations including nephritis, retinitis, interstitial pneumonitis, colitis and cytopenias (Rubin et al. 1985). Additional rare transmission of human T-lymphotropic retrovirus, human herpesvirus-8 and variant Creutzfeldt-Jakob disease has been noted (Dodd 2007). Parvovirus B19 is not routinely screened and can cause a prolonged reticulocytopenia and anemia in patients with underlying hematologic malignancies (Kaur and Basu 2005).

Bacterial infection must be considered in the patient with a new fever or fever increase $\geq 1\ ^\circ C$ from the previous 24 h during transfusion. Blood contamination can occur at the time of collection or during processing and has decreased

Table 2.3 Management guidelines for transfusion reactions and level of evidence

Type	Clinical features	Lab/imaging findings	Management	Level of evidence[a]
Acute hemolytic transfusion reaction (AHTR)	Immediate onset; fever, anxiety, hypotension, DIC, renal failure	↑Indirect bilirubin Hematuria ↑LDH/AST ↓Haptoglobin ↑Plasma-free hgb +DAT	Stop transfusion ICU support Fluid resuscitation Vasopressor support FFP, platelets for DIC Avoid PRBC transfusion Diuretics to maintain urine output once BP stabilized	1C
Febrile nonhemolytic transfusion reaction (FNHTR)	During or within 4 h of transfusion; fever, chills, rigors, nausea/vomiting, headache	None	Stop transfusion Rule out AHTR and bacterial contamination/sepsis Antipyretics Restart transfusion if serious adverse reactions ruled out	1C
Allergic transfusion reaction	Immediate for severe reaction with anaphylaxis (i.e., bronchospasm, hypotension); during or following transfusion for mild reaction (i.e., urticaria, pruritus)	None	Stop transfusion Severe reaction: epinephrine, diphenhydramine, H2 blocker, consider steroid Mild reaction: diphenhydramine	1C
Delayed hemolytic transfusion reaction (DHTR)	>24 h from transfusion and within 2 weeks; fever, chills, jaundice, malaise; can be asymptomatic	↓Hgb vs expected posttfn increment ↑Bilirubin ↑LDH +DAT +Red cell alloantibodies	Usually no treatment required Potential repeat tfn Screen for new red cell antibodies	1C
Transfusion-related acute lung injury (TRALI)	Within 6 h of transfusion; dyspnea, hypoxemia, fever, hypotension, noncardiogenic pulmonary edema	+CXR with diffuse infiltrates	Oxygen Vasopressor support Mechanical ventilation Unclear benefit for corticosteroids	1C
Bacterial sepsis	Usually of immediate onset if severe GNR; fever, chills, rigors, hypotension, DIC, oliguria, shock	+Bcx from patient and/or transfusion bag	Stop transfusion Fluid resuscitation ICU support Vasopressors Empiric antibiotics with ceftaz/tobra	1C

DIC disseminated intravascular coagulation, *bili* bilirubin, *LDH* lactate dehydrogenase, *AST* aspartate aminotransferase, *DAT* direct antiglobin test [Coombs], *ICU* intensive care unit, *FFP* fresh frozen plasma, *PRBC* packed red blood cell, *BP* blood pressure, *hgb* hemoglobin, *CXR* chest radiograph, *GNR* Gram-negative rods, *Bcx* blood culture
Adapted from Agrawal et al. (2011)
[a]Per Guyatt et al. (2006); see Preface

significantly with improved blood collection and screening procedures (Wagner 1997; Kuehnert et al. 2001; Stainsby et al. 2006; Dodd 2007). Bacterial infection is much more common with platelets compared to PRBCs since they are stored at room temperature and risk of contamination has been directly correlated to storage time (Morrow et al. 1991). Fatal infection is more likely due to Gram-negative endotoxin production as compared to the more commonly seen Gram-positive organisms (Arduino et al. 1989). Transfusion should be stopped in the event of fever or signs or symptoms of sepsis. The patient should be treated immediately with volume resuscitation, broad spectrum antibiotics and a transfusion workup commenced including blood cultures of the transfusion bag.

2.5.3 Allergic Reactions/ Anaphylaxis

Allergic reactions are common, complicating 1–5 % of transfusions and more likely with platelet or plasma transfusion (Couban et al. 2002). Reactions are type I hypersensitivity mediated and usually mild with cutaneous manifestations although systemic symptoms related to anaphylaxis are possible and usually occur within minutes of transfusion commencement. Transfusion should be held once allergic symptoms manifest; diphenhydramine is usually sufficient to manage cutaneous symptoms. In the case of systemic symptoms consistent with anaphylaxis, the transfusion should not be restarted and the patient may require additional medications including epinephrine, steroids and fluid expansion. Any patient with a systemic reaction should be evaluated for IgA deficiency. Prophylaxis with diphenhydramine in the patient with a previous reaction has not been shown beneficial although it is often utilized (Wang et al. 2002; Sanders et al. 2005; Geiger and Howard 2007; Kennedy et al. 2008). It is reasonable to consider prophylactic corticosteroids prior to transfusion in the patient with multiple reactions; if symptoms continue, or if the patient is IgA deficient, washed blood products should be utilized.

2.5.4 Febrile Nonhemolytic Transfusion Reactions

FNHTR is defined as a temperature increase of ≥1 °C associated with transfusion and not attrib-

utable to any other cause. FNHTR was common prior to the advent of leukoreduction due to pyrogenic cytokines released from leukocytes during storage (Heddle et al. 1993; King et al. 2004; Paglino et al. 2004; Yazer et al. 2004). A recent study of transfusions in a pediatric intensive care unit reported a 0.9 % rate of FNTHRs (Gauvin et al. 2006). FNHTR is a diagnosis of exclusion and therefore transfusion should be halted until an AHTR has been ruled out. Additional diagnostic considerations should include bacterial contamination and TRALI. Fever related to FNHTR can occur during or up to 4 h after the completion of transfusion and is self-limited. Antipyretics can be provided for comfort and the transfusion restarted once the patient has defervesced and more serious causes have been ruled out. The utilization of antipyretics to prevent the development of FNHTR has shown little benefit, even in the patient with a history of FNHTRs (Wang et al. 2002; Sanders et al. 2005; Geiger and Howard 2007; Kennedy et al. 2008). Notwithstanding, prophylactic antipyretics can be considered in the patient with multiple FNHTRs although may not be effectual; washed blood products can be considered with continued FNHTR.

2.5.5 Transfusion-Related Acute Lung Injury

TRALI is an increasingly recognized life-threatening complication which occurs after transfusion of plasma-containing blood products (Popovsky 2000; Bolton-Maggs and Murphy 2004; Stainsby et al. 2006). In a 2004 consensus conference, TRALI was defined as acute lung injury occurring within 6 h of transfusion without any other potential causes (Kleinman et al. 2004; Andreu 2009). Symptoms of TRALI include dyspnea, tachypnea and fever; signs include hypotension, hypoxemia and bilateral infiltrates on chest radiograph without fluid overload (Kleinman et al. 2004). A paucity of data exist in pediatric patients although it appears that the pathogenesis and course are similar to adult patients, with the majority recovering in 48–96 h after the precipitating event (Sanchez and Toy 2005; Church et al. 2006). Although the pathophysiology of TRALI is yet to be clearly delineated, passive transfer of antibody leading to neutrophil activation in the lung is thought the most likely mechanism, exacerbated in those with existing lung injury and therefore less likely in pediatric patients (Popovsky 2000; Goldman et al. 2005). Fresh frozen plasma is the most likely contributing blood product, especially when the donor is an antibody-positive multiparous female (Eder et al. 2007). Increasing platelet age at time of transfusion has also been noted as a risk factor (Silliman et al. 2003).

TRALI is a diagnosis of exclusion and patients with mild symptoms may improve without TRALI being recognized. Patients will require oxygen support and some will need mechanical ventilation and vasopressor support. Corticosteroids may be of benefit as with other causes of acute lung injury but are unproven in TRALI (Barrett and Kam 2006). Recognition of TRALI is vital in order to provide the appropriate medical management and also to potentially screen for neutrophil-specific antibodies.

2.5.6 Transfusion-Associated Circulatory Overload

TACO is also becoming increasingly recognized although is a rare phenomenon in pediatric patients with normal underlying cardiorespiratory function. TACO is defined as cardiogenic pulmonary edema and is due to too large a transfusion volume or too rapid a transfusion rate (Eder et al. 2007). Clinical signs and symptoms of TACO include dyspnea, tachypnea, hypoxemia and hypertension as compared to the hypotension seen in TRALI. Hypertension is due to a positive fluid balance with pulmonary and systemic overcirculation and therefore unlike TRALI, the patient with TACO should be managed with aggressive diuresis. In the patient not responding to diuresis, other potential diagnoses should be entertained.

2.5.7 Transfusion-Associated Graft-Versus-Host Disease

In the immunocompromised patient, nonirradiated blood and platelet products can lead to TA-GVHD, especially in the setting of histocompatible donor T cells. Manifestations of TA-GVHD are similar to GVHD seen secondary to allogeneic HSCT and include fever, anorexia, vomiting and diarrhea, and skin rash of variable presentation and severity. Pancytopenia and hepatic dysfunction may be present. The patient should be diagnosed by skin biopsy, liver biopsy or bone marrow aspirate and may require lifesaving HSCT.

2.5.8 Iron Overload

Total body iron is closely regulated in order to maintain a steady state load of 35–45 mg/kg (Shander et al. 2009). Iron absorption from food intake is extremely limited (i.e., 1 mg/day) as are mechanisms of iron excretion; therefore, when patients receive frequent PRBC transfusion with the receipt of approximately 1 mg of iron per 1 mL of transfused blood, iron overload can occur, resulting in non-transferrin-bound iron (i.e., free iron) and subsequent free iron deposition in tissues, specifically parenchymal cells of the liver, heart, pancreas and endocrine tissues (Shander et al. 2009; de Ville de Goyet et al. 2013). Free iron may also be associated with oxidative damage due to generation of free oxygen radicals, likely accentuated in the setting of concomitant chemotherapy delivery (Shander et al. 2009).

Iron overload leads to a higher incidence of organ failure and mortality in populations that are chronically transfused and has also been noted as a risk factor for mortality in oncology patients with myelodysplastic syndrome (MDS) and in those receiving HSCT (Ballas 2001; Cazzola and Malcovati 2005; Darbari et al. 2006; Malcovati et al. 2006; Armand et al. 2007; Garcia-Manero et al. 2008; Fenaux and Rose 2009; Shander et al. 2009; Alessandrino et al. 2010). In pediatric oncology, studies have shown that transfusion burden increases with increased therapy intensity in both hematologic malignancies and solid tumor patients leading to iron overload in more than half of patients although the effect of this iron overload on subsequent toxicities is poorly quantified (Emy et al. 1997; Eng and Fish 2011; Ruccione et al. 2012; de Ville de Goyet et al. 2013). Quantification of total body iron can be assessed by liver biopsy, measurement with a superconducting quantum interference device (SQUID) or more recently through proton magnetic resonance imaging (Fischer et al. 1999; Angelucci et al. 2000; Brittenham et al. 2001; St Pierre et al. 2005; Wood et al. 2005).

Iron overload may be a factor in late effects in long-term survivors of pediatric cancers and therefore all patients should be screened at the end of therapy for potential iron overload. Patients who have received >1 g of transfused iron (>4 units PRBCs) should be screened with a serum ferritin level and transferrin saturation (Halonen et al. 2003). For patients with serum ferritin levels persistently >1,000 ng/mL, measurement of total body iron stores by proton MRI should be considered. In such cases chelation therapy or serial phlebotomy should also be a consideration, especially in the adolescent male.

2.6 Summary

Blood product transfusion is a common practice in patients undergoing myelosuppressive therapy. That being said, an evidence basis for PRBC and platelet thresholds for transfusion are generally lacking and therefore consensus guidelines, assessment of each individual patient and the underlying clinical situation, as well as patient preference must all be routine considerations in the decision to transfuse. Prior to transfusion, the patient, family and practitioner must all be aware of the potential short- and long-term risks of transfusion. The practitioner should be able to determine the appropriate volume and preparative steps required for transfusion and the likely increment in hgb or platelet count after transfusion. Any potential concerning reaction during a

transfusion should be appropriately managed and assessed per standard guidelines, as described.

References

Agrawal AK, Hastings CH, Feusner J (2011) Hematologic supportive care in children with cancer. In: Pizzo PA, Poplack DG (eds) Principles and practice of pediatric oncology, 6th edn. Lippincott Williams and Wilkins, Philadelphia

Agrawal AK, Hsu E, Quirolo K et al (2012) Red blood cell transfusion in pediatric patients with severe chronic anemia: how slow is necessary. Pediatr Blood Cancer 58:466–468

Alessandrino EP, Della Porta MG, Bacigalupo A et al (2010) Prognostic impact of pre-transplantation transfusion history and secondary iron overload in patients with myelodysplastic syndrome undergoing allogeneic stem cell transplantation: a GITMO study. Haematologica 95:476–484

Almeida-Porada GD, Ascensao JL (1996) Cytomegalovirus as a cause of pancytopenia. Leuk Lymphoma 21:217–223

Alpert G, Fleisher GR (1984) Complications of infection with Epstein-Barr virus during childhood: a study of children admitted to the hospital. Pediatr Infect Dis 3:304–307

Anderson KC, Goodnough LT, Sayers M et al (1991) Variation in blood component irradiation practice: implications for prevention of transfusion-associated graft-versus-host disease. Blood 77:2096–2102

Andreu G (2009) Transfusion-associated circulatory overload and transfusion-related acute lung injury: diagnosis, pathophysiology, management and prevention. ISBT Sci Ser 4:63–71

Angelucci E, Brittenham GM, McLaren CE et al (2000) Hepatic iron concentration and total body iron stores in thalassemia major. N Engl J Med 343:327–331

Arduino MJ, Bland LA, Tipple MA et al (1989) Growth and endotoxin production of Yersinia enterocolitica and Enterobacter agglomerans in packed erythrocytes. J Clin Microbiol 27:1483–1485

Armand P, Kim HT, Cutler CS et al (2007) Prognostic impact of elevated pretransplantation serum ferritin in patients undergoing myeloablative stem cell transplantation. Blood 109:4586–4588

Athale UH, Chan AK (2007) Hemorrhagic complications in pediatric hematologic malignancies. Semin Thromb Hemost 33:408–415

Ballas SK (2001) Iron overload is a determinant of morbidity and mortality in adult patients with sickle cell disease. Semin Hematol 38:30–36

Barrera R, Mina B, Huang Y et al (1996) Acute complications of central line placement in profoundly thrombocytopenic cancer patients. Cancer 78:2025–2030

Barrett NA, Kam PC (2006) Transfusion-related acute lung injury: a literature review. Anesthesia 61:777–785

Belt RJ, Leite C, Haas CD, Stephens RL (1978) Incidence of hemorrhagic complications in patients with cancer. JAMA 239:2571–2574

Benjamin RJ, Anderson KS (2002) What is the proper threshold for platelet transfusion in patients with chemotherapy-induced thrombocytopenia? Crit Rev Oncol Hematol 42:163–171

Bishton M, Chopra R (2004) The role of granulocyte transfusions in neutropenic patients. Br J Haematol 127:501–508

Blajchman MA, Goldman M, Freedman JJ, Sher GD (2001) Proceedings of a consensus conference: prevention of post-transfusion CMV in the era of universal leukoreduction. Transfus Med Rev 15:1–20

Blumberg N, Fine L, Gettings KF, Heal JM (2005) Decreased sepsis related to indwelling venous access devices coincident with implementation of universal leukoreduction of blood transfusions. Transfusion 45:1632–1639

Bolton-Maggs PH, Murphy MF (2004) Blood transfusion. Arch Dis Child 89:4–7

Bowden RA, Slichter SJ, Sayers M et al (1995) A comparison of filtered leukocyte-reduced and cytomegalovirus (CMV) seronegative blood products for the prevention of transfusion-associated CMV infection after marrow transplant. Blood 86:3598–3603

British Committee for Standards in Hematology (BCSH) (2003) Guidelines on the use of platelet transfusions. Br J Haematol 122:10–23

Brittenham GM, Sheth S, Allen CJ et al (2001) Noninvasive methods for quantitative assessment of transfusional iron overload in sickle cell disease. Semin Hematol 38:37–56

Buchanan GR (2005) Blood transfusions in children with cancer and hematologic disorders: why, when, and how? Pediatr Blood Cancer 44:114–116

Bürger B, Zimmermann M, Mann G et al (2003) Diagnostic cerebrospinal fluid examination in children with acute lymphoblastic leukemia: significance of low leukocyte counts with blasts or traumatic lumbar puncture. J Clin Oncol 21:184–188

Busch MP, Glynn SA, Stramer SL (2005) A new strategy for estimating risks of transfusion-transmitted viral infections based on rates of detection of recently infected donors. Transfusion 45:254–264

Carr R, Hutton JL, Jenkins JA et al (1990) Transfusion of ABO-mismatched platelets leads to early platelet refractoriness. Br J Haematol 75:408–413

Cazzola M (2000) Mechanisms of anaemia in patients with malignancy: implications for the clinical use of recombinant human erythropoietin. Med Oncol 17:S11–S16

Cazzola M, Malcovati L (2005) Myelodysplastic syndromes—coping with ineffective hematopoiesis. N Engl J Med 352:536–538

Chanock SJ, Gorlin JB (1996) Granulocyte transfusions. Time for a second look. Infect Dis Clin North Am 10:327–343

Chu RW (1999) Leukocytes in blood transfusion: adverse effects and their prevention. Hong Kong Med J 5:280–284

Church GD, Price C, Sanchez R (2006) Transfusion-related acute lung injury in the paediatric patient: two case reports and a review of the literature. Transfus Med 16:343–348

Coit DB, Turnbull AD (1988) A safe technique for the placement of implantable vascular access devices in patients with thrombocytopenia. Surg Gynecol Obstet 167:429–431

Consensus Conference (1987) Platelet transfusion therapy. JAMA 257:1777–1780

Contreras M (1998) The appropriate use of platelets: an update from the Edinburgh Consensus Conference. Br J Haematol 101:10–12

Couban S, Carruthers J, Andreou P et al (2002) Platelet transfusion in children: results of a randomized, prospective, crossover trial of plasma removal and a prospective audit of WBC reduction. Transfusion 42:753–758

Cunningham RS (2003) Anemia in the oncology patient: cognitive function and cancer. Cancer Nurs 26:38S–42S

Darbari DS, Kple-Faget P, Kwagyan J et al (2006) Circumstances of death in adult sickle cell disease patients. Am J Hematol 81:858–863

Davies SC, Kinsey SE (1994) Clinical aspects of paediatric blood transfusion: cellular components. Vox Sang 67:50–53

Davies P, Robertson S, Hedge S et al (2007) Calculating the required transfusion volume in children. Transfusion 47:212–216

De Ville de Goyet M, Moniotte S, Robert A et al (2013) Iron overload in children undergoing cancer treatments. Pediatr Blood Cancer 60:1982–1987

Dodd RY (2007) Current risk for transfusion transmitted infections. Curr Opin Hematol 14:671–676

Doerfler ME, Kaufman B, Goldenberg AS (1996) Central venous catheter placement in patients with disorders of hemostasis. Chest 110:185–188

Duquesnoy RJ, Filip DJ, Rodey GE et al (1977) Successful transfusion of platelets "mis-matched" for HLA antigens to alloimmunized thrombocytopenic patients. Am J Hematol 2:219–226

Dutcher JP, Schiffer CA, Aisner J et al (1981) Alloimmunization following platelet transfusion: the absence of a dose–response relationship. Blood 57:395–398

Dwyre DM, Holland PV (2008) Transfusion-associated graft-versus-host disease. Vox Sang 95:85–93

Dwyre DM, Fernando LP, Holland PV (2011) Hepatitis B, hepatitis C and HIV transfusion-transmitted infections in the 21st century. Vox Sang 100:92–98

Dzik WH (2002) Leukoreduction of blood components. Curr Opin Hematol 9:521–526

Eder AF, Herron R, Strupp A et al (2007) Transfusion-related acute lung injury surveillance (2003–2005) and the potential impact of the selective use of plasma from male donors in the American Red Cross. Transfusion 47:599–607

Eid AJ, Brown RA, Patel R, Razonable RR (2006) Parvovirus B19 infection after transplantation: a review of 98 cases. Clin Infect Dis 43:40–48

El-Mahallawy HA, Mansour T, El-Din SE et al (2004) Parvovirus B19 infection as a cause of anemia in pediatric acute lymphoblastic leukemia patients during maintenance chemotherapy. J Pediatr Hematol Oncol 26:403–406

Emy PY, Levin TL, Sheth SS et al (1997) Iron overload in reticuloendothelial systems of pediatric oncology patients who have undergone transfusions: MR observations. Am J Radiol 168:1011–1015

Eng J, Fish JD (2011) Insidious iron burden in pediatric patients with acute lymphoblastic leukemia. Pediatr Blood Cancer 56:368–371

Fasano R, Luban NL (2008) Blood component therapy. Pediatr Clin North Am 55:421–455

Fenaux P, Rose C (2009) Impact of iron overload in myelodysplastic syndromes. Blood Rev 23:S15–S19

Fischer R, Tiemann ED, Engelhardt R et al (1999) Assessment of iron stores in children with transfusion siderosis by biomagnetic liver susceptometry. Am J Hematol 60:289–299

Friedberg RC, Donnelly SF, Boyd JC et al (1993) Clinical and blood bank factors in the management of platelet refractoriness and alloimmunization. Blood 81:3428–3434

Friedberg RC, Donnelly SF, Mintz PD (1994) Independent roles for platelet crossmatching and HLA in the selection of platelets for alloimmunized patients. Transfusion 34:215–220

Friedmann AM, Sengul H, Lehmann H et al (2002) Do basic laboratory tests or clinical observations predict bleeding in thrombocytopenic oncology patients? A reevaluation of prophylactic platelet transfusions. Transfus Med Rev 16:34–45

Gajjar A, Harrison PL, Sandlund JT et al (2000) Traumatic lumbar puncture at diagnosis adversely affects outcome in childhood acute lymphoblastic leukemia. Blood 96:3381–3384

Garcia-Manero G, Shan J, Faderl S et al (2008) A prognostic score for patients with low risk myelodysplastic syndrome. Leukemia 22:538–543

Gauvin F, Lacroix J, Robillard P et al (2006) Acute transfusion reactions in the pediatric intensive care unit. Transfusion 46:1899–1908

Geiger TL, Howard SC (2007) Acetaminophen and diphenhydramine premedication for allergic and febrile nonhemolytic transfusion reactions: good prophylaxis or bad practice? Transfus Med Rev 21:1–12

Gelb AB, Leavitt AD (1997) Crossmatch-compatible platelets improve corrected count increments in patients who are refractory to randomly selected platelets. Transfusion 37:624–630

Gibson BE, Todd A, Roberts I et al (2004) Transfusion guidelines for neonates and older children. Br J Haematol 124:433–453

Glatstein M, Oron T, Barak M et al (2005) Posttransfusion equilibration of hematocrit in hemodynamically stable neonates. Pediatr Crit Care Med 6:707–708

Gmür J, Burger J, Schanz U et al (1991) Safety of stringent prophylactic platelet transfusion policy for patients with acute leukaemia. Lancet 338:1223–1226

Goldman M, Webert KE, Arnold DM et al (2005) Proceedings of a consensus conference: towards an understanding of TRALI. Transfus Med Rev 19:2–31

Green DM, Breslow NE, Beckwith JB et al (1998) Comparison between single-dose and divided-dose administration of dactinomycin and doxorubicin for patients with Wilms' tumor: a report from the National Wilms' Tumor Study Group. J Clin Oncol 16:237–245

Grigull L, Pulver N, Goudeva L et al (2006) G-CSF mobilised granulocyte transfusions in 32 paediatric patients with neutropenic sepsis. Support Care Cancer 14:910–916

Groopman JE, Itri LM (1999) Chemotherapy-induced anemia in adults: incidence and treatment. J Natl Cancer Inst 91:1616–1634

Guyatt G, Gutterman D, Baumann MH et al (2006) Grading strength of recommendations and quality of evidence in clinical guidelines: report from an American College of Chest Physicians task force. Chest 129:174–181

Halonen P, Mattila J, Suominen P et al (2003) Iron overload in children who are treated for acute lymphoblastic leukemia estimated by liver siderosis and serum iron parameters. Pediatrics 111:91–96

Heal JM, Blumberg N, Masel D (1987) An evaluation of crossmatching, HLA, and ABO matching for platelet transfusions to refractory patients. Blood 70:23–30

Heckman KD, Weiner GJ, Davis CS et al (1997) Randomized study of prophylactic platelet transfusion threshold during induction therapy for adult acute leukemia: 10,000/microL versus 20,000/microL. J Clin Oncol 15:1143–1149

Heddle NM (2004) Universal leukoreduction and acute transfusion reactions: putting the puzzle together. Transfusion 44:1–4

Heddle NM, Klama LN, Griffith L et al (1993) A prospective study to identify the risk factors associated with acute reactions to platelet and red cell transfusion. Transfusion 33:794–797

Hillyer CD, Emmens RK, Zago-Novaretti M, Berkman EM (1994) Methods for the reduction of transfusion-transmitted cytomegalovirus infection: filtration versus the use of seronegative donor units. Transfusion 34:929–934

Hockenberry MJ, Hinds PS, Barrera P et al (2002) Incidence of anemia in children with solid tumors or Hodgkin disease. J Pediatr Hematol Oncol 24:35–37

Hockenberry-Eaton M, Hinds PS (2000) Fatigue in children and adolescents with cancer: evolution of a program of study. Semin Oncol Nurs 16:261–272

Howard JE, Perkins HA (1978) The natural history of alloimmunization to platelets. Transfusion 18:496–503

Howard SC, Gajjar AC, Ribeiro RC et al (2000) Safety of lumbar puncture for children with acute lymphoblastic leukemia and thrombocytopenia. JAMA 284:2222–2224

Howard SC, Gajjar AC, Cheng C et al (2002) Risk factors for traumatic and bloody lumbar puncture in children with acute lymphoblastic leukemia. JAMA 288:2001–2007

Jayabose S, Tugal O, Ruddy R et al (1993) Transfusion therapy for severe anemia. Am J Pediatr Hematol Oncol 15:324–327

Kaur P, Basu S (2005) Transfusion-transmitted infections: existing and emerging pathogens. J Postgrad Med 51:146–151

Kennedy LD, Case LD, Hurd DD et al (2008) A prospective, randomized, double-blind controlled trial of acetaminophen and diphenhydramine pretransfusion medication versus placebo for the prevention of transfusion reactions. Transfusion 48:2285–2291

Kickler TS, Ness PM, Baine HG (1988) Platelet crossmatching. A direct approach to the selection of platelet transfusions for the alloimmunized thrombocytopenic patient. Am J Clin Pathol 90:69–72

King KE, Shirey RS, Thoman SK et al (2004) Universal leukoreduction decreases the incidence of febrile nonhemolytic transfusion reactions to RBCs. Transfusion 44:25–29

Klein HG, Strauss RG, Schiffer CA (1996) Granulocyte transfusion therapy. Semin Hematol 33:359–368

Klein HG, Dodd RY, Ness PM et al (1997) Current status of microbial contamination of blood components: summary of a conference. Transfusion 37:95–101

Kleinman S, Caulfield T, Chan P et al (2004) Towards an understanding of transfusion-related acute lung injury: statement of a consensus panel. Transfusion 44:1774–1789

Knight K, Wade S, Balducci L (2004) Prevalence and outcomes of anemia in cancer: a systematic review of the literature. Am J Med 116:11S–26S

Kuehnert MJ, Roth VR, Haley NR et al (2001) Transfusion-transmitted bacterial infection in the United States, 1998 through 2000. Transfusion 41:1493–1499

Linden JV, Wagner K, Voytovich AE et al (2000) Transfusion errors in New York state: an analysis of 10 years' experience. Transfusion 40:1207–1213

Ljungman P (2004) Risk of cytomegalovirus transmission by blood products to immunocompromised patients and means for reduction. Br J Haematol 125:107–116

Loh AH, Chui CH (2007) Port-A-Cath insertions in acute leukemia: dose thrombocytopenia affect morbidity? J Pediatr Surg 42:1180–1184

Lowell JA, Bothe A Jr (1991) Venous access. Preoperative, operative, and postoperative dilemmas. Surg Clin North Am 71:1231–1246

Luban NL, Drothler D, Moroff G et al (2000) Irradiation of platelet components: inhibition of lymphocyte proliferation assessed by limiting-dilution analysis. Transfusion 40:348–352

Malcovati L, Della Porta MG, Cazzola M (2006) Predicting survival and leukemic evolution in patients with myelodysplastic syndrome. Haematologica 91:1588–1590

Marec-Berard P, Blay JY, Schell M et al (2003) Risk model predictive of severe anemia requiring RBC transfusion after chemotherapy in pediatric solid tumor patients. J Clin Oncol 21:4235–4238

Massey E, Paulus U, Doree C et al (2009) Granulocyte transfusions for preventing infections in patients with neutropenia or neutrophil dysfunction. Cochrane Database Syst Rev (1):CD005341

Michon J (2002) Incidence of anemia in pediatric cancer patients in Europe: results of a large, international survey. Med Pediatr Oncol 39:448–450

Mock V, Olsen M (2003) Current management of fatigue and anemia in patients with cancer. Semin Oncol Nurs 19:36–41

Moroff G, Luban NL (1992) Prevention of transfusion-associated graft-versus-host disease. Transfusion 32:102–103

Morrow JF, Braine HG, Kickler TS et al (1991) Septic reactions to platelet transfusions. A persistent problem. JAMA 266:555–558

Myhre BA, McRuer D (2000) Human error—a significant cause of transfusion mortality. Transfusion 40:879–885

Nachman J, Sather HN, Cherlow JM et al (1998) Response of children with high-risk acute lymphoblastic leukemia treated with and without cranial irradiation: a report from the Children's Cancer Group. J Clin Oncol 16:920–930

Nash T, Hoffmann S, Butch S et al (2012) Safety of leukoreduced, cytomegalovirus (CMV)-untested components in CMV-negative allogeneic human progenitor cell transplant recipients. Transfusion 52:2270–2272

Nichols WG, Price TH, Gooley T et al (2003) Transfusion-transmitted cytomegalovirus infection after receipt of leukoreduced blood products. Blood 101:4195–4200

Norfolk DR, Ancliffe PJ, Contreras M et al (1998) Consensus Conference on Platelet Transfusion, Royal College of Physicians of Edinburgh, 27–28 November 1997. Synopsis of background papers. Br J Haematol 101:609–617

Norville R, Hinds P, Wilimas J et al (1997) The effects of infusion rate on platelet outcomes and patient responses in children with cancer: an in vitro and in vivo study. Oncol Nurs Forum 24:1789–1793

O'Connell BA, Lee EJ, Rothko K et al (1992) Selection of histocompatible apheresis platelet donors by crossmatching random donor platelet concentrates. Blood 79:527–531

Paglino JC, Pomper GJ, Fisch GS et al (2004) Reduction of febrile but not allergic reactions to RBCs and platelets after conversion to universal prestorage leukoreduction. Transfusion 44:16–24

Peters C (2009) Granulocyte transfusions in neutropenic patients: beneficial effects proven? Vox Sang 96:275–283

Popovsky MA (2000) Transfusion-related acute lung injury. Curr Opin Hematol 7:402–407

Ray CE Jr, Shenoy SS (1997) Patients with thrombocytopenia: outcome of radiologic placement of central venous access devices. Radiology 204:97–99

Rebulla P (2001) Platelet transfusion trigger in difficult patients. Transfus Clin Biol 8:249–254

Rebulla P, Finazzi G, Marangoni F et al (1997) The threshold for prophylactic platelet transfusions in adults with acute myeloid leukemia. Gruppo Italiano Malattie Ematologiche Maligne dell'Adulto. N Engl J Med 337:1870–1875

Rintels PB, Kenney RM, Crowley JP (1994) Therapeutic support of the patient with thrombocytopenia. Hematol Oncol Clin North Am 8:1131–1157

Robinson SP, Marks DI (2004) Granulocyte transfusion in the G-CSF era. Where do we stand? Bone Marrow Transplant 34:839–846

Roseff SD, Luban NL, Manno CS (2002) Guidelines for assessing appropriateness of pediatric transfusion. Transfusion 42:1398–1413

Rossetto CL, McMahon JE (2000) Current and future trends in transfusion therapy. J Pediatr Oncol Nurs 17:160–170

Rubin RH, Tolkoff-Rubin NE, Oliver D et al (1985) Multicenter seroepidemiologic study of the impact of cytomegalovirus infection on renal transplantation. Transplantation 40:243–249

Ruccione KS, Midambi K, Sposto R et al (2012) Association of projected transfusional iron burden with treatment intensity in childhood cancer survivors. Pediatr Blood Cancer 59:697–702

Ruggiero A, Riccardi R (2002) Interventions for anemia in pediatric cancer patients. Med Pediatr Oncol 39:451–454

Rühl H, Bein G, Sachs UJ (2009) Transfusion-associated graft-versus-host disease. Transfus Med Rev 23: 62–71

Sachs UJ, Reiter A, Walter T et al (2006) Safety and efficacy of therapeutic early onset granulocyte transfusions in pediatric patients with neutropenia and severe infections. Transfusion 46:1909–1914

Sanchez R, Toy P (2005) Transfusion related acute lung injury: a pediatric perspective. Pediatr Blood Cancer 45:248–255

Sanders RP, Maddirala SD, Geiger TL et al (2005) Premedication with acetaminophen or diphenhydramine for transfusion with leucoreduced blood products in children. Br J Haematol 130:781–787

Schiffer CA (1991) Prevention of alloimmunization against platelets. Blood 77:1–4

Schiffer CA, Lee EJ, Ness PM et al (1986) Clinical evaluation of platelet concentrates stored for one to five days. Blood 67:1591–1594

Schiffer CA, Anderson KC, Bennett CL et al (2001) Platelet transfusion for patients with cancer: clinical practice guidelines of the American Society of Clinical Oncology. J Clin Oncol 19:1519–1538

Schrezenmeier H, Walther-Wenke G, Müller TH et al (2007) Bacterial contamination of platelet concentrates: results of a prospective multicenter study comparing pooled whole blood-derived platelets and apheresis platelets. Transfusion 47:644–652

Seidel MG, Peters C, Wacker A et al (2008) Randomized phase III study of granulocyte transfusions in neutropenic patients. Bone Marrow Transplant 42: 679–684

Shander A, Cappellini MD, Goodnough LT (2009) Iron overload and toxicity: the hidden risk of multiple blood transfusions. Vox Sang 97:185–197

Silliman CC, Boshkov LK, Mehdizadehkashi Z et al (2003) Transfusion-related acute lung injury: epidemiology and a prospective analysis of etiologic factors. Blood 101:454–462

Slichter SJ, Harker LA (1978) Thrombocytopenia: mechanisms and management of defects in platelet production. Clin Haematol 7:523–539

Sobrero A, Puglisi F, Guglielmi A et al (2001) Fatigue: a main component of anemia symptomatology. Semin Oncol 28:15–18

St Pierre TG, Clark PR, Chau-anusorn W et al (2005) Noninvasive measurement and imaging of liver iron concentrations using proton magnetic resonance. Blood 105:855–861

Stainsby D, Jones H, Asher D et al (2006) Serious hazards of transfusion: a decade of hemovigilance in the UK. Transfus Med Rev 20:273–282

Stasi R, Abriani L, Beccaglia P et al (2003) Cancer-related fatigue: evolving concepts in evaluation and treatment. Cancer 98:1786–1801

Stellato TA, Gauderer MW, Lazarus HM et al (1985) Percutaneous silastic catheter insertion in patients with thrombocytopenia. Cancer 56:2691–2693

Strauss RG, Barnes A Jr, Blanchette VS et al (1990) Directed and limited-exposure blood donations for infants and children. Transfusion 30:68–72

Tas F, Eralp Y, Basaran M et al (2002) Anemia in oncology practice: relation to diseases and their therapies. Am J Clin Oncol 25:371–379

te Loo DM, Kamps WA, van der Does-van den Berg A et al (2006) Prognostic significance of blasts in the cerebrospinal fluid without pleiocytosis or a traumatic lumbar puncture in children with acute lymphoblastic leukemia: experience of the Dutch Childhood Oncology Group. J Clin Oncol 24:2332–2336

The Trial to Reduce Alloimmunization to Platelets Study Group (1997) Leukocyte reduction and ultraviolet B irradiation of platelets to prevent alloimmunization and refractoriness to platelet transfusions. N Engl J Med 337:1861–1869

Thiele T, Krüger W, Zimmermann K et al (2011) Transmission of cytomegalovirus (CMV) infection by leukoreduced blood products not tested for CMV antibodies: a single-center prospective study in high-risk patients undergoing allogeneic hematopoietic stem cell transplantation (CME). Transfusion 51: 2620–2626

Vamvakas EC (2005) Is white blood cell reduction equivalent to antibody screening in preventing transmission of cytomegalovirus by transfusion? A review of the literature and meta-analysis. Transfus Med Rev 19:181–199

Vamvakas EC, Blajchman MA (2001) Universal WBC reduction: the case for and against. Transfusion 41:691–712

Vamvakas ED, Pineda AA (1997) Determinants of the efficacy of prophylactic granulocyte transfusions: a meta-analysis. J Clin Apher 12:74–81

van de Wetering MD, Weggelaar N, Offinga M et al (2007) Granulocyte transfusions in neutropaenic children: a systematic review of the literature. Eur J Cancer 43:2082–2092

van Marwijk Kooy M, van Prooijen HC, Moes M et al (1991) Use of leukocyte-depleted platelet concentrates for the prevention of refractoriness and primary HLA alloimmunization: a prospective, randomized trial. Blood 77:201–205

Wagner S (1997) Transfusion-related bacterial sepsis. Curr Opin Hematol 4:464–469

Wandt H, Frank M, Ehninger G et al (1998) Safety and cost effectiveness of a 10^3 x 10(9)/L trigger for prophylactic platelet transfusions compared with the traditional 20^3 x 10(9)/L trigger: a prospective comparative trial in 105 patients with acute myeloid leukemia. Blood 91:3601–3606

Wang SE, Lara PN, Lee-Ow A et al (2002) Acetaminophen and diphenhydramine as premedication for platelet transfusions: a prospective randomized double-blind placebo-controlled trial. Am J Hematol 70:191–194

Welch HG, Larson EB, Slichter SJ (1989) Providing platelets for refractory patients. Prudent strategies. Transfusion 29:193–195

Williamson LM, Lowe S, Love EM et al (1999) Serious hazards of transfusion (SHOT) initiative: analysis of the first two annual reports. BMJ 319:16–19

Wong EC, Perez-Albuerne E, Moscow JA, Luban NL (2005) Transfusion management strategies: a survey of practicing pediatric hematology/oncology specialists. Pediatr Blood Cancer 44:119–127

Wood JC, Enriquez C, Ghugre N et al (2005) MRI R2 and R2* mapping accurately estimates hepatic iron concentration in transfusion-dependent thalassemia and sickle cell disease patients. Blood 106: 1460–1465

Yazer MH, Podlosky L, Clarke G, Nahirniak SM (2004) The effect of prestorage WBC reduction on the rates of febrile nonhemolytic transfusion reactions to platelet concentrates and RBC. Transfusion 44:10–15

Tumor Lysis Syndrome

3

Anne Marsh, Anurag K. Agrawal, and James H. Feusner

Contents

Abstract

Tumor lysis syndrome (TLS) is a metabolic complication of rapid cell turnover and therefore is seen most frequently in pediatric oncology patients with large tumor burdens (often with renal parenchymal involvement), tumors with short doubling times and those exquisitely sensitive to cytotoxic therapy such as acute lymphoblastic leukemia (ALL) and non-Hodgkin lymphoma (NHL). TLS can include metabolic complications related to hyperkalemia, hyperphosphatemia (with resultant hypocalcemia) and hyperuricemia. Laboratory TLS (LTLS) should be differentiated from clinical TLS (CTLS); CTLS includes seizures, cardiac arrhythmias and acute kidney injury necessitating renal dialysis. Recognition of risk factors for LTLS and preventive therapy remain the most important management steps to minimize development of CTLS. The evidence basis behind recommendations in the management of TLS is often negligible and therefore based mostly on consensus statements; here we analyze the existing literature in relation to the consensus statements to determine and grade rational guidelines.

A. Marsh, MD • A.K. Agrawal, MD (✉)
J.H. Feusner
Department of Hematology/Oncology,
Children's Hospital and Research Center Oakland,
747 52nd Street,
Oakland, CA 94609, USA
e-mail: aagrawal@mail.cho.org

3.1 Introduction

Tumor lysis syndrome (TLS) is a metabolic complication of rapid cell turnover and therefore is seen most frequently in pediatric

J. Feusner et al. (eds.), *Supportive Care in Pediatric Oncology:
A Practical Evidence-Based Approach*, Pediatric Oncology,
DOI 10.1007/978-3-662-44317-0_3, © Springer Berlin Heidelberg 2015

oncology patients with large tumor burdens (often with renal parenchymal involvement), tumors with short doubling times and those exquisitely sensitive to cytotoxic therapy such as acute lymphoblastic leukemia (ALL) and non-Hodgkin lymphoma (NHL). TLS can include metabolic complications related to hyperkalemia, hyperphosphatemia (with resultant hypocalcemia) and hyperuricemia (HU) (Zusman et al. 1973). Laboratory TLS (LTLS) should be differentiated from clinical TLS (CTLS); CTLS includes seizures, cardiac arrhythmias and acute kidney injury (AKI) necessitating renal dialysis (Table 3.1). TLS is generally most pronounced 12–72 hours after therapy initiation (Coiffier et al. 2008). Data from German BFM ALL and NHL trials report an overall TLS incidence of 4.4–5.2 %; 66 of 78 patients with TLS in the more recent cohort had either ALL or Burkitt lymphoma (BL) (Meyer et al. 1998; Wössmann et al. 2003). Patients with ALL had a 26.4 % incidence and those with BL and lactate dehydrogenase (LDH) ≥500 U/L a 14.9 % incidence of TLS (Wössmann et al. 2003). Montesinos et al. (2008) similarly reported a high rate (17 %) of TLS in adult patients with acute myelogenous leukemia (AML) although in a consensus statement Tosi et al. (2008) note that TLS is rare in AML. Incidence has not been reported in pediatric AML. TLS has also been noted in other non-lymphomatous pediatric solid tumor types including neuroblastoma, hepatoblastoma, thymoma, Langerhans cell histiocytosis (LCH), medulloblastoma, germ cell tumors, and soft tissue sarcomas though rarely, in case reports, and specifically in those with a high tumor burden (Khan and Broadbent 1993; Hain et al. 1994; Jaing et al. 2001; Kushner et al. 2003; Trobaugh-Lotrario et al. 2004; Gemici 2006; Bercovitz et al. 2010; Bien et al. 2010). Although more likely related to chronic hypertension, TLS has also been noted to be a risk factor for the development of posterior reversible encephalopathy syndrome (PRES) (Kaito et al. 2005; Ozkan et al. 2006).

Elevated calcium phosphate product and HU increase the risk of calcium phosphate and urate precipitation in the kidneys respectively; precipitated crystals are toxic to the renal epithelium (Shimada et al. 2009). Although LTLS is quite frequent in high-risk malignancies, CTLS is uncommon (Hande and Garrow 1993; Kedar et al. 1995; Patte et al. 2002). Patte et al. (2002) reported a 1.7 % need for renal dialysis utilizing the most up to date supportive care measures in stage III/IV pediatric NHL patients. TLS can occur at diagnosis but is more common after the initiation of cytotoxic chemotherapy (Stapleton et al. 1988; Larsen and Loghman-Adham 1996; Kobayashi et al. 2010). TLS has also been noted after fever, surgical manipulation of solid tumors, after anesthesia,

Table 3.1 Parameters for laboratory and clinical tumor lysis syndrome in children

Laboratory tumor lysis syndrome (*2 or more of the following occurring from 3 days prior up to 7 days after commencement of cytotoxic therapy*)
Uric acid ≥8 mg/dL or 25 % increase from baseline
Potassium ≥6.0 mEq/L or 25 % increase from baseline
Phosphorus ≥6.5 mg/dL or 25 % increase from baseline
Calcium ≤7.0 mg/dL or 25 % decrease from baseline[a]
Clinical tumor lysis syndrome (*LTLS + 1 or more of the following*)
AKI defined as creatinine ≥1.5× ULN or GFR ≤60 mL/min[a]
Cardiac arrhythmia/sudden death
Seizure

LTLS laboratory tumor lysis syndrome, *AKI* acute kidney injury, *ULN* upper limit of normal, *GFR* glomerular filtration rate
Adapted from Coiffier et al. (2008), Tosi et al. (2008), Pession et al. (2011)
[a]Not a criterion in all consensus guidelines; GFR calculated utilizing the Schwartz et al. (1987) formula: estimated GFR (mL/min)=(0.55×length [cm])/serum creatinine (mg/dL)

and secondary to direct obstruction from retro-vesical lymphoma or massive lymphadenopathy (Lobe et al. 1990; Levin and Cho 1996, Mantadakis et al. 1999, Farley-Hills et al. 2001; Mahajan et al. 2002).

Recognition of risk factors for LTLS and preventive therapy remain the most important management steps to minimize development of CTLS. Patients who develop CTLS will require more aggressive management to prevent significant morbidity and mortality. Due to improvements in recognition and supportive care, the risk of early death from TLS is extremely low; in a survey of Dutch leukemia patients, 1 of 847 ALL and 0 of 229 AML patients suffered early death from TLS (Slats et al. 2005). Similarly, in a review of LMB89 for NHL, 0 of 561 patients suffered early death from TLS (Patte et al. 2001). HU was the most common cause of impaired renal function and two patients died secondary to metabolic complications (Meyer et al. 1998). In a cost analysis of ALL and NHL patients with TLS, Annemans et al. (2003a) reported an overall 18.9 % and 27.8 % incidence of HU and TLS respectively with costs significantly increased in those with TLS and even more so in those requiring intensive care (i.e., renal dialysis); these results were more recently corroborated by Candrilli et al. (2008). The evidence basis behind recommendations in the management of TLS is often negligible and therefore based mostly on consensus guidelines (Feusner et al. 2008). Here we analyze the existing literature in relation to the consensus guidelines to determine and grade rational recommendations.

3.2 Laboratory Risk Factors for Tumor Lysis

Determination of pretreatment risk factors for the development of CTLS would be helpful in guiding the clinician as to which patients require the most aggressive upfront therapies. Data on the utilization of such factors are mixed. In adult NHL patients, Hande and Garrow (1993) reported no difference in TLS between NHL subgroups; risk of CTLS after chemotherapy was significantly higher in those patients with pretreatment renal insufficiency (creatinine >1.5 mg/dL) and high serum LDH levels. On the other hand, in a retrospective review of children with acute leukemia, Kedar et al. (1995) found no correlation with pretreatment blast count, white blood cell (WBC) count, or LDH and the development of LTLS; Stapleton et al. (1988) similarly found no statistical difference in admission uric acid and LDH level in children with B cell ALL who did or did not subsequently develop AKI. Troung et al. (2007) found that children <10 years of age with WBC <20 × 10^9/L and no mediastinal mass or splenomegaly had a 97 % negative predictive value of developing TLS. In a study of German BFM data, Wössmann et al. (2003) found that LDH ≥500 U/L correlated with risk of both TLS and anuria in pediatric ALL and stage III/IV BL patients. In an analysis of 221 ALL patients with hyperleukocytosis (WBC ≥200 × 10^9/L) treated on the Scandinavian NOPHO trials, only initial uric acid levels (11.0 versus 7.7 mg/dL) was significant in multivariate analysis for TLS risk (WBC count and LDH were not significant) (Vaitkevičienė et al. 2013).

Mato et al. (2006) noted that LDH, uric acid and gender were LTLS predictors in multivariate analysis in adult AML patients but these factors were not specifically predictive for CTLS. Montesinos et al. (2008) found that LDH > upper limit of normal (ULN), creatinine >1.4 mg/dL, hyperuricemia (uric acid >7.5 mg/dL), and WBC >25 × 10^9/L were all significant risk factors for both LTLS and CTLS in adult AML patients and subsequently validated a risk scoring system. Whether such a scoring system can be utilized in pediatric patients is unknown. Consensus guidelines consider LDH >2× ULN and WBC >25 × 10^9/L as risk factors for the development of LTLS although it is unclear whether these factors are true measures for risk of CTLS, especially in pediatric patients (Table 3.2) (Coiffier et al. 2008; Tosi et al. 2008; Cairo et al. 2010; Agrawal and Feusner 2011; Pession et al. 2011).

Table 3.2 Risk factor stratification for clinically significant tumor lysis syndrome at disease presentation in pediatric patients[a]

High risk for CTLS
Stage III/IV Burkitt lymphoma with LDH $\geq 2\times$ ULN and/or bulky retroperitoneal disease
ALL with WBC $\geq 200\times 10^9$/L and uric acid ≥ 11.0 mg/dL[b]
Hyperphosphatemia
Hypocalcemia
Hyperkalemia
Oliguria
Renal involvement in leukemia or lymphoma
Low risk for CTLS
Non-lymphomatous solid tumors
Hodgkin lymphoma
Chronic myelogenous leukemia
Acute myelogenous leukemia
Stage I/II NHL
ALL in children <10 years of age with WBC $<20\times 10^9$/L and no mediastinal mass or splenomegaly
Intermediate risk for CTLS
All others not classified as low or high risk

CTLS clinical tumor lysis syndrome, *LDH* lactate dehydrogenase, *ULN* upper limit of normal, *ALL* acute lymphoblastic leukemia, *WBC* white blood cell, *LTLS* laboratory tumor lysis syndrome, *NHL* non-Hodgkin lymphoma
[a]See text for detail, level of evidence 1B for all categorizations (per Guyatt et al. [2006]; see Preface)
[b]WBC >25×10^9/L or LDH $\geq 2\times$ ULN without LTLS is not a risk factor for TLS in ALL patients

3.3 General Management Guidelines

Prevention is the key component of TLS management in high-risk patients and hyperhydration (i.e., 3 L/m^2/day) is the most important prophylactic intervention although randomized evidence supporting its benefit is lacking due to the risk of withholding such therapy in high-risk patients (Table 3.3) (Coiffier et al. 2008; Tosi et al. 2008). Intravenous fluids should ideally be started >24 h prior to the initiation of cytotoxic therapy. Fluid status must be monitored vigilantly taking into account the patient's daily fluid balance, urine output, laboratory evidence of renal function and physical exam evidence of fluid overload (i.e., change in weight, edema, dyspnea, rales or gallop rhythm). Dilute urine output, defined as >100 ml/m^2/h (>4 ml/kg/h for infants) with a urine specific gravity <1.010, should be established prior to the initiation of chemotherapy and should be maintained at such levels during the acute phase of therapy (Coiffier et al. 2008; Tosi et al. 2008). Loop diuretics and mannitol can be utilized to maintain good urine output but should

be avoided in patients with evidence of hypovolemia (Coiffier et al. 2008; Tosi et al. 2008).

Frequent laboratory monitoring is necessary to assess for evidence of LTLS and risk of CTLS. Uric acid, phosphate, potassium, calcium and creatinine levels should be checked prior to the initiation of cytoreductive therapy. The frequency of monitoring thereafter must be tailored to each individual patient and may be required as often as every 4–6 h in patients exhibiting significant LTLS worrisome for the development of CTLS or as infrequently as every 24 h in lower-risk patients (Coiffier et al. 2008; Tosi et al. 2008). Guidelines recommend following LDH levels as a marker of decreasing tumor burden and TLS risk although it is unclear if this is really necessary to appropriately assess the patient (Coiffier et al. 2008; Tosi et al. 2008). In addition, patients who develop hyperkalemia and hyperphosphatemia or who have poor urine output despite vigorous hydration should undergo renal ultrasound to rule out renal parenchymal involvement or obstructive uropathy.

Electrocardiographic (ECG) monitoring may be warranted if the patient has either hyperkalemia (i.e., potassium ≥ 6 mEq/L) or hypocalcemia

Table 3.3 Pharmacologic interventions for the treatment of tumor lysis syndrome[a]

Condition	Level of evidence[b]
General management	
Intravenous fluids	
D5W 1/2NS infused at 3 L/m^2/day without potassium or calcium	1C
Sodium bicarbonate 20–40 mEq/L if the patient has HU or risk for HU; can decrease to 1/4NS if on 40 mEq/L or more of sodium bicarbonate	2C
Urinary alkalinization not required if utilizing rasburicase	1B
Urinary alkalinization should not be initiated with concomitant hyperphosphatemia	1A
Laboratory monitoring	
Monitor potassium, phosphorus, calcium, uric acid, BUN/creatinine every 4–6 h in patients at high risk for tumor lysis	1C
Can wean labs to every 12–24 h as tumor burden decreases over 3–7 days	1C
Hyperuricemia	
Allopurinol[c]	1B
In all patients not receiving rasburicase; unclear evidence in low-risk patients	
10 mg/kg/day PO divided Q8h to a maximum of 800 mg/day	
Rasburicase[d]	1B
Rasburicase prophylaxis should be limited to patients with evidence-based risk factors (see Table 3.2); specifically stage III/IV BL patients with elevated LDH $\geq$2× ULN and/or bulky retroperitoneal disease, hyperleukocytic ALL (WBC $\geq$200 × 10^9/L) with severe hyperuricemia (uric acid $\geq$11.0 mg/dL) or hyperuricemia not improving with hyperhydration, urinary alkalinization and allopurinol alone	
0.03–0.05 mg/kg IV × 1; subsequent doses not usually required but can be given if uric acid again >8 mg/dL in high-risk patients	
Hyperphosphatemia	
Aluminum hydroxide	1C
Avoid in patients with renal insufficiency	
Children: 50–150 mg/kg/day PO divided Q4–6 h	
Adolescents: 300–600 mg PO TID	
Sevelamer	1C
Administer with each meal	
Children: dosing not well established	
Adolescent dosing based on phosphorus level (mg/dL):	
>5.5 and <7.5: 800 mg PO TID	
$\geq$7.5 and <9: 1200 mg PO TID	
$\geq$9: 1600 mg PO TID	
Calcium carbonate (use with caution as can increase calcium-phosphate product and risk for calcium phosphate precipitation)	1C
Children: 30–40 mg/kg/dose with each meal	
Adolescents: 1–2 g with each meal	
Hyperkalemia	
Calcium gluconate, 100–200 mg/kg IV slow infusion with ECG monitoring	1C
Sodium polystyrene sulfonate, 1 g/kg in 50 % sorbitol PO Q6h (max dose 15 g)	1C
Regular insulin + D25W, 0.1 unit/kg insulin (max 10 units) + 2 ml/kg (0.5 g/kg) D25W IV over 30 min	1C
Albuterol	1C
Inhaled via nebulizer <25 kg: 2.5 mg	
Inhaled via nebulizer 25–50 kg: 5 mg	
Inhaled via nebulizer >50 kg: 10 mg	

Table 3.3 (continued)

Condition	Level of evidence[b]
Furosemide, 0.5–1 mg/kg IV	1C
Sodium bicarbonate, 1–2 mEq/kg IV over 5–10 min (max dose 50 mEq)	1C
Hypocalcemia	
Calcium gluconate[e], 50–100 mg/kg IV slow infusion with ECG monitoring	1C

HU hyperuricemia, *BUN* blood urea nitrogen, *PO* by mouth, *TID* three times per day, *IV* intravenous, *ECG* electrocardiogram

Adapted from Coiffier et al. (2008), Tosi et al. (2008), Howard et al. (2011), Pession et al. (2011)

[a]See text for full detail

[b]Per Guyatt et al. (2006); see Preface

[c]Patients in renal failure should be dose reduced by 50%

[d]Contraindicated in patients with glucose-6-phosphate dehydrogenase (G6PD) deficiency

[e]Avoid administration unless patient has symptomatic hypocalcemia or ECG changes

(serum calcium <7 mg/dL or ionized calcium <1 mmol/L) (Coiffier et al. 2008; Tosi et al. 2008). The classic ECG findings that can be seen with mild to moderate hyperkalemia include tall peaked T-waves, prolongation of the PR interval, diminished amplitude or disappearance of the P-waves and widening of the QRS complex (Diercks et al. 2004). When severe, hyperkalemia can result in a sine-wave pattern, ventricular fibrillation or asystole (Diercks et al. 2004). The hallmark ECG finding of hypocalcemia is prolongation of the QTc interval (Diercks et al. 2004).

Management of ALL patients with severe hyperleukocytosis is not specifically addressed in the TLS guidelines; leukapheresis may be considered in ALL patients with hyperleukocytic TLS as long as delay in the initiation of induction chemotherapy can be avoided (see Chap. 6 for more detail) (Vaitkevičienė et al. 2013). Radiation therapy may additionally be considered for patients with poor urine output with evidence of obstructive uropathy or renal parenchymal disease.

3.4 Pathophysiology, Presentation and Management of Specific Metabolic Derangements

3.4.1 Hyperuricemia

Guidelines define hyperuricemia as a uric acid ≥8.0 mg/dL; a 25% increase from baseline is also considered a marker of LTLS (Table 3.1) (Coiffier et al. 2008; Pession et al. 2011).

Lysis of malignant cells leads to release of purine nucleosides adenosine and guanosine from DNA into the circulation. Upon their release into the bloodstream, purines undergo enzymatic conversion to uric acid, an insoluble metabolite not easily excreted by the kidneys. Uric acid and its precursor, xanthine, are both relatively insoluble in urine with an acidic pH. Renal precipitation of uric acid or, very rarely, xanthine (i.e., with concomitant use of allopurinol) can lead to a reversible obstructive uropathy and AKI (Rieselbach et al. 1964; Hande et al. 1981; Andreoli et al. 1986; Potter and Silvidi 1987; LaRosa et al. 2007).

3.4.1.1 Alkalinization

Urinary alkalinization has been a long-standing modality used to facilitate uric acid excretion based on the initial work by Rieselbach et al. (1964) who showed that urinary alkalinization to a goal urine pH of 7.0 in addition to hyperhydration improved urinary excretion of uric acid. Although Conger and Falk (1977) later showed in a mouse model that urine alkalinization plays only a minor role in urate excretion as compared to hyperhydration, it remains unclear if this necessarily correlates with human physiology. The solubility of uric acid increases with increasing urine pH thereby making it easier for the kidneys to excrete excess uric acid; however, the solubility of calcium phosphate decreases as the pH increases leading to potential calcium phosphate precipitation in an increasingly alkaline environment (Howard et al. 2011). Therefore, theoretical concern exists regarding routine urinary alkalinization. In consensus guidelines, Coiffier et al. (2008) recommend against routine urine alkalinization, while Tosi et al. (2008) recommend urine alkalinization in low-risk patients, highlighting the lack of evidence to make firm uniform guidance. An update of the Tosi et al. (2008) Italian guidelines recommend against alkalinization even in low-risk patients (Pession et al. 2011).

Sodium bicarbonate is generally used as the additive to intravenous fluids with a goal urine pH of 7.0. It is unlikely that patients without risk of HU benefit from urinary alkalization; those with high tumor burdens and risk for TLS may benefit from urine alkalinization although data are lacking. Additionally, with the availability of rasburicase to rapidly degrade existing uric acid to a much more soluble byproduct, the risk of hyperuricemia and subsequent urate precipitation is almost nonexistent in settings with rasburicase availability thereby negating the need for alkalinization (Tosi et al. 2008; Howard et al. 2011). Patients with hyperphosphatemia should not be alkalinized due to the increased risk of calcium phosphate precipitation and availability of rasburicase to treat concomitant hyperuricemia, if present (Howard et al. 2011). In the patient with elevated uric acid or risk of hyperuricemia without hyperphosphatemia started on alkalinization, the alkalinization can be discontinued as the uric acid normalizes and the tumor burden decreases over the first few days of therapy (Table 3.3).

3.4.1.2 Allopurinol

Allopurinol inhibits xanthine oxidase, an enzyme which converts hypoxanthine and xanthine to uric acid. Krakoff and Meyer (1965) and DeConti and Calabresi (1966) first showed that allopurinol effectively reduced serum uric acid levels without leading to significant accumulation of xanthine and hypoxanthine due to differential solubility products. Allopurinol has been noted to be quite safe and is extremely inexpensive. Xanthine nephropathy secondary to TLS and leading to AKI with concomitant allopurinol has been rarely reported in the literature (Band et al. 1970; Hande et al. 1981; Andreoli et al. 1986; Potter and Silvidi 1987; LaRosa et al. 2007). Andreoli et al. (1986) reported that although xan-

thine exceeded its solubility limit in 16 of 19 children with ALL receiving allopurinol, only 8 were noted to have precipitated xanthine in urine sediment and only half of those children developed AKI. They therefore theorized that additional factors are involved in the development of AKI during TLS. Xanthine nephropathy should be considered in the patient with AKI but appropriate TLS prophylaxis; in such cases allopurinol should be reduced or discontinued, xanthine levels should be drawn and patients should be tested for a defect in the hypoxanthine-guanine phosphoribosyl transferase (HGPRT) enzyme (LaRosa et al. 2007).

Drawbacks to allopurinol include a relatively slow onset of action (i.e., 24–72 h), the necessity of dose reduction in the setting of renal insufficiency and its inability to degrade preexisting uric acid (Howard et al. 2011). Intravenous allopurinol has been shown to be equally effective and safe as compared to oral allopurinol but comes at a much higher cost (2,000-fold) (Smalley et al. 2000; Feusner and Farber 2001; Patel et al. 2012). Prior to the advent of rasburicase, intravenous allopurinol was a potential option in patients unable to tolerate oral intake but is no longer available in Europe (Feusner and Farber 2001; Will and Tholouli 2011). Utilizing a single low dose of rasburicase, Patel et al. (2012) were able to extrapolate a significant cost savings over intravenous allopurinol. Consensus guidelines recommend allopurinol in low- and intermediate-risk patients (i.e., those patients not recommended to receive rasburicase) (Coiffier et al. 2008; Pession et al. 2011). Consensus guidelines recommend that patients who receive rasburicase should only have allopurinol initiated after rasburicase discontinuation in order to inhibit additional uric acid formation until the tumor burden is significantly decreased (i.e., usually 3–7 total days) (Coiffier et al. 2008; Tosi et al. 2008). Given the slow onset of action for allopurinol it may be more prudent to initiate allopurinol prior to this recommended time point. Similar to urine alkalinization, it is unclear if the addition of allopurinol is beneficial in patients with a low tumor burden and low risk of developing HU (Table 3.3) (Pession et al. 2011).

3.4.1.3 Rasburicase

Rasburicase, recombinant urate oxidase, converts uric acid into allantoin, a five to ten times more soluble compound, in an extremely effective manner. Due to this fact, many studies have shown that rasburicase is efficacious in correcting HU in pediatric and adult patients (Pui et al. 2001; Patte et al. 2002; Bosly et al. 2003; Coiffier et al. 2003; Jeha et al. 2005; Pession et al. 2005; Shin et al. 2006; Kikuchi et al. 2009). Follow-up studies comparing efficacy of rasburicase and allopurinol naturally show that rasburicase is much more effective in rapidly and dramatically reducing the uric acid level although such studies fail to incorporate a clinically relevant endpoint (Goldman et al. 2001; Cortes et al. 2010). Many of these studies were supported by the pharmaceutical maker of rasburicase, including grant support, providing the drug, logistic support, editorial support, and data management, and some study authors had a financial stake in the pharmaceutical company (Goldman et al. 2001; Pui et al. 2001; Patte et al. 2002; Bosly et al. 2003; Coiffier et al. 2003; Jeha et al. 2005; Shin et al. 2006; Kikuchi et al. 2009; Cortes et al. 2010). Early studies also utilized higher doses of rasburicase (i.e., 0.15–0.2 mg/kg/day) and for a longer duration (up to 7 days) based on the recommendation of the manufacturer (and what was approved by the United States Food and Drug Administration [FDA]), rather than what is more rational based on the mechanism of the drug and underlying disease process (Pui et al. 2001; Patte et al. 2002; Bosly et al. 2003; Coiffier et al. 2003; Jeha et al. 2005; Pession et al. 2005; Shin et al. 2006; Kikuchi et al. 2009).

Rasburicase doses as low as 0.017 mg/kg as a single dose have subsequently been found effective; many studies have shown that abbreviated rasburicase schedules are sufficient (Hummel et al. 2003; Lee et al. 2003; Liu et al. 2005; Ho et al. 2006; Hutcherson et al. 2006; McDonnell et al. 2006; Trifilio et al. 2006; Reeves and Bestul 2008; Campara et al. 2009; Giraldez and Puto 2010; Vadhan-Raj et al. 2012). Hummel et al. (2007) were able to utilize a low-dosing schedule resulting in an average decrease in uric acid levels by 83 % while utilizing a median total dose of rasburicase of 0.049 mg/kg, resulting in a cost reduction of 96.8 % based on manufacturer dosing recommendations. Adult patients with initial average hyperuricemia of 13.1 mg/dL were able to achieve uric acid <8.0 mg/dL with an average single rasburicase dose of 0.032 mg/kg (Hummel et al. 2007). Knoebel et al. (2011) similarly showed that most adult patients could be effectively treated with a single 0.05 mg/kg dose. Yet, recent consensus guidelines still recommend a range of 1–7 days of rasburicase at a dose of 0.1–0.2 mg/kg/dose (Coiffier et al. 2008; Tosi et al. 2008; Pession et al. 2011). Although generally safe, rasburicase must be avoided in patients with glucose-6-phosphate dehydrogenase (G6PD) deficiency and methemoglobinemia, and hemolytic anemia has been reported in childhood ALL (Bauters et al. 2011).

Even though HU is a factor in LTLS, data are less clear that rasburicase is more effective in the prevention of CTLS than allopurinol. In their analysis of BFM data, Wössmann et al. (2003) compared LTLS and anuria risk in pediatric ALL and stage III/IV BL patients with LDH $\geq$500 U/L treated with either allopurinol or rasburicase; they found that although ALL patients treated with rasburicase had a trend toward decreased LTLS, it was not clinically significant although there was a significant decrease in the incidence of anuria. LTLS or anuria risk in children with BL was not significantly different between rasburicase and allopurinol (Wössmann et al. 2003). Despite decreasing uric acid levels, Ahn et al. 2011 noted no statistical difference in LTLS, CTLS or need for renal dialysis with rasburicase compared with allopurinol. A Cochrane review of rasburicase for the prevention and treatment of TLS in children with cancer similarly showed significant reduction in uric acid levels, but the relevant analyzed studies failed to show that this equated to a significant reduction in clinically significant endpoints, specifically renal failure and mortality (Cheuk et al. 2010).

Rasburicase remains an extremely expensive drug ($535 per 1.5 mg vial) compared to allopurinol and therefore it is vital to appropriately select patients that would benefit from rasburicase through the prevention of CTLS (Goldman

2005; Patel et al. 2012). An economic analysis by Annemans et al. (2003b) reported that rasburicase is highly cost effective in the pediatric cohort, but the analysis was based on preventing/treating HU and LTLS rather than clinically significant endpoints. Another economic comparison specifically in pediatric patients showed no difference in total cost or length of stay between those treated with allopurinol and rasburicase although the number of days in critical care was significantly reduced in the rasburicase cohort (Eaddy et al. 2010). Consensus guidelines recommend rasburicase in those with "high-risk disease," defined as AML with WBC $\geq100\times10^9$/L, ALL with LDH $\geq2\times$ ULN or WBC $\geq100\times10^9$/L, BL with LDH $\geq2\times$ ULN or advanced stage (i.e., III/IV), other NHL with advanced stage and LDH $\geq2\times$ ULN, and any patient with LTLS (Cairo et al. 2010). Tosi et al. (2008) define high risk as those with renal impairment, obstructive uropathy, hyperuricemia (uric acid >8 mg/dL), bulky disease, high-grade lymphoma, T cell ALL or LDH >2× ULN. Although some of these patients will benefit from the addition of rasburicase, many of these subpopulations likely do not need rasburicase in all cases, such as ALL with solely LDH $\geq2\times$ ULN or WBC $\geq100\times10^9$/L, AML with WBC $\geq100\times10^9$/L, all T cell ALL, all LDH $\geq2\times$ ULN, and those with LTLS but without HU (Table 3.3) (Tosi et al. 2008; Agrawal and Feusner 2011).

3.4.2 Hyperkalemia

Potassium, the most abundant intracellular cation, is released into the circulation when cells lyse. The rate of release of potassium from malignant cells can exceed the excretory capacity of the kidney resulting in hyperkalemia. Dehydration, renal insufficiency and inadvertent iatrogenic administration of potassium are factors that can exacerbate the degree of hyperkalemia observed in TLS. Hyperkalemia can be acutely life threatening by precipitating cardiac arrhythmias and therefore is a medical emergency that warrants prompt intervention. Treatment of

hyperkalemia involves three main mechanisms: (1) stabilization of the resting membrane potential of cardiac myocytes, (2) transmembrane shifting of potassium from the extracellular to the intracellular compartment, and (3) enhanced excretion of potassium. Care should be taken to eliminate parenterally administered forms of potassium (e.g., intravenous fluids should not contain potassium). Enterally consumed sources of potassium should be minimized.

Administration of calcium gluconate helps stabilize the resting membrane potential of the myocardium. Calcium gluconate should be given to any patient with a serum potassium level >7.0 mEq/L or any patient with evidence of an arrhythmia (Coiffier et al. 2008). Calcium gluconate has an onset of action within minutes with a duration of effect of about 30 min. Due to the short half-life, the dose may need to be repeated until more definitive measures to reduce the potassium have been initiated. The translocation of potassium from the extracellular compartment to the intracellular compartment is an effective, albeit, temporary management strategy. Drugs that can be used to shift potassium into the intracellular compartment include the combination of insulin and glucose, β-agonists such as albuterol, and sodium bicarbonate. The combination of insulin and glucose shifts potassium into cells within 10–20 min, has a duration of effect that lasts 2–3 h and can lower serum potassium by 0.5–1.5 mEq/L (Gennari 2002). Continuous inhalation of albuterol is equally effective compared to insulin and glucose with a similar duration of effect; however the onset of action is slightly longer at 20–30 min (Gennari 2002). Sodium bicarbonate can be used to shift potassium intracellularly when an acidosis is present but is felt to be somewhat less effective than insulin and glucose or albuterol (Gennari 2002).

The definitive treatment of hyperkalemia involves enhancing the excretion of potassium in order to lower body levels. Ion-exchange resins such as sodium polystyrene sulfonate (Kayexalate®) administered orally along with the laxative sorbitol bind to potassium in the colon and enhance excretion of potassium in the stool. The onset of action of sodium polystyrene sulfonate is delayed and can take up to 4–6 h, necessitating the administration of more temporizing measures in the interim (Gennari 2002). Potassium-wasting loop diuretics such as furosemide can be used to enhance renal excretion of potassium. Furosemide should be used with caution in patients with renal insufficiency (i.e., estimated GFR <35 mL/min/1.73 m^2 using the Schwartz formula) and should be avoided in patients with hypovolemia (Schwartz et al. 1987). Dialysis should be considered in the patient with hyperkalemia not improving with the above therapies, at risk for continued significant cell lysis or with oliguria/anuria. See Table 3.3 for a summary of recommendations, dosing and grading.

3.4.3 Hyperphosphatemia

The backbone of DNA is abundantly rich in phosphate and tumor cells have been noted to have significantly increased phosphate concentrations (Traut 1994). Therefore, actively dividing malignant cells are a risk for hyperphosphatemia with rapid cell lysis. Hyperphosphatemia in and of itself rarely leads to clinical symptoms; however, significant complications can arise if calcium phosphate precipitates in the kidneys leading to nephrocalcinosis and AKI.

The treatment of hyperphosphatemia includes hyperhydration, limiting enteral intake of phosphate, utilization of phosphate binders, and, when severe, initiation of dialysis. Phosphate binders used in the treatment of TLS include aluminum hydroxide, sevelamer and calcium carbonate (Abdullah et al. 2008). Prolonged use of aluminum hydroxide beyond 1–2 days has been cautioned against in order to avoid the potential for aluminum toxicity (Coiffier et al. 2008). Patients with hyperphosphatemia should not receive urinary alkalinization as described. Calcium carbonate should be utilized with caution due to the potential for calcium phosphate precipitation. See Table 3.3 for a summary of recommendations, dosing and grading.

3.4.4 Hypocalcemia

In order to maintain a steady level of calcium relative to phosphorus (i.e., calcium-phosphate product), calcium and phosphate have an inverse homeostatic relationship. Therefore the hypocalcemia seen in TLS is a direct consequence of hyperphosphatemia. Clinical symptoms of hypocalcemia include neuromuscular irritability (e.g., muscle cramps, tetany, carpopedal spasms, seizure) and cardiac arrhythmias, and can range in severity from relatively minor to potentially life-threatening (Diercks et al. 2004). Accurate measurement of serum calcium levels is dependent upon albumin levels. When the patient is hypoalbuminemic, an ionized calcium level should be measured to confirm the degree of hypocalcemia.

No intervention is needed for the patient with asymptomatic hypocalcemia. For patients who are symptomatic, calcium gluconate may be administered. The lowest dose required to alleviate symptoms should be given in order to minimize the risk for calcium phosphate precipitation. The risk for precipitation is not insignificant and can be estimated by calculating the calcium-phosphate product (serum calcium multiplied by serum phosphate). Risk for nephrocalcinosis increases as the calcium-phosphate product increasingly exceeds 60 mg^2/dL^2 (Howard et al. 2011). See Table 3.3 for a summary of recommendations, dosing and grading.

3.5 Renal Interventions

No clear evidence-based guidelines exist as to when dialysis should be implemented for TLS. Coiffier et al. (2008) suggest renal consultation in patients with decreased urine output and in those with persistent hyperphosphatemia or hypocalcemia. Tosi et al. (2008) suggest renal replacement therapy in those with persistent hyperkalemia, severe metabolic acidosis, volume overload not responding to diuresis, and uremic symptoms such as pericarditis and encephalopathy. The need for dialysis with hyperuricemia is unlikely other than in settings without access to rasburicase (Howard et al. 2011). Continuous arteriovenous and venovenous hemofiltration, continuous venovenous hemodialysis, and continuous venovenous hemodiafiltration have all been found safe and effective in CTLS (Bishof et al. 1990; Heney et al. 1990; Sakarcan and Quigley 1994; Saccente et al. 1995; Howard et al. 2011). Long-term renal function in pediatric patients who suffer from TLS has been reported to be normal (Stapleton et al. 1988).

3.6 Summary

TLS risk factor stratification is vital for determining which preventative measures are appropriate for each individual patient. Although guidelines exist, the risk stratification provided is based on consensus statements and adult data and does not extrapolate to all pediatric oncology populations. Subsequently such stratification may lead to increased utilization of expensive medications such as rasburicase in situations where it is not justified based on the existing evidence. Although urinary alkalinization may not be recommended in some guidelines, it may still be beneficial in situations where the uric acid level is not high enough to justify rasburicase. The practitioner should be aware of true high-risk scenarios in which rasburicase should be utilized and the patient monitored extremely carefully for metabolic complications related to hyperkalemia, hypocalcemia and AKI secondary to calcium phosphate precipitation. Early consultation with nephrology and intensive care should be considered in such high-risk situations.

References

Abdullah S, Diezi M, Sung L et al (2008) Sevelamer hydrochloride: a novel treatment of hyperphosphatemia associated with tumor lysis syndrome in children. Pediatr Blood Cancer 51:59–61

Agrawal AK, Feusner JH (2011) Management of tumour lysis syndrome in children: what is the evidence for prophylactic rasburicase in non-hyperleucocytic leukaemia? Br J Haematol 153:275–276

Ahn YH, Kang HJ, Shin HY et al (2011) Tumour lysis syndrome in children: experience of last decade. Hematol Oncol 29:196–201

Andreoli SP, Clark JH, McGuire WA et al (1986) Purine excretion during tumor lysis in children with acute lymphocytic leukemia receiving allopurinol: relationship to acute renal failure. J Pediatr 109: 292–298

Annemans L, Moeremans K, Lamotte M et al (2003a) Incidence, medical resource utilization and costs of hyperuricemia and tumour lysis syndrome in patients with acute leukaemia and non-Hodgkin's lymphoma in four European countries. Leuk Lymphoma 44:77–83

Annemans L, Moeremans K, Lamotte M et al (2003b) Pan-European multicentre economic evaluation of recombinant urate oxidase (rasburicase) in prevention and treatment of hyperuricaemia and tumour lysis syndrome in haematological cancer patients. Support Care Cancer 11:249–257

Band PR, Silverberg DS, Henderson JF et al (1970) Xanthine nephropathy in a patient with lymphosarcoma treated with allopurinol. N Engl J Med 283: 354–357

Bauters T, Mondelaers V, Robays H et al (2011) Methemoglobinemia and hemolytic anemia after rasburicase administration in a child with leukemia. Int J Clin Pharm 33:58–60

Bercovitz RS, Greffe BS, Hunger SP (2010) Acute tumor lysis syndrome in a 7-month-old with hepatoblastoma. Curr Opin Pediatr 22:113–116

Bien E, Maciejka-Kapuscinska L, Niedzwiekci M et al (2010) Childhood rhabdomyosarcoma metastatic to the bone marrow presenting with disseminated intravascular coagulation and acute tumour lysis syndrome: review of the literature apropos of two cases. Clin Exp Metastasis 27:399–407

Bishof NA, Welch TR, Strife F et al (1990) Continuous hemodiafiltration in children. Pediatrics 85:819–823

Bosly A, Sonet A, Pinkerton CR et al (2003) Rasburicase (recombinant urate oxidase) for the management of hyperuricemia in patients with cancer. Report of an international compassionate use study. Cancer 98:1048–1054

Cairo MS, Coiffier B, Reiter A et al (2010) Recommendations for the evaluation of risk and prophylaxis of tumour lysis syndrome (TLS) in adults and children with malignant diseases: an expert TLS panel consensus. Br J Haematol 149:578–586

Campara M, Shord SS, Haaf CM (2009) Single-dose rasburicase for tumour lysis syndrome in adults: weight-based approach. J Clin Pharm Ther 34: 207–213

Candrilli S, Bell T, Irish W et al (2008) A comparison of inpatient length of stay and costs among patients with hematologic malignancies (excluding Hodgkin disease) associated with and without acute renal failure. Clin Lymphoma Myeloma 8:44–51

Cheuk DK, Chiang AK, Chan GC et al (2010) Urate oxidase for the prevention and treatment of tumor lysis syndrome in children with cancer. Cochrane Database Syst Rev (6):CD006945

Coiffier B, Altman A, Pui CH et al (2008) Guidelines for the management of pediatric and adult tumor lysis syndrome: an evidence-based review. J Clin Oncol 26:2767–2778

Coiffier B, Mounier N, Bologna S et al (2003) Efficacy and safety of rasburicase (recombinant urate oxidase) for the prevention and treatment of hyperuricemia during induction chemotherapy of aggressive non-Hodgkin's lymphoma: results of the GRAAL1 (Groupe d'Etude des Lymphomes de l'Adulte Trial on Rasburicase Activity in Adult Lymphoma) study. J Clin Oncol 21:4402–4406

Conger JD, Falk SA (1977) Intrarenal dynamics in the pathogenesis and prevention of acute urate nephropathy. J Clin Invest 59:786–793

Cortes J, Moore JO, Maziarz RT et al (2010) Control of plasma uric acid in adults at risk for tumor lysis syndrome: efficacy and safety of rasburicase alone and rasburicase followed by allopurinol compared with allopurinol alone—results of a multicenter phase III study. J Clin Oncol 28:4207–4213

DeConti RC, Calabresi P (1966) Use of allopurinol for prevention and control of hyperuricemia in patients with neoplastic disease. N Engl J Med 274:481–486

Diercks DB, Shumaik GM, Harrigan RA et al (2004) Electrocardiographic manifestations: electrolyte abnormalities. J Emerg Med 27:153–160

Eaddy M, Seal B, Tangirala M et al (2010) Economic comparison of rasburicase and allopurinol for treatment of tumor lysis syndrome in pediatric patients. Am J Health Syst Pharm 67:2110–2114

Farley-Hills E, Byrne AJ, Brennan L et al (2001) Tumour lysis syndrome during anaesthesia. Paediatr Anaesth 11:233–236

Feusner J, Farber MS (2001) Role of intravenous allopurinol in the management of acute tumor lysis syndrome. Semin Oncol 28:13–18

Feusner JH, Ritchey AK, Cohn SL et al (2008) Management of tumor lysis syndrome: need for evidence-based guidelines. J Clin Oncol 26:5657–5658

Gemici C (2006) Tumour lysis syndrome in solid tumors. Clin Oncol 18:773–780

Gennari FJ (2002) Disorders of potassium homeostasis: hypokalemia and hyperkalemia. Crit Care Clin 18:273–288

Giraldez M, Puto K (2010) A single, fixed dose of rasburicase (6 mg maximum) for treatment of tumor lysis syndrome in adults. Eur J Haematol 85:177–179

Goldman SC, Holcenberg JS, Finklestein JZ et al (2001) A randomized comparison between rasburicase and allopurinol in children with lymphoma or leukemia at high risk for tumor lysis. Blood 97:2998–3003

Goldman SC (2005) Patient selection and treatment of tumor lysis syndrome in adults with hematologic malignancies. Support Cancer Ther 2:167

Guyatt G, Gutterman D, Baumann MH et al (2006) Grading strength of recommendations and quality of evidence in clinical guidelines: report from an American College of Chest Physicians task force. Chest 129:174–181

Hain RD, Rayner L, Weitzman S et al (1994) Acute tumour lysis syndrome complicating treatment of stage IVS neuroblastoma in infants under six months of age. Med Pediatr Oncol 23:136–139

Hande KR, Hixson CV, Chabner BA (1981) Postchemotherapy purine excretion in lymphoma patients receiving allopurinol. Cancer Res 41:2273–2279

Hande KR, Garrow GC (1993) Acute tumor lysis syndrome in patients with high-grade non-Hodgkin's lymphoma. Am J Med 94:133–139

Heney D, Essex-Cater A, Brocklebank JT et al (1990) Continuous arteriovenous haemofiltration in the treatment of tumour lysis syndrome. Pediatr Nephrol 4:245–247

Ho VQ, Wetzstein GA, Patterson SG et al (2006) Abbreviated rasburicase dosing for the prevention and treatment of hyperuricemia in adults at risk for tumor lysis syndrome. Support Cancer Ther 3:178–182

Howard SC, Jones DP, Pui CH (2011) The tumor lysis syndrome. N Engl J Med 364:1844–1854

Hummel M, Buchheidt D, Reiter S et al (2003) Successful treatment of hyperuricemia with low doses of recombinant urate oxidase in four patients with hematologic malignancy and tumor lysis syndrome. Leukemia 17:2542–2544

Hummel M, Reiter S, Adam K et al (2007) Effective treatment and prophylaxis of hyperuricemia and impaired renal function in tumor lysis syndrome with low doses of rasburicase. Eur J Haematol 80:331–336

Hutcherson DA, Gammon DC, Bhatt MS et al (2006) Reduced-dose rasburicase in the treatment of adults with hyperuricemia associated with malignancy. Pharmacotherapy 26:242–247

Jaing TH, Hsueh C, Tain YL et al (2001) Tumor lysis syndrome in an infant with Langerhans Cell Histiocytosis successfully treated using continuous arteriovenous hemofiltration. J Pediatr Hematol Oncol 23:142–144

Jeha S, Kantarjian H, Irwin D et al (2005) Efficacy and safety of rasburicase, a recombinant urate oxidase (Elitek™), in the management of malignancy-associated hyperuricemia in pediatric and adult patients: final results of a multicenter compassionate use trial. Leukemia 19:34–38

Kaito E, Terae S, Kobayashi R et al (2005) The role of tumor lysis in reversible posterior leukoencephalopathy syndrome. Pediatr Radiol 35:722–727

Kedar A, Grow W, Neiberger RE (1995) Clinical versus laboratory tumor lysis syndrome in children with acute leukemia. Pediatr Hematol Oncol 12:129–134

Khan J, Broadbent VA (1993) Tumor lysis syndrome complicating treatment of widespread metastatic abdominal rhabdomyosarcoma. Pediatr Hematol Oncol 10:151–155

Kikuchi A, Kigasawa H, Tsurusawa M et al (2009) A study of rasburicase for the management of hyperuricemia in pediatric patients with newly diagnosed hematologic malignancies at high risk for tumor lysis syndrome. Int J Hematol 90:492–5000

Knoebel RW, Lo M, Crank CW (2011) Evaluation of a low, weight-based dose of rasburicase in adult patients for the treatment or prophylaxis of tumor lysis syndrome. J Oncol Pharm Pract 17:147–154

Kobayashi D, Wofford MM, McLean TW et al (2010) Spontaneous tumor lysis syndrome in a child with T-cell acute lymphoblastic leukemia. Pediatr Blood Cancer 54:773–775

Krakoff IH, Meyer RL (1965) Prevention of hyperuricemia in leukemia and lymphoma: use of allopurinol, a xanthine oxidase inhibitor. JAMA 193:1–6

Kushner BH, LaQuaglia MP, Modak S et al (2003) Tumor lysis syndrome, neuroblastoma, and correlation between serum lactate dehydrogenase levels and MYCN-amplification. Med Pediatr Oncol 41:80–82

Larsen G, Loghman-Adham M (1996) Acute renal failure with hyperuricemia as initial presentation of leukemia in children. J Pediatr Hematol Oncol 18:191–194

LaRosa C, McMullen L, Bakdash S et al (2007) Acute renal failure from xanthine nephropathy during management of acute leukemia. Pediatr Nephrol 22:132–135

Lee AC, Li CH, So KT et al (2003) Treatment of impending tumor lysis with single-dose rasburicase. Ann Pharmacother 37:1614–1617

Levin M, Cho S (1996) Acute tumor lysis syndrome in high grade lymphoblastic lymphoma after a prolonged episode of fever. Med Pediatr Oncol 26:417–418

Liu CY, Sims-McCallum RP, Schiffer CA (2005) A single dose of rasburicase is sufficient for the treatment of hyperuricemia in patients receiving chemotherapy. Leuk Res 29:463–465

Lobe TE, Karkera MS, Custer MD et al (1990) Fatal refractory hyperkalemia due to tumor lysis during primary resection for hepatoblastoma. J Pediatr Surg 25:249–250

Mahajan A, Nirmal S, English MW et al (2002) Acute tumor lysis syndrome in Hodgkin disease. Med Pediatr Oncol 39:69–70

Mantadakis E, Aquino VM, Strand WR et al (1999) Acute renal failure due to obstruction in Burkitt lymphoma. Pediatr Nephrol 13:237–240

Mato AR, Riccioi BE, Qin L et al (2006) A predictive model for the detection of tumor lysis syndrome during AML induction therapy. Leuk Lymphoma 47:877–883

McDonnell AM, Lenz KL, Frei-Lahr D et al (2006) Single-dose rasburicase 6 mg in the management of tumor lysis syndrome in adults. Pharmacotherapy 26:806–812

Meyer U, Jansen P, Yakisan E et al (1998) Impaired renal function and tumor lysis syndrome in pediatric patients with Non-Hodgkin's Lymphoma and B-ALL. Observations from the BFM-trials. Klin Padiatr 210:279–284

Montesinos P, Lorenzo I, Martím G et al (2008) Tumor lysis syndrome in patients with acute myeloid leukemia: identification of risk factors and development of a predictive model. Haematologica 93:67–74

Ozkan A, Hakyemez B, Ozkalemkas F et al (2006) Tumor lysis syndrome as a contributory factor to the development of reversible posterior leukoencephalopathy. Neuroradiology 48:887–892

Patel S, Le A, Gascon S (2012) Cost-effectiveness of rasburicase over i.v. allopurinol for treatment of tumor lysis syndrome. Am J Health Syst Pharm 69:1015–1016

Patte C, Auperin A, Michon J et al (2001) The Société Française d'Oncologie Pédiatrique LMB89 protocol: highly effective multiagent chemotherapy tailored to the tumor burden and initial response in 561 unselected children with B-cell lymphomas and L3 leukemia. Blood 97:3370–3379

Patte C, Sakiroglu C, Ansoborlo S et al (2002) Urate-oxidase in the prevention and treatment of metabolic complications in patients with B-cell lymphoma and leukemia, treated in the Société Française d'Oncologie Pédiatrique LMB89 protocol. Ann Oncol 13:789–795

Pession A, Barbieri E, Santoro N et al (2005) Efficacy and safety of recombinant urate oxidase (rasburicase) for treatment and prophylaxis of hyperuricemia in children undergoing chemotherapy. Haematolgica 90:141–142

Pession A, Masetti R, Gaidano G et al (2011) Risk evaluation, prophylaxis, and treatment of tumor lysis syndrome: consensus of an Italian expert panel. Adv Ther 28:684–697

Potter JL, Silvidi AA (1987) Xanthine lithiasis, nephrocalcinosis, and renal failure in a leukemia patient treated with allopurinol. Clin Chem 33:2314–2316

Pui CH, Mahmoud HH, Wiley JM et al (2001) Recombinant urate oxidase for the prophylaxis or treatment of hyperuricemia in patients with leukemia or lymphoma. J Clin Oncol 19:697–704

Reeves DJ, Bestul DJ (2008) Evaluation of a single fixed dose of rasburicase 7.5 mg for the treatment of hyperuricemia in adults with cancer. Pharmacotherapy 28:685–690

Rieselbach RE, Bentzel CJ, Cotlove E et al (1964) Uric acid excretion and renal function in the acute hyperuricemia of leukemia. Pathogenesis and therapy of uric acid nephropathy. Am J Med 37:872–884

Saccente SL, Kohaut EC, Berkow RL (1995) Prevention of tumor lysis syndrome using continuous venovenous hemofiltration. Pediatr Nephrol 9:569–573

Sakarcan A, Quigley R (1994) Hyperphosphatemia in tumor lysis syndrome: the role of hemodialysis and continuous veno-venous hemofiltration. Pediatr Nephrol 8:351–353

Schwartz GJ, Brion LP, Spitzer A (1987) The use of plasma creatinine concentration for estimating glomerular filtration ration in infants, children, and adolescents. Pediatr Clin North Am 34:571–590

Shimada M, Johnson RJ, May WS Jr et al (2009) A novel role for uric acid in acute kidney injury association with tumour lysis syndrome. Nephrol Dial Transplant 24:2960–2964

Shin HY, Kang HJ, Park ES et al (2006) Recombinant urate oxidase (rasburicase) for the treatment of hyperuricemia in pediatric patients with hematologic malignancies: results of a compassionate prospective multicenter study in Korea. Pediatr Blood Cancer 46: 439–445

Slats AM, Egeler RM, van der Does-van den Berg A et al (2005) Causes of death—other than progressive leukemia—in childhood acute lymphoblastic (ALL) and myeloid leukemia (AML): the Dutch Childhood Oncology Group experience. Leukemia 19: 537–544

Smalley RV, Guaspari A, Haase-Statz S et al (2000) Allopurinol: intravenous use for prevention and treatment of hyperuricemia. J Clin Oncol 18: 1758–1763

Stapleton FB, Strother DR, Roy S 3rd et al (1988) Acute renal failure at onset of therapy for advanced stage Burkitt lymphoma and B cell acute lymphoblastic lymphoma. Pediatrics 82:863–869

Tosi P, Barosi G, Lazzaro C et al (2008) Consensus conference on the management of tumor lysis syndrome. Haematologica 93:1877–1885

Traut TW (1994) Physiological concentrations of purines and pyrimidines. Mol Cell Biochem 140:1–22

Trifilio S, Gordon L, Singhal S et al (2006) Reduced-dose rasburicase (recombinant xanthine oxidase) in adult cancer patients with hyperuricemia. Bone Marrow Transplant 37:997–1001

Trobaugh-Lotrario AD, Liang X, Janik JS et al (2004) Thymoma and tumor lysis syndrome in an adolescent. J Clin Oncol 22:955–957

Troung TH, Beyene J, Hitzler J et al (2007) Features at presentation predict children with acute lymphoblastic leukemia at low risk for tumor lysis syndrome. Cancer 110:1832–1839

Vadhan-Raj S, Fayad LE, Fanale MA et al (2012) A randomized trial of a single-dose rasburicase versus five-daily doses in patients at risk for tumor lysis syndrome. Ann Oncol 23:1640–1645

Vaitkevičienė G, Heyman M, Jonsson OG et al (2013) Early morbidity and mortality in childhood acute lymphoblastic leukemia with very high white blood cell count. Leukemia 27:2259–2262

Will A, Tholouli E (2011) The clinical management of tumour lysis syndrome in haematological malignancies. Br J Haematol 154:3–13

Wössmann W, Schrappe M, Meyer U et al (2003) Incidence of tumor lysis syndrome in children with advanced stage Burkitt's lymphoma/leukemia before and after introduction of prophylactic use of urate oxidase. Ann Hematol 82:160–165

Zusman J, Brown DM, Nesbit ME (1973) Hyperphosphatemia, hyperphosphaturia and hypocalcemia in acute lymphoblastic leukemia. N Engl J Med 289: 1335–1340

Cardiopulmonary Emergencies

4

Jennifer Michlitsch

Contents

Abstract

Children with malignancies are at risk for a number of cardiopulmonary complications. These are most frequently seen at the time of initial presentation but can also be seen in the setting of progressive disease or relapse. When severe, these complications require prompt evaluation and may require emergency intervention. This chapter reviews the pathophysiology, clinical presentation, diagnosis and treatment of the most common cardiopulmonary emergencies seen in the pediatric oncology population: superior vena cava and superior mediastinal syndromes, pericardial effusion and tamponade, pleural effusion, hypertensive emergencies, and pulmonary leukostasis. Recommendations for management are included and graded based on a review of the existing available evidence.

4.1   Introduction

Children with malignancies are at risk for a number of cardiopulmonary complications. These are most frequently seen at the time of initial presentation but can also be seen in the setting of progressive disease or relapse. When severe, these complications require prompt evaluation and may require emergency intervention. This chapter reviews the pathophysiology, clinical presentation, diagnosis and treatment of

J. Michlitsch, MD
Department of Hematology/Oncology,
Children's Hospital and Research Center Oakland,
747 52nd Street, Oakland, CA 94609, USA
e-mail: jmichlitsch@mail.cho.org

J. Feusner et al. (eds.), *Supportive Care in Pediatric Oncology:
A Practical Evidence-Based Approach*, Pediatric Oncology,
DOI 10.1007/978-3-662-44317-0_4, © Springer Berlin Heidelberg 2015

Table 4.1 Summary of recommendations for management of cardiopulmonary emergencies

Clinical scenario	Recommendations	Level of evidence[a]
SVCS/SMS	Elevate head of the bed	1C
	Place all IV lines in lower extremities	2C
	Consider use of loop diuretics	2C
	Remove indwelling catheter if associated with thrombosis	1C
	Avoid sedation with general anesthesia if possible	1B
	Consider use of pre-biopsy steroids to shrink tumor	2C
	Consider pre-biopsy radiation therapy to shrink tumor	2C
Malignancy-associated pericardial effusions	Close observation only if patient is asymptomatic	1C
	Emergent pericardiocentesis under echocardiographic guidance if patient is symptomatic	1C
	Consider pigtail drainage catheter for prolonged drainage	2C
	Surgical management if not controlled by above methods	1C
	Volume resuscitation to elevate intracardiac pressures	2C
	Avoid mechanical ventilation with positive airway pressure	2C
Malignancy-associated pleural effusions	Close observation only if patient is asymptomatic	1B
	Thoracentesis if patient is symptomatic (send fluid for evaluation, including cytology)	1B
	Consider indwelling catheter for prolonged drainage	2C
	Intrapleural fibrinolysis for loculated effusion	1A
	VATS for early organizing empyema	1C
	Thoracotomy with decortication for advanced organizing empyema	1C
	Consider pleurodesis for refractory and recurrent effusion	2C
Hypertensive emergencies	Immediate intravenous therapy for severe hypertension	1C
	Rapid bolus of phentolamine	
	Continuous infusion of phentolamine or sodium nitroprusside	
	Avoid β-blocking agents initially	
	Oral therapy for less severe hypertension	1C
	α-blocking agent (i.e., doxazosin)	
	Calcium channel blocker	
	Consider addition of β-blocker after α-adrenoreceptor blockade	
	Prevention of hypertensive crisis if marked catecholamine release anticipated	1C
	α-adrenoreceptor blockade with phenoxybenzamine	
	Subsequent addition of β-blockade to prevent reflex tachycardia	

SVCS superior vena cava syndrome, *SMS* superior mediastinal syndrome, *IV* intravenous, *VATS* video-assisted thoracoscopic surgery
[a]Per Guyatt et al. (2006); see Preface

the most common cardiopulmonary emergencies seen in the pediatric oncology population: superior vena cava and superior mediastinal syndromes, pericardial effusion and tamponade, pleural effusion, hypertensive emergencies, and pulmonary leukostasis. Recommendations for management are included and graded based on a review of the existing available evidence (Table 4.1).

4.2 Superior Vena Cava and Superior Mediastinal Syndromes

Superior vena cava syndrome (SVCS) occurs when the superior vena cava is obstructed, thereby restricting blood return to the heart. Superior mediastinal syndrome (SMS) is the term used when SVCS coexists with obstruction of the trachea. The terms are sometimes used interchangeably in children, in whom mediastinal pathology frequently involves compression of both the SVC and the trachea. Malignancies are the most common cause of this condition. The most common pediatric malignancy associated with SVCS is lymphoma, but it can also be seen in other solid tumors such as germ cell tumors, neuroblastoma, Ewing sarcoma, and soft tissue sarcoma, as well as leukemia (Ingram et al. 1990; Halfdanarson et al. 2006).

4.2.1 Pathophysiology

The superior vena cava carries blood from the head, arms and upper torso to the heart. This thin-walled vessel is easily compressed by tumors or other pathology in the mediastinum leading to impedance in venous return. If the occlusion occurs gradually, collaterals may form thereby mitigating the symptoms. Airway compromise results from both direct compression of the tracheobronchial tree and edema of these airways due to venous engorgement.

4.2.2 Clinical Presentation and Diagnosis

4.2.2.1 History and Physical Exam
SVCS/SMS should be suspected in a patient with engorgement of the veins in the head, face and neck. The most common presenting signs and symptoms are facial swelling and plethora, distended neck and chest wall veins, and upper extremity edema. Respiratory symptoms include dyspnea and cough. Less frequently seen are central nervous system (CNS) symptoms caused by impeded venous return and subsequent cerebral edema. These can include headache, dizziness, confusion, syncope and even obtundation (Wilson et al. 2007a). The onset of symptoms is usually insidious but may occur rapidly especially when the underlying cause is a rapidly growing tumor.

4.2.2.2 Imaging Studies
The diagnosis of SVCS/SMS is often made on the basis of clinical signs and symptoms but imaging studies are helpful in determining the underlying etiology. A chest radiograph is easy to obtain and can confirm the presence of a mediastinal mass. A computed tomography (CT) scan of the chest is typically the most useful imaging study and should be obtained after the administration of intravenous (IV) contrast to best evaluate the SVC. CT can provide information regarding the exact size and location of the mass (which can provide clues regarding its etiology), as well as infiltration into surrounding structures and vascularity. It is important to keep in mind that patients with SMS are at high risk for adverse cardiorespiratory events if sedated. Ultrasonography can be performed when sedation is not possible or if the patient cannot lie supine. Echocardiography may be required if there is suspicion of infiltration by the mass into the pericardial cavity or pericardial effusion, based on physical exam or CT scan findings.

4.2.2.3 Other Studies
Tissue is required to make a definitive diagnosis and should be obtained by the least invasive procedure possible to reduce the possibility of an adverse cardiorespiratory event. If there is an associated pleural or pericardial effusion, thoracentesis or pericardiocentesis respectively may be not only therapeutic but also diagnostic in approximately 50 % of cases (Rice et al. 2006). An enlarged palpable lymph node may be more easily biopsied than a mediastinal mass. Mediastinoscopy is more invasive but has the highest diagnostic yield, and some studies have reported low complication rates even in the presence of SMS (Dosios et al. 2005).

4.2.3 Treatment

SVCS/SMS is not typically considered to be a true medical emergency unless airway compromise or neurologic symptoms are present (Yellin et al. 1990). However, tumors with rapid growth can lead to a rapid progression of symptoms. Management consists of both relief of the obstructive symptoms and treatment of the underlying malignancy (Table 4.1). Most data regarding management of SVCS come from case series as there have not been many randomized controlled trials; such studies comparing management options for patients with SVCS/SMS have had difficulty accruing patients (Wilson et al. 2007b). Elevation of the head of the bed can assist in venous drainage and decreasing edema (Cheng 2009). All IV lines should be placed in the lower extremities, so as to prevent further raised hydrostatic pressure in the SVC. Loop diuretics are sometimes used, although it is unclear whether these agents have a significant effect on the rate of clinical improvement (Schraufnagel et al. 1981). In patients with SVC obstruction resulting from intravascular thrombosis associated with an indwelling catheter, removal of the catheter should be strongly considered.

Sedation should be avoided as much as possible, as sedative medications result in reduced respiratory drive and relaxation of bronchial muscles. When a biopsy is required, obtaining tissue under local anesthesia should be the goal. The indicators of risk for general anesthesia in such patients are controversial. Large retrospective reviews have not identified any single clinical sign or test that can accurately predict which patients with a mediastinal mass will experience complications under general anesthesia (Hack et al. 2008). Patients with stridor, orthopnea, wheezing, SVC obstruction, CNS symptoms, pericardial effusion, tracheal or bronchial compression >50–70 %, pulmonary artery outflow obstruction, or peak expiratory flow rate (PEFR) of <50 % are considered to be at higher anesthetic risk (Hack et al. 2008). Others have suggested that PEFR and tracheal cross-sectional area seem to be the most reliable criteria in identifying children at greatest risk for anesthetic complications, and that if both the PEFR and the tracheal cross-sectional area are >50 % of predicted values general anesthesia can be administered safely (Ricketts 2001). If general anesthesia is considered necessary, spontaneous ventilation should be maintained if possible.

As lymphoma and leukemia are among the most common causes of a mediastinal mass and resultant SVCS in children, many centers recommend delaying diagnostic biopsy in symptomatic patients for 24–48 h while emergent corticosteroids or radiation are given in an effort to shrink the tumor size. However, there is concern that such pretreatment can distort cellular morphology and thereby adversely affect the ability to make a histologic diagnosis (Ferrari and Bedford 1990). Retrospective reviews have found that pre-biopsy steroid or radiation treatment caused delay or failure of definitive diagnosis or staging in a minority of children; fortunately many of these patients who were empirically treated did well and have remained disease-free at last follow-up (Loeffler et al. 1986; Borenstein et al. 2000). In an effort to preserve tumor histology for diagnostic purposes, radiation oncologists should attempt to spare radiation to a limited portion of the tumor, with the later goal of obtaining untreated biopsy tissue from that region. This limited "postage stamp" approach to the radiation field is also used to safely treat various types of tumors (Slotman et al. 1996; Hayakawa et al. 1999). Alternate tissue sources from which to make the diagnosis should be considered when possible, including pleural or pericardial effusions and enlarged palpable lymph nodes (see Sect. 4.2.2.3). Ultimately, the decision to treat such a patient prior to obtaining tissue for biopsy should depend on the patient's clinical status and severity of cardiorespiratory symptoms.

4.3 Pericardial Effusion and Cardiac Tamponade

Pericardial effusions are common in adult malignancy, with some series reporting this condition in up to one-third of patients with cancer (Wilkes et al. 1995; McCurdy and Shanholtz 2012). Such effusion can be caused by direct tumor invasion into the pericardium or, rarely, by metastases from other locations. While frequently asymptomatic, severe cases can lead to compression of the heart chambers and cardiac tamponade (Medary et al. 1996).

4.3.1 Pathophysiology

The pericardium is composed of a serous layer of mesothelial cells adherent to the surface of the heart and a fibrous parietal layer formed by the pericardium and reflecting back on itself. The space between these two layers contains up to 50 mL of fluid which serves as a lubricant. Excess fluid can accumulate in this space without affecting the pericardial pressure until it reaches the volume that begins to distend the pericardium, termed the pericardial reserve volume. Once this reserve volume is reached, pressure begins to rise sharply due to the relative inextensibility of the pericardium. The heart is then forced to compete with the increased pericardial contents for the fixed intrapericardial volume which in turn leads to an impaired filling of the cardiac chambers and hemodynamic compromise. This compression of the heart due to the pericardial accumulation of fluid is termed cardiac tamponade and can be life threatening (Spodick 2003).

4.3.2 Clinical Presentation and Diagnosis

4.3.2.1 History and Physical Exam

Small pericardial effusions are frequently asymptomatic (Maher et al. 1996). The amount of pericardial fluid that causes tamponade is related to the rate of fluid accumulation. Rapidly accumulating effusions can cause symptoms with as little as 200 mL of fluid, whereas if fluid accumulates over weeks to months, the pericardial tissue can stretch and may hold >2 L or more before tamponade develops (Karam et al. 2001). In the case of malignancy, the onset is more often insidious.

The most common presenting symptom is exertional dyspnea (Wilkes et al. 1995). Other symptoms include cough, chest pain, dysphagia, hoarseness and hiccups (Karam et al. 2001). The most common sign is pulsus paradoxus, which is defined as a decrease in systolic blood pressure of more than 10 mmHg during inspiration. Tachycardia is frequently seen. The classic description of cardiac tamponade is Beck's triad: hypotension, increased jugular venous pressure

and quiet heart sounds. However, this is seen mostly in rapidly forming effusions and acute tamponade, and only infrequently in patients with chronic pericardial effusion (Tseng et al. 1999).

4.3.2.2 Imaging and Other Studies

The presence of a pericardial effusion can be suspected based on chest radiograph findings which classically show an enlarged cardiac silhouette. The classic appearance of a "water bottle heart" that is globular in appearance is a sensitive but nonspecific finding (Fig. 4.1). An electrocardiogram may reveal low-voltage waveforms and less frequently electrical alternans, a condition where consecutive QRS complexes alternate in height between beats (Karam et al. 2001). Echocardiography, however, has become the preferred diagnostic test for assessing pericardial effusion and cardiac tamponade. It should be ordered when there is a significant pericardial effusion suspected, as it can not only define the size and location of an effusion but also assess the hemodynamic significance and help guide pericardiocentesis (Tseng et al. 1999).

4.3.3 Treatment

The timing and type of treatment for pericardial effusion depend on the severity of symptoms

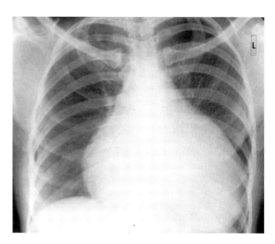

Fig. 4.1 Enlarged ("water bottle") silhouette of the heart on chest radiograph in a patient with pericardial effusion

(Table 4.1). If the effusion is asymptomatic, continued close observation for hemodynamic complications is required but the effusion generally resolves with treatment of the underlying malignancy (Bashir et al. 2007). In the case of tamponade or if the pericardial effusion is otherwise hemodynamically significant, the fluid should be drained emergently. Pericardiocentesis under echocardiographic guidance is the therapy of choice and has been shown to be a safe and effective treatment for pediatric oncology patients with symptomatic pericardial effusion or tamponade (Medary et al. 1996). In addition to relieving symptoms related to the effusion, this procedure can be used to determine the etiology of a malignant effusion. As the recurrence rate of pericardial effusions after initial drainage can be as high as 50 %, consideration should be given to introducing an indwelling pigtail drainage catheter at the time of pericardiocentesis to allow for prolonged drainage (Tsang et al. 1999). Surgical management of malignant pericardial effusion should be reserved for the rare case that cannot be controlled by this method (Maher et al. 1996). In the case of acute cardiac tamponade, the patient should receive volume resuscitation to elevate intracardiac pressures to greater than pericardial pressures. Mechanical ventilation with positive airway pressure should be avoided in these patients because it can further decrease cardiac output (Spodick 2003).

4.4   Pleural Effusion

A pleural effusion is a collection of fluid that accumulates between the visceral and parietal pleurae. Excessive amounts of such fluid can impair breathing by limiting lung expansion during ventilation. In the pediatric population, the most common cause of a pleural effusion is an underlying pneumonia, followed by congenital heart disease and less commonly malignancy (Beers and Abramo 2007). Severe cases can lead to significant respiratory compromise and may require emergent management.

4.4.1   Pathophysiology

The pleural space is bordered by the parietal pleura which covers the inner surface of the thoracic cavity and the visceral pleura which covers the lung surfaces. Like the pericardial space, there is normally a small amount of lubricating fluid between these two layers, but this fluid can increase secondary to underlying pathology. Pleural effusions are classified as either transudates or exudates. Exudates are typically of infectious etiology and result from inflammation on the pleural surface. Transudates, on the other hand, are generally of noninfectious etiology and result from an imbalance between the rate of pleural fluid formation and its reabsorption as the distribution of hydrostatic and oncotic pressure across the pleura is altered.

Malignancy can cause pleural effusion in a number of different ways. A malignant pleural effusion is defined by the presence of cancer cells in the pleural space. This can result from direct extension of tumor cells from an adjacent cancer (such as cancers of the chest wall, lung or breast), hematogenous metastases to the parietal pleura, or invasion of the pulmonary vessels with embolization of tumor cells to the visceral pleural. Tumor deposits spread along the pleural membranes and obstruct lymphatic stomata (small openings of lymphatic capillaries on the free surface of the mesothelium), thereby impairing the drainage of intrapleural fluid. In addition, pleural tumor deposits stimulate the release of cytokines that lead to increased vascular and pleural membrane permeability (Das 2006). Malignancy can also cause pleural effusions indirectly. Such effusions can result from mediastinal lymph node tumor infiltration, superior vena cava syndrome, bronchial obstruction, or decreased oncotic pressure and are termed paraneoplastic or paramalignant effusions (Rice et al. 2006; Heffner and Klein 2008). Paraneoplastic pleural effusions are seen in up to 30 % of adult patients with lymphoma. Most effusions seen with Hodgkin disease are paraneoplastic and result from thoracic duct obstruction, while most effusions seen with non-Hodgkin lymphoma develop as a direct result of pleural infiltration with tumor cells (Das 2006). Pleural effusions can be the initial presentation of a malignancy, a delayed complication in a patient with a known malignancy or the first sign of tumor recurrence following therapy (Heffner and Klein 2008).

4.4.2 Clinical Presentation and Diagnosis

4.4.2.1 History and Physical Exam
Many patients with small pleural effusions are asymptomatic. Larger effusions can cause respiratory signs and symptoms such as tachypnea, cough, dyspnea, orthopnea and retractions. Fever may also be present. Patients can develop pleuritic chest pain which is often described as sharp and worse with deep inspiration. Physical examination often reveals decreased or absent breath sounds on the side of the effusion, dullness on chest percussion and egophony. It should be noted that these physical findings are not always seen in infants (Beers and Abramo 2007).

4.4.2.2 Imaging Studies
When a pleural effusion is suspected, a chest radiograph is the first study to obtain. In the adult, about 200 mL of fluid must be present to be visible on a PA view, while just 50 mL will cause costophrenic blunting on the lateral view (Blackmore et al. 1996). A lateral decubitus chest radiograph can help establish whether the effusion is free flowing or loculated; free-flowing fluid will layer out in a dependent fashion when the affected side is placed down. Ultrasonography is useful to distinguish solid versus liquid lesions and to evaluate for the presence of loculations. CT is helpful in visualizing the underlying lung parenchyma and can also help visualize loculations although not with the same degree of certainty as ultrasound (Cassina et al. 1999). Magnetic resonance imaging (MRI) provides better imaging of soft tissues than chest CT and can detect tumor invasion into the chest wall and diaphragm (Lorigan and Libshitz 1989).

4.4.3 Treatment

Treatment of a pleural effusion depends on the size of the effusion and patient symptoms; not all effusions require drainage (Table 4.1). If the patient is symptomatic, pleural aspiration (thoracentesis) can be both diagnostic and therapeutic. When done under ultrasound guidance, this procedure is associated with a low complication rate (Jones et al. 2003). Once obtained, the fluid should be analyzed to determine whether it is a transudate or exudate. Transudates are generally pale yellow and serous in appearance and have lower protein and lactate dehydrogenase (LDH) concentrations compared with the serum. Exudates are more often cloudy or frankly purulent and contain protein and LDH concentrations that are greater than 50 % and 60 % of the serum concentrations respectively. A milky color to the fluid suggests a chylothorax, and triglyceride and cholesterol levels should be measured in these cases. When malignancy is suspected, the fluid should be sent for cytology as diagnosis has been shown possible in up to 65 % of cases in adults (Ong et al. 2000). The fluid can also be used to look for tumor markers such as α-fetoprotein (AFP), β-human chorionic gonadotropin (β-HCG) and others, depending on the type of tumor suspected. Flow cytometry and cytogenetics can also be performed on the pleural fluid (Das 2006).

Care must be taken when performing thoracentesis as the removal of large volumes of pleural fluid can lead to reexpansion pulmonary edema (RPE). RPE occurs when atelectatic lung regions are rapidly expanded beyond their capacity to reinflate, thus causing alveolar capillary injury. It has been suggested that intrapleural pressure be monitored during thoracentesis and the procedure discontinued when a certain threshold pressure has been reached or 1 L of fluid has been removed, but this is controversial. Others suggest that patients' symptoms during the procedure correlate with intrapleural pressure and that RPE can be avoided if thoracentesis is discontinued when patients experience nonspecific chest discomfort (Jones et al. 2003;

Feller-Kopman et al. 2006). Patients with malignancy-related pleural effusions and recalcitrant tumors may experience reaccumulation of fluid and recurrence of symptoms within 30 days following thoracentesis; therefore, the placement of an indwelling catheter should be considered to allow for prolonged drainage and longer-term relief of symptoms in such cases. Once the diagnosis of a new or recurrent malignancy is made, tumor-specific therapy should be initiated, as possible.

If the pleural effusion is complicated or has evolved to an empyema (an effusion that becomes infected), further intervention may be warranted. Fibrinolytic agents have been shown to be effective therapy in loculated pleural effusions in the pediatric population (Thomson et al. 2002; Cochran et al. 2003). These work by decreasing fibrinous strands and reopening pleural pores blocked by fibrinous debris, thereby increasing the reabsorption of pleural fluid. Intrapleural streptokinase and urokinase have been used in the past but carry a risk of hypersensitivity reactions. Many centers are now administering intrapleural tissue plasminogen activator (tPA) to assist with drainage of loculated pleural effusions in pediatric patients (Feola et al. 2003). When chest tube drainage and fibrinolytics have failed to alleviate a complicated effusion, more invasive surgical intervention is required. Video-assisted thoracoscopic surgery (VATS) is generally considered the procedure of choice for early organizing empyemas as it is less invasive than thoracotomy and has been shown to have significant success. For more advanced organizing empyemas, thoracotomy with decortication remains the treatment of choice (Cassina et al. 1999).

In select patients with refractory and severe recurrent effusions, pleurodesis may be considered. In pleurodesis the pleural space is artificially obliterated by injecting an irritant (such as talc) into the pleural space thus creating inflammation that then tacks the two pleura together. This permanently obliterates the pleural space and prevents reaccumulation of fluid. Pleurodesis is most often used in adults with advanced-stage cancer but has been shown beneficial in pediatric onco-

logy patients with intractable effusions as part of palliative end of life care (Hoffer et al. 2007).

4.5 Hypertensive Emergencies

Severe hypertension has been noted in pediatric oncology patients with neuroblastoma, renal tumors including Wilms tumor and rhabdoid tumor, and, rarely, non-Hodgkin lymphoma involving the kidney, pheochromocytoma, and paraganglioma (Manger and Gifford 2002; Madre et al. 2006). Hypertension can be secondary to catecholamine release in neuroblastoma, pheochromocytoma or paraganglioma, from renal parenchymal tumor involvement, from compression of the renal arteries, or from renal vein thrombosis (Madre et al. 2006). Hypertensive emergency is generally seen secondary to catecholamine release and is a rare finding in neuroblastoma (Manger and Gifford 2002, Seefelder et al. 2005). Pheochromocytoma and paraganglioma are rare catecholamine-producing tumors of chromaffin cells that produce catecholamines which cause some degree of hypertension in most cases (Manger and Gifford 2002). When there is a rapid and marked release of catecholamines, a hypertensive crisis can be precipitated which can be life threatening if not treated emergently.

4.5.1 Pathophysiology

Tumor secretion of catecholamines is responsible for the majority of signs and symptoms associated with pheochromocytoma. These tumors usually secrete predominantly norepinephrine, but in some cases epinephrine and rarely dopamine are secreted. Patients with neuroblastoma and severe hypertension have been similarly noted to have release of norepinephrine and dopamine (Seefelder et al. 2005). Some pheochromocytomas secrete catecholamines intermittently and cause paroxysmal hypertension, while others constantly secrete catecholamines and cause sustained hypertension. Physiologically, norepinephrine increases peripheral vascular resistance with a consequent increase in both systolic and diastolic blood pressure. Epinephrine increases cardiac output and systolic blood pressure but has no major effect on diastolic blood pressure (Prejbisz et al. 2011).

Hypovolemia also occurs in the majority of patients, primarily those with sustained hypertension. In addition, many peptide substances have been identified in these tumors, including vasoactive intestinal peptide (a potent vasodilator), neuropeptide Y (a potent vasoconstrictor), calcitonin, serotonin and others.

4.5.2 Clinical Presentation and Diagnosis

4.5.2.1 History and Physical Exam

Patients with pheochromocytoma typically have "attacks" precipitated by hypercatecholaminemia, and these can occur as often as several times daily. Attacks tend to occur abruptly and subside slowly and are often precipitated by palpation of the tumor, postural changes, exertion, anxiety, pain, or ingestion of certain drugs or foods containing tyramine.

During paroxysmal hypertension, headaches are common and are usually severe and throbbing. They are often accompanied by nausea and vomiting. Palpitations with tachycardia occur frequently as does generalized sweating. Many patients experience acute anxiety with fear of impending death. Other symptoms include tremulousness, pain in the chest, abdomen, lower back or groin, weakness, fatigue, severe weight loss, and heat intolerance (Manger and Gifford 2002).

4.5.2.2 Laboratory Studies

The diagnosis of pheochromocytoma is best made by measuring plasma free metanephrines or catecholamines and 24 h urine fractionated metanephrines. Urinary catecholamines, total metanephrines and vanillylmandelic acid (VMA) measurements are less reliable in pheochromocytoma as compared to neuroblastoma. Rarely patients with essential or neurogenic hypertension will have moderate elevations of plasma catecholamines. In these cases the clonidine suppression test is used to differentiate etiologies of hypertension. Clonidine suppresses sympathetic nerve

activity and plasma norepinephrine by >50 % in patients with neurogenic hypertension, but not in patients with pheochromocytoma. This is because the catecholamine release from pheochromocytoma is believed to be "autonomous" and not responsive to the normal physiological suppressive effect of clonidine (Karlberg et al. 1986).

4.5.2.3 Imaging Studies

When the clinical presentation and laboratory studies are suggestive of pheochromocytoma, imaging is necessary to establish the tumor location. CT identifies 95 % of adrenal pheochromocytomas that are ≥ 1 cm and about 90 % of extra-adrenal abdominal locations ≥ 2 cm. However, MRI is more sensitive and specific than CT for detecting these tumors. MIBG (I-meta-iodobenzylguanidine) scanning is highly specific for diagnosis and localization as this radiopharmaceutical agent concentrates in approximately 85 % of pheochromocytomas. It can be especially helpful in detecting metastases, very small tumors or those in unusual extra-adrenal locations. Additionally, bone scanning with technitium-99m may demonstrate metastatic lesions missed by MIBG (Manger and Gifford 2002).

4.5.3 Treatment

In the case of very severe hypertension, immediate and proper antihypertensive therapy is needed (Table 4.1). There are no official guidelines, but consensus recommends phentolamine as a rapid IV bolus. Phentolamine is a nonselective α-adrenergic antagonist and works primarily by causing vasodilation by α_1 blockade. It has a short half-life so may need to be repeated at 5 min intervals until hypertension is adequately controlled. It can also be given as a continuous infusion, with the infusion rate adjusted for the patient's blood pressure. Alternatively, sodium nitroprusside can be given by continuous infusion. This agent is broken down to release nitric oxide in the circulation which initiates a cascade of reactions resulting in vascular smooth muscle relaxation and vasodilation. β-blocking agents should not be used initially as this can result in unopposed stimulation of α-adrenoreceptors thereby leading to a rise in blood pressure (Boutros et al. 1990; Manger and Gifford 2002; Darr et al. 2012).

If hypertension is less severe, treatment should include an α-blocking agent that can be given orally, such as doxazosin. Calcium channel blockers have also been used successfully in these patients, although diltiazem fails to prevent uncontrolled blood pressure during surgery for pheochromocytoma, and verapamil has been associated with the development of pulmonary edema in the postsurgical period. If tachycardia or arrhythmias are present, β-blockers such as propranolol or atenolol are indicated after appropriate α-adrenoreceptor blockade (Brouwers et al. 2003; Seefelder et al. 2005).

When marked catecholamine release is anticipated (such as with direct manipulation of tumor during surgery), caution must be taken to prevent hypertensive crises. The patient must be prepared using pharmacological blockade of α-adrenoreceptors, ideally with phenoxybenzamine (Seefelder et al. 2005). Phenoxybenzamine is usually given at a starting dose of 10 mg twice a day (or 0.2 mg per kg per day in pediatric patients), and then gradually increased up to 0.4–1.2 mg per kg per day, divided into 3–4 separate doses. With this regimen adequate α-receptor blockade is generally achieved within 14 days. Once α-blockade is achieved, β-blockade is added to prevent reflex tachycardia. Atenolol is frequently used in this scenario (Witteles et al. 2000; Brouwers et al. 2003).

4.6 Pulmonary Leukostasis

Hyperleukocytosis is defined as a white blood cell (WBC) count >100×10^9/L and is associated with increased morbidity and mortality in patients with acute myelogenous leukemia. Hyperleukocytosis can cause pulmonary leukostasis which may lead to severe respiratory compromise and even death. Pulmonary leukostasis can present with hypoxia, dyspnea and tachypnea. Chest radiography and CT scan often reveal bilateral parenchymal infiltrates as well as diffuse ground glass opacities (Piro et al. 2011). Other organs can be involved

as well, such as the CNS. Please refer to Chap. 6 for a discussion of the pathophysiology and management of hyperleukocytosis.

4.7 Summary

Cardiopulmonary emergencies compromise many etiologies in the broader category of oncologic emergencies and often present at initial oncologic diagnosis. The practitioner must be aware of potential tumor pathology that can lead to such emergent situations and how best to manage such patients during the acute period. The evidence basis for management in these circumstances is often based on best practice and consensus statements rather than controlled trials as it is difficult to conduct interventional trials in such emergency situations.

References

Bashir H, Hudson MM, Kaste SC et al (2007) Pericardial involvement at diagnosis in pediatric hodgkin lymphoma patients. Pediatr Blood Cancer 49:666–671
Beers SL, Abramo TJ (2007) Pleural effusions. Pediatr Emerg Care 23:330–338
Blackmore CC, Black WC, Dallas RV et al (1996) Pleural fluid volume estimation: a chest radiograph prediction rule. Acad Radiol 3:103–109
Borenstein SH, Gerstle T, Malkin D et al (2000) The effects of prebiopsy corticosteroid treatment on the diagnosis of mediastinal lymphoma. J Pediatr Surg 35:973–976
Boutros AR, Bravo EL, Zanettin G et al (1990) Perioperative management of 63 patients with pheochromocytoma. Cleve Clin J Med 57:613–617
Brouwers FM, Lenders JWM, Eisenhofer G et al (2003) Pheochromocytoma as an endocrine emergency. Rev Endocr Metab Disord 4:121–128
Cassina P, Hauser M, Hillejan L (1999) Video-assisted thorascopy in the treatment of pleural empyema: stage-based management and outcome. J Thorac Cardiovasc Surg 117:234–238
Cheng S (2009) Superior vena cava syndrome: a contemporary review of a historic disease. Cardiol Rev 17:16–23
Cochran JB, Tecklenburg FW, Turner RB (2003) Intrapleural instillation of fibrinolytic agents for treatment of pleural empyema. Pediatr Crit Care Med 4:39–43
Darr R, Lenders JW, Hofbauer LC et al (2012) Pheochromocytoma – update on disease management. Ther Adv Endocrinol Metab 3:11–26

Das DK (2006) Serous effusions in malignant lymphomas: a review. Diagn Cytopathol 34:335–347

Dosios T, Theakos N, Chatziantoniou C (2005) Cervical mediastinoscopy and anterior mediastinotomy in superior vena cava obstruction. Chest 128:1551–1556

Feller-Kopman D, Walkey A, Berkowitz D et al (2006) The relationship of pleural pressure to symptom development during therapeutic thoracentesis. Chest 129:1556–1560

Feola G, Shaw C, Coburn L (2003) Management of complicated parapneumonic effusions in children. Tech Vasc Interv Radiol 6:197–204

Ferrari LR, Bedford RF (1990) General anesthesia prior to treatment of anterior mediastinal masses in pediatric cancer patients. Anesthesiology 72:991–995

Guyatt G, Gutterman D, Baumann MH et al (2006) Grading strength of recommendations and quality of evidence in clinical guidelines: report from an American College of Chest Physicians task force. Chest 129:174–181

Hack HA, Wright NB, Wynn RF (2008) The anaesthetic management of children with anterior mediastinal masses. Anaesthesia 63:837–846

Halfdanarson TR, Hogan WJ, Moynihan TJ (2006) Oncologic emergencies: diagnosis and treatment. Mayo Clin Proc 81:835–848

Hayakawa K, Mitsuhashi N, Yoshihiro S et al (1999) Limited field irradiation for medically inoperable patients with peripheral stage I non-small cell lung cancer. Lung Cancer 26:137–142

Heffner JE, Klein JS (2008) Recent advances in the diagnosis and management of malignant pleural effusions. Mayo Clin Proc 83:235–250

Hoffer FA, Hancock ML, Hinds PS et al (2007) Pleurodesis for effusions in pediatric oncology patients at end of life. Pediatr Radiol 37:269–273

Ingram L, Rivera GK, Shapiro DN (1990) Superior vena cava syndrome associated with childhood malignancy: analysis of 24 cases. Med Pediatr Oncol 18:476–481

Jones PW, Moyers JP, Rogers JT et al (2003) Ultrasound-guided thoracentesis: is it a safer method? Chest 123:418–423

Karam N, Patel P, deFilippi C (2001) Diagnosis and management of chronic pericardial effusions. Am J Med Sci 322:79–87

Karlberg BE, Hedman L, Lennquist S et al (1986) The value of the clonidine-suppression test in the diagnosis of pheochromocytoma. World J Surg 10:753–761

Loeffler JS, Leopold KA, Recht A et al (1986) Emergency prebiopsy radiation for mediastinal masses: impact on subsequent pathologic diagnosis and outcome. J Clin Oncol 4:716–721

Lorigan JG, Libshitz HI (1989) MR imaging of malignant pleural mesothelioma. J Comput Assist Tomogr 13:617–620

Madre C, Orbach D, Baudouin V et al (2006) Hypertension in childhood cancer: a frequent complication of certain tumor sites. J Pediatr Hematol Oncol 28:659–664

Maher EA, Shepherd FA, Todd TJ (1996) Pericardial sclerosis as the primary management of malignant pericardial effusion and cardiac tamponade. J Thorac Cardiovasc Surg 112:637–643

Manger WM, Gifford RW (2002) Pheochromocytoma. J Clin Hypertens 4:62–72

McCurdy MT, Shanholtz CB (2012) Oncologic emergencies. Crit Care Med 40:2212–2222

Medary I, Steinherz LJ, Aronson DC et al (1996) Cardiac tamponade in the pediatric oncology population: treatment by percutaneous catheter drainage. J Pediatr Surg 31:197–200

Ong KC, Indumathi V, Poh WT et al (2000) The diagnostic yield of pleural fluid cytology in malignant pleural effusions. Singapore Med J 41:19–23

Piro E, Carillo G, Levato L et al (2011) Reversal of leukostasis-related pulmonary distress syndrome after leukapheresis and low-dose chemotherapy in acute myeloid leukemia. J Clin Oncol 29:e725–e726

Prejbisz A, Lenders JW, Eisenhofer G et al (2011) Cardiovascular manifestations of pheochromocytoma. J Hypertens 29:2049–2060

Rice TW, Rodriguez RM, Barnette R et al (2006) Prevalence and characteristics of pleural effusions in superior vena cava syndrome. Respirology 11:299–305

Ricketts RR (2001) Clinical management of anterior mediastinal tumors in children. Semin Pediatr Surg 10:161–168

Schraufnagel DE, Hill R, Leech JA et al (1981) Superior vena cava obstruction: is it a medical emergency? Am J Med 70:1169–1174

Seefelder C, Sparks JW, Chirnomas D et al (2005) Perioperative management of a child with severe hypertension from a catecholamine secreting neuroblastoma. Paediatr Anaesth 15:606–610

Slotman BJ, Antonisse IE, Njo KH (1996) Limited field irradiation in early stage (T1–2, N0) non-small cell lung cancer. Radiother Oncol 41:41–44

Spodick DH (2003) Acute cardiac tamponade. N Engl J Med 349:684–690

Thomson AH, Hull J, Kumar MR et al (2002) A randomized trial of intrapleural urokinase in the treatment of childhood empyema. Thorax 57:343–347

Tsang TS, Oh JK, Seward JB (1999) Diagnosis and management of cardiac tamponade in the era of echocardiography. Clin Cardiol 22:446–452

Wilkes JD, Fidias P, Vaickus L et al (1995) Malignancy-related pericardial effusion. Cancer 76:1377–1387

Wilson LD, Detterbeck FC, Yahalom J (2007a) Superior vena cava syndrome with malignant causes. N Engl J Med 356:1862–1869

Wilson P, Bezjak A, Asch M et al (2007b) The difficulties of a randomized study in superior vena caval obstruction. J Thorac Oncol 2:514–519

Witteles RM, Kaplan EL, Roizen MF (2000) Safe and cost-effective preoperative preparation of patients with pheochromocytoma. Anesth Analg 91:302–304

Yellin A, Rosen A, Reichert N et al (1990) Superior vena cava syndrome. The myth – the facts. Am Rev Respir Dis 141:1114–1118

Neurologic Emergencies

5

Amit Sabnis, Jonathan L. Finlay, and Sabine Mueller

Contents

A. Sabnis, MD (✉)
Division of Hematology/Oncology,
Department of Pediatrics,
Benioff Children's Hospital,
University of California-San Francisco,
505 Parnassus Avenue,
San Francisco, CA 94143, USA
e-mail: sabnisa@peds.ucsf.edu

J.L. Finlay, MB, ChB, FRCP
Department of Hematology/Oncology/BMT,
Nationwide Children's Hospital,
Columbus, OH, USA

S. Mueller, MD, PhD
Division of Hematology/Oncology,
Department of Pediatrics,
Neurology and Neurosurgery,
Benioff Children's Hospital,
University of California-San Francisco,
San Francisco, CA, USA

Abstract

Neurologic complications of cancer and cancer therapy are common and can arise rapidly in pediatric oncology patients. Some of these complications can present as emergent situations that require rapid diagnosis and treatment; familiarity with these conditions and a low index of suspicion are absolutely necessary in caring for such patients. The emergencies of spinal cord compression, acute alteration in mental status, increased intracranial pressure and stroke are addressed in this chapter. Specific attention is given to the acute neurotoxic effects of common chemotherapeutic agents. In addition to background regarding possible etiologies that are unique

J. Feusner et al. (eds.), *Supportive Care in Pediatric Oncology:
A Practical Evidence-Based Approach*, Pediatric Oncology,
DOI 10.1007/978-3-662-44317-0_5, © Springer Berlin Heidelberg 2015

to the child with cancer, the evidence bases for diagnostic steps and management are discussed. This chapter provides the necessary framework to recognize potential neurologic emergencies in pediatric oncology patients and highlights when to utilize a multidisciplinary team approach including pediatric oncologists and neuro-oncologists, intensivists, neurologists, radiation oncologists, and neurosurgeons to provide optimal care.

5.1 Introduction

Neurologic complications of cancer and cancer therapy are common and can arise rapidly in pediatric oncology patients. Some of these complications can present as emergent situations that require rapid diagnosis and treatment; familiarity with these conditions and a low index of suspicion are absolutely necessary in caring for such patients. The emergencies of spinal cord compression, acute alteration in mental status, increased intracranial pressure and stroke are addressed in this chapter. Specific attention is given to the acute neurotoxic effects of common chemotherapeutic agents. In addition to background regarding possible etiologies that are unique to the child with cancer, the evidence bases for diagnostic steps and management are discussed and graded (Table 5.1). This chapter provides the necessary framework to recognize potential neurologic emergencies in pediatric oncology patients and highlights when to utilize a multidisciplinary team approach including pediatric oncologists and neuro-oncologists, intensivists, neurologists, radiation oncologists, and neurosurgeons to provide optimal care.

5.2 Spinal Cord Compression

Compression of the spinal cord can be caused by mass effect from either extradural or intradural tumors. Presenting symptoms can initially be nonspecific, and the diagnosis can be missed if the index of suspicion on the part of the examiner is not sufficiently high. Cord compression may herald a new diagnosis of cancer, be a sign of treatment failure or relapse, or indicate a complication of treatment such as a post-lumbar puncture hematoma. In addition to spinal cord compression, this section describes conus medullaris and cauda equina syndromes.

5.2.1 Presentation

Back pain is a presenting symptom in 80–90 % of patients presenting with malignant spinal cord compression (Pollono et al. 2003). In patients old enough to describe their symptoms, this pain is classically radicular, radiating to the legs, sharp, and described as electric. Non-radicular pain may be also reported. However, younger patients may not be able to localize pain or provide any description of its quality.

Weakness is present in similar numbers of patients at presentation, but again can be difficult to elicit in the young child. Increased "clumsiness," particularly affecting gait, or refusal to walk, can be manifestations of neurologic weakness. In patients who are able to comply with examination, localization of the weakness can help identify the level of compression (Table 5.2). Weakness may initially be flaccid, with subsequent hyperreflexia in extremities distal to the site of compression. Compression at the level of the cauda equina causes absent reflexes due to the peripheral nature of the injury.

Isolated bowel or bladder dysfunction with perineal anesthesia suggests compression of either the conus medullaris or cauda equina, but sympathetic denervation from a higher compression can reproduce symptoms of urinary retention. A history of progressive constipation or abdominal pain with a full bladder should therefore warrant further investigation. Sensory changes (paresthesias or anesthesia) should be carefully investigated to determine patterns of distribution. The presence of any sensory level of such findings is a very concerning sign and can additionally help localize a lesion.

Table 5.1 Summary of recommendations for management of neurologic emergencies[a]

Clinical scenario	Recommendations	Level of evidence[b]
Spinal cord compression	Corticosteroids: decadron 1–2 mg/kg (max 10 mg) followed by 0.25–0.5 mg/kg (max 4 mg) Q6h—may complicate ability to make a diagnosis	1C
	Surgery: rapid progression of symptoms or total plegia are indications for emergent surgical management	1B
	Radiation therapy: radiosensitive tumors (i.e., lymphoma, leukemia) while leaving additional diagnostic sites; patients who are too unstable for surgery; for palliation	1C
Altered mental status	Workup to include structural, metabolic and infectious causes	1C
	Antiepileptics (benzodiazepines first-line) for acute seizure management with AMS	1B
	Hypertonic saline for seizures secondary to hyponatremia, then slow correction to avoid central pontine myelinolysis	1B
Increased intracranial pressure	Acute evaluation and management of airway, breathing and circulation in the intensive care setting	1C
	Consideration for intubation	1C
	Elevate head of bed	1C
	Treatment of hyperthermia with antipyretics and cooling	1C
	Head CT or MRI prior to LP	1C
	Measurement of LP opening pressure	1B
	Consideration for hyperosmolar therapy with mannitol or hypertonic saline	1C
Cerebrovascular accident	MRI preferred over CT; CT can be done acutely to rule out hemorrhage	1C
	Treatment with a specialized team including pediatric stroke specialist, neurosurgeon, interventional radiologist	1C
	Permissive hypertension in ischemic stroke	1C
	tPA if no contraindications in ischemic stroke	2C
	Assessment for underlying prothrombotic state	2C
	Neurosurgical intervention for hemorrhagic stroke	1C
	Assessment of coagulopathy and FFP therapy if coagulopathic	1C
	Utilization of recombinant factor VII in hemorrhagic stroke	2C
Sinovenous thrombosis secondary to asparaginase therapy	Measurement and repletion of antithrombin (with pooled or recombinant product) and plasminogen	1B
	Repletion of fibrinogen with cryoprecipitate to normal levels (i.e., >150 mg/dL)	1C
	Anticoagulation if without a severe hemorrhagic component (i.e., unfractionated heparin)	1C
	Reinstitution of asparaginase after recovery	1B
	Prophylaxis with antithrombin is not currently recommended	2C
Neurosurgery	Prophylactic antiepileptics after neurosurgical intervention	2C
IT neurotoxicity	Dextromethorphan in the acute phase of IT MTX neurotoxicity	2C
	Aminophylline in the acute phase of IT MTX neurotoxicity	2C
	Leucovorin rescue for patients who have had IT MTX neurotoxicity in the past	2C
	Rechallenging with IT MTX or substituting with IT HC/Ara-C for future IT therapy	2C
Ifosfamide-induced encephalopathy	Methylene blue for acute treatment or future prophylaxis if with IIE	2C
	Thiamine for acute treatment or future prophylaxis if with IIE	2C

(continued)

Table 5.1 (continued)

Clinical scenario	Recommendations	Level of evidence[b]
Posterior reversible encephalopathy syndrome	Acute seizure management (if present) as above	1B
	Controlling of blood pressure with calcium channel blockers or β-blockers	1B
	MRI imaging with FLAIR and DWI	1B

AMS altered mental status, *CT* computed tomography, *MRI* magnetic resonance imaging, *LP* lumbar puncture, *tPA* tissue plasminogen activator, *FFP* fresh frozen plasma, *IT* intrathecal, *MTX* methotrexate, *HC* hydrocortisone, *IIE* ifosfamide-induced encephalopathy, *FLAIR* fluid attenuated inversion recovery, *DWI* diffusion-weighted imaging
[a]See text for full detail
[b]Per Guyatt et al. (2006); see Preface

Table 5.2 Localization of spinal cord compression by weakness

Nerve roots	Muscle action and deep tendon reflexes (DTRs)
C3–C5	Diaphragmatic excursion
C5–C6	Biceps and brachioradialis DTRs
C6–C7	Triceps DTR
C8–T1	Hand function
L2–L3	Hip flexion
L3–L4	Patellar DTR
L4–L5	Ankle dorsiflexion
L5–S1	Knee flexion
S1–S2	Ankle plantarflexion; S1 mediates Achilles DTR

5.2.2 Differential Diagnosis

Cord compression can be the presenting feature of a new malignancy and patients may have either acute or subacute presentations. Of tumors arising from the extradural space, paravertebral Ewing sarcoma is the most frequent malignancy to cause cord compression (Klein et al. 1991; Pollono et al. 2003). Neuroblastoma can also present with cord compression given their origin in the prevertebral sympathetic chain. While less common, primary or metastatic vertebral bone lesions such as osteosarcoma or Langerhans cell histiocytosis have also been associated with cord compression. Pathologic fracture complicating a primary bone lesion may cause the presenting symptoms. Both acute lymphoblastic leukemia (ALL) and acute myelogenous leukemia (AML) can present with extramedullary disease that can cause cord compression. Discrete masses composed of leukemic cells (chloromas or granulocytic sarcomas), are more commonly observed in AML than ALL (Mantadakis et al. 2008; Olcay et al. 2009; Isome et al. 2011). Both Hodgkin and non-Hodgkin lymphoma can similarly lead to cord compression through direct mass effect (Acquaviva et al. 2003; Daley et al. 2003; Gupta et al. 2009).

Intraspinal tumors in children (Fig. 5.1) are most commonly gliomas or ependymomas (Huisman 2009; Benesch et al. 2010). Drop metastases from posterior fossa tumors, most notably primitive neuroectodermal tumors (PNET; medulloblastoma), can also cause cord compression. Patients with neurocutaneous syndromes such as neurofibromatosis type-1 (NF-1) and NF-2, von Hippel-Lindau disease, and tuberous sclerosis warrant special consideration when presenting with signs of spinal cord compression given their propensity for various intraspinal tumors such as malignant peripheral nerve sheath tumor, ependymoma, hemangioblastoma and astrocytoma, respectively.

In the patient with known tumor, new symptoms of cord compression should raise concern for development of metastatic disease. Patients who have recently undergone a lumbar puncture, particularly in the setting of low platelets or coagulopathy, are at risk for an epidural hematoma that may require emergent evacuation. A potential mimic of cord compression in the pediatric oncology patient is acute onset transverse myelitis. This entity can present with symptoms of weakness, bowel and bladder dysfunction, and a sensory level; magnetic resonance imaging (MRI) may demonstrate inflammatory changes

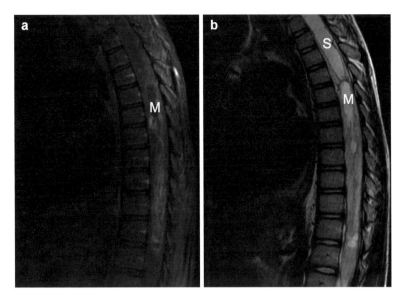

Fig. 5.1 Intraspinal glioma. This 10-year-old patient presented with several weeks of progressive bilateral lower extremity weakness. The T1-weighted gadolinium-enhanced MRI shown in Panel **a** demonstrates a cystic mass ("M") in the upper thoracic spinal cord. The T2-weighted image in Panel **b** highlights the development of syrinx ("S"), seen as bright cerebrospinal fluid in this sequence, cranial to the mass. Pathology from a biopsy specimen taken at the time of diagnosis was consistent with pilocytic astrocytoma

within the cord, but no compressive mass. Transverse myelitis has been reported in patients following either intrathecal or high-dose intravenous cytarabine (Schwenn et al. 1991).

5.2.3 Management

The first step in managing a patient with suspected cord compression is involvement of a multidisciplinary team including neurosurgery, neurology, oncology, intensivists and radiation oncology. Frequent monitoring for progression of symptoms is vital, as this can rapidly change the therapeutic plan. Initial steps should be aimed at verifying the diagnosis and attempting to alleviate compressive symptoms medically while a more definitive treatment plan is formulated.

5.2.3.1 Imaging
MRI of the spine can help narrow the differential diagnosis, allow for surgical planning and identify potential sites of multifocal disease. The entire spine should be imaged with pre- and post-

gadolinium contrast to maximize yield. Brain imaging may also be warranted if the lesions are suspicious for drop metastases or if the patient presents with signs or symptoms of increased intracranial pressure such as headache, emesis, hypertension with bradycardia, or cranial nerve palsies.

5.2.3.2 Corticosteroids
Steroid treatment is employed to relieve any vasogenic edema that may be contributing to cord compression. In the case of ALL and lymphoma, corticosteroids also have a direct antitumor effect that may benefit the patient in the short term, but ultimately make diagnosis of the underlying malignancy much more challenging. If a hematopoietic malignancy is likely, steroids should be given only when urgent diagnostic procedures have been scheduled (e.g., bone marrow aspiration and biopsy, lymph node excisional biopsy).

Outside of this scenario, the benefits of steroids are thought to outweigh their risks and are routinely used when cord compression is diagnosed, although clinical trials in children are lacking. In adults there is no evidence supporting high-dose dexamethasone; an initial dose of 1–2 mg/kg (max 10 mg) followed by 0.25–0.5 mg/kg (max 4 mg) every 6 h can be considered while awaiting further therapy (Kaal and Vecht 2004; Loblaw et al. 2005; George et al. 2008).

5.2.3.3 Surgery

Surgery in spinal cord compression can be utilized for tumor debulking with spinal cord stabilization or for diagnostic biopsy in the highly chemotherapy- or radiotherapy-sensitive tumor. Prospective studies in adult patients with cord compression have favored early laminectomy and debulking over radiation therapy alone although more recent retrospective studies have called this into question (Patchell et al. 2005; Rades et al. 2010). Laminectomy in the young child can lead to spinal deformities requiring future surgical intervention and therefore pediatric retrospective studies argue against an early surgical approach (Parikh and Crawford 2003). Recovery from surgery can also lead to delays in instituting definitive chemoradiotherapy.

An early case series from St. Jude Children's Research Hospital suggested that initial debulking is warranted for sarcomas, whereas biopsy with chemotherapy or radiotherapy should be considered for patients with neuroblastoma, germ cell tumors and lymphomas (Klein et al. 1991). Patients presenting with rapid evolution of symptoms or complete loss of motor function were treated with urgent surgical decompression regardless of tumor histology. Smaller case series have supported the use of initial chemotherapy in neuroblastoma, Ewing sarcoma and germ cell tumors (Hayes et al. 1984). A study of 76 children with neuroblastoma from Italy found no difference in the success rates of chemotherapy, radiotherapy or surgical debulking in improvement of neurological signs, but noted that patients receiving radiotherapy or surgical debulking all went on to receive additional therapy for cord compression, whereas chemotherapy patients did not (De Bernardi et al. 2001). A follow-up study from this same group also noted a higher incidence of spinal deformities in the group receiving surgical intervention with a trend towards worse neurologic outcomes. As with the St. Jude data, patients with rapidly progressive symptoms or severe presentations were all treated with emergent surgery, making that group much higher risk than those treated with chemotherapy or radiotherapy (Angelini et al. 2011). A more contemporary study of 122 patients did not find any difference in spinal outcomes in patients treated with chemotherapy or surgery which the authors attribute to improvement in surgical technique (Simon et al. 2012).

In summary, each case of cord compression warrants individual consideration before a decision to proceed with debulking or biopsy can be made. Rapid progression of symptoms and total plegia are indications for emergent surgical management. Spinal column instability, which warrants surgical intervention, will also often necessitate surgical debulking. If the malignancy is known to be chemotherapy sensitive (i.e., hematopoietic malignancies, neuroblastoma, Ewing sarcoma, germ cell tumors), biopsy either at the site of cord compression or at another more easily accessible site can be considered prior to institution of chemotherapy. The timely availability of these options may also influence the treatment decision.

5.2.3.4 Radiation Therapy

The advantages of external beam radiation therapy include rapid onset of action and minimal invasiveness making radiation therapy an attractive option for patients who are too unstable to be considered surgical candidates, or in the palliative setting. Tumors that are radiosensitive such as hematologic malignancies (i.e., chloromas) and lymphoma may benefit from urgent radiotherapy while leaving additional diagnostic disease sites intact. Extensive metastatic disease may similarly be more amenable to radiation therapy than a surgical approach; when surgery is the primary therapeutic modality, adjunctive radiation may have a role in local control.

A case series from Children's Hospital of Philadelphia demonstrated the benefit of urgent radiation therapy in combination with chemotherapy in a pediatric population with a

variety of tumor types: of 33 patients presenting with cord compression, 55 % demonstrated
improvement following chemoradiotherapy
and 30 % had stabilization of their neurologic
symptoms (Bertsch et al. 1998).

Dose-dependent long-term complications
arising from radiation therapy can include future
growth complications such as scoliosis as well as
risk of secondary malignancy, particularly
meningioma (Hoffman and Yock 2009).
Stereotactic radiosurgery can deliver a single
treatment dose up to 13 Gy to localized tumors
without exceeding spinal cord tolerance; additionally, the spinal cord can tolerate high total
doses, with a risk of myelopathy of <1 % at
54 Gy in adult patients (Kirkpatrick et al. 2010).

5.2.4 Outcomes

The best predictor of outcome in multiple studies
has been the degree of neurologic disability at the
time of presentation. One large cohort study suggested that only approximately 50 % of patients
with paraplegia at the time of presentation
improved despite treatment whereas close to
90 % of patients without paraplegia had improvement in their symptoms (Pollono et al. 2003).
Published outcomes data are from small cohort
studies with a variety of pathologic diagnoses
and treatments, making any broad interpretation
difficult. There is a general consensus, however,
that outcomes for pediatric cord compression are
significantly better than in adult patients.

5.3 Altered Mental Status

For the purposes of this chapter, altered mental
status (AMS) includes patients with symptoms of
encephalopathy (confusion, somnolence or
coma) and those with seizures (which often,
though not always, alter the level of consciousness). Although there are often distinct differential diagnoses for encephalopathy and seizure,
many conditions unique to the pediatric oncology
patient can predispose to either presentation.
Additionally, subclinical seizure is a diagnostic

consideration in any patient with altered
mentation. For these reasons, we suggest a common approach to the differential diagnosis and
initial management of such patients.

5.3.1 Presentation

Confusion or somnolence in an oncology patient
should prompt a thorough neurologic examination and review of recent medications.
Nonresponsive patients require urgent steps to
secure the airway, breathing and circulation prior
to additional diagnostic interventions. AMS may
be due to a diffuse process affecting the brain,
such as medication effect or subclinical seizure,
or be due to direct involvement of the brainstem,
increased intracranial pressure (ICP), or impending herniation. Ruling out the latter by means of
neurologic assessment is of utmost importance.
Details in the management of increased ICP are
discussed in Sect. 5.4.

5.3.2 Initial Management

The first goal in a seizing patient is to stop the
seizures. Benzodiazepines are often used as
first-line medications in this setting. Lorazepam
can be given intravenously if access is available;
otherwise intranasal, buccal, or rectal formulations of diazepam or lorazepam can be
employed. It is important to anticipate and treat
the adverse effects of these medications including respiratory depression or hypotension, as
repeated dosing may be required to halt seizure
activity. Failure to respond to benzodiazepines
(or recurrent seizures after initial response)
should prompt escalation to additional antiepi-
leptics such as phenobarbital or fosphenytoin.
Levetiracetam is another antiepileptic that has
the advantage of not inducing hepatic enzyme
activity and thus has fewer interactions with
chemotherapy. Seizures refractory to these
interventions can be treated with intravenous
loading with either valproic acid or levetiracetam and necessitate urgent determination of the
underlying etiology.

Initial diagnostic workup should include serum chemistries, especially sodium, calcium, magnesium, phosphorus, and glucose, and head imaging. CT is often the easiest imaging to obtain in this setting and can rule out emergent, life-threatening causes of seizure. If there are concerns for cerebrovascular accident, a stroke-protocol MRI with diffusion-weighted imaging or magnetic resonance angiography should be considered. The seizing oncology patient should be managed in consultation with neurology; early neurosurgical involvement is also imperative for patients with known or suspected intra-cranial processes.

Continuous electroencephalography (EEG) monitoring should be strongly considered for any patient with persistent AMS or concerns for sub-clinical seizure. Lumbar puncture and MRI may be indicated when the patient is stabilized to look for evidence of progressive malignancy, infection or demyelination. Further treatment is dependent on the results of these initial diagnostic studies, as discussed below.

5.3.3 Differential Diagnosis

The differential diagnosis of seizure or AMS can be broadly divided into structural causes, including primary CNS or metastatic disease; metabolic derangements resulting in hyponatremia, hypocalcemia or hypoglycemia; infectious complications; toxic effects of chemotherapy; or stroke (ischemic or hemorrhagic). Posterior reversible encephalopathy syndrome (PRES) can also present with seizure. Seizures secondary to neurologic emergencies such as stroke are discussed in greater detail in Sect. 5.5.

5.3.3.1 Structural

Primary CNS tumors can directly lead to seizures. Oligodendrogliomas and gangliogliomas are common causes of brain tumor-induced seizure, though other low-grade gliomas and dysembryoblastic neuroepithelial tumors (DNETs) can be associated with seizures as well (Ogiwara et al. 2010). Such low-grade lesions may be surgically resected to provide relief from symptom-

atic seizures. Extracranial tumors can invade the CNS either by direct invasion, as with paramningeal rhabdomyosarcoma, or by hematogenous metastasis, as in Ewing sarcoma (the most common cause of pediatric CNS parenchymal metastasis), extracranial germ cell tumors, and leukemias.

Intracranial hemorrhage is another consideration in the seizing patient. Intratumoral hemorrhage has been variably reported in adults receiving the monoclonal antibody bevacizumab for primary CNS tumors (Seet et al. 2011; Khasraw et al. 2012). Certain primary childhood CNS tumors have a high proclivity for spontaneous intratumoral hemorrhage due to their intrinsic high vascularity; notorious examples are primary CNS choriocarcinoma, choroid plexus carcinoma and malignant gliomas. Derangement of the hemostatic system as seen in acute promyelocytic leukemia or after asparaginase therapy can also lead to intracranial hemorrhage in a patient without CNS disease.

Patients who have undergone resection of CNS tumors may develop postoperative seizures. No clear consensus exists regarding the use of prophylactic antiepileptic therapy in the postoperative setting. The American Academy of Neurology recommends tapering antiepileptic drugs (AEDs) within the first postoperative week, though it does not make a recommendation regarding AED initiation due to a lack of evidence even in the adult setting (Glantz et al. 2000). A retrospective study of 223 patients from Children's Hospital of Philadelphia found that age younger than 2 years, supratentorial location of tumor and postoperative hyponatremia were the only independent predictors of postoperative seizure (Hardesty et al. 2011). Of the 229 operations reviewed, 7.4 % of patients seized and only 4.4 % received routine postoperative AEDs (Hardesty et al. 2011). Due to insufficient evidence, the use of prophylactic AEDs should be determined under consultation with the patient's neurosurgeon and intensive care team. Given the low incidence of unprovoked postoperative seizure, workup of new seizures following tumor resection is warranted to exclude alternative etiologies.

5.3.3.2 Metabolic

The metabolic causes of AMS or seizure in pediatric oncology are similar to other pediatric patients: hyponatremia, hypoglycemia, and, less frequently, hypocalcemia secondary to hyperphosphatemia in severe tumor lysis syndrome (discussed in Chap. 3).

Iatrogenic Hyponatremia

Hyponatremia severe enough to provoke seizures warrants urgent correction though overly rapid correction can lead to central pontine myelinolysis. The risks of this complication are greater in chronic hyponatremia and in adult patients. A reasonable goal is to raise the sodium by ≤10 mEq/L in the first 24 h and then slowly normalize the serum sodium over the next 48 h. Hypertonic saline should be used in the seizing patient as it allows for more rapid correction than isotonic fluids which can be accomplished by calculation of the sodium deficit and either a subsequent fluid infusion rate or bolus therapy (Adrogue and Madias 2000; Sterns et al. 2009; Moritz and Ayus 2010).

Syndrome of Inappropriate Antidiuretic Hormone (SIADH) Release

The syndrome of inappropriate antidiuretic hormone (SIADH) secretion leads to dilutional hyponatremia due to inappropriate resorption of free water in the renal collecting tubules. SIADH has a multitude of causes including poorly understood effects of CNS or intrapulmonary lesions as well as secondary to chemotherapeutic agents including vincristine, cyclophosphamide, cisplatin and melphalan (Lim et al. 2010). The diagnosis of SIADH relies on the combined laboratory findings of low serum osmolarity (i.e., <290 mOsm/L) with inappropriately concentrated urine osmolality (i.e., >100 mOsm/kg).

Treatment of SIADH depends on: (1) removing the causative agent when possible; (2) restricting free water intake to ≤urine output (±insensible losses); and (3) correction with hypertonic saline, if indicated. Hypertonic saline is generally avoided in patients with asymptomatic SIADH and in those presenting solely with AMS but may be necessary to control seizures. Free water restriction is difficult in situations where hyperhydration is necessary to avoid chemotherapeutic toxicity as with cyclophosphamide administration. In these situations, using normal saline as opposed to hypotonic fluids and checking serum sodium levels frequently is warranted. Chronic SIADH can be managed with oral urea and fluid restriction (Huang et al. 2006). The oral vasopressin receptor antagonist tolvaptan has been shown to be effective in adult patients with paraneoplastic SIADH, but data on broader use in cancer patients and the safety in pediatrics are not yet available (Kenz et al. 2011).

Cerebral Salt Wasting

Cerebral salt wasting (CSW) is a controversial diagnosis of unclear etiology; some authors suggest CSW does not exist or is exceedingly rare, while others suggest it is not cerebral in origin (Singh et al. 2002; Rivkees 2008). Nonetheless, CSW is a consideration in the pediatric neuro-oncology patient with hyponatremia and seizures. In reviewing children recovering from craniotomy for tumor resection, Hardesty et al. (2011) found that nearly half the patients with laboratory identified CSW developed postoperative seizures. The main clinical distinction between patients with SIADH and CSW is volume status; CSW represents hypovolemic hyponatremia, while patients with SIADH are either slightly hypervolemic or euvolemic. As in patients with SIADH, CSW patients will have hyponatremia, low serum osmolarity and relatively concentrated urine with high urine sodium excretion. The patient with CSW will often respond to isotonic fluid infusion, whereas normal saline frequently worsens hyponatremia in patients with SIADH. Correction of hypovolemia is the main therapy in CSW. Patients with chronic hyponatremia may require oral supplementation with salt tablets.

5.3.3.3 Infection

Patients receiving immunosuppressive chemotherapy have an increased risk for CNS infection which may present with AMS or seizure. Lumbar puncture is a helpful diagnostic tool in this setting, but should be deferred until the patient has been stabilized and CT imaging performed. Institution of broad antimicrobial coverage should not be delayed to obtain cerebrospinal fluid (CSF); cell counts can be informative in non-cytopenic patients even after sterilization of CSF and polymerase chain reaction (PCR)-based assays for viruses can remain positive after antiviral therapy has been instituted.

Infectious studies should include cultures of blood and CSF. Enterovirus, herpes simplex virus (HSV) and human herpesvirus-6 (HHV6) can be detected by CSF PCR. Culture or direct fluorescence antibody (DFA) testing of oropharyngeal lesions should also be considered. Treatment with high-dose acyclovir should be initiated urgently if viral meningoencephalitis is suspected.

A study of 40 cases of bacterial and fungal meningitis in pediatric oncology patients found that recent neurosurgery or a CNS device was present in the majority of cases (Sommers and Hawkins 1999). Among patients without neurosurgical intervention, those with hematologic malignancies and prolonged neutropenia were at the highest risk for infection.

5.3.3.4 Chemotherapy-Associated Neurotoxicity

Methotrexate, ifosfamide, and cytarabine (Ara-C) are commonly used pediatric chemotherapeutic agents that can provoke seizures and encephalopathy. Transverse myelitis is a peculiar complication described following the combined intravenous and intrathecal administration of cytarabine. Vincristine is most commonly known for its associated peripheral neuropathies, but medical errors in administration have highlighted its extreme neurotoxicity when introduced into the CNS or given at erroneously high doses systemically. Thiotepa, carmustine (BCNU) and busulfan are myeloablative agents used at high doses in stem cell transplant with neurologic dose-limiting toxicities (Papadopoulos et al. 1998). Other less commonly used agents such as nelarabine (a prometabolite of Ara-G) have simi-

larly been implicated in patients developing new encephalopathy or seizures.

Methotrexate

Acute neurotoxicity has been described within 24 h of intravenous or intrathecal methotrexate administration, consisting of confusion, seizures, or encephalopathy. Methotrexate neurotoxicity is frequently self-resolving and is not related to drug levels (Rubnitz et al. 1998). By contrast, acute neurotoxicity following a methotrexate overdose can be very severe. Symptoms include myelopathy, seizures, encephalopathy and death from progressive necrotizing leukoencephalopathy. Published experience in overdose suggests benefit from high-dose intravenous (IV) leucovorin, IV carboxypeptidase G2 and alkalinization of the urine, with hemodialysis if renal insufficiency develops. If the overdose was administered intrathecally, the addition of CSF lavage or exchange and intrathecal administration of carboxypeptidase G2 have been used with good outcomes (Spiegel et al. 1984; Widemann et al. 2004).

Subacute methotrexate neurotoxicity includes a constellation of neurologic symptoms, often reversible, that occur after either IV or IT methotrexate. Symptoms include severe headache, focal or generalized seizures, AMS ranging from confusion to coma, and sensory and motor findings consistent with cerebrovascular accident. Aphasia is commonly reported (Dufourg et al. 2007). The median time from methotrexate administration to symptom development is consistently reported to be 10 days (Mahoney et al. 1998). The risk of developing methotrexate neurotoxicity increases with combination IV/IT therapy, increasing total cumulative administered methotrexate dose and cranial irradiation (Land et al. 1994; Reddick et al. 2005).

There is no single diagnostic test for methotrexate neurotoxicity; therefore recognizing the clinical scenario is vital to making the diagnosis. MRI can support the diagnosis (Fig. 5.2), as patients have characteristic changes on diffusion-weighted imaging that mimic ischemia (Reddick et al. 2005). However, unlike true ischemic changes, there is rapid normalization within sev-

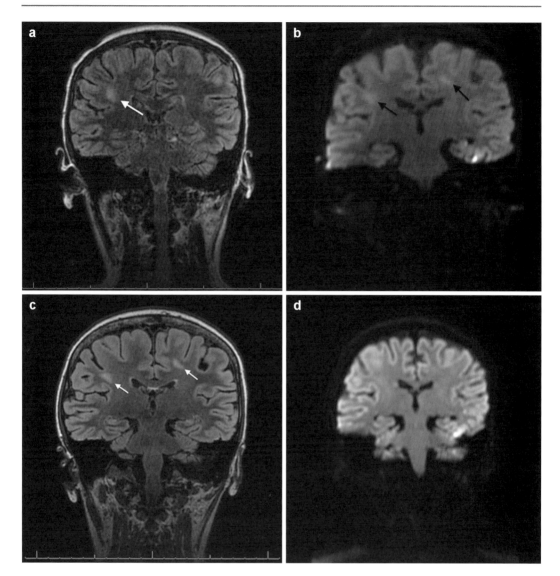

Fig. 5.2 Subacute methotrexate neurotoxicity. This 12-year-old patient with acute lymphoblastic leukemia developed symptoms of aphasia and lethargy approximately 10 days following combined intrathecal and high-dose intravenous (5 g/m²) methotrexate during delayed intensification. The T2-FLAIR MRI shown in Panel **a** demonstrates the development of ill-defined patches of hyperintensity within the white matter (*white arrow*). Diffusion-weighted imaging taken concurrently, shown in Panel **b**, shows restricted diffusion (*black arrows*). Although the pattern is not consistent with any one vascular territory, infarct is on the differential diagnosis with such findings. Fortunately, the patient's symptoms resolved over 48 h, and while repeat scans taken 1 month later demonstrate continuation and evolution of the T2-FLAIR changes (Panel **c**, *white arrows*), the diffusion changes have now completely resolved (Panel **d**). The patient has continued to be completely asymptomatic but has not yet been rechallenged with intrathecal methotrexate

eral weeks (Sandoval et al. 2003). MRI findings are frequently multifocal and do not fit vascular distribution patterns. These MRI changes can also be seen in asymptomatic patients receiving methotrexate. Therefore, more extensive investi-gation to rule out other causes of seizure or AMS is often necessary.

As mentioned, the majority of cases of metho-trexate neurotoxicity are self-resolving. There are varying amounts of preclinical data and published case series that support the use of aminophylline or dextromethorphan in the acute phase and leucovorin rescue with future IT methotrexate in patients who have developed neurotoxicity in the past (Winick et al. 1992; Drachtman et al. 2002; Inaba et al. 2008). Aminophylline can be considered for patients who have acute obtundation after methotrexate. If toxicity is thought secondary to IT therapy, one can consider postponing the next scheduled IT methotrexate or substituting IT Ara-C and hydrocortisone, though there are very limited data to show this is an effective IT therapy in ALL. Patients can be safely rechallenged with IT methotrexate, either with or without leucovorin or aminophylline rescue, and not redevelop neurotoxicity (Rollins et al. 2004; Inaba et al. 2008). Thus, completely eliminating methotrexate from future therapy is not usually indicated.

Ifosfamide

Patients receiving ifosfamide may develop encephalopathy that can range from sleepiness and confusion to seizures or coma, starting several hours after infusion commencement. The reported frequency of this side effect is as high as 22 % in pediatric patients (Pratt et al. 1986). Although there is no clear dose-dependence, studies have suggested that hypoalbuminemia and renal dysfunction are risk factors (David and Picus 2005). The exact mechanism for ifosfamide-induced encephalopathy (IIE) is unclear although it is thought secondary to high levels of urine glutaric acid which is linked to one particular metabolite of ifosfamide, chloroethylamine (Kupfer et al. 1994). Methylene blue has been reported to successfully treat IIE and may also be effective as prophylaxis through unclear mechanisms, possibly by correcting derangement in mitochondrial flavoproteins (Pelgrims et al. 2000; Hamadani and Awan 2006). A review by Patel (2006) found that a lack of controlled evidence makes the effectiveness of methylene blue unclear. Thiamine has also been reported to be an effective treatment and prophylaxis for IIE through unclear mechanisms and also with a lack of controlled data (Hamadani and Awan 2006).

Cytarabine

The pyrimidine analog cytarabine is frequently used in the treatment of pediatric leukemia and lymphoma. There is a wide range of employed dosages and at lower doses neurologic toxicity is uncommon. Higher doses, however, are associated with an acute cerebellar syndrome in ≥ 10 % of patients (Baker et al. 1991). There is a clear dose-dependence of this side effect and it is generally seen at doses ≥ 3 g/m^2/day; spacing administration from twice daily to once daily has been shown to reduce the incidence of cerebellar toxicity (Smith et al. 1997).

The clinical manifestations of cytarabine-induced cerebellar toxicity include the classic cerebellar signs of dysarthria, dysdiadochokinesia and ataxia (Smith et al. 1997). Cerebral dysfunction can also be seen in a subset of cases, with manifestations including encephalopathy, seizures and coma. Histopathologic changes seen in the cerebellar syndrome include loss of Purkinje cells in the cerebellar hemispheres and vermis along with a proliferation of glial cells known as Bergmann's gliosis (Baker et al. 1991).

Symptoms often resolve following discontinuation of cytarabine; however some patients will have permanent neurologic damage. One large case series of adults and children receiving high-dose cytarabine found that approximately 1 % of patients who developed severe cerebellar symptoms had an irreversible or fatal course (Herzig et al. 1987). Although this same report demonstrated that some patients may be rechallenged without permanent neurologic damage, the decision to proceed with additional cytarabine is a difficult one. Identified risk factors for cerebellar syndrome include dose and timing as discussed above as well as hepatic or renal insufficiency and older age (Herzig et al. 1987; Baker et al. 1991; Rubin et al. 1992). No potential genetic modifiers have been reported in the literature.

IT cytarabine can be administered in its standard formulation or as a slow-release liposomal formulation (DepoCyt). The liposomal formulation appears to have a higher incidence of arachnoiditis; prophylactic corticosteroids may be beneficial in this situation (Glantz et al. 1999). As discussed, concomitant administration of IT and high-dose IV cytarabine is associated with the development of transverse myelitis presenting as bowel and bladder dysfunction with lower extremity weakness and should be avoided (Dunton et al. 1986; Schwenn et al. 1991).

5.3.3.5 Posterior Reversible Encephalopathy Syndrome

Posterior reversible encephalopathy syndrome (PRES, also called RPLS, reversible posterior leukoencephalopathy syndrome) was first described as a syndrome of encephalopathy accompanied by transient subcortical white matter changes on T2-weighted MRI (Hinchey et al. 1996). The clinical manifestations of PRES include headaches, seizures, AMS and cortical blindness. Hypertension is a clear antecedent and most significant risk factor in the development of PRES. Hypertension may be secondary to medications, such as corticosteroids, or concurrent medical conditions such as renal failure from tumor lysis syndrome (Greenwood et al. 2003). Retrospective studies also suggest a higher incidence of PRES during induction chemotherapy, independent of tumor lysis syndrome or hyperleukocytosis (Norman et al. 2007).

Since its initial description, PRES has been recognized to not be limited to the posterior circulation of the brain nor to white matter exclusively nor be fully reversible in all cases (Lucchini et al. 2008). While the initial report postulated a role for immunosuppression in the pathogenesis of PRES, it has been subsequently described in non-immunocompromised patients such as in pregnancy-induced hypertension. Specific immunosuppressive medications, such as tacrolimus and cyclosporine, continue to be implicated in case reports in part due to their effect on blood pressure.

PRES has been noted in pediatric malignancies including ALL, AML, non-Hodgkin lymphoma, and solid tumors including neuroblastoma, osteosarcoma, and Ewing sarcoma. Hypertension was a clearly identified preceding event in the majority of cases. Seizures were the most common clinical manifestation, with AMS, headache and some form of visual disturbance occurring in 30–40 % of cases (de Laat et al. 2011). While the majority of patients had a reversible course, 12 % had persistent neurologic symptoms.

Brain MRI is required to make the diagnosis of PRES. Vasogenic edema most often symmetrically affects the parietal and occipital subcortical white matter. Cortex, basal ganglia, and posterior fossa structures such as cerebellum and brainstem can also be involved.

Treatment of PRES begins with aborting seizures, if present, and decreasing the patient's blood pressure using calcium channel blockers such as nifedipine or ß-blockers such as labetalol. Ongoing antiepileptic therapy is often warranted in the acute setting. While many studies suggest that AEDs may be tapered when neuroimaging normalizes, multiple retrospective reviews of pediatric oncology patients with PRES have found high rates of ongoing epilepsy (Morris et al. 2007; de Laat et al. 2011). Chemotherapy is often held while the patient is symptomatic and there are multiple reports of safe resumption of antineoplastic therapy, including any possible offending agents, with no recurrence of symptoms (Morris et al. 2007; Norman et al. 2007; de Laat et al. 2011).

5.3.4 Outcomes

While many of the described causes of seizures are temporary, some patients with childhood cancer will require long-term prophylactic AEDs. Data from the Childhood Cancer Survivor Study showed that 6 % of childhood ALL survivors were identified as having a seizure disorder with at least half developing this as a late effect of therapy (Goldsby et al. 2010). The choice of prophylactic AED is made based on seizure etiology and response to therapy, but drug-drug interactions with chemotherapeutics is an important consideration as well.

In a retrospective study of ALL patients, treatment with phenytoin, phenobarbital or carbamazepine for at least 1 month duration was associated with an increased risk of relapse in patients with B cell, though not T cell, ALL (Relling et al. 2000). The investigators showed that the use of these enzyme-inducing antiepileptic medications led to increased clearance of some chemotherapeutic agents.

Levetiracetam is an AED that is not metabolized through the CYP450 system, making it a safer choice for prolonged therapy. Although considered efficacious without affecting relapse risk, studies in pediatric ALL are minimal (Ruggiero et al. 2010). Regardless of the choice of agent, the practitioner should be aware of the high potential for altered drug metabolism in patients receiving cytochrome P450-inducing or P450-inhibiting AEDs.

5.4   Increased Intracranial Pressure

Increased ICP is due to an increase in the volume of one of three constituents of the intracranial space: blood, CSF or soft tissue. In infants whose fontanels are still open there is a greater capacity for an increase in any one of these compartments prior to the development of symptoms.

Intracranial hypertension can lead to a loss of cerebral perfusion pressure (CPP), defined as the mean arterial pressure less the intracranial pressure (CPP=MAP–ICP). Insufficient CPP will produce secondary ischemia due to a lack of forward blood flow. Even more concerning, intracranial hypertension can lead to herniation syndromes wherein brain parenchyma is pushed downward below the tentorium cerebelli, through the foramen magnum, or transversely across the falx cerebri, in all cases leading to potentially irreversible neurologic damage or death. Early diagnosis, stabilization and institution of therapy appropriate to the cause of increased ICP are essential in preventing these outcomes.

5.4.1   Presentation

Headache is one of the most common, and unfortunately least specific, features that can herald increased ICP. In a retrospective review of 315 pediatric patients with headache who had neuroimaging, headache awakening the patient from sleep and a negative family history for migraine were the strongest individual predictors of a mass lesion (Medina et al. 1997). Confusion and abnormal neurologic examination were also risk factors in that study. Vomiting is another common presenting sign; this is classically worst in the morning, due to increasing ICP while sleeping in the supine position relative to standing. Rapidly increasing ICP may present with a short interval of headache or constitutional symptoms that precedes coma or death due to pressure on the reticular activating system in the midbrain.

In infants, irritability may be the only presenting symptom. Physical examination may reveal a wide, tense fontanel with split sutures. Measuring head circumference should be a standard part of the neurologic examination in an infant, and discordance between circumference and weight or length should prompt closer investigation. Sundowning, a downward gaze preference at rest, may also be seen.

Focal neurologic features of increased ICP depend on the location of the mass or the progression of any herniation. Optic nerve swelling in response to intracranial hypertension can lead to papilledema. However, papilledema may not develop for weeks after the onset of increased ICP and therefore a normal fundoscopic exam does not rule out intracranial hypertension. Cranial nerves III, IV and VI can also be affected leading to paralysis of gaze or complaints of diplopia. Ipsilateral mydriasis with poor pupillary response to light can be seen due to the effect of increased ICP on CN III or from direct impingement in uncal herniation. Finally, a localized mass or ischemia from decreased CPP can lead to focal deficits of strength or sensation. Cushing's triad, the combination of hypertension, bradycardia, and an irregular respiratory pattern, is a late manifestation of increased ICP and an ominous sign of impending herniation.

5.4.2   Initial Management

The patient with suspected increased ICP should have their airway, breathing and circulation secured before proceeding with diagnostic evaluation. A normal arterial partial pressure of carbon dioxide (P_aCO_2) will prevent hypercapnea-induced vasodilation with subsequent spikes in ICP; intubation should be instituted in the patient with hypoxia, hypoventilation, excessive sedation or loss of protective airway reflexes. Hypotension will lead to a drop in CPP with attendant ischemia and should be treated with normal saline infusion to attain euvolemia. Additional measures to decrease ICP such as elevating the head of the bed and keeping the patient's head at midline should be commenced emergently. Hyperthermia should be treated with antipyretics or cooling measures to decrease metabolic demand. Pain should be aggressively treated to prevent spikes in blood pressure or ICP.

Patients who are stabilized with these measures should undergo emergent head imaging. A noncontrast head CT or rapid-sequence MRI can quickly identify a new mass lesion, obstructive hydrocephalus, or hemorrhage. Negative head imaging should prompt further workup. MR angiography and venography can be helpful in finding occult thrombosis. Mass lesions may warrant MRI for further evaluation prior to operative intervention. A lumbar puncture should not be performed without confirmatory negative head imaging to rule out the risk of downward herniation with CSF release. Opening pressure should ideally be measured with the patient's legs extended or with the patient in the sitting position. Although there are not clear guidelines for normal ICP in children, values >20 mmHg are considered elevated in adults.

Patients who have progressively worsening neurologic exams or clear signs of herniation on physical examination or imaging require more aggressive interventions. Hyperosmolar therapy with mannitol or hypertonic saline can be used to decrease the total brain water content. Mannitol is started at doses of 0.25–1 g/kg of a 20 % solution and repeated every 6 h until serum osmolarity is raised to between 300 and 320 mOsm/L (Pitfield et al. 2012). Hypertonic saline has the advantage of not causing osmotic diuresis so may be preferred in the hypovolemic patient (Khanna et al. 2000). Additional treatment measures will generally be tailored to the underlying etiology.

5.4.3 Differential Diagnosis

5.4.3.1 Soft Tissue

A large meta-analysis of published data suggests that signs of increased ICP such as headache and vomiting are the most common presenting features in patients with newly diagnosed brain tumors, whether located supratentorially or in the posterior fossa (Wilne et al. 2007). In the patient with a known CNS lesion, development of new symptoms of increased ICP should raise concern for tumor progression leading to obstructive hydrocephalus. While corticosteroids are not standard therapy for increased ICP, the vasogenic edema associated with a mass lesion can be reduced with dexamethasone and should be considered in patients with primary brain lesions causing increased ICP (Andersen and Jensen 1998). Additional treatment may include surgical resection with or without placement of a ventriculoperitoneal shunt (VPS). For patients with unresectable disease, either due to multifocality or other comorbidities, radiation therapy or stereotactic radiosurgery can be considered.

5.4.3.2 Cerebrospinal Fluid

Hydrocephalus is an excess of CSF within the skull. Increased production of CSF is relatively rare, but can be seen in patients with choroid plexus papilloma (Eisenberg et al. 1974). More commonly, drainage of CSF is obstructed due to mass effect on the ventricular system. Cranial venous drainage can also be impeded by obstruction of the great vessels in superior vena cava syndrome, which is discussed in detail in Chap. 4. CNS tumors arising from the third and fourth ventricles can easily block the flow of CSF and produce symptoms of obstructive hydrocephalus (Fig. 5.3). An external ventricular drain (EVD) may help relieve the pressure from such an obstruction in the short term, allowing for attempted total resection in a more controlled fashion. Unfortunately, up to one-third of patients with posterior fossa masses will develop postoperative hydrocephalus requiring long-term shunting (Culley et al. 1994). Based on this statistic, some neurosurgeons

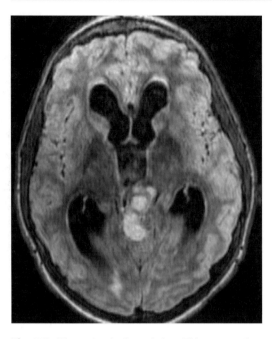

Fig. 5.3 Obstructive hydrocephalus. This teenage boy presented with a gradual history of headaches, ataxia and progressively worsening vomiting. T2-weighted MRI taken at the time of his presentation to medical care demonstrates a cystic mass arising in the posterior fossa. The lateral ventricles and third ventricle, seen with dark CSF on this sequence, are massively dilated in this example of obstructive hydrocephalus. Pathology after gross total resection was consistent with low-grade glioma

will opt for preemptive VPS placement. A recent retrospective review of children with posterior fossa masses identified several risk factors to predict the need for a VPS: age <2 years, papilledema, severity of preoperative hydrocephalus and cerebral metastases (Riva-Cambrin et al. 2009).

Malignant leptomeningeal involvement, as seen in leukemia as well as primary CNS tumors such as medulloblastoma, can occasionally be severe enough to block resorption of CSF through the arachnoid granulations. This condition can be treated by VPS placement while systemic therapy is instituted though the shunt may become clogged by extensive cellular material.

Finally, malfunction or infection of a previously placed VPS is an important diagnostic consideration. Diagnosis via VPS tapping and need for externalization or revision should be established based on neurosurgical consultation.

5.4.3.3 Hemorrhage and Thrombosis

An excess of blood in the cranial vault can be caused by hemorrhage (e.g., within the tumor or tumor bed) or by thrombosis with poor venous drainage. Thrombosis is a well-described complication of asparaginase therapy in ALL. L-asparaginase has been shown to decrease levels of antithrombin and plasminogen leading to a prothrombotic state (Leone et al. 1993). Simultaneous depletion of fibrinogen can also predispose to hemorrhage. Thrombosis in childhood ALL patients is not uncommon; one meta-analysis reported a prevalence of 3.2 %, with roughly half of the events CNS thromboembolic events, and the majority of those sinovenous thromboses (Athale and Chan 2003).

Sinovenous thrombosis should be treated with anticoagulation to prevent clot extension. Repletion of antithrombin using pooled human concentrate (Thrombate) or recombinant antithrombin (ATryn) is required to achieve therapeutic anticoagulation with either unfractionated or low molecular weight heparin. In addition, cryoprecipitate can be used to replete fibrinogen up to normal levels (i.e., >150 mg/dL), treating ongoing coagulopathy and decreasing the risk of bleeding. Fresh frozen plasma can be used in lieu of these products, but has limited amounts of antithrombin and fibrinogen, which are the most consistently decreased in studies of asparaginase therapy. Minor hemorrhages seen in association with sinovenous thrombosis may make the decision to anticoagulate more difficult, but the use of a reversible agent (unfractionated heparin), frequent monitoring of hemostatic parameters, and careful neurologic monitoring in an intensive care unit can decrease the risks associated with this strategy. Without treatment, sinovenous thrombosis can progress to infarction with worsened hemorrhagic complications.

In the event of anaphylaxis to *E. coli* asparaginase, *Erwinia* asparaginase is often substituted as an alternative therapy. Giving equivalent doses, a European trial did find a reduced incidence of coagulation abnormalities with *Erwinia* asparaginase compared to *E. coli*, though the frequency of thrombotic events was not reported (Duval et al. 2002). The same study was stopped early, however, due to superior survival in the *E. coli* asparaginase arm, and so routine substitution of *Erwinia* asparaginase for concerns of thrombosis is not recommended. The frequency of thrombotic events appears to be similar in patients treated with the longer-acting PEG-asparaginase as compared to those treated with L-asparaginase (Silverman et al. 2010).

The decision to restart asparaginase following sinovenous thrombosis is a complex one; limited data suggest that asparaginase can be safely restarted (Grace et al. 2011). The recurrence risk was higher in adults, consistent with the observation that the overall risk of venous thromboembolism increases from puberty throughout adulthood (White 2003).

Prophylaxis with purified antithrombin is not recommended in pediatric oncology (Mattioli Belmonte et al. 1991). The PARKAA (Prophylactic Antithrombin Replacement in Kids with Acute Lymphoblastic Leukemia Treated with Asparaginase) study, a randomized trial comparing prophylactic antithrombin repletion to observation, found a nonstatistical trend towards fewer thromboses in the prophylaxis group but lacked power to make conclusive recommendations (Mitchell et al. 2003).

5.4.3.4 Idiopathic Intracranial Hypertension

Idiopathic intracranial hypertension (IIH), previously termed pseudotumor cerebri, is a poorly understood syndrome characterized by elevated ICP without any obvious structural cause. Several chemotherapeutic agents can predispose the pediatric oncology patient to IIH. Corticosteroids, and specifically their withdrawal, have been associated with the development of IIH in children (Neville and Wilson 1970). IIH is also a commonly reported side effect of treatment with vitamin A analogs, including all-trans retinoic acid (ATRA) in the treatment of acute promyelocytic leukemia and isotretinoin and fenretinide in the treatment of neuroblastoma (Bigby and Stern 1988; Smith et al. 1992; Children's Oncology Group [CCG 09709] et al. 2006).

Treatment of IIH can include serial large-volume CSF drainage through lumbar punctures

or the use of acetazolamide. In cases of ATRA-related IIH, ATRA is often held with additional supportive steps to help alleviate symptoms (Holmes et al. 2012). Rechallenge with ATRA can be attempted if symptoms subside. The most severe complication of IIH is visual loss due to optic nerve ischemia; patients should therefore have routine ophthalmologic follow-up. Occasionally IIH is severe enough to require surgical CSF shunting to prevent further optic nerve damage (Chern et al. 2012).

5.5 Cerebrovascular Disease in Pediatric Cancer Patients

Cerebrovascular disease is one of the most devastating disorders and can present as either cerebrovascular accident (CVA, also referred to as stroke) or cerebrovascular malformations such as aneurysms. For the pediatric oncology patient, we will focus on stroke as the manifestation of cerebrovascular disease. Stroke is a disabling consequence of childhood cancer—and childhood cancer treatment—that remains poorly understood. Stroke can occur in the perioperative setting or may be treatment related and is broadly classified as hemorrhagic or ischemic. Ischemic stroke, which represents about 55 % of pediatric CVA, is further subdivided into large and small vessel stroke.

Stroke is generally defined as the abrupt onset of focal neurologic deficits referable to a vascular distribution and lasting >24 h. In children, especially the very young, stroke can also present as AMS or seizures (Zimmer et al. 2007; Hartman et al. 2009; Beslow et al. 2010). A recent retrospective analysis reported that children <1 year of age ($n = 11$) commonly presented with AMS or seizures, whereas older children ($n = 65$) commonly presented with focal weakness in ischemic stroke (Abend et al. 2011). Neurologic deficits that last <24 h are generally classified as a transient ischemic attack (TIA). Thus, the diagnosis of stroke is made based on the patient's clinical presentation with laboratory studies and brain imaging as diagnostic correlates. Silent strokes seen on imaging alone are referred to as infarcts.

Cerebral ischemia is caused by a reduction in blood flow to the brain. Clinical symptoms occur within seconds to minutes due to the lack of glycogen storage in neurons, leading to energy failure. If blood flow is not restored quickly, infarction or death of brain tissue occurs. A generalized reduction in blood flow due to hypotension usually produces syncope. If the blood flow is not restored quickly, infarction between the border zones of major cerebral artery distribution occurs, referred to as a "watershed infarct," presenting with proximal arm and leg weakness. Focal ischemia is often due to thrombosis of cerebral vessels or by emboli from other sources (e.g., the heart). Hemorrhagic stroke causes symptoms due to mass effect on surrounding brain structures and by direct toxic effect of blood. Pediatric stroke research has mainly focused on ischemic stroke, and therefore our knowledge of pediatric hemorrhagic stroke remains limited (Zimmer et al. 2007). In cases where bleeding occurs within a brain lesion (such as a primary brain tumor), pediatric oncologists often refer to this as intratumoral bleeding rather than hemorrhagic stroke. Here, for consistency, intratumoral hemorrhage is included within the category of hemorrhagic stroke.

5.5.1 Presentation of Stroke in Pediatric Patients

The clinical presentation of a CVA depends on the territory of brain involved. Table 5.3 lists key clinical findings based on the vascular territory, mainly attributable to ischemic stroke. In young children focal neurological deficits can be more subtle and harder to elicit.

Hemorrhagic stroke in children, especially the very young, often presents with nonspecific signs and symptoms such as AMS or seizures; headache is often reported in older children. One study assessed the clinical presentation of 51 children ≥6 years of age and found that 73 % presented with headache, 57 % with AMS, 39 % with focal neurological signs, 33 % with nausea/vomiting, and 16 % with seizures or other symptoms such as dysphasia and abnormal gait (Lo 2011).

Table 5.3 Symptoms of cerebrovascular accident by vascular territory

	Artery	Key signs and symptoms
Anterior circulation	Middle cerebral artery	Contralateral hemiplegia
		Contralateral hemianesthesia
		Contralateral homonymous hemianopia
		If dominant hemisphere:
		Global aphasia
		If nondominant hemisphere:
		Neglect
		Anosognosia[a]
		Constructional apraxia[b]
	Anterior cerebral artery	Contralateral paralysis of foot and leg
		Contralateral sensory loss of leg and toes
		Urinary incontinence
		Abulia[c]
		Gait apraxia
Posterior circulation	Posterior cerebral artery	Contralateral homonymous hemianopia with macular sparing
		If thalamus and internal capsule involved: contralateral hemisensory loss and hemiparesis
		Visual and color agnosias
		Prosopagnosia[d]
		Claude's syndrome (3rd nerve palsy with contralateral ataxia)
		Weber's syndrome (3rd nerve palsy with contralateral hemiplegia)
	Basilar artery	Bilateral long tract signs (sensory and motor)
		Cranial nerve dysfunctions
		Cerebellar dysfunction

[a]Anosognosia: Unawareness of neurologic deficit
[b]Construction apraxia: Inability to copy simple line drawings
[c]Abulia: Akinetic mutism
[d]Prosopagnosia: Impairment in facial recognition

5.5.2 Differential Diagnosis of Stroke

In the child with acute onset of new neurologic symptoms, the initial differential diagnosis is broad and includes limited focal movement secondary to pain, Todd's paralysis after seizure, complex migraines, intoxication presenting as AMS or ataxia, medication side effects, and peripheral nerve injuries, among others. Despite increasing stroke awareness in the adult population, the diagnosis of stroke in children continues to be significantly delayed (McGlennan and Ganesan 2008; Rafay et al. 2009; Srinivasan et al. 2009). A recent report of children suffering from arterial ischemic stroke documented a median time >24 h between clinical onset and imaging confirmation.

5.5.3 Etiology of Stroke in Pediatric Cancer Patients

The underlying etiology of stroke in pediatric cancer patients is complex and poorly studied. In about 30 % of children presenting with an acute ischemic stroke, no cause could be elucidated despite extensive investigations (Roach 2000). No long-term, prospective study is available to better define the risk and underlying mechanisms of stroke in pediatric cancer patients. Current studies lack rigorous imaging correlates of stroke symptoms and are often based on self-reports from patients or their caregivers.

Stroke can occur during neurosurgery in pediatric intracranial tumors with close proximity of tumor and intracranial vessels. Further, several chemotherapeutic agents have been associated with increased risk of stroke such as mentioned with asparaginase and notably with the monoclonal antibody bevacizumab, which is directed against vascular endothelial growth factor receptor (VEGFR). In adult patients bevacizumab has been associated with a small but significant increase in arterial thrombotic events as well as risk for intracerebral hemorrhage (Taugourdeau-Raymond et al. 2012). The incidence of bevacizumab-associated cerebral hemorrhage in children is unknown.

Previous studies have shown that children treated for CNS tumors, leukemia, Hodgkin lymphoma, and other cancers carry a significantly increased stroke risk (Fig. 5.4), with cranial radiation therapy (CRT) a particularly strong risk factor (Bowers et al. 2005, 2006; Haddy et al. 2011). How CRT increases stroke risk in cancer survivors is not well understood. Few risk factors for stroke and arteriopathy in children treated with

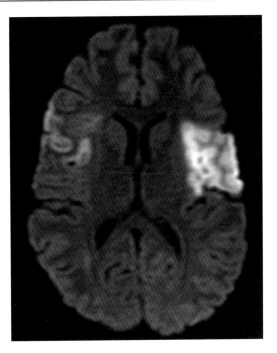

Fig. 5.4 Ischemic stroke. This 19-year-old young woman, whose MRI is shown in this figure, presented with acute dysarthria and right-handed sensory changes. The diffusion-weighted images shown here demonstrate bilateral strokes with restricted diffusion, which appear bright in this sequence. The patient had a history of Hodgkin lymphoma diagnosed 4 years prior which had relapsed and subsequently treated with an autologous and then allogeneic hematopoietic stem cell transplant. Although the patient did have irradiation as part of her therapy, no arteriopathy could be detected on magnetic resonance angiography to explain the origin of her stroke

CRT have been described and include optic pathway tumors associated with NF-1, younger age and higher radiation dose to the circle of Willis (Grill et al. 1999). Current literature has focused on arteriopathies that develop within a relative short time following CRT (Bitzer and Topka 1995; Laitt et al. 1995; Omura et al. 1997; Grill et al. 1999; Fouladi et al. 2000). Moyamoya, a specific type of cerebral arteriopathy characterized by progressive stenosis of the terminal internal carotid arteries, has been shown more prevalent in children who undergo CRT for ALL and brain tumors as compared to children who do not receive CRT (Kikuchi et al. 2007; Ullrich et al. 2007). Others have shown that children treated with CRT are at increased risk for lacunar strokes, thought secondary to small vessel vasculopathy (Fouladi et al. 2000).

There is an additional body of literature that raises concern for long-term effects of radiation therapy by accelerating atherosclerosis, the most common etiology of stroke in adults (Dorresteijn et al. 2005). In pediatric and adult cancer patients, neck irradiation increased cervical carotid artery wall thickness, a marker for atherosclerosis (O'Leary et al. 1999; Hollander et al. 2002; Dorresteijn et al. 2005; Meeske et al. 2009). In a retrospective cohort study of 367 adult patients with head and neck tumors, neck irradiation increased risk of carotid artery-related strokes by almost tenfold compared to normal adults, and that risk was enhanced by hypertension (Dorresteijn et al. 2002). In animal models, irradiation of hypercholesterolemic mice and rabbits leads to accelerated atherosclerotic plaque formation (Vos et al. 1983). Hence, it is plausible that CRT leads to accelerated intracranial atherosclerosis and thereby increases long-term stroke risk as childhood cancer survivors become young adults.

5.5.4 Management of Acute Stroke

In the child with acute neurologic deficits, the initial evaluation should include a detailed neurologic examination to localize the site of stroke as well as careful review of the prior history and current medications. Brain imaging studies should be performed at the time of presentation if the onset of symptoms is acute. The type of imaging used will depend on availability and on the age of the child. MRI is preferred over CT given the radiation exposure associated with CT as well as the differences in time delay and resolution. CT will reliably identify hemorrhage as the cause of stroke but may fail to show ischemic stroke if the images are obtained within the first hours of presentation, if the stroke is small, and especially if located within the posterior fossa, due to bone artifact. MRI will detect hemorrhage and small strokes even in the early hours after onset of symptoms. MR angiography can identify stenosis of large intracranial vessels as well as arterial dissection. Transcranial Doppler

(TCD) is another method to noninvasively assess and follow narrowing of intracranial vessels. Additional imaging with conventional angiography might be indicated depending on severity. Children with stroke should be treated by a specialized team including a pediatric stroke specialist, a pediatric neurosurgeon, an interventional radiologist and a rehabilitation team to ensure the best possible outcome.

5.5.4.1 Ischemic Stroke

After an ischemic stroke is diagnosed, the patient should be monitored and treated in a pediatric intensive care unit. Treatment is mainly supportive. Similar to hemorrhagic stroke, the first steps are to stabilize the child and assess the airway, breathing and circulation. Permissive hypertension is indicated to assure collateral flow to the area of ischemia and minimize injury. Fever is detrimental and children should be treated with antipyretics to achieve normothermia. Glucose levels should be carefully monitored and normalized as needed. Intravenous recombinant tissue plasminogen activator (tPA) is used in the acute setting in patients ≥ 18 years of age within the first 4.5 h after onset of symptoms if no contraindications to tPA are present. There is limited understanding of the safety and efficacy of tPA in pediatric patients, and therefore it is not yet the standard of care in this patient population. The Thrombolysis in Pediatric Stroke Study (TIPS) is a multicenter trial with the goal to assess the safety and efficacy of tPA in children with ischemic stroke; results from this study are pending (Amlie-Lefond et al. 2009). To assess the underlying etiology of ischemic stroke, children often have vascular imaging performed, particularly MR angiography. The necessity of assessment of an underlying prothrombotic state in pediatric stroke is unclear, and testing has not been shown useful in improving clinical outcomes (Raffini 2008). For all pediatric stroke cases, the reported prevalence of prothrombotic conditions ranges from 20–50 % (Mackay and Monagle 2008). Assessment of the most common thrombophilias including antithrombin deficiency, protein C or protein S deficiency, hyperhomocysteinemia, prothrombin 20210 gene mutation, elevated

FVIII, factor V Leiden mutation, elevated lipoprotein(a) and antiphospholipid antibodies can be considered (Raffini 2008; Roach et al. 2008). Pregnancy should be excluded in teenage girls presenting with stroke and discontinuation of estrogen-containing contraceptives should be considered (Roach et al. 2008).

Prior studies have shown that the risk of stroke recurrence in children with an underlying arteriopathy is high and therefore these children should be prophylaxed with either antiplatelet agents or anticoagulation (Fullerton et al. 2007). However, systematic studies of secondary stroke prevention in children with arteriopathies, including children with irradiation-induced vasculopathies, are not available in the literature. A special writing group of the American Heart Association Council and the Council on Cardiovascular Disease in the Young has issued consensus guidelines for management of infants and children with stroke (Roach et al 2008). These guidelines outline specific treatment recommendations for children with an ischemic stroke based on the underlying condition including Moyamoya syndrome which can be associated with CRT in pediatric cancer patients.

5.5.4.2 Hemorrhagic Stroke

Hematomas can expand over several hours from initial presentation and monitoring in the pediatric intensive care unit is indicated. The initial management of the child with hemorrhagic stroke should include assessment of the airway, breathing and circulation. Blood pressure management is directed towards normal blood pressure values for age. Children are at risk to develop hydrocephalus and placement of an EVD may be required. A Camino® bolt can be used to monitor ICP if no hydrocephalus is present. Awake patients can be monitored with serial examinations, whereas children with depressed level of consciousness will benefit from invasive ICP monitoring to maintain adequate CPP. The use of recombinant factor VII (rFVIIa) to halt hemorrhage in pediatric patients is still under investigation and currently not considered standard therapy (McQuilten et al. 2012). Pediatric neurosurgery should be consulted immediately for cerebellar hemorrhage, as evacuation is often indicated. Patients with thrombocytopenia should be treated with platelet transfusions to maintain a platelet count $\geq 100 \times 10^9$/L. The role of routine seizure prophylaxis in the absence of seizures is unclear. Adult patients with hemorrhagic strokes who were treated with prophylactic AEDs had worse outcome than those who were just monitored (Messe et al. 2009). Currently there are no data available for children. A special writing group of the American Heart Association Council and the Council on Cardiovascular Disease in the Young has issued consensus guidelines for management of infants and children with stroke; potential relevant recommendations in pediatric nontraumatic hemorrhagic stroke include utilization of cerebral angiography if MR angiography is nondiagnostic, adequate factor replacement in children with coagulopathy, and optimization of respiratory effort, control of hypertension, control of seizures, and management of ICP to help stabilize the patient (Roach et al. 2008).

5.5.5 Outcome of Acute Stroke

Currently there are no reported data that address the outcome of pediatric cancer patients after stroke. However, stroke is an important cause of disability in the general pediatric population. After stroke, children suffer from motor and sensory deficits, cognitive decline and epilepsy. Outcome research in pediatric stroke has been hampered by the lack of validated and standardized outcome measures (Engelmann and Jordan 2012). Recently the Pediatric Stroke Outcome Measure (PSOM) was published with a reported inter-rater variability of 0.93 (95 % CI 0.76–0.98) (Kitchen et al. 2012). Development and systematic use of such validated assessments will be important to fully understand the impact of stroke on pediatric patient as well as assess efficacy of current treatment modalities.

5.6 Summary

The diversity of neurologic complications in pediatric oncology, and the frequency with which they occur, demand a careful awareness on the part of physicians caring for these patients. The approaches described above highlight the unique effects of cancer and cancer treatment on the nervous system as well as the lack of evidence basis for much of the current standards of care.

References

Abend NS, Beslow LA, Smith SE et al (2011) Seizures as a presenting symptom of acute arterial ischemic stroke in childhood. J Pediatr 159:479–483

Acquaviva A, Marconcini S, Municchi G et al (2003) Non-Hodgkin lymphoma in a child presenting with acute paraplegia: a case report. Pediatr Hematol Oncol 20:245–251

Adrogue HJ, Madias NE (2000) Hyponatremia. N Engl J Med 342:1581–1589

Amlie-Lefond C, Chan AK, Kirton A et al (2009) Thrombolysis in acute childhood stroke: design and challenges of the thrombolysis in pediatric stroke clinical trial. Neuroepidemiology 32:279–286

Andersen C, Jensen FT (1998) Differences in blood-tumour-barrier leakage of human intracranial tumours: quantitative monitoring of vasogenic oedema and its response to glucocorticoid treatment. Acta Neurochir (Wien) 140:919–924

Angelini P, Plantaz D, De Bernardi B et al (2011) Late sequelae of symptomatic epidural compression in children with localized neuroblastoma. Pediatr Blood Cancer 57:473–480

Athale UH, Chan AK (2003) Thrombosis in children with acute lymphoblastic leukemia: part I. Epidemiology of thrombosis in children with acute lymphoblastic leukemia. Thromb Res 111:125–131

Baker WJ, Royer GL Jr, Weiss RB (1991) Cytarabine and neurologic toxicity. J Clin Oncol 9:679–693

Benesch M, Weber-Mzell D, Gerber NU et al (2010) Ependymoma of the spinal cord in children and adolescents: a retrospective series from the HIT database. J Neurosurg Pediatr 6:137–144

Bertsch H, Rudoler S, Needle MN et al (1998) Emergent/urgent therapeutic irradiation in pediatric oncology: patterns of presentation, treatment, and outcome. Med Pediatr Oncol 30:101–105

Beslow LA, Licht DJ, Smith SE et al (2010) Predictors of outcome in childhood intracerebral hemorrhage: a prospective consecutive cohort study. Stroke 41:313–318

Bigby M, Stern RS (1988) Adverse reactions to isotretinoin. A report from the Adverse Drug Reaction Reporting System. J Am Acad Dermatol 18:543–552

Bitzer M, Topka H (1995) Progressive cerebral occlusive disease after radiation therapy. Stroke 26:131–136

Bowers DC, McNeil DE, Liu Y et al (2005) Stroke as a late treatment effect of Hodgkin's Disease: a report from the Childhood Cancer Survivor Study. J Clin Oncol 23:6508–6515

Bowers DC, Liu Y, Leisenring W et al (2006) Late-occurring stroke among long-term survivors of childhood leukemia and brain tumors: a report from the Childhood Cancer Survivor Study. J Clin Oncol 24:5277–5282

Chern JJ, Tubbs RS, Gordon AS et al (2012) Management of pediatric patients with pseudotumor cerebri. Childs Nerv Syst 28:575–578

Children's Oncology Group (CCG 09709), Villablanca JG, Krailo MD et al (2006) Phase I trial of oral fenretinide in children with high-risk solid tumors: a report from the Children's Oncology Group (CCG 09709). J Clin Oncol 24:3423–3430

Culley DJ, Berger MS, Shaw D et al (1994) An analysis of factors determining the need for ventriculoperitoneal shunts after posterior fossa tumor surgery in children. Neurosurgery 34:402407; discussion 407–408

Daley MF, Partington MD, Kadan-Lottick N et al (2003) Primary epidural burkitt lymphoma in a child: case presentation and literature review. Pediatr Hematol Oncol 20:333–338

David KA, Picus J (2005) Evaluating risk factors for the development of ifosfamide encephalopathy. Am J Clin Oncol 28:277–280

De Bernardi B, Pianca C, Pistamiglio P et al (2001) Neuroblastoma with symptomatic spinal cord compression at diagnosis: treatment and results with 76 cases. J Clin Oncol 19:183–190

de Laat P, Te Winkel ML, Devos AS et al (2011) Posterior reversible encephalopathy syndrome in childhood cancer. Ann Oncol 22:472–478

Dorresteijn LD, Kappelle AC, Boogerd W et al (2002) Increased risk of ischemic stroke after radiotherapy on the neck in patients younger than 60 years. J Clin Oncol 20:282–288

Dorresteijn LD, Kappelle AC, Scholz NM et al (2005) Increased carotid wall thickening after radiotherapy on the neck. Eur J Cancer 41:1026–1030

Drachtman RA, Cole PD, Golden CB et al (2002) Dextromethorphan is effective in the treatment of subacute methotrexate neurotoxicity. Pediatr Hematol Oncol 19:319–327

Dufour MN, Landman-Parker J, Auclerc MF et al (2007) Age and high-dose methotrexate are associated to clinical acute encephalopathy in FRALLE 93 trial for acute lymphoblastic leukemia in children. Leukemia 21:238–247

Dunton SF, Nitschke R, Spruce WE et al (1986) Progressive ascending paralysis following administration of intrathecal and intravenous cytosine arabinoside. A Pediatric Oncology Group study. Cancer 57:1083–1088

Duval M, Suciu S, Ferster A et al (2002) Comparison of Escherichia coli-asparaginase with Erwinia-asparaginase in the treatment of childhood lymphoid malignancies: results of a randomized European Organisation for Research and Treatment of Cancer-

Children's Leukemia Group phase 3 trial. Blood 99:2734–2739

Eisenberg HM, McComb JG, Lorenzo AV (1974) Cerebrospinal fluid overproduction and hydrocephalus associated with choroid plexus papilloma. J Neurosurg 40:381–385

Engelmann KA, Jordan LC (2012) Outcome measures used in pediatric stroke studies: a systematic review. Arch Neurol 69:23–27

Fouladi M, Langston J, Mulhern R et al (2000) Silent lacunar lesions detected by magnetic resonance imaging of children with brain tumors: a late sequela of therapy. J Clin Oncol 18:824–831

Fullerton HJ, Wu YW, Sidney S et al (2007) Risk of recurrent childhood arterial ischemic stroke in a population-based cohort: the importance of cerebrovascular imaging. Pediatrics 119:495–501

George R, Jeba J, Ramkumar G et al (2008) Interventions for the treatment of metastatic extradural spinal cord compression in adults. Cochrane Database Syst Rev (4):CD006716

Glantz MJ, LaFollette S, Jaeckle KA et al (1999) Randomized trial of a slow-release versus a standard formulation of cytarabine for the intrathecal treatment of lymphomatous meningitis. J Clin Oncol 17:3110–3116

Glantz MJ, Cole BF, Forsyth PA et al (2000) Practice parameter: anticonvulsant prophylaxis in patients with newly diagnosed brain tumors. Report of the Quality Standards Subcommittee of the American Academy of Neurology. Neurology 54:1886–1893

Goldsby RE, Liu Q, Nathan PC et al (2010) Late-occurring neurologic sequelae in adult survivors of childhood acute lymphoblastic leukemia: a report from the Childhood Cancer Survivor Study. J Clin Oncol 28:324–331

Grace RF, Dahlberg SE, Neuberg D et al (2011) The frequency and management of asparaginase-related thrombosis in paediatric and adult patients with acute lymphoblastic leukaemia treated on Dana-Farber Cancer Institute consortium protocols. Br J Haematol 152:452–459

Greenwood MJ, Dodds AJ, Garricik R et al (2003) Posterior leukoencephalopathy in association with the tumour lysis syndrome in acute lymphoblastic leukaemia–a case with clinicopathological correlation. Leuk Lymphoma 44:719–721

Grill J, Couanet D, Cappelli C et al (1999) Radiation-induced cerebral vasculopathy in children with neurofibromatosis and optic pathway glioma. Ann Neurol 45:393–396

Gupta V, Srivastava A, Bhatia B (2009) Hodgkin disease with spinal cord compression. J Pediatr Hematol Oncol 31:771–773

Guyatt G, Gutterman D, Baumann MH et al (2006) Grading strength of recommendations and quality of evidence in clinical guidelines: report from an American College of Chest Physicians task force. Chest 129:174–181

Haddy N, Mousannif A, Tukenova M et al (2011) Relationship between the brain radiation dose for the treatment of childhood cancer and the risk of long-term cerebrovascular mortality. Brain 134:1362–1367

Hamadani M, Awan F (2006) Role of thiamine in managing ifosfamide-induced encephalopathy. J Oncol Pharm Pract 12:237–239

Hardesty DA, Sanborn MR, Parker WE et al (2011) Perioperative seizure incidence and risk factors in 223 pediatric brain tumor patients without prior seizures. J Neurosurg Pediatr 7:609–615

Hartman AL, Lunney KM, Serena JE (2009) Pediatric stroke: do clinical factors predict delays in presentation? J Pediatr 154:727–732

Hayes FA, Thompson EI, Hvizdala E et al (1984) Chemotherapy as an alternative to laminectomy and radiation in the management of epidural tumor. J Pediatr 104:221–224

Herzig RH, Hines JD, Herzig GP et al (1987) Cerebellar toxicity with high-dose cytosine arabinoside. J Clin Oncol 5:927–932

Hinchey J, Chaves C, Appignani B et al (1996) A reversible posterior leukoencephalopathy syndrome. N Engl J Med 334:494–500

Hoffman KE, Yock TI (2009) Radiation therapy for pediatric central nervous system tumors. J Child Neurol 24:1387–1396

Hollander M, Bots ML, Del Sol AI et al (2002) Carotid plaques increase the risk of stroke and subtypes of cerebral infarction in asymptomatic elderly: the Rotterdam study. Circulation 105:2872–2877

Holmes D, Vishnu P, Dorer RK et al (2012) All-trans retinoic acid-induced pseudotumor cerebri during induction therapy for acute promyelocytic leukemia: a case report and literature review. Case Rep Oncol Med 2012:313057

Huang EA, Feldman BJ, Schwartz ID et al (2006) Oral urea for the treatment of chronic syndrome of inappropriate antidiuresis in children. J Pediatr 148:128–131

Huisman TA (2009) Pediatric tumors of the spine. Cancer Imaging 9:S45–S48

Inaba H, Khan RB, Laningham FH et al (2008) Clinical and radiological characteristics of methotrexate-induced acute encephalopathy in pediatric patients with cancer. Ann Oncol 19:178–184

Isome K, Matsubara K, Taki T et al (2011) Spinal cord compression by epidural involvement over 21 vertebral levels in acute lymphoblastic leukemia. J Pediatr Hematol Oncol 33:153–157

Kaal EC, Vecht CJ (2004) The management of brain edema in brain tumors. Curr Opin Oncol 16:593–600

Kenz S, Haas CS, Werth SC et al (2011) High sensitivity to tolvaptan in paraneoplastic syndrome of inappropriate ADH secretion (SIADH). Ann Oncol 22:2696

Khanna S, Davis D, Peterson B et al (2000) Use of hypertonic saline in the treatment of severe refractory post-traumatic intracranial hypertension in pediatric traumatic brain injury. Crit Care Med 28:1144–1151

Khasraw M, Holodny A, Goldlust SA et al (2012) Intracranial hemorrhage in patients with cancer treated with bevacizumab: the Memorial Sloan-Kettering experience. Ann Oncol 23:458–463

Kikuchi A, Maeda M, Hanada R et al (2007) Moyamoya syndrome following childhood acute lymphoblastic leukemia. Pediatr Blood Cancer 48:268–272

Kirkpatrick JP, van der Kogel AJ, Schultheiss TE (2010) Radiation dose-volume effects in the spinal cord. Int J Radiat Oncol Biol Phys 76:S42–S49

Kitchen L, Westmacott R, Friefeld S et al (2012) The pediatric stroke outcome measure: a validation and reliability study. Stroke 43:1602–1608

Klein SL, Sanford RA, Muhlbauer MS (1991) Pediatric spinal epidural metastases. J Neurosurg 74:70–75

Kupfer A, Aeschlimann C, Wermuth B et al (1994) Prophylaxis and reversal of ifosfamide encephalopathy with methylene-blue. Lancet 343:763–764

Laitt RD, Chambers EJ, Goddard PR et al (1995) Magnetic resonance imaging and magnetic resonance angiography in long term survivors of acute lymphoblastic leukemia treated with cranial irradiation. Cancer 76: 1846–1852

Land VJ, Shuster JJ, Crist WM et al (1994) Comparison of two schedules of intermediate-dose methotrexate and cytarabine consolidation therapy for childhood B-precursor cell acute lymphoblastic leukemia: a Pediatric Oncology Group study. J Clin Oncol 12: 1939–1945

Leone G, Gugliotta L, Mazzucconi MG et al (1993) Evidence of a hypercoagulable state in patients with acute lymphoblastic leukemia treated with low dose of E. coli L-asparaginase: a GIMEMA study. Thromb Haemost 69:12–15

Lim YJ, Park EK, Koh HC et al (2010) Syndrome of inappropriate secretion of antidiuretic hormone as a leading cause of hyponatremia in children who underwent chemotherapy or stem cell transplantation. Pediatr Blood Cancer 54:734–737

Lo WD (2011) Childhood hemorrhagic stroke: an important but understudied problem. J Child Neurol 26:1174–1185

Loblaw DA, Perry J, Chambers A, Laperriere NJ (2005) Systematic review of the diagnosis and management of malignant extradural spinal cord compression: the Cancer Care Ontario Practice Guidelines Initiative's Neuro-Oncology Disease Site Group. J Clin Oncol 23:2028–2037

Lucchini G, Grioni D, Colombini A et al (2008) Encephalopathy syndrome in children with hemato-oncological disorders is not always posterior and reversible. Pediatr Blood Cancer 51:629–633

Mackay MT, Monagle P (2008) Perinatal and early childhood stroke and thrombophilia. Pathology 40:116–123

Mahoney DH Jr, Shuster JJ, Nitschke R et al (1998) Acute neurotoxicity in children with B-precursor acute lymphoid leukemia: an association with intermediate-dose intravenous methotrexate and intrathecal triple therapy–a Pediatric Oncology Group study. J Clin Oncol 16:1712–1722

Mantadakis E, Katragkou A, Papadaki E et al (2008) Spinal cord compression in an adolescent with relapsed B-precursor acute lymphoblastic leukemia and mental neuropathy. Int J Hematol 88:294–298

Mattioli Belmonte M, Gugliotta L, Delvos U et al (1991) A regimen for antithrombin III substitution in patients with acute lymphoblastic leukemia under treatment with L-asparaginase. Haematologica 76:209–214

McGlennan C, Ganesan V (2008) Delays in investigation and management of acute arterial ischaemic stroke in children. Dev Med Child Neurol 50:537–540

McQuilten ZK, Barnes C, Zatta A et al (2012) Off-label use of recombinant factor VIIa in pediatric patients. Pediatrics 129:e1533–e1540

Medina LS, Pinter JD, Zurakowski D et al (1997) Children with headache: clinical predictors of surgical space-occupying lesions and the role of neuroimaging. Radiology 202:819–824

Meeske KA, Siegel SE, Gilsanz V et al (2009) Premature carotid artery disease in pediatric cancer survivors treated with neck irradiation. Pediatr Blood Cancer 53:615–621

Messe SR, Sansing LH, Cucchiara BL et al (2009) Prophylactic antiepileptic drug use is associated with poor outcome following ICH. Neurocrit Care 11:38–44

Mitchell L, Andrew M, Hanna K et al (2003) Trend to efficacy and safety using antithrombin concentrate in prevention of thrombosis in children receiving l-asparaginase for acute lymphoblastic leukemia. Results of the PAARKA study. Thromb Haemost 90:235–244

Moritz ML, Ayus JC (2010) New aspects in the pathogenesis, prevention, and treatment of hyponatremic encephalopathy in children. Pediatr Nephrol 25:1225–1238

Morris EB, Laningham FH, Sandlund JT et al (2007) Posterior reversible encephalopathy syndrome in children with cancer. Pediatr Blood Cancer 48:152–159

Neville BG, Wilson J (1970) Benign intracranial hypertension following corticosteroid withdrawal in childhood. Br Med J 3:554–556

Norman JK, Parke JT, Wilson DA et al (2007) Reversible posterior leukoencephalopathy syndrome in children undergoing induction therapy for acute lymphoblastic leukemia. Pediatr Blood Cancer 49:198–203

O'Leary DH, Polak JF, Kronmal RA et al (1999) Carotid-artery intima and media thickness as a risk factor for myocardial infarction and stroke in older adults. Cardiovascular Health Study Collaborative Research Group. N Engl J Med 340:14–22

Ogiwara H, Nordli DR, DiPatri AJ et al (2010) Pediatric epileptogenic gangliogliomas: seizure outcome and surgical results. J Neurosurg Pediatr 5:271–276

Olcay L, Aribas BK, Gokce M (2009) A patient with acute myeloblastic leukemia who presented with conus medullaris syndrome and review of the literature. J Pediatr Hematol Oncol 31:440–447

Omura M, Aida N, Sekido K et al (1997) Large intracranial vessel occlusive vasculopathy after radiation therapy in children: clinical features and usefulness of magnetic resonance imaging. Int J Radiat Oncol Biol Phys 38:241–249

Papadopoulos KP, Garvin JH, Fetell M et al (1998) High-dose thiotepa and etoposide-based regimens with autologous hematopoietic support for high-risk or recurrent CNS tumors in children and adults. Bone Marrow Transplant 22:661–667

Parikh SN, Crawford AH (2003) Orthopaedic implications in the management of pediatric vertebral and spinal cord tumors: a retrospective review. Spine (Phila Pa 1976) 28:2390–2396

Patchell RA, Tibbs PA, Regine WF et al (2005) Direct decompressive surgical resection in the treatment of spinal cord compression caused by metastatic cancer: a randomised trial. Lancet 366:643–648

Patel PN (2006) Methylene blue for management of ifosfamide-induced encephalopathy. Ann Pharmacother 40:299–303

Pelgrims J, De Vos F, Van den Brande J et al (2000) Methylene blue in the treatment and prevention of ifosfamide-induced encephalopathy: report of 12 cases and a review of the literature. Br J Cancer 82:291–294

Pitfield AF, Carroll AB, Kissoon N (2012) Emergency management of increased intracranial pressure. Pediatr Emerg Care 28:200–204; quiz 205–207

Pollono D, Tomarchia S, Drut R et al (2003) Spinal cord compression: a review of 70 pediatric patients. Pediatr Hematol Oncol 20:457–466

Pratt CB, Green AA, Horowitz ME et al (1986) Central nervous system toxicity following the treatment of pediatric patients with ifosfamide/mesna. J Clin Oncol 4:1253–1261

Rades D, Huttenlocher S, Dunst J et al (2010) Matched pair analysis comparing surgery followed by radiotherapy and radiotherapy alone for metastatic spinal cord compression. J Clin Oncol 28:3597–3604

Rafay MF, Pontigon AM, Chiang J et al (2009) Delay to diagnosis in acute pediatric arterial ischemic stroke. Stroke 40:58–64

Raffini L (2008) Thrombophilia in children: who to test, how, when, and why? Hematology Am Soc Hematol Educ Program 228–235

Reddick WE, Glass JO, Helton KJ et al (2005) Prevalence of leukoencephalopathy in children treated for acute lymphoblastic leukemia with high-dose methotrexate. AJNR Am J Neuroradiol 26:1263–1269

Relling MV, Pui CH, Sandlund JT et al (2000) Adverse effect of anticonvulsants on efficacy of chemotherapy for acute lymphoblastic leukaemia. Lancet 356:285–290

Riva-Cambrin J, Detsky AS, Lamberti-Pasculli M et al (2009) Predicting postresection hydrocephalus in pediatric patients with posterior fossa tumors. J Neurosurg Pediatr 3:378–385

Rivkees SA (2008) Differentiating appropriate antidiuretic hormone secretion, inappropriate antidiuretic hormone secretion and cerebral salt wasting: the common, uncommon, and misnamed. Curr Opin Pediatr 20:448–452

Roach ES (2000) Etiology of stroke in children. Semin Pediatr Neurol 7:244–260

Roach ES, Golomb MR, Adams R et al (2008) Management of stroke in infants and children: a scientific statement from a Special Writing Group of the American Heart Association Stroke Council and the Council on Cardiovascular Disease in the Young. Stroke 39:2644–2691

Rollins N, Winick N, Bash R et al (2004) Acute methotrexate neurotoxicity: findings on diffusion-weighted imaging and correlation with clinical outcome. AJNR Am J Neuroradiol 25:1688–1695

Rubin EH, Andersen JW, Berg DT et al (1992) Risk factors for high-dose cytarabine neurotoxicity: an analysis of a cancer and leukemia group B trial in patients with acute myeloid leukemia. J Clin Oncol 10:948–953

Rubnitz JE, Relling MV, Harrison PL et al (1998) Transient encephalopathy following high-dose methotrexate treatment in childhood acute lymphoblastic leukemia. Leukemia 12:1176–1181

Ruggiero A, Rizzo D, Mastrangelo S et al (2010) Interactions between antiepileptic and chemotherapeutic drugs in children with brain tumors: is it time to change treatment? Pediatr Blood Cancer 54:193–198

Sandoval C, Kutscher M, Jayabose S et al (2003) Neurotoxicity of intrathecal methotrexate: MR imaging findings. AJNR Am J Neuroradiol 24:1887–1890

Schwenn MR, Blattner SR, Lynch E et al (1991) HiC-COM: a 2-month intensive chemotherapy regimen for children with stage III and IV Burkitt's lymphoma and B-cell acute lymphoblastic leukemia. J Clin Oncol 9:133–138

Seet RC, Rabinstein AA, Lindell PE et al (2011) Cerebrovascular events after bevacizumab treatment: an early and severe complication. Neurocrit Care 15:421–427

Silverman LB, Supko JG, Stevenson KE et al (2010) Intravenous PEG-asparaginase during remission induction in children and adolescents with newly diagnosed acute lymphoblastic leukemia. Blood 115:1351–1353

Simon T, Niemann CA, Hero B et al (2012) Short- and long-term outcome of patients with symptoms of spinal cord compression by neuroblastoma. Dev Med Child Neurol 54:347–352

Singh S, Bohn D, Carlotti AP et al (2002) Cerebral salt wasting: truths, fallacies, theories, and challenges. Crit Care Med 30:2575–2579

Smith MA, Adamson PC, Balis FM et al (1992) Phase I and pharmacokinetic evaluation of all-trans-retinoic acid in pediatric patients with cancer. J Clin Oncol 10:1666–1673

Smith GA, Damon LE, Rugo HS et al (1997) High-dose cytarabine dose modification reduces the incidence of neurotoxicity in patients with renal insufficiency. J Clin Oncol 15:833–839

Sommers LM, Hawkins DS (1999) Meningitis in pediatric cancer patients: a review of forty cases from a single institution. Pediatr Infect Dis J 18:902–907

Spiegel RJ, Cooper PR, Blum RH et al (1984) Treatment of massive intrathecal methotrexate overdose by ventriculolumbar perfusion. N Engl J Med 311:386–388

Srinivasan J, Miller SP, Phan TG et al (2009) Delayed recognition of initial stroke in children: need for increased awareness. Pediatrics 124:e227–e234

Sterns RH, Nigwekar SU, Hix JK (2009) The treatment of hyponatremia. Semin Nephrol 29:282–299

Taugourdeau-Raymond S, Rouby F, Default A et al (2012) Bevacizumab-induced serious side-effects: a review of the French pharmacovigilance database. Eur J Clin Pharmacol 68:1103–1107

Ullrich NJ, Robertson R, Kinnamon DD et al (2007) Moyamoya following cranial irradiation for primary brain tumors in children. Neurology 68:932–938

Vos J, Aarnoudse MW, Dijk F et al (1983) On the cellular origin and development of atheromatous plaques. A light and electron microscopic study of combined X-ray and hypercholesterolemia-induced atheromatosis in the carotid artery of the rabbit. Virchows Arch B Cell Pathol Incl Mol Pathol 43:1–16

White RH (2003) The epidemiology of venous thromboembolism. Circulation 107:I4–I8

Widemann BC, Balis FM, Shalabi A et al (2004) Treatment of accidental intrathecal methotrexate overdose with intrathecal carboxypeptidase G2. J Natl Cancer Inst 96:1557–1559

Wilne S, Collier J, Kennedy C et al (2007) Presentation of childhood CNS tumours: a systematic review and meta-analysis. Lancet Oncol 8:685–689

Winick NJ, Bowman WP, Kamen BA et al (1992) Unexpected acute neurologic toxicity in the treatment of children with acute lymphoblastic leukemia. J Natl Cancer Inst 84:252–256

Zimmer JA, Garg BP, Williams LS et al (2007) Age-related variation in presenting signs of childhood arterial ischemic stroke. Pediatr Neurol 37:171–175

Hyperleukocytosis

6

Ana E. Aguilar, Anurag K. Agrawal,
and James H. Feusner

Contents

A.E. Aguilar, MD
Department of Hematology/Oncology and BMT,
Children's Hospital of Los Angeles,
Los Angeles, CA, USA

A.K. Agrawal, MD (✉) • J.H. Feusner, MD
Department of Hematology/Oncology,
Children's Hospital and Research Center Oakland,
747 52nd Street, Oakland, CA 94609, USA
e-mail: aagrawal@mail.cho.org

Abstract

Hyperleukocytosis (HL) is defined as a white blood cell (WBC) count $>100\times10^9$/L and in pediatric patients is typically seen in acute lymphoblastic leukemia (ALL), acute myelogenous leukemia (AML) and chronic myelogenous leukemia (CML). Although significant gains have been made in the treatment of pediatric leukemia, HL continues to pose risk both in regard to early death and decreased overall survival. Patients with HL are at risk for acute complications due to rapid proliferation of leukemic blasts resulting in leukostasis and tumor lysis syndrome (TLS) as well as blast cell lysis leading to the release of anti- and procoagulant factors. The degree of HL that is clinically significant in pediatric ALL and AML is controversial. Here we consider the differing presentations in patients with HL and concomitant ALL, AML, and CML and potential WBC thresholds at which patients require supplementary supportive care measures in an attempt to reduce early morbidity and mortality. In addition to an analysis of the evidence behind standard care measures, the potential benefit of leukapheresis will be examined and recommendations given.

J. Feusner et al. (eds.), *Supportive Care in Pediatric Oncology:
A Practical Evidence-Based Approach*, Pediatric Oncology,
DOI 10.1007/978-3-662-44317-0_6, © Springer Berlin Heidelberg 2015

6.1   Introduction

Hyperleukocytosis (HL) is defined as a white blood cell (WBC) count >100×10⁹/L and in pediatric patients is typically seen in acute lymphoblastic leukemia (ALL), acute myelogenous leukemia (AML) and chronic myelogenous leukemia (CML) (Porcu et al. 2000). Recent pediatric studies have noted an HL incidence of 10.9–13.1 % in ALL and 18.3–19.1 % in AML patients with early death rates of 2.7 % in ALL (WBC >200×10⁹/L) and 2.8–3.9 % in AML (WBC >100×10⁹/L) (Creutzig et al. 2004; Inaba et al. 2008; Möricke et al. 2008; Gaynon et al. 2010; Sung et al. 2012; Vaitkevičienė et al. 2013). The degree of HL that is clinically significant in pediatric ALL and AML is controversial.

Patients with HL are at risk for acute complications due to rapid proliferation of leukemic blasts resulting in leukostasis and tumor lysis syndrome (TLS) as well as blast cell lysis leading to the release of anti- and procoagulant factors. In a pathologic survey of 206 adult leukemia patients at autopsy, McKee and Collins (1974) noted leukemic thrombi aggregates in pulmonary and central nervous system (CNS) vasculature in AML and CML but not in ALL patients. In studying the rheology of myeloblasts and lymphoblasts, Lichtman (1973) importantly noted that total blood viscosity (cytocrit) is rarely altered in HL due to a concomitant decrease in red cell mass (erythrocrit) and that deformability of both myeloblasts and lymphoblasts is decreased, thus theoretically allowing for aggregation in small vessels, especially for the larger myeloblasts. Stucki et al. (2001) showed that myeloblasts are able to adhere to vascular endothelium through cytokine secretion. Thus, decreased deformability and endothelial myeloblast interaction are likely more important mechanisms for leukostasis than plasma viscosity (Porcu et al. 2000).

High blast counts, especially in AML, are related to increased risk of early mortality secondary to leukostasis and leukemic cell lysis both before and after commencement of chemotherapy (Wald et al. 1982, Hug et al. 1983, Bunin and Pui 1985; Dutcher et al. 1987; Würthner et al. 1999; Porcu et al. 2000;

Novotny et al. 2005). In both pediatric and adult AML patients, leukostasis has been reported with WBC >50×10⁹/L as well as <50×10⁹/L (Soares et al. 1992; Creutzig et al. 2004). The most severe complications of leukostasis and blast cell lysis are respiratory failure, pulmonary hemorrhage, and intracranial hemorrhage (ICH). ICH often presents at diagnosis in patients with ALL, AML as well as specifically AML M3 subtype (acute promyelocytic leukemia; APL) (Kim et al. 2006; Sung et al. 2012; Vaitkevičienė et al. 2013). Neurologic manifestations can range from headache and confusion to somnolence, stupor, and coma. Additional potential manifestations include priapism, dactylitis, retinal hemorrhage, renal infiltration/failure, bowel ischemia, congestive heart failure and cardiac tamponade (Rowe and Lichtman 1984; da Costa et al. 1999; Lowe et al. 2005; Novotny et al. 2005; Vaitkevičienė et al. 2013).

Here we consider the differing presentations in patients with HL and concomitant ALL, AML, APL, and CML and potential WBC thresholds at which patients require supplementary supportive care measures in an attempt to reduce early morbidity and mortality. In addition to an analysis of the evidence behind standard care measures, the potential benefit of leukapheresis will be examined. Recommendations are summarized in Table 6.1.

6.2   Acute Lymphoblastic Leukemia

Risk factors for HL in pediatric ALL patients include age <1 year, T-cell phenotype, MLL (11q23) rearrangement, Philadelphia chromosome t(9;22) and leukemic cell ploidy ≤50 (Pui et al. 1990; Eguiguren et al. 1992; Vaitkevičienė et al. 2009). Historically, long-term outcomes in ALL patients with HL have been lowest, likely due to these underlying disease characteristics (Möricke et al. 2008; Vaitkevičienė et al. 2009; Gaynon et al. 2010). In ALL cooperative group studies, 10.9–13.1 % of patients had initial WBC ≥100×10⁹/L and 4.8–5.8 % had initial WBC

$\geq 200 \times 10^9$/L (Möricke et al. 2008; Gaynon et al. 2010; Lund et al. 2011). For the 132 patients with initial WBC $\geq 200 \times 10^9$/L in the Scandinavian NOPHO ALL-92 and ALL-2000 protocols, 7 (5.3 %) suffered early death, 6 secondary to neurologic complications, and none secondary to TLS with 5 dying prior to therapy initiation (Lund et al. 2011).

Table 6.1 Summary of management strategies and level of evidence for management of pediatric leukemic hyperleukocytosis[a]

Disease	Potential side effect	Treatment	Level of evidence[b]
Acute lymphoblastic leukemia	Leukostasis	Rapid initiation of chemotherapy	1A
		Hyperhydration	1C
		Consider leukapheresis for WBC >400–600 × 10⁹/L if no delay in antileukemic chemotherapy initiation	2C
	Tumor lysis syndrome	Hyperhydration	1B
		One dose of rasburicase prior to antileukemic chemotherapy initiation; see Chap. 3 for more detail	1A
	Isolated hyperuricemia	One dose of prophylactic rasburicase	1B
		Follow with alkalinization and allopurinol	2C
		Consider additional rasburicase doses if repeat uric acid >7.5 mg/dL	2C
	DIC/coagulopathy	FFP to keep PT/PTT WNL	1C
		Fibrinogen (concentrate or cryo) to keep fibrinogen >150 mg/dL	1C
	Thrombocytopenia	Platelet transfusion to keep platelets >50 × 10⁹/L if WBC >300–400 × 10⁹/L	1C
	Symptomatic anemia	Transfuse small aliquots (e.g., 5 mL/kg) and keep hgb <10 g/dL	1C
Acute myelogenous leukemia (except APL)	Leukostasis	Rapid initiation of chemotherapy	1A
		Careful hydration	1C
		Consider leukapheresis	2C
		Consider HU	2C
	Tumor lysis syndrome	Hyperhydration	1C
		One dose of rasburicase if uric acid >7.5 mg/dL; see Chap. 3 for more detail	2C
	DIC/coagulopathy	FFP to keep PT/PTT WNL	1C
		Fibrinogen (concentrate or cryo) to keep fibrinogen >150 mg/dL	1C
	Thrombocytopenia	Platelet transfusion to keep platelets >50 × 10⁹/L	1C
	Isolated hyperuricemia	One dose of prophylactic rasburicase	1B
		Follow with alkalinization and allopurinol	2C
		Consider additional rasburicase doses if repeat uric acid >7.5 mg/dL	2C
	Symptomatic anemia	Transfuse small aliquots (e.g., 5 mL/kg) and keep hgb <10 g/dL	1C
Acute promyelocytic leukemia	DIC/coagulopathy	Rapid initiation of ATRA or ATO	1A
		FFP to keep PT/PTT WNL	1C
		Fibrinogen (concentrate or cryo) to keep fibrinogen >150 mg/dL	1C
		Avoid invasive procedures	1C
		Unclear benefit of leukapheresis	2C
	Thrombocytopenia	Platelet transfusion to keep platelets >50 × 10⁹/L at the minimum	1C
	APL differentiation syndrome/RAS	Dexamethasone	1B
	Leukocytosis with ATRA or ATO	HU	1B
		Consider holding ATRA or ATO	1C

(continued)

Table 6.1 (continued)

Disease	Potential side effect	Treatment	Level of evidence[b]
Chronic myelogenous leukemia	Leukostasis	Hyperhydration	1C
		HU	1C
		Consider leukapheresis	2C
	Priapism	Hyperhydration	1C
		HU	1C
		Consider leukapheresis	2C
		Urologic consultation for therapeutic aspiration and possible intracavernous sympathomimetic therapy	1C
		Pain management	1C

WBC white blood cell, *DIC* disseminated intravascular coagulation, *FFP* fresh frozen plasma, *PT* prothrombin time, *PTT* partial thromboplastin time, *WNL* within normal limits, *cryo* cryoprecipitate, *hgb* hemoglobin, *APL* acute promyelocytic leukemia, *HU* hydroxyurea, *RAS* retinoic acid syndrome, *ATRA* all-trans retinoic acid, *ATO* arsenic trioxide
[a]See text for full detail
[b]Per Guyatt et al. (2006); see Preface

In a follow-up study of 221 NOPHO patients with WBC $\geq 200 \times 10^9/L$, Vaitkevičienė et al. (2013) importantly note that all complications secondary to HL, except the need for dialysis, occurred at significantly higher median WBC counts: neurologic (WBC $530 \times 10^9/L$ vs. $327 \times 10^9/L$), respiratory (WBC $620 \times 10^9/L$ vs. $336 \times 10^9/L$), bleeding (WBC $420 \times 10^9/L$ vs. $327 \times 10^9/L$), and dialysis (WBC $310 \times 10^9/L$ vs. $357 \times 10^9/L$). Neurologic and bleeding complications occurred at a significantly higher age, while respiratory distress occurred at a significantly younger age. In multivariate analysis, only WBC count and neurologic symptoms at admission were significantly associated with risk of early death; timing of administration of antileukemic therapy, admission hemoglobin level and administration of packed red blood cells (PRBCs) were not significant. Six patients (2.7 %) died within 2 weeks of presentation, all secondary to neurologic complications, with 4 of the 6 presenting with severe symptoms. Patients receiving mechanical cytoreduction (leukapheresis or exchange transfusion) prior to chemotherapy initiation had significant delay in antileukemic therapy initiation with no noted survival benefit. TLS occurred in 12 % of patients with statistically higher initial uric acid levels (11.0 vs. 7.7 mg/dL). Patients with T-cell and infant ALL were at increased risk of TLS, rasburicase significantly reduced the risk of TLS and no patient died from TLS. Initial uric acid level

was the only significant factor for the development of TLS on multivariate analysis (WBC count, lactate dehydrogenase, corticosteroid dose and mechanical cytoreduction were not significant). In their supplemental HL guidelines, Vaitkevičienė et al. (2013) recommend prompt initiation of antileukemic therapy after diagnostic evaluations and rasburicase administration with no recommendation for leukapheresis or exchange transfusion.

Maurer et al. (1988) similarly reported an 8.4 % incidence of WBC $>200 \times 10^9/L$ in a pediatric ALL cohort. Early death occurred in 7 of 124 (5.6 %) patients, 4 from sepsis, 1 from pneumonia, 1 from GI hemorrhage and 1 from ICH. Four (3.2 %) patients suffered ICH with 3 occurring at presentation and all with WBC $>600 \times 10^9/L$. Although electrolyte abnormalities were decreased in those undergoing leukapheresis, risk of renal dysfunction requiring dialysis was low, occurring in only 3 (2.4 %) patients, all of whom had received low-dose prednisone pretreatment. WBC $>600 \times 10^9/L$ and massive splenomegaly were the only significant adverse prognostic factors on multivariate analysis.

In a comprehensive study of HL over a 40-year period at St. Jude Children's Research Hospital, Lowe et al. (2005) reported 178 of 2,288 (7.8 %) children with ALL presenting with WBC $>200 \times 10^9/L$. Early death occurred in 7 (3.9 %), 3 from sepsis and 2 each from ICH and respiratory failure. Cytoreduction was performed in those with a median initial leukocyte count of $416 \times 10^9/L$ vs. $295 \times 10^9/L$ in the nonreduced cohort. The time to initiate chemotherapy was significantly longer in the cytoreduced cohort. Neurologic and respiratory complications were statistically more likely with WBC $>400 \times 10^9/L$. Older age was also significant for neurologic complications. Four patients suffered from ICH (2.2 %), all with initial WBC $>400 \times 10^9/L$ and 3 at initial presentation to the tertiary care institution. Two of the 4 received PRBC transfusion prior to ICH, while the other 2 had initial hemoglobin of 10.1 and 10.2 g/dL. The majority of neurologic complications (13 of 16; 81 %) occurred at presentation; the additional 3 occurred 24 h after presentation, 1 in the cytoreduced group and 2 in the nonreduced cohort. Pulmonary complications occurred more commonly in the cytoreduced cohort and were equally common before and after cytoreduction. Metabolic complications were common, with hyperkalemia in 10 % and hyperphosphatemia in 20 %, but only 1 patient died secondary to metabolic dysfunction (hyperkalemia) and overt renal dysfunction was rare. Although it was unclear if cytoreduction was beneficial in the prevention of TLS or leukostasis symptoms and did not impact early mortality, Lowe et al. (2005) recommend cytoreduction for WBC $>400 \times 10^9/L$. Again, early initiation of chemotherapy in pediatric ALL seems most important although it is unlikely to impact those presenting with severe neurologic dysfunction and may not impact early death.

6.3 Acute Myelogenous Leukemia

Like ALL, HL has been shown to be a negative prognostic factor in long-term outcome in pediatric AML patients (Inaba et al. 2008; Lange et al. 2008). In analysis of AML-BFM 93 and AML-BFM 98, Creutzig et al. (2004) reported a 19.1 % incidence of HL with significantly increased risk of early death with WBC $\geq 100 \times 10^9/L$ (9.9 % vs. 2.1 % with WBC $<100 \times 10^9/L$) and even more so with WBC $\geq 200 \times 10^9/L$ (16.9 % vs. 2.4 % with WBC $<200 \times 10^9/L$). Multivariate analysis found

HL, FAB M5 and low-performance status as significant independent prognostic factors. A recent analysis of COG AML studies AAML03P1 and AAML0531 reported an 18.8 % incidence of HL with independent risk factors including age ≤ 1 year, FAB M1, M4, and M5, inv(16), and FLT3-ITD+ (Sung et al. 2012). These findings have been corroborated by other studies (Creutzig et al. 1987; Meshinchi et al. 2001; Inaba et al. 2008). TLS was rare although hyperphosphatemia and hyperuricemia were significantly associated with increased initial WBC count. Initial WBC count was significantly associated with hypoxia, pulmonary hemorrhage, CNS ischemia, CNS hemorrhage and death (Sung et al. 2012). Patients with the highest WBC counts ($\geq 400 \times 10^9/L$) were at greatest risk for early death and leukapheresis did not appear to impact early death: 1 of 16 (6.3 %) receiving leukapheresis experienced early death as compared to 3 of 73 (4.1 %) who were not leukapheresed (Sung et al. 2012). Overall, the induction death rate was 3.9 % for WBC $\geq 100 \times 10^9/L$ vs. 1.3 % for WBC $<100 \times 10^9/L$. In a comprehensive review of retrospective AML studies in both pediatric and adult patients with HL, Oberoi et al. (2014) reported an overall early death rate of 20.1 % which was not significantly influenced by the use of leukapheresis. Hemorrhage and bleeding (75 %) was the most common cause of early death followed by leukostasis (9.1 %); APL patients constituted only 2–5.5 % of all studied patients and pediatric data were not separately analyzed (Oberoi et al. 2014).

Inaba et al. (2008) studied newly diagnosed AML patients at St. Jude Children's Research Hospital and found an 18.3 % incidence of HL; in the most recent period, the early death rate was 2.8 % as compared to a previous time period with an early death rate of 22.9 %. Complications secondary to HL were similar in both time periods and significantly correlated with median WBC count: neurologic (WBC $221 \times 10^9/L$ vs. $158 \times 10^9/L$), pulmonary ($240 \times 10^9/L$ vs. $155 \times 10^9/L$), and renal (WBC $275 \times 10^9/L$ vs. $159 \times 10^9/L$). Leukoreduction was utilized in the later time period at the discretion of the treating physician; early death occurred in 1 of 20 patients leukoreduced and 0 of 16 not leukoreduced although those leukoreduced had a significantly higher admission WBC count

(206×10^9/L vs. 116×10^9/L). Metabolic complications were uncommon although more prevalent in those with FAB M4/M5 subtypes. Twelve of the 17 deaths occurred due to hemorrhage (gastrointestinal, pulmonary or intracranial).

Earlier studies have reported a much higher death rate, likely due in part to less intensive supportive care measures (Wald et al. 1982; Bunin and Pui 1985; Creutzig et al. 2004; Inaba et al. 2008). Although significant data are lacking, one study in adult AML M5 patients with HL and pulmonary symptoms has shown potential benefit with the addition of dexamethasone to improve lung function in the acute period (Azoulay et al. 2012). The utilization of leukapheresis in AML is controversial and discussed further in Sect. 6.7.

6.4   Acute Promyelocytic Leukemia

HL is an uncommon presenting feature in APL although pediatric patients have an increased incidence of microgranular APL (M3v) with concomitant HL (Rovelli et al. 1992; Guglielmi et al. 1998; de Botton et al. 2004). HL can more commonly be seen as part of APL differentiation syndrome (previously called retinoic acid syndrome) after commencement of either all-trans retinoic acid (ATRA) or arsenic trioxide (ATO) therapy (Vahdat et al. 1994; Camacho et al. 2000; Levy et al. 2008; Zhang et al. 2008; Sanz et al. 2009; Zhou et al. 2010). In some studies, increasing leukocytosis (WBC $>10\times10^9$/L) was a risk factor for the development of the clinical findings of APL differentiation syndrome such as unexplained fever, weight gain, respiratory distress, pulmonary infiltrates, pleural effusions or pericarditis (Frankel et al. 1992; Vahdat et al. 1994; Camacho et al. 2000). HL either at diagnosis or after initiation of differentiating therapy is a risk factor for early death, especially from ICH secondary to disseminated intravascular coagulation (DIC) (Rovelli et al. 1992; Roberts et al. 2000; Zhang et al. 2008; Zhou et al. 2010).

Due to the risk of early death from DIC and hemorrhage, especially in those with the highest WBC counts, it is vital to initiate supportive care and induction therapy with ATRA and/or ATO emergently (Sanz et al. 2005, 2009; Tallman and Altman 2009). In lieu of randomized data, expert guidelines recommend treatment of coagulopathy with fresh frozen plasma, fibrinogen (fibrinogen concentrate or cryoprecipitate), and platelet transfusion to maintain fibrinogen >150 mg/dL and platelets $>50\times10^9$/L at the minimum in those with HL, with frequent (i.e., every 6–8 h) monitoring and correction (Sanz et al. 2005, 2009; Tallman and Altman 2009). Studies on the complementary use of antifibrinolytics such as tranexamic acid have not shown benefit (Sanz et al. 2009). Diagnostic lumbar puncture and placement of a central venous catheter should be avoided until the coagulopathy has resolved (Sanz et al. 2005, 2009; Tallman and Altman 2009). Initiation of treatment with a differentiating agent should start prior to genetic confirmation of diagnosis in those cases with sufficient clinical suspicion (Sanz et al. 2005, 2009; Tallman and Altman 2009). The clinician should be cognizant of the risk for HL development and concomitant DIC after initiation of either ATRA or ATO.

In the pediatric North American INT0129 APL trial, hydroxyurea was initiated at a dose of 1 g/m^2 and ATRA held if the WBC rose to $>30\times10^9$/L during ATRA therapy until the WBC count was $<10\times10^9$/L (Gregory et al. 2009). In a Chinese study of 19 children with APL who received single-agent ATO, all developed an increase in WBC count with induction ATO with 5 having WBC $>100\times10^9$/L (Zhou et al. 2010). The two children with the highest WBC counts, 178×10^9/L and 252×10^9/L after ATO initiation, both died from ICH. Zhou et al. (2010) initiated hydroxyurea for all WBC $>20\times10^9$/L while also decreasing the ATO dose or even holding it in patients with severe leukocytosis. The benefit of holding ATO therapy with HL is unclear (Levy et al. 2008; Sanz et al. 2009). Oral corticosteroids, which are utilized as treatment for APL differentiation syndrome, have also been suggested as a prophylactic agent with WBC >5–50×10^9/L or with the initiation of induction therapy in all patients to prevent the development of subsequent HL as well as severe pulmonary or CNS symptoms (Wiley and Firkin 1995; Sanz et al. 2005, 2009; Tallman and Altman 2009) Randomized data are lacking. The use of leukapheresis in APL with HL is controversial and discussed in Sect. 6.7.

6.5 Chronic Myelogenous Leukemia

HL is reported to be more common in pediatric patients with CML as compared to adults (Rowe and Lichtman 1984; Millot et al. 2005). Even with the high WBC counts at presentation, prevalence of leukostasis secondary to pediatric CML is thought to be uncommon although it was seen frequently in the small review by Rowe and Lichtman (1984). Symptoms of leukostasis in CML patients can include neurologic complaints such as papilledema, cranial nerve defects, and tinnitus, respiratory complaints, and priapism (Rowe and Lichtman 1984). Priapism has been noted in pediatric ALL and CML (Castagnetti et al. 2008; Vaitkevičienė et al. 2013). Management of HL in CML prior to the initiation of tyrosine kinase inhibitor therapy can be accomplished with hydroxyurea (Schwartz and Canellos 1975). Management of pediatric patients with signs and symptoms of leukostasis lacks an evidence basis in the literature although sources recommend utilization of chemotherapy in addition to leukapheresis (Rowe and Lichtman 1984; Castagnetti et al. 2008). For low-flow (ischemic) priapism in particular, adult guidelines recommend chemotherapy, leukapheresis, and urologic therapy with therapeutic aspiration and intracavernous sympathomimetics if aspiration alone is not successful (Montague et al. 2003; Rogers et al. 2012). Castagnetti et al. (2008) suggest patients can be managed without invasive urologic procedures utilizing chemotherapy and leukapheresis alone; however, their small cohort required a long period of time to recover from priapism and half did not receive leukapheresis. In addition they recommend the use of anticoagulation with low-molecular-weight heparin (especially with concomitant thrombocytosis) although significant evidence on utility is lacking. On long-term follow-up, none of their patient cohort had developed clinical evidence of erectile dysfunction.

6.6 Management of Tumor Lysis Syndrome

The general management of tumor lysis syndrome (TLS) is discussed in Chap. 3. Patients with HL are at increased risk of both laboratory and clinical TLS, especially those with ALL. Truong et al. (2007) showed that WBC $>20 \times 10^9$/L was an independent risk factor for the development of TLS in pediatric ALL. Montesinos et al. (2008) similarly reported that WBC $>25 \times 10^9$/L was an independent risk factor for TLS in adult AML patients, but it is unclear if TLS is a significant issue in pediatric AML even with HL (Inaba et al. 2008; Sung et al. 2012). Prevention through the utilization of hyperhydration, urine alkalinization, and allopurinol are all proven methods to reduce the risk of metabolic complications in pediatric patients with HL and ALL (Maurer et al. 1988; Lascari 1991). Maurer et al. (1988) showed no benefit in preventing metabolic derangement through the use of low-dose prednisone prior to initiation of induction chemotherapy in pediatric ALL patients with WBC $>200 \times 10^9$/L.

The most recent expert TLS guidelines list both ALL and AML with concomitant HL as high-risk for the development of TLS and recommend prophylactic use of rasburicase in addition to aggressive hydration to prevent hyperuricemia (Cairo et al. 2010). These recommendations concurred with the Italian consensus guidelines for ALL, although in the Italian opinion TLS was rare in AML even with HL and therefore should not be considered high-risk (Tosi et al. 2008). Cairo et al. (2010) recommend one dose of rasburicase at a dose of 0.1–0.2 mg/kg prior to the initiation of therapy, while Tosi et al. (2008) recommend continuing daily therapy at a dose of 0.2 mg/kg/day for 3–5 days. Additionally, the concomitant use of allopurinol (due to the very rarely reported precipitation of uric acid precursor xanthine) and alkalinization (due to potential risk of calcium phosphate precipitation) are not recommended (Coiffier et al. 2008; Tosi et al. 2008; Howard et al. 2011; Vaitkevičienė et al. 2013). Rasburicase is contraindicated in patients with glucose-6-phosphate dehydrogenase (G6PD) deficiency and methemoglobinemia (Tosi et al. 2008; Cairo et al. 2010; Howard et al. 2011; Vaitkevičienė et al. 2013).

6.7   Leukapheresis

The most recent recommendations by the American Society for Apheresis (ASFA) suggest leukapheresis as first-line therapy for patients with leukostasis secondary to HL due to the potential to impact early death, although long-term outcome is unaffected (Schwartz et al. 2013). However, the potential to impact early death through leukapheresis was not shown in a meta-analysis of AML studies by Oberoi et al. (2014). The role of apheresis as leukostasis prophylaxis with HL is not established but may be considered (Schwartz et al. 2013). Per the ASFA guidelines, the utilization of leukapheresis is listed as a strong recommendation with moderate-quality evidence for treatment of leukostasis symptoms and should be considered as a weak recommendation for leukostasis prophylaxis in higher-risk AML patients (e.g., M4/M5 subtypes, rapidly rising blast count) with WBC $>100 \times 10^9$/L and ALL patients with WBC $>400 \times 10^9$/L (Schwartz et al. 2013). Per the ASFA guidelines, leukapheresis should not be utilized solely for the prevention or treatment of TLS in patients with HL (Schwartz et al. 2013). These recommendations are unchanged from the previous 2007 and 2010 ASFA guidelines (Szczepiorkowski et al. 2007, 2010). No specific contraindication to the use of leukapheresis in APL patients is included in these guidelines although it is mentioned as a relative contraindication in other guidelines due to the theoretical risk of worsening DIC and the increasing risk of ICH with lysis of leukemic promyelocytes (Blum and Porcu 2007; Szczepiorkowski et al. 2007; Sanz et al. 2009; Szczepiorkowski et al.

2010; Zuckerman et al. 2012; Kim and Sloan 2013; Schwartz et al. 2013). Data to support this contraindication are limited to one small study in which a majority of patients undergoing leukapheresis for HL had an adverse event that was not temporally related to the leukapheresis procedure (Vahdat et al. 1994; Tallman and Altman 2009). Strauss et al. (1985) successfully performed exchange transfusion on a 2-year-old child with APL and a presenting WBC count of 617×10^9/L. Zuckerman et al. (2012) recommend leukapheresis in symptomatic adult AML patients with WBC $>50 \times 10^9$/L and in symptomatic ALL and CML adult patients with WBC $>150 \times 10^9$/L. Additionally, although stating a lack of evidence, they recommend leukapheresis in asymptomatic adult AML patients with WBC $>100 \times 10^9$/L to prevent leukostasis and asymptomatic adult ALL patients with WBC $>300 \times 10^9$/L to prevent TLS.

Whether leukapheresis is an effective modality to reduce early mortality is controversial. McCarthy et al. (1997) studied 48 unselected adult and pediatric patients with WBC $>100 \times 10^9$/L who were leukoreduced and found no statistical difference in early mortality rate compared with similar unselected patients who were not leukoreduced. Porcu et al. (1997) similarly showed that effective leukapheresis did not impact early mortality in adult patients, especially those presenting with symptoms of leukostasis. Additional adult studies, mainly with AML patients, have had similar findings (Tan et al. 2005; Chang et al. 2007; De Santis et al. 2011). Others have found a significant improvement in early death rate in adult AML cohorts receiving leukapheresis without impact on overall survival (Thiébaut et al. 2000; Giles et al. 2001; Bug et al. 2007). Although multiple case reports and case series are available in the pediatric literature in regard to the effectiveness of exchange transfusion and leukapheresis in HL, significant pediatric data on resultant early mortality and long-term outcomes, especially in AML, are lacking (Carpentieri et al. 1979; Kamen et al. 1980; Shende et al. 1981; Warrier et al. 1981; Del Vasto et al. 1982; Strauss et al. 1985; Bunin et al. 1987; Sykes et al. 2011). Potential complications from apheresis procedures, especially in children, must also be considered, and such procedures should only be performed in specialized centers (Michon et al. 2007).

6.8 Other Treatment Modalities for Cytoreduction

Many older studies have utilized more conservative measures with success in cytoreduction for patients with HL. Such interventions may have a non-inferior impact on early death as compared to more invasive and expensive interventions such as leukapheresis.

6.8.1 Hyperhydration

Randomized controlled trials are lacking in regard to the benefits of hyperhydration although multiple small studies, especially in pediatric ALL, have shown significant decrement in the WBC count with hydration alone, obviating the need for leukapheresis (Maurer et al. 1988; Lascari 1991; Nelson et al. 1993; Basade et al. 1995).

6.8.2 Hydroxyurea

Berg et al. (1979) reported on an adult cohort of 87 AML patients who were pretreated with large doses of hydroxyurea and found no difference in early death or long-term outcome in those with and without HL. Hydroxyurea was effective in rapidly lowering the WBC count in the majority of patients. Grund et al. (1977) similarly showed that hydroxyurea was effective in decreasing WBC count in a small cohort of adult patients with acute leukemia.

6.8.3 Cranial Irradiation

Cranial radiotherapy has been noted as an effective cytoreductive technique for intracerebral leukostasis in both children and adult patients (Gilchrist et al. 1981; Ferro et al. 2014). Ferro et al. (2014) successfully utilized whole-brain radiation therapy to alleviate neurologic symptoms in an adult cohort with AML and HL. Maurer et al. (1988) showed no benefit of cranial irradiation in a pediatric ALL cohort with WBC $>200 \times 10^9$/L. Chang et al. (2007) utilized cranial irradiation and leukapheresis in adult patients with AML and HL and found no decrease in acute ICH or improved survival. Due to long-term neurologic sequelae, especially in young patients (i.e., <6 years), and risk for secondary malignancy, cranial irradiation has fallen out of favor (New 2001).

6.9 Other Supportive Care Considerations

6.9.1 Potential Laboratory Discrepancies

6.9.1.1 Pseudohyperkalemia
Hyperleukocytosis has been noted to cause pseudohyperkalemia due to increased fragility of blasts leading to cell rupture and increased potassium in the plasma sample. Cell lysis can occur secondary to minor mechanical stress such as pneumatic tube transport, prolonged tourniquet placement, vacutainer collection, manual shaking or centrifugation. Delayed analysis can also lead to hyperkalemia. Venous blood gas samples are a simple way to avoid such spurious results (Dimeski and Bird 2009).

6.9.1.2 Pseudohypoxemia
Due to the rapid consumption of oxygen by leukemic blasts, it is vital that blood gas samples be kept on ice and analyzed immediately to prevent spurious results (Fox et al. 1979; Hess et al. 1979; Shohat et al. 1988; Charoenratanakul and Loasuthi 1997). Generally the patient's clinical condition and pulse oximetry reading will correlate, obviating the need for blood gas measurement. Gartrell and Rosenstrauch (1993) note that methemoglobinemia may be underreported at diagnosis in patients with HL; modern pulse oximetry should correlate with blood gas results in these cases.

6.9.1.3 Pseudohypoglycemia

Consumption of glucose by excess leukocytes can lead to pseudohypoglycemia in patients with HL (Elrishi et al. 2010). Samples that are kept cold and run promptly can avoid this potential spurious result.

6.9.1.4 Pseudothrombocytosis

Leukemic blast lysis can lead to cell fragmentation which automated counters may read as platelets leading to an artificial increase in the platelet count. Since DIC is a common presentation with HL and platelet transfusion may be required to prevent bleeding with underlying true thrombocytopenia, it is important to examine the peripheral smear if the automated platelet count reading does not correlate with previous values or the status of the patient.

6.9.2 Transfusion Practice with Underlying Hyperleukocytosis

As described by Lichtman (1973), blood viscosity is usually unaltered in HL secondary to a decrease in the erythrocrit concomitant with the increased leukocrit. Therefore, blood transfusion should be avoided as it can lead to increased risk of leukostasis by increasing blood viscosity. Harris (1978) noted that the mean hemoglobin concentration was significantly higher in adult AML patients who suffered an early death with three patients dying soon after blood transfusion. Therefore, asymptomatic patients should not be transfused and in general hemoglobin concentration should be maintained below 10 g/dL (Harris 1978). Evidence regarding this recommendation in ALL patients is less clear (Lowe et al. 2005; Vaitkevičienė et al. 2013).

6.9.3 Anesthetic Procedures

Due to the risk of pulmonary complications, anesthesia should be undertaken with extreme care in the patient with HL but is often required due to the need for diagnostic procedures such as lumbar puncture and bone marrow aspiration. Fong et al. (2009) retrospectively reviewed 52

pediatric cases with HL that required anesthesia; 3 children required postanesthesia intensive care and 13 had less serious adverse events, all of a respiratory nature. In patients with respiratory distress or mediastinal mass at presentation, consideration should be given for utilizing peripheral blood for leukemia cytomorphology and cytogenetics rather than bone marrow aspiration (Vaitkevičienė et al. 2013).

6.10 Summary

Although significant gains have been made in the treatment of pediatric leukemia, notably ALL, APL, and CML, HL continues to pose risk both in regard to early death and decreased long-term survival. An evidence basis for supportive care guidelines is lacking in HL; yet, even without such consensus, intensive supportive care has significantly improved early death, especially in AML patients. Many patients who ultimately have early death present with features, chiefly ICH, for which no intervention will likely improve survival. Additionally, many therapies that have been suggested have no impact on overall survival; in fact, secondary to the underlying aggressive phenotypes, the overall survival is often shorter with HL. Based on the available evidence, we present our recommendations in Table 6.1. In general, prompt correction of coagulopathy, hypofibrinogenemia, thrombocytopenia, and hyperuricemia and rapid initiation of hydration and antileukemic therapy are vital management strategies for all patients with HL.

References

Azoulay É, Canet E, Raffoux E et al (2012) Dexamethasone in patients with acute lung injury from acute monocytic leukaemia. Eur Respir J 39:648–653

Basade M, Dhar AK, Kulkarni SS et al (1995) Rapid cytoreduction in childhood leukemic hyperleukocytosis by conservative therapy. Med Pediatr Oncol 25:204–207

Berg J, Vincent PC, Gunz FW (1979) Extreme leucocytosis and prognosis of newly diagnosed patients with acute non-lymphocytic leukaemia. Med J Aust 1: 480–482

Blum W, Porcu P (2007) Therapeutic apheresis in hyper-leukocytosis and hyperviscosity syndrome. Semin Thromb Hemost 33:350–354

Bug G, Anargyrou K, Tonn T et al (2007) Impact of leu-kapheresis on early death rate in adult acute myeloge-nous leukemia presenting with hyperleukocytosis. Transfusion 47:1843–1850

Bunin NJ, Pui CH (1985) Differing complications of hyperleukocytosis in children with acute lymphoblas-tic or acute nonlymphoblastic leukemia. J Clin Oncol 3:1590–1595

Bunin NJ, Kunkel K, Callihan TR (1987) Cytoreductive procedures in the early management in cases of leuke-mia and hyperleukocytosis in children. Med Pediatr Oncol 15:232–235

Cairo MS, Coiffier B, Reiter A et al (2010) Recommendations for the evaluation of risk and pro-phylaxis of tumour lysis syndrome (TLS) in adults and children with malignant diseases: an expert TLS panel consensus. Br J Haematol 149:578–586

Camacho LH, Soignet SL, Chanel S et al (2000) Leukocytosis and the retinoic acid syndrome in patients with acute promyelocytic leukemia treated with arsenic trioxide. J Clin Oncol 18:2620–2625

Carpentieri U, Patten EV, Chamberlin PA et al (1979) Leukapheresis in a 3-year-old with lymphoma in leu-kemic transformation. J Pediatr 94:919–921

Castagnetti M, Sainati L, Giona F et al (2008) Conservative management of priapism secondary to leukemia. Pediatr Blood Cancer 51:420–423

Chang MC, Chen TY, Tang JL et al (2007) Leukapheresis and cranial irradiation in patients with hyperleuko-cytic acute myeloid leukemia: no impact on early mor-tality and intracranial hemorrhage. Am J Hematol 82:976–980

Charoenratanakul S, Loasuthi K (1997) Pseudohypoxaemia in a patient with acute leukaemia. Thorax 52:394–395

Coiffier B, Altman A, Pui CH et al (2008) Guidelines for the management of pediatric and adult tumor lysis syndrome: an evidence-based review. J Clin Oncol 26:2767–2778

Creutzig U, Ritter J, Budde M et al (1987) Early deaths due to hemorrhage and leukostasis in childhood acute myelog-enous leukemia: associations with hyperleukocytosis and acute monocytic leukemia. Cancer 60:3071–3079

Creutzig U, Zimmermann M, Reinhardt D et al (2004) Early deaths and treatment-related mortality in chil-dren undergoing therapy for acute myeloid leukemia: analysis of the multicenter clinical trials AML-BFM 93 and AML-BFM 98. J Clin Oncol 22:4384–4393

da Costa CM, de Carmargo B, Gutierrez y Lamelas R et al (1999) Cardiac tamponade complicating hyperleuko-cytosis in a child with leukemia. Med Pediatr Oncol 32:120–123

de Botton S, Coiteux V, Chevret S et al (2004) Outcome of childhood acute promyelocytic leukemia with all-trans-retinoic acid and chemotherapy. J Clin Oncol 22:1404–1412

De Santis GC, de Oliveira LC, Romano LG et al (2011) Therapeutic leukapheresis in patients with leukostasis secondary to acute myelogenous leukemia. J Clin Apher 26:181–185

Del Vasto F, Caldore M, Russo F et al (1982) Exchange transfusion in leukemia with hyperleukocytosis. J Pediatr 100:1000

Dimeski G, Bird R (2009) Hyperleukocytosis: pseudohy-perkalemia and other biochemical abnormalities in hyperleukocytosis. Clin Chem Lab Med 47:880–881

Dutcher JP, Schiffer CA, Wiernik PH (1987) Hyperleukocytosis in adult acute nonlymphocytic leu-kemia: impact on remission rate and duration, and sur-vival. J Clin Oncol 5:1364–1372

Eguiguren JM, Schell MJ, Crist WM et al (1992) Complications and outcome in childhood acute lym-phoblastic leukemia with hyperleukocytosis. Blood 79:871–875

Elrishi MA, Simpson AI, Bradley EJ et al (2010) Artifactual hypoglycaemia secondary to leukaemoid reaction. Pract Diab Int 27:62–63

Ferro A, Jabbour SK, Taunk NK et al (2014) Cranial irra-diation in adults diagnosed with acute myelogenous leukemia presenting with hyperleukocytosis and neu-rologic dysfunction. Leuk Lymphoma 55:105–109

Fong C, Fung W, McDonald J et al (2009) Anesthesia for children with hyperleukocytosis a retrospective review. Paediatr Anaesth 19:1191–1198

Fox MJ, Brody JS, Weintraub LR (1979) Leukocyte lar-ceny: a cause of spurious hypoxemia. Am J Med 67:742–746

Frankel SR, Eardley A, Lauwers G et al (1992) The "reti-noic acid syndrome" in acute promyelocytic leukemia. Ann Intern Med 117:292–296

Gartrell K, Rosenstrauch W (1993) Hypoxaemia in patients with hyperleukocytosis: true or spurious, and clinical implications. Leuk Res 17:915–919

Gaynon PS, Angiolillo AL, Carroll WL et al (2010) Long-term results of the children's cancer group studies for childhood acute lymphoblastic leukemia 1983–2002: a Children's Oncology Group Report. Leukemia 24:285–297

Gilchrist GS, Fountain KS, Dearth JC et al (1981) Cranial irradiation in the management of extreme leukemic leukocytosis complicating childhood acute lympho-cytic leukemia. J Pediatr 98:257–259

Giles FJ, Shen Y, Kantarijian HM et al (2001) Leukapheresis reduces early mortality in patients with acute myeloid leukemia with high white cell counts but does not improve long term survival. Leuk Lymphoma 42:67–73

Gregory J, Kim H, Alonzo T et al (2009) Treatment of children with acute promyelocytic leukemia: results of the first North American intergroup trial INT0129. Pediatr Blood Cancer 53:1005–1010

Grund FM, Armitage JO, Burns CP (1977) Hydroxyurea in the prevention of the effects of leukostasis in acute leukemia. Arch Intern Med 137:1246–1247

Guglielmi C, Martelli MP, Diverio D et al (1998) Immunophenotype of adult and childhood acute pro-myelocytic leukaemia: correlation with morphology, type of PML gene breakpoint and clinical outcome. A cooperative Italian study on 196 cases. Br J Haematol 102:1035–1041

Guyatt G, Gutterman D, Baumann MH et al (2006) Grading strength of recommendations and quality of evidence in clinical guidelines: report from an American College of Chest Physicians Task Force. Chest 129:174–181

Harris AL (1978) Leukostasis associated with blood transfusion in acute myeloid leukaemia. Br Med J 1: 1169–1171

Hess CE, Nichols AB, Hunt WB et al (1979) Pseudohypoxemia secondary to leukemia and thrombocytosis. N Engl J Med 301:361–363

Howard SC, Jones DP, Pui CH (2011) The tumor lysis syndrome. N Engl J Med 364:1844–1854

Hug V, Keating M, McCredie K et al (1983) Clinical course and response to treatment of patients with acute myelogenous leukemia presenting with a high leukocyte count. Cancer 52:773–779

Inaba H, Fan Y, Pounds S et al (2008) Clinical and biologic features and treatment outcome of children with newly diagnosed acute myeloid leukemia and hyperleukocytosis. Cancer 113:522–529

Kamen BA, Summers CP, Pearson HA (1980) Exchange transfusion as a treatment for hyperleukocytosis, anemia, and metabolic abnormalities in a patient with leukemia. J Pediatr 96:1045–1046

Kim YA, Sloan SR (2013) Pediatric therapeutic apheresis: rationale and indications for plasmapheresis, cytapheresis, extracorporeal photopheresis, and LDL apheresis. Pediatr Clin N Am 60:1569–1580

Kim H, Lee JH, Choi SJ et al (2006) Risk score model for fatal intracranial hemorrhage in acute leukemia. Leukemia 20:770–776

Lange BJ, Smith FO, Feusner J et al (2008) Outcomes in CCG-2961, a Children's Oncology Group Phase 3 Trial for untreated pediatric acute myeloid leukemia: a report from the Children's Oncology Group. Blood 111:1044–1053

Lascari AD (1991) Improvement of leukemic hyperleukocytosis with only fluid and allopurinol therapy. Am J Dis Child 145:969–970

Levy M, Wofford MM, Powell BL et al (2008) Hyperleukocytosis from arsenic trioxide. Pediatr Blood Cancer 50:1265–1267

Lichtman MA (1973) Rheology of leukocytes, leukocyte suspensions, and blood in leukemia. J Clin Invest 52:350–358

Lowe EJ, Pui CH, Hancock ML et al (2005) Early complications in children with acute lymphoblastic leukemia presenting with hyperleukocytosis. Pediatr Blood Cancer 45:10–15

Lund B, Åsberg A, Heyman M et al (2011) Risk factors for treatment related mortality in childhood acute lymphoblastic leukaemia. Pediatr Blood Cancer 56: 551–559

Maurer HS, Steinherz PG, Gaynon PS et al (1988) The effect of initial management of hyperleukocytosis on early complications and outcome of children with acute lymphoblastic leukemia. J Clin Oncol 6:1425–1432

McCarthy LJ, Danielson CF, Rothenberger SS (1997) Indications for emergency apheresis procedures. Crit Rev Clin Lab Sci 34:573–610

McKee LC Jr, Collins RD (1974) Intravascular leukocyte thrombi and aggregates as a cause of morbidity and mortality in leukemia. Medicine (Baltimore) 53:463–478

Meshinchi S, Woods WG, Stirewalt DL et al (2001) Prevalence and prognostic significance of Flt3 internal tandem duplication in pediatric acute myeloid leukemia. Blood 97:89–94

Michon B, Moghrabi A, Winikoff R et al (2007) Complications of apheresis in children. Transfusion 47:1837–1842

Millot F, Traore P, Guilhot J et al (2005) Clinical and biological features at diagnosis in 40 children with chronic myeloid leukemia. Pediatrics 116:140–143

Montague DK, Jarow J, Broderick GA et al (2003) American Urological Association guideline on the management of priapism. J Urol 170:1318–1324

Montesinos P, Lorenzo I, Martín G et al (2008) Tumor lysis syndrome in patients with acute myeloid leukemia: identification of risk factors and development of a predictive model. Haematologica 93:67–74

Möricke A, Reiter A, Zimmermann M et al (2008) Risk-adjusted therapy of acute lymphoblastic leukemia can decrease treatment burden and improve survival: treatment results of 2169 unselected pediatric and adolescent patients enrolled in the trial ALL-BFM 95. Blood 111:4477–4489

Nelson SC, Bruggers CS, Kurtzberg J et al (1993) Management of leukemic hyperleukocytosis with hydration, urinary alkalinization, and allopurinol. Are cranial irradiation and invasive cytoreduction necessary? Am J Pediatr Hematol Oncol 15:351–355

New P (2001) Radiation injury to the nervous system. Curr Opin Neurol 14:725–734

Novotny JR, Müller-Beissenhirtz H, Herget-Rosenthal S et al (2005) Grading of symptoms in hyperleukocytic leukaemia: a clinical model for the role of different blast types and promyelocytes in the development of leukostasis syndrome. Eur J Haematol 74:501–510

Oberoi S, Lehrnbecher T, Phillips B et al (2014) Leukapheresis and low-dose chemotherapy do not reduce early mortality in acute myeloid leukemia hyperleukocytosis: a systematic review and meta-analysis. Leuk Res 38:460–468

Porcu P, Danielson CF, Orazi A et al (1997) Therapeutic leukapheresis in hyperleucocytic leukaemias: lack of correlation between degree of cytoreduction and early mortality rate. Br J Haematol 98:433–436

Porcu P, Cripe LD, Ng EW et al (2000) Hyperleukocytic leukemias and leukostasis: a review of pathophysiology, clinical presentation and management. Leuk Lymphoma 39:1–18

Pui CH, Behm FG, Singh B et al (1990) Heterogeneity of presenting features and their relation to treatment outcome in 120 children with T-cell acute lymphoblastic leukemia. Blood 75:174–179

Roberts TF, Sprague K, Schenkein D et al (2000) Hyperleukocytosis during induction therapy with arsenic trioxide for relapsed acute promyelocytic leukemia associated with central nervous system infarction. Blood 96:4000–4001

Rogers R, Latif Z, Copland M (2012) How I manage priapism in chronic myeloid leukemia patients. Br J Haematol 158:155–164

Rovelli A, Biondi A, Rajnoldi AC et al (1992) Microgranular variant of acute promyelocytic leukemia in children. J Clin Oncol 10:1413–1418

Rowe JM, Lichtman MA (1984) Hyperleukocytosis and leukostasis: common features of childhood chronic myelogenous leukemia. Blood 63:1230–1234

Sanz MA, Tallman MS, Lo-Coco F (2005) Tricks of the trade for the appropriate management of newly diagnosed acute promyelocytic leukemia. Blood 105: 3019–3025

Sanz MA, Grimwade D, Tallman MS et al (2009) Management of acute promyelocytic leukemia: recommendations from an expert panel on behalf of the European LeukemiaNet. Blood 113:1875–1891

Schwartz JH, Canellos GP (1975) Hydroxyurea in the management of the hematologic complications of chronic granulocytic leukemia. Blood 46:11–16

Schwartz J, Winters JL, Padmanabhan A et al (2013) Guidelines on the use of therapeutic apheresis in clinical practice—evidence-based approach from the Writing Committee of the American Society for Apheresis: the sixth Special Issue. J Clin Apher 28:145–284

Shende A, Festa R, Honigman R et al (1981) Exchange transfusion as a treatment for hyperleukocytosis, anemia, and metabolic abnormalities in patients with leukemia. J Pediatr 98:851–852

Shohat M, Schonfeld T, Zaizoz T et al (1988) Determination of blood gases in children with extreme leukocytosis. Crit Care Med 16:787–788

Soares FA, Landell GA, Cardoso MC (1992) Pulmonary leukostasis without hyperleukocytosis: a clinicopathologic study of 16 cases. Am J Hematol 40:28–32

Strauss RA, Gloster DS, McCallister JA et al (1985) Acute cytoreduction techniques in the early treatment of hyperleukocytosis associated with childhood hematologic malignancies. Med Pediatr Oncol 13:346–351

Stucki A, Rivier AS, Gikic M et al (2001) Endothelial cell activation by myeloblasts: molecular mechanisms of leukostasis and leukemic cell dissemination. Blood 97:2121–2129

Sung L, Aplenc R, Alonzo TA et al (2012) Predictors and short-term outcomes of hyperleukocytosis in children with acute myeloid leukemia: a report from the Children's Oncology Group. Haematologica 97: 1770–1773

Sykes JA, Kalyanaraman M, Kamalakar P et al (2011) Acute lymphoblastic leukemia with hyperleukocytosis, sinus pauses, and hypoxemic respiratory failure in an infant. Pediatr Emerg Care 27:212–214

Szczepiorkowski ZM, Bandarenko N, Kim HC et al (2007) Guidelines on the use of therapeutic apheresis in clinical practice—evidence-based approach from the Apheresis Applications Committee of the American Society for Apheresis. J Clin Apher 22:106–175

Szczepiorkowski ZM, Winters JL, Bandarenko N et al (2010) Guidelines on the use of therapeutic apheresis in clinical practice—evidence-based approach from the Apheresis Applications Committee of the American Society for Apheresis. J Clin Apher 25:83–177

Tallman MS, Altman JK (2009) How I treat acute promyelocytic leukemia. Blood 114:5126–5135

Tan D, Hwang W, Goh YT (2005) Therapeutic leukapheresis in hyperleukocytic leukemias—the experience of a tertiary institution in Singapore. Ann Acad Med Singapore 34:229–234

Thiébaut A, Thomas X, Belhabri A et al (2000) Impact of pre-induction therapy leukapheresis on treatment outcome in adult acute myelogenous leukemia presenting with hyperleukocytosis. Ann Hematol 79: 501–506

Tosi P, Barosi G, Lazzaro C et al (2008) Consensus conference on the management of tumor lysis syndrome. Haematologica 93:1877–1885

Truong TH, Beyene J, Hitzler J et al (2007) Features at presentation predict children with acute lymphoblastic leukemia at low risk for tumor lysis syndrome. Cancer 110:1832–1839

Vahdat L, Maslak P, Miller WH Jr et al (1994) Early mortality and the retinoic acid syndrome in acute promyelocytic leukemia: impact of leukocytosis, low-dose chemotherapy, PMN/RAR-alpha isoform, and CD13 expression in patients treated with all-trans retinoic acid. Blood 84:3843–3849

Vaitkevičienė G, Forestier E, Hellebostad M et al (2009) High white blood cell count at diagnosis of childhood acute lymphoblastic leukaemia: biological background and prognostic impact. Results from the NOPHO ALL-92 and ALL-2000 studies. Eur J Haematol 86:38–46

Vaitkevičienė G, Heyman M, Jonsson OG et al (2013) Early morbidity and mortality in childhood acute lymphoblastic leukemia with very high white blood cell count. Leukemia 27:2259–2262

Wald BR, Heisel MA, Ortega JA (1982) Frequency of early death in children with acute leukemia presenting with hyperleukocytosis. Cancer 50:150–153

Warrier RP, Ravindranath Y, Emami A et al (1981) Exchange transfusion for hyperleukocytosis, anemia, and metabolic abnormalities in leukemia. J Pediatr 98:338–339

Wiley JS, Firkin FC (1995) Reduction of pulmonary toxicity by prednisolone prophylaxis during all-trans retinoic acid treatment of acute promyelocytic leukemia. Australian Leukaemia Study Group. Leukemia 9:774–778

Würthner JU, Köhler G, Behringer D et al (1999) Leukostasis followed by hemorrhage complicating the initiation of chemotherapy in patients with acute myeloid leukemia and hyperleukocytosis. Cancer 85:368–374

Zhang L, Zhao H, Zhu X et al (2008) Retrospective analysis of 65 Chinese children with acute promyelocytic leukemia: a single center experience. Pediatr Blood Cancer 51:210–215

Zhou J, Zhang Y, Li J et al (2010) Single-agent arsenic trioxide in the treatment of children with newly diagnosed acute promyelocytic leukemia. Blood 115:1697–1702

Zuckerman T, Ganzel C, Tallman MS et al (2012) How I treat hematologic emergencies in adults with acute leukemia. Blood 120:1993–2002

The Acute Abdomen

7

Monica Khurana and Wendy Su

Contents

M. Khurana
Division of Hematology/Oncology,
Riley Children's Hospital,
Indianapolis, IN, USA

W. Su (✉)
Division of Pediatric Surgery,
Children's Hospital and Research Center Oakland,
747 52nd Street, Oakland, CA 94609, USA
e-mail: wsu@mail.cho.org

Abstract

Pediatric oncology patients develop similar abdominal emergencies as immunocompetent children in addition to acute abdomen from malignancy or secondary to treatment. Cytotoxic chemotherapy, radiotherapy and extensive surgical resection all contribute to the risk of gastrointestinal symptoms. Immunocompromised children may lack the inflammatory signs of acute abdomen making prompt diagnosis of pediatric oncologic abdominal emergencies challenging. Here we review the most common abdominal emergencies secondary to malignancy including gastrointestinal hemorrhage, infection, mechanical obstruction, and perforation as well as management strategies for these conditions. A high index of suspicion and a prompt multidisciplinary approach are essential for optimal patient care. Early initiation of aggressive medical management reduces the need for invasive surgical treatment and concomitantly improves mortality rates. As there is a lack of evidence-based guidelines, the reviewed recommendations for supportive care and treatment of pediatric oncologic abdominal emergencies predominantly stem from expert opinion.

J. Feusner et al. (eds.), *Supportive Care in Pediatric Oncology:
A Practical Evidence-Based Approach*, Pediatric Oncology,
DOI 10.1007/978-3-662-44317-0_7, © Springer Berlin Heidelberg 2015

7.1 Introduction

Pediatric oncology patients develop similar abdominal emergencies as immunocompetent children in addition to acute abdomen from malignancy or secondary to treatment (Fisher and Rheingold 2011). Cytotoxic chemotherapy, radiotherapy and extensive surgical resection all contribute to the risk of gastrointestinal (GI) symptoms. Pain is the most common and sensitive clinical symptom of an abdominal emergency; however, immunocompromised patients often lack the inflammatory response needed to elicit and localize signs of an acute abdomen making prompt diagnosis of pediatric oncologic abdominal emergencies challenging (Silliman et al. 1994; Fisher and Rheingold 2011; Andreyev et al. 2012).

In general, the most common abdominal emergencies secondary to malignancy are GI hemorrhage, infection, mechanical obstruction and perforation (Haut 2005; Pizzo 2011). Table 7.1 outlines the causes of abdominal pain in children with cancer and Table 7.2 the most common diagnoses associated with acute abdomen. A high index of suspicion and prompt multidisciplinary approach including surgical consultation are essential for optimal patient care (Arul and Spicer 2008; Fisher and Rheingold 2011). Detailed history and physical examination are of paramount importance to aid in establishing the differential diagnosis. Appropriate laboratory studies and diagnostic imaging can provide clues to etiology and location of pathology. Early initiation of aggressive medical management reduces the need for invasive measures and improves mortality rates (Yip and Goddard 2010). However, given the lack of randomized therapeutic trials, current recommendations for supportive care and treatment of pediatric oncologic abdominal emergencies stem from expert opinion and are summarized and graded in Table 7.3.

Table 7.1 Gastrointestinal side effects of cancer therapy

Treatment modality	Potential side effects
Chemotherapy	Bacterial overgrowth
	Bile acid malabsorption
	Pancreatic insufficiency
	Neutropenic enterocolitis
	Edema, ulceration, atrophy
	Increased bowel permeability
	Transmural infection
Radiation therapy	Radiation enteritis
	Stricture
	Inflammation/cell death
	Progressive ischemia
	Fibrosis
	Loss of stem cells
Surgery	Ileus
	Adhesion formation
	Postoperative intussusception

Table 7.2 Etiology of acute abdomen in pediatric oncology patients

Clinical scenario	Underlying etiologies
Infection	Bacterial
	Viral
	Fungal
	Opportunistic
Inflammation (acute)	Neutropenic enterocolitis
	Perforation
	Graft-versus-host disease
	Pancreatitis
	Perirectal abscess
	Appendicitis
Inflammation (chronic)	Bowel obstruction
	Adhesions/strictures
	Intussusception
	Graft-versus-host disease
	Pancreatitis
Ischemia	Mesenteric ischemia
Metabolic	Malabsorption
	Hepatic insufficiency
	VIP secretion
Vascular	Mesenteric vascular insufficiency
	Mesenteric thrombosis
	Venoocclusive disease/sinusoidal obstructive syndrome
Primary tumor/secondary malignancy	Obstruction
	Perforation
	Hemorrhage
	Abdominal compartment syndrome
	Pancreatitis
Congenital/anatomic	Meckel's diverticulum
	Intestinal duplication

VIP vasoactive intestinal peptide

7.2   Gastrointestinal Infection

Infection is a common complication of children undergoing cancer treatment; nearly one-third of these infections originate from the GI tract (Hobson et al. 2005). GI tract infection results from direct chemotherapeutic toxicity, opportunistic infections, and common conditions such as rotavirus or *Clostridium difficile* that also affect healthy children. Typhlitis and appendicitis were the most common surgical complications

in pediatric leukemia patients, occurring at frequencies of 1.7 % and 1.5 %, respectively, among children treated at a single institution (Hobson et al. 2005). Detailed history and physical exam, neutrophil count, stool cultures, and appropriate diagnostic imaging studies are necessary to establish the correct diagnosis and guide treatment. When the etiology remains unclear, diagnostic laparoscopy offers a minimally invasive approach to visually inspect the peritoneal cavity.

Table 7.3 Summary of treatment strategies and level of evidence for management of acute abdomen[a]

Clinical scenario	Recommendations	Level of evidence[b]
Neutropenic enterocolitis/typhlitis	Initial evaluation with ultrasound	1C
	CT if high clinical suspicion and US nondiagnostic	1C
	Initial complete gut rest (NPO)	2C
	Parenteral nutrition while NPO	1C
	Nasogastric suction for decompression	2C
	Narcotics for analgesia	1C
	Consideration for GCSF utilization	2C
	Broad antimicrobial coverage	1C
	Surgery only if supportive care fails to improve clinical picture	1C
Appendicitis	Initial evaluation with US	1C
	CT if US equivocal	1C
	Surgical management if strong concern for appendicitis based on exam or imaging findings	1C
Perirectal abscess	Sitz baths for symptomatic relief	1C
	Laxatives and stool softeners to minimize painful defecation and prevent trauma	1C
	Broad-spectrum antibiotics	1C
	Surgery only if supportive care fails to improve clinical picture	1C
GI hemorrhage	Acute stabilization; fluid support, PRBC transfusion, vasopressors	1C
	Elevate head of bed to 30–45°	2C
	Keep hemoglobin >8 g/dL and platelets >75 × 10⁹/L	1C
	Correction of coagulopathy with FFP	1C
	Consideration for gastric lavage	2C
	Endoscopic evaluation and management	1C
Pancreatitis	CT with IV contrast for evaluation	1C
	Consideration for US as primary imaging modality	2C
	Early introduction of enteral feeding	1C
	Early oral refeeding in those with mild pancreatitis	2C
	Narcotics for analgesia	1C
	Antiemetics as needed	1C
	Broad-spectrum antibiotics in the patient with necrotic pancreatitis and clinical deterioration	1B
	Consideration for octreotide	2C

(continued)

Table 7.3 (continued)

Clinical scenario	Recommendations	Level of evidence[b]
Bowel obstruction	Initial evaluation with KUB followed by abdominal CT	1C
	Avoidance of barium in neutropenic patients	1C
	Initial complete gut rest (NPO)	1C
	Parenteral nutrition while NPO	1C
	Nasogastric suction for decompression	1C
	Narcotics for analgesia	1C
	Antiemetics as needed	1C
	Surgery if with persistent bleeding, intraperitoneal perforation, clinical deterioration, or presence of a mass	1C
Tumor rupture/organ perforation	Acute stabilization; fluid support, PRBC transfusion, vasopressors	1C
	Initial complete gut rest (NPO)	1C
	Nasogastric suction for decompression	1C
	Broad-spectrum antibiotics	1C
	Surgical evaluation/intervention	1C
Abdominal compartment syndrome	Diagnosis based on IAP $\geq$20 mmHg	2C
	Nasogastric suction for decompression	1C
	Avoidance of elevation of head of bed, sedatives, and analgesics which may all increase IAP	2C
	Percutaneous catheter decompression of intraperitoneal air or fluid	1C
	Optimize fluid balance with hypertonic crystalloids and colloids	1C

CT computed tomography, *US* ultrasound, *NPO* nothing by mouth, *GCSF* granulocyte colony-stimulating factor, *GI* gastrointestinal, *PRBC* packed red blood cell, *FFP* fresh frozen plasma, *IV* intravenous, *KUB* kidney, ureter, bladder, *IAP* intra-abdominal pressure
[a]See text for full detail
[b]Per Guyatt et al. (2006); see Preface

7.2.1 Neutropenic Enterocolitis

Neutropenic enterocolitis refers to necrotizing inflammation of the small or large intestine that occurs in the setting of neutropenia. Typhlitis specifically refers to necrotizing inflammation of the cecum, the most commonly affected bowel segment (Arul and Spicer 2008). Though usually seen with prolonged neutropenia (i.e., >7 days), typhlitis has been reported without neutropenia (McCarville et al. 2005). The watershed vasculature and distensibility of the cecum may explain its predilection for infection compared to other bowel segments. With earlier diagnosis and intervention, current mortality rates for typhlitis are approximately 2.5 % (Haut 2005; Pizzo 2011). Factors that may contribute to the development of neutropenic enterocolitis include: (1) prophylactic antibiotics which alter normal

colonic flora; (2) cytotoxic chemotherapy which disrupts the bowel mucosal barrier permitting microbial and fungal invasion which may lead to hemorrhage and necrosis; and (3) prolonged neutropenia which prevents adequate infection clearance and predisposes to sepsis (Arul and Spicer 2008).

Bacterial pathogens account for >90 % of enterocolitic infection. The most common bacterial pathogens include *Escherichia coli*, *Pseudomonas aeruginosa* and *Clostridium difficile* (Haut 2005). Less common bacterial pathogens include coagulase-negative staphylococcus and alpha-hemolytic streptococcus. The most common fungal pathogens are *Candida* spp. (Albano and Sandler 2004; Fisher and Rheingold 2011; Pizzo 2011). Typhlitis typically develops in patients >10 years of age and within 2–3 weeks of receiving intensive chemotherapy (McCarville et al. 2005; Sundell et al. 2012). Case series suggest that patients with acute myelogenous leukemia (AML) are at high risk for typhlitis in any phase of therapy (Gray et al. 2010).

Symptoms of neutropenic enterocolitis are nonspecific and highly variable and include abdominal pain, vomiting, diarrhea and GI bleeding (McCarville et al. 2005; Sundell et al. 2012). Signs can include fever, abdominal distension, tachycardia, hypotension, sepsis, and peritoneal irritation that can be diffuse or localized to the right lower quadrant (Sundell et al. 2012). Uncommonly a cecal mass is palpable (Haut 2005; Gray et al. 2010). Appendicitis, pancreatitis, pseudomembranous colitis, intussusception, and pelvic or peritoneal abscess should be considered in the differential diagnosis.

In the neutropenic patient with acute abdominal pain, a two-view plain radiograph should first be obtained as it may show an appendicolith, pneumatosis, or free air. Plain radiographs may support the diagnosis of enterocolitis with findings of pneumatosis and bowel wall thickening although most findings are nonspecific (Fisher and Rheingold 2011; Pizzo 2011; Sundell et al. 2012). Presence of free air will require immediate surgical consultation and intervention. Contrast enema is contraindicated if neutropenic enterocolitis is suspected as it may lead to perforation (Arul and Spicer 2008; Morgan et al. 2011). Ultrasound (US) is the preferred imaging modality for demonstrating bowel wall thickening (McCarville et al. 2005). A diagnosis of enterocolitis consists of bowel wall thickening >3 mm, and mortality rates increase when bowel wall thickening exceeds 10 mm (Pizzo 2011; Sundell et al. 2012). If US results are inconclusive, computed tomography (CT) is the current definitive imaging study (Cloutier 2010; Pizzo 2011). CT is very sensitive for identifying cecal wall thickening, transmural inflammation, soft tissue masses and pneumatosis. A characteristic feature of typhlitis on CT is necrosis localized to the cecum. Both US and CT may reveal a target sign, an echogenic center with a wide hypoechogenic periphery, at the cecum in typhlitis. CT may overestimate bowel wall thickening leading to false-positive diagnoses of enterocolitis and

typhlitis. Magnetic resonance imaging (MRI) for the diagnosis of neutropenic enterocolitis has not been reported in the medical literature.

Supportive management of enterocolitis has typically included complete gut rest (NPO) during the acute phase of symptomatic pain, parenteral nutrition while NPO and nasogastric suctioning for decompression (Sundell et al. 2012). However, evidence regarding the benefit of these interventions is lacking. Narcotics should be utilized for analgesia. Vasopressor support may be required; hypotension is associated with poor outcome. Patients may require packed red blood cell and platelet transfusions (Albano and Sandler 2004; Pizzo 2011). The utility of granulocyte colony-stimulating factor (GCSF) in patients with enterocolitis is unclear, and the use of GCSF is discussed in more detail in Chap. 15. A non-evidence-based argument to support GCSF use is generally that resolution of neutropenia parallels resolution of typhlitis (Fisher and Rheingold 2011). On the other hand, GCSF could theoretically increase inflammation and cause obstruction.

Early imaging and rapid initiation of antimicrobials are vital, as these interventions may decrease mortality in neutropenic enterocolitis. Antibacterial therapy should be broad to cover for enteric pathogens, especially Gram-negative and anaerobic microbes in addition to Gram-positive enterococcal species. Cloutier (2010) suggests that monotherapy with piperacillin-tazobactam or imipenem-cilastatin or dual therapy with either ceftazidime or cefepime with metronidazole is sufficient initial coverage for neutropenic enterocolitis. Metronidazole is the generally preferred anaerobic coverage given the similar clinical features of typhlitis and pseudomembranous enterocolitis due to *C. difficile* (Sundell et al. 2012). Such regimens have not been specifically studied in pediatric neutropenic enterocolitis.

Typhlitis is an oncologic emergency because it may lead to bowel obstruction or perforation requiring surgical intervention (Haut 2005). Consultation with surgery should be requested early, even if surgery is not anticipated. Surgery should be deferred until supportive therapy has clearly failed or the following complications develop: perforation, hemorrhage despite correction of thrombocytopenia and coagulopathies, obstruction, necrosis, abscess or peritonitis requiring drainage, fistula, toxic megacolon, or septic shock (Gray et al. 2010; Morgan et al. 2011; Sundell et al. 2012). Surgery consists of visualization and management of bleeding, resecting necrotic portions of the bowel, and possible transient diversion via colostomy (Pizzo 2011).

7.2.2 Appendicitis

Incidence of appendicitis in pediatric leukemia and lymphoma is the same as the general population, ranging from 0.5–1.5 % (Hobson et al. 2005; Fisher and Rheingold 2011). Signs and symptoms of appendicitis may overlap with neutropenic colitis; in the patient who does not improve with medical management for enterocolitis, the physician should consider appendicitis (Albano and Sandler 2004). In the review by Hobson et al. (2005), they found that pediatric oncology patients had inconsistent clinical signs and symptoms of appendicitis, routinely lacked fever and often lacked localizing signs on abdominal exam. However, in a similar cohort, Chui et al. (2008) reported that fever was common and the majority presented with localizing abdominal signs prior to surgery. In both cohorts, a delay in diagnosis was common (Hobson et al. 2005; Chui et al. 2008).

Although a KUB may show an appendicolith to diagnosis appendicitis, a staged protocol with US followed by CT in those patients with an equivocal US has been found accurate and cost-efficient in the regular pediatric population while reducing radiation exposure (Wan et al. 2009; Krishnamoorthi et al. 2011). Whether this methodology is effective for pediatric oncology patients is unknown. Hobson et al. (2005) noted that CT evaluation was not accurate in their cohort of pediatric oncology patients, with only 2 of 7 patients having classic CT findings. Again, Chui et al. (2008) reported dissimilar results as 8 of 10 patients had CT imaging consistent with appendicitis. Additionally, patients with typhlitis

have been noted to have appendiceal thickening of uncertain significance in a small percentage of cases and not correlated with development of appendicitis (McCarville et al. 2004). Isolated appendiceal typhlitis has also been noted in case reports (McAteer et al. 2014).

Management of acute appendicitis during neutropenic episodes remains somewhat controversial. Small case series have shown that medical management with broad spectrum antibiotics has resulted in resolution of symptoms without recurrence (Wiegering et al. 2008). Others suggest that surgery remains the definitive treatment modality even in the presence of neutropenia, with the antecedent potential for infectious complications and delayed wound healing, given the potential risks of ruptured appendicitis (Hobson et al. 2005; Chui et al. 2008). It is unclear if those patients who were medically managed had appendicitis or rather isolated appendiceal typhlitis. It has also been argued that pediatric oncology patients undergoing a primary abdominal operation have incidental appendectomy to decrease future risk of appendicitis especially during periods of neutropenia (Steinberg et al. 1999).

7.2.3 Perirectal Abscess

Prolonged severe neutropenia can also lead to the development of perirectal abscess. Most abscesses are polymicrobial, including Gram-negative, Gram-positive and anaerobic organisms. Commonly seen microbes are *E. coli*, *P. aeruginosa*, and staphylococcal and streptococcal species (Pizzo 2011). Perirectal abscesses are often occult. Patients infrequently complain of anorectal pain, which can be independent of defecation. Since neutropenia precludes the development of purulence, exam may yield only erythema, tenderness to anorectal palpation, edema or cellulitis (Pizzo 2011). Perianal examination is essential in the neutropenic patient to monitor for this potential complication; rectal examination should be avoided due to concern for damaging friable mucosa and introducing bacteria (Büyükaşik et al. 1988; Wolfe and Kennedy 2011; Mercer-Falkoff and Lacy 2013).

Initial medical management of perirectal abscess includes sitz baths to provide symptomatic relief as well as laxatives and stool softeners to minimize painful defecation and prevent fissures and tears. As with enterocolitis, broad-spectrum parenteral antibiotics should be utilized. GCSF can be considered in the neutropenic patient although there is no evidence to support its usage. Surgical management may include incision and drainage, debridement, or further intervention but only if there is a fluctuant mass, large amounts of necrotic tissue, progression to necrotizing fasciitis, or a persistent fistula (Arul and Spicer 2008; Pizzo 2011).

7.3 Gastrointestinal Hemorrhage

Severe GI hemorrhage requires immediate medical, and potentially, surgical intervention. Common etiologies include gastritis or esophagitis, ulcers, necrotizing pancreatitis, primary GI tumors, infection, and radiation-induced inflammation and microvascular damage (i.e., mucosal telangiectasias). Hemorrhagic gastritis of varying severity may occur in almost half of pediatric oncology patients (Kaste et al. 1999). Common etiologies of ulcer formation include peptic ulcer disease, infection, increased intracranial pressure stimulating the vagal nerve and parietal cells (Cushing's ulcer), and steroids. Esophageal bleeding results from progressive esophageal varices associated with portal hypertension or Mallory-Weiss tears with repeated emesis. Tumors precipitate bleeding by vascular infiltration or abnormal tumor vessel growth (direct damage) as well as infarctions and lacerations via mass effect (indirect damage). Common infectious agents that may trigger significant bleeding include fungi such as *Candida* spp., viral pathogens including *Herpesviridae*, *C. difficile*, and the opportunistic protozoan cryptosporidium (Kaste et al. 1999; Fisher and Rheingold 2011). Sepsis and disseminated intravascular coagulation can exacerbate bleeding. Anti-angiogenic chemotherapeutic agents such as bevacizumab, sunitinib, and sorafenib can cause severe

bleeding, poor wound healing, and gastric perforation; such adverse manifestations should prompt immediate discontinuation. Ginkgo biloba, a commonly utilized nutritional supplement for fatigue, depression and memory loss, has been associated with an increased bleeding risk (Demshar et al. 2011). Oncology patients should avoid aspirin and nonsteroidal anti-inflammatory drugs (NSAIDs) to reduce bleeding risk.

Signs and symptoms of GI hemorrhage vary. Symptoms include pain, hematemesis, melena or hematochezia, and anemia-induced symptoms and signs such as fatigue, headache, dizziness, syncope, dyspnea, pallor, and oliguria. To prevent aspiration, the patient's head of the bed should be at an angle of 30–45° (Fisher and Rheingold 2011). In the patient with signs or symptoms of volume depletion, immediate bolus intravenous isotonic crystalloid fluids should be initiated and type O⁻ red blood cells considered while awaiting results of blood counts and for preparation of crossmatched packed red blood cells. If thrombocytopenia is suspected, empiric platelet transfusion can also be considered. If hypotension persists despite appropriate fluids and blood products, vasopressors are indicated. The initial emergent laboratory workup includes: (1) complete blood count (CBC) to evaluate severity of anemia and thrombocytopenia; (2) coagulation evaluation with prothrombin, partial thromboplastin time and fibrinogen; and (3) type and cross in preparation for blood products. Setting goals and anticipating blood loss will maximize safety. Goals include: (1) correction of anemia, with maintenance of hemoglobin ≥ 8 g/dL; (2) correction of thrombocytopenia, with maintenance of platelets $\geq 75 \times 10^9$/L; and (3) correction of any coagulopathy with either fresh frozen plasma or fibrinogen. Complete gut rest may be augmented with histamine blockers or proton pump inhibitors.

The necessity of gastric lavage remains unclear. In non-oncology adult patients, the aspirate results determine an individual's pre-endoscopic risk stratification. A high-risk lesion consists of a bleeding lesion or visible vessel on endoscopy. A bloody (versus "coffee-ground" or bilious) aspirate is 75 % specific for an active upper GI bleed (Abdulrahman et al. 2004). Less is known about the utility of gastric lavage in pediatric oncology patients. In children with bright red blood or evidence of brisk bleeding during gastric lavage, management includes prompt endoscopic ligation or sclerotherapy. If the patient has esophageal varices, systemic infusion of vasopressin for 24 h may decrease portal circulation enough to halt bleeding without endoscopic intervention.

Although endoscopy potentially increases the risk of infection in neutropenic patients, it is the standard method to identify and control both upper and lower GI hemorrhage. If endoscopy fails to identify the origin of the bleed, angiography or radionuclide scans may help localize the source, assuming that the rate of bleeding exceeds 1 or 0.5 mL/min for these different diagnostic methodologies, respectively. If hemorrhage persists or recurs, management includes reevaluation and treatment of anemia, thrombocytopenia, and coagulopathies followed by repeat endoscopy or surgical intervention (Arul and Spicer 2008). Surgical intervention should precede endoscopic hemostasis if bleeding is associated with tumor. Figure 7.1 outlines the algorithmic approach to the management of acute GI bleeding in pediatric oncology patients.

7.4 Pancreatitis

Pancreatitis represents a rare but well-known complication of multiple chemotherapeutic agents, most notably asparaginase, steroids, mercaptopurine and cytarabine (Haut 2005; Trivedi and Pichumoni 2005; Garg et al. 2010). L-asparaginase and PEG-asparaginase derived from *E. coli* are well described for inducing acute pancreatitis of all degrees of severity with a reported incidence of 2–18 % (Knoderer et al. 2007; Kearney et al. 2009). Although suggested in some studies, it is not clear that PEG-asparaginase leads to an increased risk of pancreatitis as compared to L-asparaginase (Silverman et al. 2001; Knoderer et al. 2007). Older patients (i.e. >9 years) have been noted to have a significantly increased risk of pancreatitis with

pancreatitis occurring early after asparaginase introduction and typically days after L-asparaginase and weeks after PEG-asparaginase secondary to differences in drug half-life (Silverman et al. 2001; Knoderer et al. 2007; Kearney et al. 2009). No difference in pancreatits incidence has been noted with intramuscular versus intravenous PEG-asparaginase to date (Silverman et al. 2010). In their retrospective review, Knoderer et al. (2007) note that asparaginase-associated pancreatitis was significantly correlated with concomitant prednisone and daunomycin and significantly less likely with dexamethasone. Reintroduction of asparaginase after pancreatitis is controversial. In their review, Kearney et al. (2009) did not show a significant difference in outcome in those patients with and without pancreatitis although their general practice was to rechallenge patients. Knoderer et al. (2007) reported a 7.7 % incidence of pancreatitis with rechallenge as compared to Kearney et al. (2009) who reported a 63 % recurrence rate. Clinical diagnosis of asparaginase-associated pancreatitis is relatively straightforward; Kearney et al. (2009) note that all patients presented with abdominal or back pain and the majority had nausea or emesis. Severity of pancreatitis was not noted to correlate with degree of elevation of amylase and lipase (Kearney et al. 2009).

Laboratory workup merely supports the clinical suspicion of acute pancreatitis. Initial laboratory tests should include: (1) electrolytes to evaluate for hypocalcemia secondary to its precipitation; (2) renal and liver function tests to monitor for multiorgan failure secondary to cytokine release from the inflamed or necrotic pancreas; (3) triglycerides, inciting agents that when hydrolyzed to free fatty acids lead to free radical damage; and (4) the exocrine enzymes amylase and lipase, which when elevated suggest pancreatic autodigestion and are the hallmark of diagnosis (Tsuang et al. 2009). Of note, amylase and lipase may not be significantly elevated. Excessive cytokine release can lead to respiratory distress and therefore arterial blood gas and chest radiography may be clinically indicated for proper management (Arul and Spicer 2008).

In general, the preferred abdominal imaging modality to identify the extent of pancreatic edema, hemorrhage, necrosis, and other abnormalities is CT with IV contrast although Kearney et al. (2009) note significant correlation between US and CT when utilizing US as the primary imaging modality in patients with asparaginase-associated pancreatitis. Plain film is usually unremarkable although abdominal radiography (i.e., kidney, ureter, bladder; KUB) may show a sentinel loop in the left upper abdomen representing a localized ileus as a result of peripancreatic inflammation.

Treatment of acute pancreatitis has historically included nasogastric decompression, gut rest, hydration with electrolyte replacement or parenteral nutrition for prolonged gut rest, analgesia that usually includes opioids, and antiemetics. Whether nasogastric decompression is necessary is unclear; Kearney et al. (2009) reported that only 29 % of pediatric patients with asparaginase-associated pancreatitis were treated with nasogastric decompression with no difference in outcome. Additional pediatric data are lacking. Similarly, the need for gut rest has recently come into question. In adult patients with severe acute pancreatitis, Kumar et al. (2006) showed that enteral nutrition via both nasogastric and nasojejunal routes was well

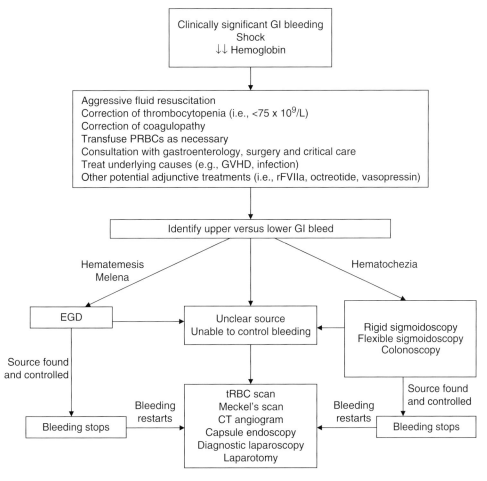

Fig. 7.1 Algorithm for management of clinically significant gastrointestinal bleeding in pediatric oncology patients. *GI* gastrointestinal, *PRBC* packed red blood cell, *GVHD* graft-versus-host disease, *rFVIIa* recombinant factor VIIa, *EGD* esophagogastroduodenoscopy, *tRBC* technetium-99m-tagged red blood cell, *CT* computed tomography

tolerated, while in a meta-analysis Petrov et al. (2007) reported that oral refeeding in adults was significantly associated with pain relapse. In a review by Kumar and Gariepy (2013) they conclude that early introduction of enteral feeding should be strongly considered in pediatric patients no matter the severity of the pancreatitis while early oral refeeding can be considered in those with mild disease although pediatric data are lacking. Despite its theoretical association with reduced sphincter of Oddi spasms, no clinical studies support meperidine over other narcotics (Thompson 2001). Potential complications include development of an abscess, pseudocyst, necrosis or hemorrhage. Most cases of pancreatitis resolve spontaneously and complications are rare; incidence of asparaginase-induced hemorrhagic pancreatitis in pediatric oncology is <0.5 % (Top et al. 2005). Unlike uncomplicated acute pancreatitis, hemorrhagic pancreatitis is a medical emergency with mortality rates approaching 100 % if untreated (Top et al. 2005). Hypovolemic shock is common and initial management parallels that of any GI bleed.

Pediatric oncology patients are generally placed on an empiric antibiotic regimen as utilized in neutropenic enterocolitis at the time of pancreatitis diagnosis. Procurement of cultures to guide antibiotic therapy can be accomplished via CT-guided fine-needle aspiration (Tenner et al. 2013). Duration of antimicrobial coverage is generally 10–14 days, depending on the patient's clinical status. Surgical debridement becomes necessary only when clinical deterioration persists despite adequate antibiotic coverage; percutaneous catheter drainage to irrigate the necrosis can be considered prior to surgical debridement (Top et al. 2005). The synthetic somatostatin octreotide, which inhibits exocrine pancreatic enzyme production, represents a promising experimental option in pediatrics but is still investigational (Wu et al. 2008).

7.5   Bowel Obstruction

Bowel obstruction results from luminal obstruction, lesions within the bowel wall, extrinsic bowel compression, dysfunctional motility, and radiation-induced enteritis (Arul and Spicer 2008; Yip and Goddard 2010). Primary tumors that invade through the GI mucosa and contribute to luminal or intrinsic obstruction include non-Hodgkin lymphoma (especially Burkitt lymphoma), rhabdomyosarcoma and teratoma. In patients with primary abdominal Burkitt lymphoma, almost a fifth of patients present with small bowel intussusception at the time of diagnosis (Gupta et al. 2007). Tumors that contribute to extrinsic compression include neuroblastoma and peritoneal metastases of Wilms tumor. Postoperative complications after tumor resection may also contribute to GI luminal obstruction; these include stricture formation, intussusception, and, less frequently, hernia. Although postoperative adhesions are the most common cause of extrinsic bowel compression, these generally present as obstruction months to years later. In contrast, postoperative small bowel intussusception usually occurs within 2 weeks of surgery. Functional motility obstruction commonly follows administration of vinca alkaloids and opiates as well as after any abdominal surgical procedure. Of note, fecal impaction is a common cause of obstruction in both immunocompetent and immunocompromised pediatric patients. The risk of radiation-induced bowel obstruction increases with prior abdominal surgery, treatment with concomitant radiation-sensitizing chemotherapy, radiation doses >45 Gy to the bowel and young age at time of therapy (Silliman et al. 1994; Kaste et al. 1999). Radiation-induced bowel injury leading to obstruction occurs within 6–24 months after completion of radiotherapy (Kaste et al. 1999).

Although the etiologies differ, the symptoms, signs, laboratory results and imaging suggestive of mechanical obstruction in pediatric oncology patients mimic any patient with an abdominal mechanical obstruction. Patients may have intermittent abdominal pain, intractable nausea or bilious emesis, constipation, hematochezia, or abdominal distension. Physical exam consistent with obstruction includes hyperactive or high-pitched bowel sounds, peritoneal signs and a palpable mass. In contrast, absent bowel sounds suggest an ileus or functional obstruction. Due to emesis and decreased oral intake, patients often present dehydrated on exam and laboratory assessment; patients may have a relative increase from baseline white blood count with evidence of hemoconcentration as well as hypochloremic metabolic alkalosis. Imaging studies begin with supine, upright and decubitus abdominal radiographs. Although not pathognomonic, air-fluid levels in dilated bowel loops and pneumatosis intestinalis on KUB are strongly supportive of obstruction. Dilated and contracted bowel loops may be appreciated proximal and distal to the obstruction, respectively. Abdominal CT with oral contrast will best localize the obstruction and identify the etiology (Silliman et al. 1994; Yip and Goddard 2010). Patients with neutropenia or necrotic bowel are at high risk of infection and perforation of the thinned intestinal mucosa and should not undergo small bowel follow-through exam using barium.

Management of obstruction includes bowel rest, decompression via nasogastric tube, and intravenous fluids to resolve electrolyte derangements and treat dehydration. Additional supportive care measures include antiemetics, anticholinergics and analgesics. As bowel cleansing preparations are contraindicated in gastrointestinal obstruction, enemas and suppositories are suggested to resolve fecal impaction and can be used with caution in immunocompromised patients (Arul and Spicer 2008; Yip and Goddard 2010). Indications for surgical intervention include: (1) persistent bleeding in the absence of neutropenia, thrombocytopenia or coagulopathy; (2) intraperitoneal perforation; (3) clinical deterioration of unknown etiology, especially if requiring blood pressure support with either colloids or vasopressors; and (4) any abdominal process that would require surgery in an immunocompetent host such as a mass lesion (Silliman et al. 1994). In contrast to non-oncologic episodes of intussusception, children with intussusception caused by tumor require surgical reduction rather than air-contrast or barium enema (Fisher and Rheingold 2011).

7.6 Tumor Rupture and Organ Perforation

Tumor rupture and organ perforation are surgical emergencies. Etiologies include the malignancy itself, treatment sequelae, iatrogenic intervention and unresolved obstruction. The most common cause of GI perforation is iatrogenic intervention, specifically endoscopy (Gagneja and Sinicrope 2002). Tumors at risk for spontaneous rupture include Wilms tumor, hepatoblastoma, neuroblastoma and B-cell lymphoma (Arul and Spicer 2008). Tumor rupture in patients with Burkitt lymphoma may occur at presentation, during surgical intervention or steroid therapy, or with tumor necrosis (Fisher and Rheingold 2011). If lymphoma erodes the intestinal wall, it can cause GI perforation at the site of transmural invasion. Tumor rupture and organ perforation are not limited to solid tumors or bowel; leukemic patients with splenomegaly have a small risk for splenic rupture, either spontaneously or with trivial trauma (Gagneja and Sinicrope 2002). In addition, therapy with prolonged corticosteroids, bevacizumab or radiation disrupts the GI mucosal epithelium. As previously mentioned, bevacizumab potentially increases the risk of gastric perforation (Demshar et al. 2011). Sequelae like peptic ulcer disease and adhesions, acting as lead points for mesenteric twisting, represent conditions that further weaken the intestinal wall. Frequent endoscopic procedures, unresolved obstruction or infection, or medically refractory conditions such as gastritis and ulcers predispose to perforation (Yip and Goddard 2010; Fisher and Rheingold 2011).

Although shock and peritoneal signs strongly suggest perforation, presentation varies considerably in immunocompromised pediatric oncology patients. Exam may reveal the classic acute abdomen with the patient rigid in a flexed position and exhibiting rebound tenderness or, in contrast, display only mild evidence of discomfort, tenderness, or distension. Intestinal distension usually results from the patient swallowing excessive amounts of air or from excessive gas production from bacterial overgrowth. Cecal diameters >13 cm dramatically increase the risk of perforation. Occasionally subcutaneous emphysema may be appreciated. Bowel sounds range from absent to hyperactive. Gastric perforation commonly presents with acute onset of severe abdominal pain that is often associated with nausea and vomiting, including hematemesis. Patients may complain of shoulder pain, which is referred pain from an irritated diaphragm (Gagneja and Sinicrope 2002; Yip and Goddard 2010).

Laboratory workup may reveal relative leukocytosis, neutrophilia, and anemia due to peritonitis and hemorrhage as well as electrolyte imbalances that need correction prior to surgery (Gagneja and Sinicrope 2002). Initial imaging consists of an upright KUB to evaluate for air under the diaphragm that may extend into the liver, enabling visualization of the hepatic ligament, and decubitus KUB to evaluate for air along the flank. Another clue to the presence of perforation is visualization of both sides of the bowel wall. In the setting of an indeterminate KUB, CT scan should be utilized (Gagneja and Sinicrope 2002).

Surgical consultation is paramount with suspicion of tumor rupture or organ perforation. Pending surgical intervention, immediate management includes making the patient NPO with nasogastric tube placement with suction to evacuate the stomach and protect the airway. In addition, urinary catheterization and analgesics may be necessary to monitor fluid status and control pain, respectively. Given the risk of infection, adequate coverage for Gram-negative enteric and anaerobic organisms should be implemented similar to treatment for neutropenic enterocolitis. Laparoscopy should be utilized when possible, with surgery consisting of bowel resection of the affected area followed by reanastomosis. Patients with excessive tumor burden, such as those with disseminated Burkitt lymphoma, require reduction by chemotherapy prior to surgical intervention (Gagneja and Sinicrope 2002; Fisher and Rheingold 2011).

7.7 Abdominal Compartment Syndrome

Although mostly seen in adult patients who have sustained trauma, abdominal compartment syndrome (ACS) may occur in pediatric patients, including those with large tumor masses at presentation or as a postoperative complication (Fisher and Rheingold 2011; Terpe et al. 2012). The mechanism of ACS appears to be ischemia-reperfusion injury with associated bowel isch-

emia or necrosis (Beck et al. 2001). Two large prospective studies report the incidence of ACS among children admitted to the intensive care unit to be <1 %, irrespective of an oncologic diagnosis and with high risk of mortality (Cheatham et al. 2007). Increased intra-abdominal pressure (IAP) leads to multiorgan compromise by initially impairing respiratory mechanics which alter cardiac output leading to organ hypoperfusion and subsequent renal and cerebral insufficiency (De Backer 1999).

Although no definitive ACS diagnostic criteria exist for the pediatric population, children are thought to require an IAP of ≥20 mmHg with associated organ compromise (Beck et al. 2001; Cheatham et al. 2007; Fisher and Rheingold 2011). Patients with ACS will present with a tense and distended abdomen with associated hypotension, oliguria or anuria and respiratory compromise (Beck et al. 2011). The aims of ACS management are to: (1) improve abdominal wall compliance with positioning and medications; (2) decrease intraluminal content with nasogastric suction; (3) decrease extraluminal content with percutaneous catheter decompression of intraperitoneal air or fluid; and (4) optimize fluid balance to reduce end-organ hypoperfusion without worsening IAH. Elevating the head of the bed increases IAP and should be avoided; similarly, sedatives and analgesics will increase abdominal muscle tone and should be minimized, as possible. Studies in adults with ACS are investigating neuromuscular blockade as a means to decrease IAP. Careful aggressive fluid resuscitation with hypertonic crystalloids and colloids should be attempted although refractory IAH or end-organ damage requires immediate surgical decompression (Cheatham et al. 2007).

7.8 Summary

Prompt identification of abdominal emergencies in pediatric oncology patients can be a challenge due to decreased signs and symptoms of inflammation in the immunocompromised host. Successful outcomes require vigilance for atypical presentations in immunocompromised children; early initiation of broad-spectrum, empiric antibiotics to reduce infection-related mortality; supportive care measures such as volume resuscitation and bleeding control; identification of inciting chemotherapeutic agents as well as radiation therapy; appropriate utilization of imaging modalities; and a multidisciplinary team approach with oncology, surgery, and radiology to accelerate diagnosis and treatment. Prompt diagnosis and early medical management reduces the necessity of invasive measures. The majority of guidelines for care of these emergent issues are based on consensus panels and expert opinion due to a lack of randomized controlled trial data.

References

Abdulrahman MA, Fallone CA, Barkun AN (2004) Nasogastric aspirate predicts high-risk endoscopic lesions in patients with acute upper GI bleeding. Gastrointest Endosc 59:172–178

Albano EA, Sandler E (2004) Oncologic emergencies. In: Altman AJ, Reaman GH (eds) Supportive care of children with cancer: current therapy and guidelines from the children's oncology group, 3rd edn. The John Hopkins University Press, Baltimore

Andreyev HJ, Davison SE, Gillespie C et al (2012) Practice guidance on the management of acute and chronic gastrointestinal problems arising as a result of treatment for cancer. Gut 61:179–192

Arul GS, Spicer RD (2008) Gastrointestinal complications. In: Carachi R, Grosfeld JL, Azmy AF (eds) The surgery of childhood tumors, 2nd edn. Springer, New York

Beck R, Halberthal M, Zonis Z et al (2001) Abdominal compartment syndrome in children. Pediatr Crit Care Med 2:51–56

Büyükaşik Y, Ozcebe OI, Sayinalp N et al (1988) Perianal infections in patients with leukemia: importance of the course of neutrophil count. Dis Colon Rectum 41:81–85

Cheatham ML, Malbrain ML, Kirkpatrick A et al (2007) Results from the International Conference of Experts on intra-abdominal hypertension and abdominal compartment syndrome. II. Recommendations. Intensive Care Med 33:951–962

Chui CH, Chan MY, Tan AM et al (2008) Appendicitis in immunocompromised children: still a diagnostic and therapeutic dilemma? Pediatr Blood Cancer 50:1282–1283

Cloutier RL (2010) Neutropenic enterocolitis. Hematol Oncol Clin North Am 24:577–584

De Backer D (1999) Abdominal compartment syndrome. Crit Care 3:R103–R104

Demshar R, Vanek R, Mazanec P (2011) Oncologic emergencies: new decade, new perspectives. AACN Adv Crit Care 22:337–348

Fisher MJ, Rheingold SR (2011) Oncologic emergencies. In: Pizzo PA, Poplack DG (eds) Principles and practice of pediatric oncology, 6th edn. Lippincott Williams & Wilkins, Pennsylvania

Gagneja HK, Sinicrope FA (2002) Gastrointestinal emergencies. In: Yeung SJ, Escalante CP (eds) Oncologic emergencies. BC Decker Inc, Hamilton

Garg R, Agarwala S, Bhatnagar V (2010) Acute pancreatitis induced by ifosfamide therapy. J Pediatr Surg 45:2071–2073

Gray TL, Ooi CY, Tran D et al (2010) Gastrointestinal complications in children with acute myeloid leukemia. Leuk Lymphoma 51:768–777

Gupta H, Davidoff AM, Pui CH et al (2007) Clinical implications and surgical management of intussusception in pediatric patients with Burkitt lymphoma. J Pediatr Surg 42:998–1001

Guyatt G, Gutterman D, Baumann MH et al (2006) Grading strength of recommendations and quality of evidence in clinical guidelines: report from an American College of Chest Physicians Task Force. Chest 129:174–181

Haut C (2005) Oncological emergencies in the pediatric intensive care unit. AACN Clin Issues 16: 232–245

Hobson MJ, Carney DE, Molik KA et al (2005) Appendicitis in childhood hematologic malignancies: analysis and comparison with typhlitis. J Pediatr Surg 40:214–220

Kaste SC, Rodriguez-Galindo C, Furman WL (1999) Pictorial essay: imaging pediatric oncologic emergencies of the abdomen. AJR Am J Roentgenol 173:729–736

Kearney SL, Dahlberg SE, Levy DE et al (2009) Clinical course and outcome in children with acute lymphoblastic leukemia and asparaginase-associated pancreatitis. Pediatr Blood Cancer 53:162–167

Knoderer HM, Robarge J, Flockhart DA (2007) Predicting asparaginase-associated pancreatitis. Pediatr Blood Cancer 49:634–639

Krishnamoorthi R, Ramarajan N, Wang NE et al (2011) Effectiveness of a staged US and CT protocol for the diagnosis of pediatric appendicitis: reducing radiation exposure in the age of ALARA. Radiology 259:231–239

Kumar A, Singh N, Prakash S et al (2006) Early enteral nutrition in severe acute pancreatitis: a prospective randomized controlled trial comparing nasojejunal and nasogastric routes. J Clin Gastroenterol 40: 431–434

Kumar S, Gariepy CD (2013) Nutrition and acute pancreatitis: review of the literature and pediatric perspectives. Curr Gastroenterol Rep 15:338

McAteer JP, Sanchez SE, Rutledge JC, Waldhausen JH (2014) Isolated appendiceal typhlitis masquerading as perforated appendicitis in the setting of acute lymphoblastic leukemia. Pediatr Surg Int 30:561–564

McCarville MB, Thompson J, Li C et al (2004) Significance of appendiceal thickening in association with typhlitiis in pediatric oncology patients. Pediatr Radiol 34:245–249

McCarville MB, Adelman CS, Li C et al (2005) Typhlitis in childhood cancer. Cancer 104:380–387

Mercer-Falkoff A, Lacy J (2013) Oncologic emergencies. In: Rose MG, Devita VT Jr, Lawrence TS, Rosenberg SA (eds) Oncology in primary care. Lippincott Williams & Wilkins, Philadelphia

Morgan C, Tillett T, Braybrooke J et al (2011) Management of uncommon chemotherapy-induced emergencies. Lancet Oncol 12:806–814

Petrov MS, van Santvoort HC, Besselink MG et al (2007) Oral refeeding after onset of acute pancreatitis: a review of literature. Am J Gastroenterol 102: 2079–2084

Pizzo PA (2011) Management of oncologic emergencies. In: Lanzkowsky P (ed) Manual of pediatric hematology and oncology, 5th edn. Elsevier, San Francisco

Silliman CC, Haase GM, Strain JD et al (1994) Indications for surgical intervention for gastrointestinal emergencies in children receiving chemotherapy. Cancer 74:203–216

Silverman LB, Gelber RD, Dalton VK et al (2001) Improved outcome for children with acute lymphoblastic leukemia: results of Dana-Farber Consortium Protocol 91-01. Blood 97:1211–1218

Silverman LB, Supko JG, Stevenson KE et al (2010) Intravenous PEG-asparaginase during remission induction in children and adolescents with newly diagnosed acute lymphoblastic leukemia. Blood 115: 1351–1353

Steinberg R, Freud E, Yaniv I, Katz J, Zer M (1999) A plea for incidental appendectomy in pediatric patients with malignancy. Pediatr Hematol Oncol 16:431–435

Sundell N, Boström H, Edenholm M et al (2012) Management of neutropenic enterocolitis in children with cancer. Acta Paediatr 101:308–312

Tenner S, Baillie J, DeWitt J et al (2013) American College of Gastroenterology guideline: management of acute pancreatitis. Am J Gastroenterol 108: 1400–1415

Terpe F, Siekmeyer M, Bierbach U et al (2012) Fulminant and fatal course of acute lymphoblastic leukemia due to lactic acidosis and suspected abdominal compartment syndrome. J Pediatr Hematol Oncol 34:e80–e83

Thompson DR (2001) Narcotic analgesic effects on the sphincter of Oddi: a review of the data and therapeutic implications in treating pancreatitis. Am J Gastroenterol 96:1266–1272

Top PC, Tissing JW, Kuiper JW et al (2005) L-asparaginase-induced severe necrotizing pancreatitis successfully treated with percutaneous drainage. Pediatr Blood Cancer 44:95–97

Trivedi C, Pichumoni CS (2005) Drug-induced pancreatitis: an update. J Clin Gastroenterol 39:709–716

Tsuang W, Navaneethan U, Ruiz L et al (2009) Hypertriglyceridemic pancreatitis: presentation and management. Am J Gastroenterol 104:984–991

Wolfe RE, Kennedy ES (2011) Granulocytopenia. In: Schaider JJ, Barkin RM, Hayden SR, Wolfe RE, Barkin AZ, Shayne P, Rosen P (eds) Rosen & Barkin's 5-minute emergency medicine consult, 4th edn. Lippincott Williams & Wilkins, Philadelphia

Wan MJ, Krahn M, Ungar WJ et al (2009) Acute appendicitis in young children: cost-effectiveness of US versus CT in diagnosis–a Markov decision analytic model. Radiology 250:378–386

Wiegering VA, Kellenberger CJ, Bodmer N et al (2008) Conservative management of acute appendicitis in children with hematologic malignancies during chemotherapy-induced neutropenia. J Pediatr Hematol Oncol 30:464–467

Wu SF, Chen AC, Peng CT et al (2008) Octreotide therapy in asparaginase-associated pancreatitis in childhood acute lymphoblastic leukemia. Pediatr Blood Cancer 51:824–825

Yip D, Goddard N (2010) Oncological emergencies: diagnosis and management. In: Robotin M, Olver I, Girgis A (eds) When cancer crosses disciplines: a physician's handbook. Imperial College Press, London

Thrombotic Disorders

8

Nahal Lalefar and Robert Raphael

Contents

N. Lalefar, MD (✉) • R. Raphael, MD
Department of Hematology/Oncology,
Children's Hospital and Research Center Oakland,
747 52nd Street, Oakland, CA 94609, USA
e-mail: nlalefar@mail.cho.org

Abstract

Thromboembolism is a well-recognized complication of cancer in children, with important clinical and therapeutic implications. The exact incidence is unknown, with wide variation in reported rates. Thromboembolism has been most extensively studied in acute lymphoblastic leukemia but also affects children with other malignancies. Risk factors include the presence or dysfunction of a central venous catheter, inherited thrombophilia, use of asparaginase and steroids, older age, and intrathoracic or metastatic disease. The most commonly affected sites are the central nervous system in acute lymphoblastic leukemia and the upper extremity veins which are often associated with a central venous catheter. Current evidence does not support screening asymptomatic patients or providing routine prophylactic anticoagulation in pediatric cancer patients. For patients with symptomatic thromboembolism, a review of the evidence for different therapeutic anticoagulation modalities is discussed with graded recommendations; due to a lack of reported data, much of the guidelines are based on expert opinion or consensus statements. The necessary duration of therapy is unknown but generally depends on clinical response and the presence of ongoing risk factors for bleeding or thrombosis. Additional research is needed to better understand the epidemiology of thrombosis in childhood cancer and to optimize both therapy and prevention.

J. Feusner et al. (eds.), *Supportive Care in Pediatric Oncology:*
A Practical Evidence-Based Approach, Pediatric Oncology,
DOI 10.1007/978-3-662-44317-0_8, © Springer Berlin Heidelberg 2015

8.1 Introduction

Thrombosis is a well-recognized complication of cancer and its treatment in both adults and children. The etiology of thrombosis in cancer is complex and multifactorial but generally involves all three elements of Virchow's triad: venous stasis, hypercoagulability and endothelial damage. Malignant cells may alter hemostasis by producing inflammatory cytokines and procoagulant molecules. Humoral coagulation abnormalities are common in cancer patients including increased fibrin formation and degradation as well as altered (i.e., increased or decreased) levels of fibrinogen and other clotting factors. Tumor cells may express tissue factor and cancer procoagulants on their surface, upregulate plasminogen activation inhibitor-1 (PAI-1), and secrete prostaglandins and thromboxanes which promote platelet activation and aggregation (Dipasco et al. 2012). Thrombin generation is also increased in patients with acute lymphoblastic leukemia (ALL) at diagnosis and early in treatment (Athale and Chan 2003b). Vascular endothelium may be activated or damaged through complex interactions with tumor cells and leukocytes, as well as by surgical interventions and indwelling central venous catheters (CVCs). The result of these pathophysiologic changes is essentially an acquired thrombophilia, similar to chronic low-grade disseminated intravascular coagulation (Dipasco et al. 2011).

Adults with cancer have a four- to sixfold increase in the risk of thromboembolism (TE), the second most common proximate cause of death in this patient population (Athale et al. 2007; Dipasco et al. 2011). Thrombosis in childhood is much less common than in adults among the general population, with an estimated prevalence of 0.6–1.1 per 10,000 in the United States (Boulet et al. 2011). Over 70 % of TE in children occurs in the setting of chronic disease, including cancer (Kerlin 2012). Malignancy accounts for 25–40 % of all pediatric thromboses, and children with cancer are at least 600 times more likely to develop TE than healthy children (Athale et al. 2008b).

Relatively little is known about the epidemiology of thrombosis in pediatric oncology. The majority of data derive from children with ALL, with a paucity of information regarding other malignancies. In a retrospective study of 726 patients consecutively diagnosed with cancer at McMaster Children's Hospital from 1990 to 2006, 57 patients were diagnosed with TE for an overall prevalence of 7.9 % (Athale et al. 2008b). In this study, the prevalence of thrombosis varied by underlying malignancy: 14.2 % in ALL, 13.2 % in sarcoma, 11.9 % in lymphoma, 5.9 % in acute myeloid leukemia (AML), 2.4 % in Wilms tumor, 2.3 % in neuroblastoma and 0.5 % in central nervous system (CNS) tumors. For all non-CNS malignancies, the overall prevalence of TE was 10.7 %. Significant reported risk factors for TE in children with cancer include the presence of a CVC, older age, treatment with asparaginase or corticosteroids, the presence of metastases, CVC dysfunction, blood vessel compression by a bulky solid tumor, particularly with intrathoracic disease, and in some studies, inherited thrombophilia (Nowak-Göttl et al. 1999; Nowak-Göttl et al. 2003; Athale et al. 2005; Caruso et al. 2006; Paz-Priel et al. 2007; Athale et al. 2008). Clinical manifestations are similar to those of TE in children without malignancy and vary with the location and extent of thrombosis. The risk of recurrent TE in childhood cancer is not known, but recurrence rate of TE in children generally is estimated to be 5–10 % and may be higher for those with ongoing risk factors such as a CVC, malignancy and asparaginase treatment (Kerlin 2012). The impact of thrombosis on morbidity, mortality, and outcome in childhood cancer is unknown, and management recommendations are generally extrapolated from the adult literature; graded guidelines based on reported evidence are presented in Table 8.1.

8.2 Acute Lymphoblastic Leukemia (ALL)

The incidence of thromboembolism in children with ALL is estimated to be between 1.1 and 36.7 % (Athale and Chan 2003a). This wide variation is likely due to differences in the definition of TE (symptomatic versus occult), diagnostic methods, study design, reporting period and treatment regimens. The true incidence is likely underestimated because patients are generally not screened for asymptomatic TE. The Prophylactic Antithrombin Replacement in Kids with ALL treated with Asparaginase (PARKAA) study reported a TE incidence of 36.7 % with prospective screening radiography after induction therapy; only 5 % were clinically symptomatic (Mitchell et al. 2003b). A meta-analysis estimated the rate of symptomatic thrombosis in 1,752 children with ALL from 17 prospective studies to be 5.2 % (Caruso et al. 2006). The risk is highest during induction, with an incidence rate more than double that in later phases of therapy. Although rare, thrombosis can also occur prior to the start of ALL treatment (Payne and Vora 2007).

The CNS is by far the most common location of thrombosis in ALL, accounting for 54 % of events in the meta-analysis by Caruso et al. (2006). Twenty-nine percent of these were cerebral sinovenous thromboses (CSVT), while other types of CNS events were less clearly defined (Caruso et al. 2006). In their review, Athale and Chan (2003a) reported that 52 % of CNS events were CSVT, with 43.7 % parenchymal lesions and 4.3 % combined. The etiology of CNS thrombosis in children with cancer is likely multifactorial and related to direct tumor invasion, chemotherapy-induced hypercoagulability, and associated complications like dehydration and infection (Wiernikowski and Athale 2006). Non-CNS events in the meta-analysis by Caruso et al. (2006) included deep vein thrombosis (DVT, 43 %), pulmonary emboli (PE, 2 %) and right atrial thromboses (2 %). DVT was noted to be more common in upper than lower extremities, most in association with a CVC (Caruso et al. 2006). The majority of thromboses are venous, with only 3 % of events reported as arterial in the review by Athale and Chan (2003a). In 5 % of cases, thromboses were multifocal and 50 % of TE occurred in potentially life-threatening locations (Caruso et al. 2006). Thrombosis accounts for a relatively small fraction of treatment-related mortality, with reports ranging from 0 to 4.8 %, largely from PE and CNS events (Athale and Chan 2003a). Very little evidence exists about morbidity from TE in pediatric ALL; one study of pediatric ALL survivors reported a 50 % prevalence of post-thrombotic syndrome (PTS) following a symptomatic TE (Kuhle et al. 2008). PTS includes symptoms of pain, swelling and skin changes to the affected limb. For patients with CNS TE, reports suggest that up to 15–20 % will have residual neurologic deficits, while the effect on neurocognitive outcome is unknown (Athale and Chan 2003a). Others report that full neurologic recovery is the norm (Payne and Vora 2007). Qureshi et al. (2010) reported no permanent sequelae of TE among 59 children with ALL, including those with CSVT who presented with neurologic deficits.

8.3 ALL Risk Factors

Several studies have identified older age as a significant risk factor for TE among children treated for ALL (Athale and Chan 2003a). An analysis of 91 patients treated at McMaster Children's Hospital following Dana Farber Cancer Institute (DFCI) protocols for ALL found that 7 of 16 patients ≥10 years (44 %) developed symptomatic TE versus 3 of 75 (4 %) in younger patients (Athale et al. 2005). Patients classified with high-risk ALL also appear more likely to develop TE, though this is confounded by the effect of age, as older children are considered high-risk by definition. In the same McMaster study, 26 % of the 35 high-risk patients developed TE (11 % of those <10 years) versus 2 % of 56 standard-risk patients. The effect of gender on the risk of TE has been less clear, with contradictory reports published; in the McMaster study, gender did not influence risk of TE (Athale and Chan 2003a; Athale et al. 2005). The presence of a CVC is a well-established risk factor for TE in the general pediatric population as well as in ALL; half of all symptomatic DVT in children with ALL are associated with a CVC (Athale and Chan 2003a).

Table 8.1 Summary of treatment strategies and level of evidence for the management of thrombosis in pediatric oncology patients[a]

Clinical scenario	Recommendations	Level of evidence[b]
Primary thromboprophylaxis	Not recommended (including LMWH, warfarin, FFP)	1B
	Routine screening with coagulation studies or for thrombophilia not recommended	2C
	Thrombophilia screening can be considered for patients with known TE risk factors	2C
Development of a non-CVC-related thrombosis	Thrombophilia screening	2C
Thromboembolism	Treatment with LMWH	2B
	Thrombolysis with tPA or thrombectomy for life- or limb-threatening thrombosis	2C
	Warfarin generally not recommended but can be considered with long-term anticoagulation	2B
	Treatment for a minimum of 3 months and until the precipitating factor has resolved	2C
	Consideration for holding asparaginase therapy during acute TE	2C
	If nonfunctioning or no longer needed, the CVC should be removed after 3–5 days of anticoagulation	1B
	If functioning and clinically necessary, the CVC can remain with continuing anticoagulation	2C
Cerebral sinovenous thrombosis	Total anticoagulation for at least 3 months	1B
	Continued anticoagulation for 3 additional months if with persistent occlusion or symptoms	2C
	If with hemorrhage, anticoagulation can be reserved for cases with thrombus extension	2C
	Prophylactic anticoagulation should be given with subsequent asparaginase doses	2C
Thrombocytopenia with anticoagulation	Initially transfuse to keep platelets >20–50×10^9/L	2C
	Subsequently, hold anticoagulation for platelets <20–50×10^9/L	2C
Lumbar puncture with concomitant anticoagulation	LMWH should be held 24 h prior and resumed 12 h after LP	1C

LMWH low-molecular-weight heparin, *FFP* fresh frozen plasma, *TE* thromboembolism, *CVC* central venous catheter, *tPA* tissue plasminogen activator, *LP* lumbar puncture
[a]See text for full detail
[b]Per Guyatt et al. (2006); see Preface

Multiple studies have reported the association of genetic prothrombotic defects and ALL, including factor V Leiden, prothrombin gene G20210A mutation, MTHFR C677T and A1298 mutations, deficiencies of protein C, protein S, or antithrombin (AT), and high lipoprotein (a) levels. In the largest study, Nowak-Göttl et al. (1999) prospectively evaluated inherited thrombophilia traits in 301 children enrolled on ALL Berlin-Frankfurt-Muenster (BFM) 90/95 protocols. Eleven percent of patients with complete follow-up experienced a symptomatic TE, and the presence of an inherited thrombophilia significantly increased the risk: 46.5 % with an identified prothrombotic defect experienced a TE versus 2.2 % without such a defect. The greatest risk was associated with protein C, protein S and AT deficiency (Nowak-Göttl et al. 1999). In contrast, the North American PARKAA study prospectively evaluated the prothrombin 20210A mutation and factor V Leiden in 60 children with ALL and correlated with screening radiography but found no association with TE (occult or symptomatic), though four of eight patients with antiphospholipid antibodies did experience thrombosis (Mitchell et al. 2003b). Caruso et al. (2006) reviewed five prospective studies reporting prothrombotic genetic defects; the prevalence of mutations was similar to the general population and the pooled relative risk of TE with thrombophilia was 8.5. It remains unclear as to why studies of risk in children with thrombophilia have shown such variable conclusions (Raffini and Thornburg 2009).

Much of the literature regarding thrombosis in ALL patients centers on the use of L-asparaginase. Asparaginase catalyzes the hydrolysis of the amino acid asparagine to aspartic acid and ammonia. The rapid depletion of the circulating pool of asparagine reduces hepatic protein synthesis, which in turn causes a decrease in natural anticoagulants such as AT, fibrinogen, and plasminogen, as well as protein C and S. The coagulopathy associated with asparaginase may result in both thrombosis and hemorrhage, although the former is much more common (Athale and Chan 2003b). The pharmacology of asparaginase is affected by its source (*Escherichia coli* or *Erwinia chrysanthemi*), different commercial manufacturers (European, Japanese, American), and modifications (polyethylene glycosylated; PEG-asparaginase), with profound effects on half-life, asparagine depletion and protein synthesis inhibition. Comparison of published rates of TE associated with asparaginase is hampered by this variability as well as by variations in dosage, timing of administration, and concomitant chemotherapy. In the meta-analysis by Caruso et al. (2006), the rate of TE was significantly decreased with doses of $\geq$10,000 units/m^2 vs. $\leq$6,000 units/m^2 and with <9 days of asparaginase exposure; type of asparaginase or manufacturer did not show significant differences.

PEG-asparaginase, formed by covalently attaching polyethylene glycol to the native *E. coli* asparaginase enzyme, is now more commonly used in ALL therapy protocols and was associated with a 2 % risk of thrombosis in a study of 197 patients treated from 2005 to 2007 following a DFCI protocol including prednisone during induction (Silverman et al. 2010). Qureshi et al. (2010) reported venous thrombosis in 3.2 % of 1,824 patients treated on the British UK ALL 2003 protocol using PEG-asparaginase and dexamethasone during induction and delayed intensification. Ninety percent of events occurred during PEG-asparaginase exposure, 70 % of which were during induction. Although CVC placement was deferred to the end of induction on this protocol to reduce the risk of CVC-associated TE, 50 % of events were CVC related, while 36 % involved the CNS and the remainder were DVTs (Qureshi et al. 2010). All patients recovered completely without clinical sequelae, and 73 % received subsequent asparaginase (the majority with prophylactic LMWH) with no recurrent TE or excess bleeding. Intravenous PEG-asparaginase has been reported to have a similar rate of thrombotic complications as intramuscular administration (Silverman et al. 2010).

The effect of asparaginase may be further augmented by the concurrent use of corticosteroids during ALL induction, which can also increase the VTE risk eight to tenfold (Nowak-Göttl et al. 2009; Mitchell et al. 2010). In a prospective cohort study of 420 ALL patients enrolled on separate German cooperative protocols, symptomatic TE occurred in 11.6 % of those treated with concurrent prednisone and *E. coli* asparaginase in induction versus 2.5 % among those who received asparaginase in consolidation without prednisone (Nowak-Göttl et al. 2001). Steroids increase the level of prothrombin as well as factor VIII, von Willebrand factor, PAI-1 and AT (Harlev et al. 2010). Some evidence exists for a lower risk of TE with prednisone versus dexamethasone; 10.4 % of children receiving dexamethasone during induction on the BFM 2000 protocol developed TE compared with 1.8 % of those who received prednisone on the earlier BFM 90/95 protocols despite similar asparaginase dose and schedule (Nowak-Göttl et al. 2003). Caruso et al. (2006), however, showed no difference in rate of TE between prednisone and dexamethasone in induction although prednisone led to a significant increased risk in postinduction phases. Further data are required to make firm conclusions regarding the effect of steroids on thrombosis risk in pediatric ALL patients.

8.4   Other Malignancies

Data regarding TE in pediatric malignancies other than ALL are limited. Overall, more than 40 % of pediatric oncology patients with TE have a diagnosis other than ALL, and the prevalence among non-ALL cancers is about 16 % (Wiernikowski and Athale 2006). Lymphoma and sarcoma have an increased risk of TE, while brain tumors do not (Athale et al. 2008b). As in children with ALL, children with other malignancies are at significantly increased risk of TE if older and if with CVC dysfunction; mediastinal disease is a significant risk factor in children with lymphoma with a trend toward increased risk in patients with more extensive disease (Athale et al. 2007; Athale et al. 2008a).

A 2008 retrospective study of 75 children diagnosed between 1999 and 2004 with Hodgkin lymphoma (HL) or non-Hodgkin lymphoma (NHL) reported 9 patients (12 %) with 16 thrombotic events (Athale et al. 2008a). Twelve of these events were venous and there was a 2.6 % rate of PE (Athale et al. 2008a). Sixty-nine percent were associated with a CVC and none were CNS events, in contrast with the distribution in ALL patients. However, it has been reported separately that 1–3 % of patients with advanced NHL develop CSVT (Wiernikowski and Athale 2006). In multivariate analysis, mediastinal involvement increased the risk of thrombosis; 9 of 51 patients with mediastinal lymphadenopathy developed TE versus none of 21 patients without mediastinal involvement (Athale et al. 2008a). Lymphoma type, gender, presence of B-symptoms, age and stage were not risk factors for TE in lymphoma patients. Notably, despite the use of asparaginase, children with NHL did not appear to be at higher risk for TE than children with HL, contrasting results in adults (Wiernikowski and Athale 2006; Athale et al. 2008a). The meta-analysis additionally noted a 40 % recurrence rate (four patients); of these patients, only two had received secondary thromboprophylaxis with coumadin or LMWH and both had TE recurrence while on coumadin.

A retrospective cohort study investigated thromboses in 122 children and adolescents with soft tissue sarcoma treated at the National Cancer Institute from 1980 to 2002 (Paz-Priel et al. 2007). The authors reported 23 thromboembolic events in 19 patients and an overall TE incidence of 16 %. Over 50 % of the TE were detected at the time of initial cancer evaluation and 57 % were symptomatic. Thirty-five percent of thromboses were related to tumor compression and 13 % CVC associated. Involved sites included extremity DVT (43 %), PE (22 %) and inferior vena cava (17 %). Patients with distant metastasis were 2.5 times more likely to have a clot, 23 % vs. 10 %, with a trend towards significance (Paz-Priel et al. 2007). The rate of TE was similar for all types of sarcoma and between children and young adults. Though thrombophilia was infrequently investigated, four patients had lupus anticoagulant detected. In another single-institution retrospective analysis of pediatric sarcoma patients treated between 1990 and 2005, 10 of 70 patients (14.3 %) developed symptomatic TE (all DVTs), six of which were CVC associated (Athale et al. 2007). CVC dysfunction significantly increased the risk of TE: 55 % of those with CVC problems developed TE versus 8.2 % in those without. Prevalence of TE was increased in patients with pulmonary disease, metastases, older age and Ewing sarcoma, but these factors failed to reach statistical significance. Relapse and death were more common in patients with symptomatic TE but again without reaching statistical significance.

In adults with malignant brain tumors, the risk of TE is 20 % in the perioperative period without prophylaxis and risk remains high throughout treatment, reaching 28 %, particularly in adult patients with malignant gliomas (Wiernikowski and Athale 2006). TE is comparatively much less common in children with CNS tumors (Athale et al. 2008b). Tabori et al. (2004) reviewed 462 pediatric patients with malignant brain tumors over 14 years in Israel and only three (0.6 %) had symptomatic VTE. All were severely debilitated at the time of TE diagnosis, likely stemming from complications of their underlying malignancy (Tabori et al. 2004). In a report of 253 patients treated at St. Jude Children's Research Hospital, the frequency of symptomatic TE was 2.8 %, with increased risk associated with CVC dysfunction (Deitcher et al. 2004). Athale et al. (2008b) reported a significantly lower prevalence of TE in patients with CNS tumors than other groups, with

Table 8.2 Summary of known and presumed risk factors for thromboembolism in pediatric oncology patients[a]

Known risk factors[b]	Type of malignancy
	ALL
	AML
	Lymphoma
	Sarcoma
	Older age
	Presence of central venous cathether
	Dysfunction of central venous catheter
	Asparaginase therapy in ALL
	Steroid therapy in ALL
	Blood vessel compression by bulky solid tumor
Presumed risk factors[c]	Type of malignancy
	Other solid tumors including Wilms tumor and neuroblastoma
	Thrombophilia
	History of thromboembolism
	Concomitant asparaginase and steroids in ALL
	Mediastinal involvement in lymphoma patients
	Solid tumor patients with extensive metastatic disease
	Sepsis
	Surgery
	Immobilization
Not risk factors[d]	CNS tumors
	Gender

ALL acute lymphoblastic leukemia, *AML* acute myelogenous leukemia, *CNS* central nervous system
[a]See text for detail
[b]Consistent significant multivariate analysis proving risk
[c]Inconsistent results; trend towards significance
[d]Consistent significant analyses proving not a risk factor

one event among 201 children with CNS tumors. A summary of known and presumed risk factors for TE is presented in Table 8.2.

8.5 Central Venous Catheters

CVCs are essential in pediatric oncology but associated with risk of infection and thrombosis. The actual incidence of TE in children with CVCs for cancer treatment is unknown, with a wide range in reported rates due to variation in definitions, diagnostic methods and populations studied (Wiernikowski and Athale 2006). Most CVC-related thromboses are asymptomatic and located at the entry site of the catheter into the vein (Nowak-Göttl et al. 2009). The morbidity of these asymptomatic catheter-associated thromboses is unknown. Glaser et al. (2001) reported evidence of thrombosis in 12 of 24 asymptomatic pediatric oncology patients with implantable CVCs (ports) screened by contrast venography. As mentioned, the PARKAA study reported a prevalence of 37 % in children with ALL and indwelling CVCs screened radiographically after induction therapy, but only 5 % had clinical symptoms (Mitchell et al. 2003b). Symptoms may include swelling, pain, tenderness, erythema or discoloration of the affected limb, or dilated vessels. CVC-related TE can lead to recurrent TE (4–19 %), PE (8–15 %), PTS (5–25 %), and death (2–4 %) (Nowak-Göttl et al. 2009). The mechanisms by which CVCs may lead to TE include changes to venous flow dynamics, trauma to the vessel wall, or hyperosmolar substances such as parenteral nutrition or chemotherapy (Wiernikowski and Athale 2006). External tunneled CVCs are more likely to develop thrombosis than implanted catheters (ports); a retrospective analysis of 362 patients with ALL enrolled on a Pediatric Oncology Group (POG) protocol noted that external CVCs were 3.9 times more likely to be associated with thrombosis than internal catheters (McLean et al. 2005). In a prospective study, Male et al. (2003) showed significantly increased risk of TE with CVC placement on the left side, in the subclavian vein and when inserted percutaneously. Some institutions and protocols have recommended delaying the insertion of a CVC until the end of induction therapy for ALL to minimize risk, but acceptance of this policy has been variable and it remains unclear if timing of CVC insertion is a risk factor for TE (McLean et al. 2005; Astwood and Vora 2011).

8.6 Diagnosis

The medical complexity of pediatric oncology patients and the often subtle or nonspecific signs and symptoms of TE mandate a high index of suspicion. Although the "gold standard" for diagnosis of DVT in adults is bilateral venography, in clinical practice it is infrequently used in children due to technical difficulties, the need for iodinated contrast, and the possibility of inducing or extending thrombus (Manco-Johnson 2006). Doppler ultrasound is useful for assessment of lower extremity DVT and for jugular and distal upper extremity veins, but is less sensitive for proximal upper system thrombosis. The PARKAA study documented low sensitivity (20 %) of ultrasound for superior vena cava (SVC) and proximal subclavian thrombosis compared to venography, though the latter was inferior for internal jugular thrombosis (Mitchell et al. 2003b). Magnetic resonance imaging (MRI) with angiography/venography (MRA/MRV) or computed tomography (CT) with intravenous contrast are useful when ultrasound cannot be reliably performed. MRI with MRA/MRV is the modality of choice for evaluating CNS thrombosis. Echocardiogram may be used for evaluation of proximal SVC and cardiac thrombosis. High-resolution spiral CT scan with contrast is most commonly used for diagnosis of PE in children, but ventilation/perfusion (V/Q) scans may be used as well (Wiernikowski and Athale 2006).

8.7   Management

8.7.1   Prevention

Although several professional organizations have published guidelines for VTE prophylaxis in adult oncology patients, evidence-based guidelines for prevention in children with cancer are lacking. The American Society of Clinical Oncology (ASCO), the National Comprehensive Cancer Network (NCCN), and others have recommended prophylactic anticoagulation for all hospitalized oncology patients and for high-risk surgical oncology patients, but not for ambulatory cancer patients with or without CVCs (Khorana et al. 2009). These guidelines, developed for adults with a very different range of malignancies, comorbidities, and treatments than seen in children, are clearly not directly applicable to the pediatric oncology population.

Evidence from clinical trials of thromboprophylaxis in children with cancer is limited and generally

inconclusive. The Prophylaxis of Thromboembolism in Kids (PROTEKT) trial randomized 186 children with CVCs, half with cancer, to receive reviparin LMWH prophylaxis or standard care. There was no difference in the rate of TE or adverse events, but the study was underpowered and terminated early due to slow accrual (Massicotte et al. 2003). The PARKAA trial randomly assigned 85 patients treated for ALL on contemporary North American protocols to receive weekly infusions of AT during induction with asparaginase. Twenty-eight percent of patients treated with AT developed TE versus 37 % in the control group, but the study was underpowered to show a significant difference, and no difference was seen in markers of endogenous thrombin generation (Mitchell et al. 2003a). Supplementation with fresh frozen plasma (FFP) has been shown to be ineffective in correcting hemostatic parameters in children treated with asparaginase (Nowak-Göttl et al. 2009). Ruud et al. (2006) reported no reduction in the incidence of CVC-related jugular thrombosis among 62 children with cancer in a randomized, placebo-controlled study of low-dose warfarin prophylaxis.

Several small cohort studies and case series have reported various methods of thromboprophylaxis. Harlev et al. (2010) screened 80 children with ALL for inherited thrombophilia and provided enoxaparin prophylaxis during induction for 18 patients with prothrombin gene mutation or factor V Leiden heterozygosity. Six patients (7.5 %) developed TE, half of whom had PT mutation and were receiving prophylaxis. Elhasid et al. (2001) prescribed enoxaparin prophylaxis during asparaginase treatment to 41 consecutive children with ALL and reported no episodes of TE and no bleeding but with no comparative control group. Meister et al. (2008) reported no episodes of TE in 41 children treated on BFM ALL trials with AT supplementation and enoxaparin prophylaxis in induction and reduction versus 13 % of 71 patients in an earlier cohort treated on the same protocol with AT supplementation alone. Mitchell et al. (2010) recently reported validation of a predictive model for identifying the risk of TE in children with ALL treated on Berlin-Frankfurt-Munster (BFM), Cooperative Acute Lymphoblastic Leukemia (COALL) and French Acute

Lymphoblastic Leukemia (FRALLE) induction protocols. The model incorporates factors including concomitant asparaginase with steroids, presence of a CVC and genetic thrombophilia. Eight high-risk patients received enoxaparin prophylaxis during induction at their physicians' discretion and one developed TE as compared with eight events among 11 high-risk patients who received no thromboprophylaxis (Mitchell et al. 2010). Of note, this predictive model was protocol specific (no high-risk patients on the FRALLE protocol experienced TE) and would require further study before application in the context of current North American or other protocols.

The small size, variability and design of these studies constitute significant limitations. At this time, there is insufficient evidence to recommend routine thromboprophylaxis in children with cancer. The American College of Chest Physicians (ACCP), in its 2012 clinical practice guidelines for antithrombotic therapy in children and neonates, recommends against the use of routine systemic thromboprophylaxis for children with short- or medium-term CVCs (Monagle et al. 2012). Without evidence to support any benefit of prophylactic FFP or AT replacement, routine screening of coagulation tests during ALL induction therapy is not recommended. Similarly, routine screening of children with ALL (or other malignancies) for inherited thrombophilia is not currently advised outside of a clinical trial, but may be appropriate for patients with a confirmed family history of a high-risk genetic defect (Astwood and Vora 2011). Secondary screening may be considered for patients at the time of diagnosis with symptomatic TE. At our institution, patients who develop a non-CVC-associated thrombosis are usually tested for factor V Leiden, prothrombin G20210A mutation, protein C and S deficiency, AT deficiency, lipoprotein (a), fasting serum homocysteine, factor VIII, and antiphospholipid antibodies.

Prophylaxis may be considered for select groups of patients at increased risk, including those with known inherited prothrombotic defects who are receiving asparaginase, adolescents undergoing major surgery or prolonged immobilization, and patients with a previous history of TE

with other risk factors such as surgery or disease relapse (Wiernikowski and Athale 2006). Evidence-based data to support these considerations in pediatric patients are lacking.

8.7.2 Treatment

LMWH is the anticoagulant of choice for most pediatric patients, offering advantages of reduced monitoring, minimal drug or diet interactions, and a favorable safety profile (Monagle et al. 2012). The REVIVE (reviparin in childhood venous thromboembolism) trial is the only randomized study of LMWH in pediatrics (Massicotte et al. 2003). This trial compared reviparin to unfractionated heparin (UH) and oral anticoagulation in children with TE but terminated early due to slow enrollment. Though underpowered, it contributed to other accumulating evidence that LMWH is safe and effective treatment for TE in pediatrics (Massicotte et al. 2003). Alternatives include UH, which may be preferred initially over LMWH in circumstances of increased bleeding risk where rapid reversal may be necessary. Systemic or catheter-directed thrombolysis with tissue plasminogen activator (tPA) may be considered in some cases of high-risk thrombosis, though experience in children, particularly in the setting of malignancy, is very limited. The 2012 ACCP guidelines suggest tPA use only for life- or limb-threatening thrombosis in children (Monagle et al. 2012). Warfarin is often problematic in children with cancer because of problems related to dosing, drug interactions, vitamin K variability, and difficulty of oral administration during episodes of nausea and mucositis. It is generally not recommended for children during treatment for cancer, but can be considered for long-term or indefinite anticoagulation, when required.

In their 2012 guidelines, the ACCP suggests that children with cancer who develop TE follow the general recommendations for children with TE, using LMWH for a minimum of 3 months and until the precipitating factor has resolved (Monagle et al. 2012). In the acute setting of symptomatic TE, LMWH such as enoxaparin should be initiated twice daily at 1–1.5 mg/kg/ dose subcutaneously and adjusted to maintain an anti-Xa level of 0.5–1.0 units/mL in a sample taken 4 h after injection (Manco-Johnson 2006). Whether a minimum of 3 months of LMWH treatment is necessary in a TE that resolves quickly is unknown and more rapid transition to prophylactic dosing may be reasonable (Manco-Johnson 2006).

Patients may transition to once-daily pro- phylactic dosing (although ideal prophylactic dosing remains q12 h), with a target anti-Xa level of 0.1–0.3 units/mL (although anti-Xa levels do not generally need to be followed with prophy- lactic dosing), upon recanalization or after 3–6 months (Manco-Johnson 2006; Nowak-Göttl et al. 2009). Prophylaxis should continue throughout asparaginase therapy until 48 h after the last dose or 2 weeks after PEG-asparaginase (Payne and Vora 2007). Due to noted worse outcomes in patients receiving less asparagi- nase, the general recommendation is to tempo- rarily suspend asparaginase after TE diagnosis and restart at a later point with concomitant anticoagulation (Silverman et al. 2001; Grace et al. 2011). In the analysis of Dana Farber Cancer Institute (DFCI) consortium data, Grace et al. (2011) reported that 77 % of patients restarted asparaginase with 17 % of pediatric patients having recurrent TE following this methodology. The ACCP guidelines also recom- mend continuing prophylactic dosing of antico- agulation until CVC removal, with therapeutic dosing if there is a recurrence of TE until 3 months after CVC removal. Clinicians will need to take into consideration the need for surgery, chemotherapy and other treatments that may modify the risk-benefit ratio for the treatment of TE during this period. If nonfunctioning or no longer needed, the CVC should be removed after at least 3–5 days of anticoagulation, but if func- tional and still clinically necessary, the CVC can remain in situ with anticoagulation as described above (Monagle et al. 2012).

Optimal dosing of unfractionated heparin (UH) is poorly defined in children and has been extrapolated from adult data. If UH is initially used, the ACCP recommendation is to bolus with 75 units/kg IV over 10 min, then start an initial maintenance dose of 20 units/kg/h for patients >1 year of age (28 units/kg/h for infants). Activated PTT should be monitored 4 h after the loading dose and 4 h after every change in infusion rate. The rate should be adjusted to maintain an aPTT of 60–85 s (2–3 times upper limit of normal; unfractionated anti-Xa level of 0.35–0.7 units/mL). Once therapeutic aPTT levels are obtained, monitoring requires a daily CBC and aPTT. Plasminogen and antithrombin should be monitored and repleted to ensure hepa- rin efficacy; D-dimers can be measured to moni- tor response and fibrinogen should be followed and repleted to prevent bleeding complications. Boluses should be withheld if there is a signifi- cant bleeding risk (Monagle et al. 2012).

In the case of life-threatening TE, the ACCP recommends thrombectomy along with thera- peutic anticoagulation. In the setting of lower extremity VTE where anticoagulation is contra- indicated, a retrievable IVC filter may be placed temporarily. For children with CVC-associated right atrial thrombosis, catheter removal with or without anticoagulation is recommended, while anticoagulation is encouraged and, potentially, if the thrombus is large (i.e., >2 cm) and mobile, with CVC removal and consideration for surgi- cal intervention or thrombolysis as indicated (Monagle et al. 2012). For children with CSVT without significant intracranial hemorrhage, the ACCP recommends initial anticoagulation with UH or LMWH and total anticoagulation for at least 3 months, continuing for 3 additional months for persistent occlusion or symptoms. If there is significant hemorrhage, anticoagulation may either be initiated or reserved for cases with thrombus extension after 5–7 days. Surgical inter- vention or thrombolysis is reserved for patients who show no improvement on initial anticoagu- lation therapy (Monagle et al. 2012).

Necessity of reduction or cessation of antico- agulation during periods of thrombocytopenia is unstudied, and decisions should be tailored to individual circumstances. During initial therapeu- tic anticoagulation, platelets may be transfused to maintain a platelet count of $>20–50 \times 10^9$/L (Manco-Johnson 2006; Nowak-Göttl et al. 2009).

Safe LMWH dosing in the stable pediatric oncology patient with thrombocytopenia is unclear; our institutional practice is to hold LMWH with platelet counts $<50 \times 10^9$/L although other treatment strategies may be equally valid. Enoxaparin should be held 24 h before lumbar punctures or other procedures and resumed 12 h later or 24 h after neurosurgery (Manco-Johnson 2006; Wiernikowski and Athale 2006).

8.8 Summary

TE is a common and significant complication of childhood cancer, though the exact incidence remains unknown. Most evidence pertains to children with ALL, but those with solid tumors and other hematologic malignancies are also affected. The most important risk factors include older age, presence of a CVC, CVC dysfunction, asparaginase treatment, and intrathoracic or metastatic disease in solid tumors. Clinical features and diagnosis of TE are similar in cancer to the general pediatric population, with a predominance of catheter-associated venous thromboses and, in ALL, sinovenous thrombosis. Screening for inherited thrombophilia or for asymptomatic TE is not recommended, and there is insufficient evidence to support primary prophylaxis with anticoagulation or clotting factor support. Management of symptomatic TE in children with cancer should follow established general pediatric guidelines but presents particular challenges due to the additional risks of bleeding, ongoing therapy and underlying malignancy. LMWH is the treatment of choice for TE in pediatric oncology with anticoagulation continuing while risk factors, such as a CVC or asparaginase therapy, persist. Dose adjustment during periods of thrombocytopenia or with invasive procedures may be required. Despite an abundance of data regarding thrombosis in adults with cancer, there is relatively little evidence to guide the management of TE in children with malignancy. More research is urgently needed to better understand the epidemiology and risk factors for thrombosis in these children and to develop strategies for prevention and optimal therapy.

References

Astwood E, Vora A (2011) Personal practice: how we manage the risk of bleeding and thrombosis in children and young adults with acute lymphoblastic leukaemia. Br J Haematol 152:505–511

Athale UH, Chan AK (2003a) Thrombosis in children with acute lymphoblastic leukemia: part I. Epidemiology of thrombosis in children with acute lymphoblastic leukemia. Thromb Res 111:125–131

Athale UH, Chan AK (2003b) Thrombosis in children with acute lymphoblastic leukemia. Part II. Pathogenesis of thrombosis in children with acute lymphoblastic leukemia: effects of the disease and therapy. Thromb Res 111:199–212

Athale UH, Siciliano SA, Crowther M et al (2005) Thromboembolism in children with acute lymphoblastic leukaemia treated on Dana-Farber Cancer Institute protocols: effect of age and risk stratification of disease. Br J Haematol 129:803–810

Athale U, Cox S, Siciliano S, Chan AK (2007) Thromboembolism in children with sarcoma. Pediatr Blood Cancer 49:171–176

Athale UH, Nagel K, Khan AA, Chan AK (2008a) Thromboembolism in children with lymphoma. Thromb Res 122:459–465

Athale U, Siciliano S, Thabane L et al (2008b) Epidemiology and clinical risk factors predisposing to thromboembolism in children with cancer. Pediatr Blood Cancer 51:792–797

Boulet SL, Amenda D, Gross SC, Hooper WC (2011) Health care expenditures associated with venous thromboembolism among children. Thromb Res 129: 583–587

Caruso V, Iacoviello L, Di Castelnuovo A et al (2006) Thrombotic complications in childhood acute lymphoblastic leukemia: a meta-analysis of 17 prospective studies comprising 1752 pediatric patients. Blood 108:2216–2222

Deitcher SR, Gajjar A, Kun L, Heideman RL (2004) Clinically evident venous thromboembolic events in children with brain tumors. J Pediatr 145:848–850

Dipasco PJ, Misra S, Koniaris LG, Moffat FL Jr (2011) Thrombophilic state in cancer, part I: biology, incidence, and risk factors. J Surg Oncol 104:316–322

Dipasco PJ, Misra S, Koniaris LG, Moffat FL Jr (2012) The thrombophilic state in cancer part II: cancer outcomes, occult malignancy, and cancer suppression. J Surg Oncol 106:517–523

Elhasid R, Lanir N, Sharon R et al (2001) Prophylactic therapy with enoxaparin during L-asparaginase treatment in children with acute lymphoblastic leukemia. Blood Coagul Fibrinolysis 12:367–370

Glaser DW, Medeiros D, Rollins N, Buchanan GR (2001) Catheter-related thrombosis in children with cancer. J Pediatr 138:255–259

Grace RF, Dahlberg SE, Neuberg D et al (2011) The frequency and management of asparaginase-related thrombosis in paediatric and adult patients with acute lymphoblastic leukaemia treated on Dana-Farber Cancer Institute consortium protocols. Br J Haematol 152:452–459

Guyatt G, Gutterman D, Baumann MH et al (2006) Grading strength of recommendations and quality of evidence in clinical guidelines: report from an American College of Chest Physicians Task Force. Chest 129:174–181

Harlev D, Zaidman I, Sarig G et al (2010) Prophylactic therapy with enoxaparin in children with acute lymphoblastic leukemia and inherited thrombophilia during L-asparaginase treatment. Thromb Res 126:93–97

Kerlin BA (2012) Current and future management of pediatric venous thromboembolism. Am J Hematol 87:S68–S74

Khorana AA, Streiff MB, Farge D et al (2009) Venous thromboembolism prophylaxis and treatment in cancer: a consensus statement of major guidelines panels and call to action. J Clin Oncol 27:4919–4926

Kuhle S, Spavor M, Massicotte P et al (2008) Prevalence of post-thrombotic syndrome following asymptomatic thrombosis in survivors of acute lymphoblastic leukemia. J Thromb Haemost 6:589–594

Male C, Chait P, Andrew M et al (2003) Central venous line-related thrombosis in children: association with central venous line location and insertion technique. Blood 101:4273–4278

Manco-Johnson MJ (2006) How I treat venous thrombosis in children. Blood 107:21–29

Massicotte P, Julian JA, Gent M et al (2003) An open-label randomized controlled trial of low molecular weight heparin for the prevention of central venous line-related thrombotic complications in children: the PROTEKT trial. Thromb Res 109:101–108

McLean TW, Fisher CJ, Snively BM, Chauvenet AR (2005) Central venous lines in children with lesser risk acute lymphoblastic leukemia: optimal type and timing of placement. J Clin Oncol 23:3024–3029

Meister B, Kropshofer G, Klein-Franke A et al (2008) Comparison of low-molecular-weight heparin and antithrombin versus antithrombin alone for the prevention of symptomatic venous thromboembolism in children with acute lymphoblastic leukemia. Pediatr Blood Cancer 50:298–303

Mitchell L, Andrew M, Hanna K et al (2003a) Trend to efficacy and safety using antithrombin concentrate in prevention of thrombosis in children receiving l-asparaginase for acute lymphoblastic leukemia. Results of the PAARKA study. Thromb Haemost 90:235–244

Mitchell LG, Andrew M, Hanna K et al (2003b) A prospective cohort study determining the prevalence of thrombotic events in children with acute lymphoblastic leukemia and a central venous line who are treated with L-asparaginase: results of the Prophylactic Antithrombin Replacement in Kids with Acute Lymphoblastic Leukemia Treated with Asparaginase (PARKAA) Study. Cancer 97:508–516

Mitchell L, Lambers M, Flege S et al (2010) Validation of a predictive model for identifying an increased risk for

thromboembolism in children with acute lymphoblastic leukemia: results of a multicenter cohort study. Blood 115:4999–5004

Monagle P, Chan AK, Goldenberg NA et al (2012) Antithrombotic therapy in neonates and children: Antithrombotic Therapy and Prevention of Thrombosis, 9th ed: American College of Chest Physicians Evidence-Based Clinical Practice Guidelines. Chest 141:e737S–e801S

Nowak-Göttl U, Wermes C, Junker R et al (1999) Prospective evaluation of the thrombotic risk in children with acute lymphoblastic leukemia carrying the MTHFR TT 677 genotype, the prothrombin G20210A variant, and further prothrombotic risk factors. Blood 93:1595–1599

Nowak-Göttl U, Heinecke A, von Kries R et al (2001) Thrombotic events revisited in children with acute lymphoblastic leukemia: impact of concomitant Escherichia coli asparaginase/prednisone administration. Thromb Res 103:165–172

Nowak-Göttl U, Ahlke E, Fleischhack G et al (2003) Thromboembolic events in children with acute lymphoblastic leukemia (BFM protocols): prednisone versus dexamethasone administration. Blood 101:2529–2533

Nowak-Göttl U, Kenet G, Mitchell LG (2009) Thrombosis in childhood acute lymphoblastic leukaemia: epidemiology, aetiology, diagnosis, prevention and treatment. Best Pract Res Clin Haematol 22:103–114

Payne JH, Vora AJ (2007) Thrombosis and acute lymphoblastic leukaemia. Br J Haematol 138:430–445

Paz-Priel I, Long L, Helman LJ et al (2007) Thromboembolic events in children and young adults with pediatric sarcoma. J Clin Oncol 25:1519–1524

Qureshi A, Mitchell C, Richards S et al (2010) Asparaginase-related venous thrombosis in UKALL 2003—re-exposure to asparaginase is feasible and safe. Br J Haematol 149:410–413

Raffini L, Thornburg C (2009) Testing children for inherited thrombophilia: more questions than answers. Br J Haematol 147:277–288

Ruud E, Holmstrøm H, De Lange C et al (2006) Low-dose warfarin for the prevention of central line-associated thromboses in children with malignancies—a randomized, controlled study. Acta Paediatr 95:1053–1059

Silverman LB, Gelber RD, Dalton VK et al (2001) Improved outcome for children with acute lymphoblastic leukemia: results of Dana-Farber Consortium Protocol 91-01. Blood 97:1211–1218

Silverman LB, Supko JG, Stevenson KE et al (2010) Intravenous PEG-asparaginase during remission induction in children and adolescents with newly diagnosed acute lymphoblastic leukemia. Blood 115:1351–1353

Tabori U, Beni-Adani L, Dvir R et al (2004) Risk of venous thromboembolism in pediatric patients with brain tumors. Pediatr Blood Cancer 43:633–636

Wiernikowski JT, Athale UH (2006) Thromboembolic complications in children with cancer. Thromb Res 118:137–152

Pain Management

9

Sonia Malhotra and Scott Maurer

Contents

S. Malhotra, MD
Section of Palliative Care and Medical Ethics,
Division of General Internal Medicine,
University of Pittsburgh School of Medicine,
Pittsburgh, PA, USA

S. Maurer, MD (✉)
Division of Pediatric Hematology/Oncology
and Department of Supportive Care,
Children's Hospital of Pittsburgh,
University of Pittsburgh School of Medicine,
4401 Penn Avenue, 5th Floor PL,
Pittsburgh, PA 15224, USA
e-mail: scott.maurer@chp.edu

Abstract

Pain is a common and often underreported and undertreated symptom in children with cancer. Recognition of pain and prompt and vigilant treatment are essential facets of high quality patient care. This chapter serves to provide an overview of the assessment and management of pain in pediatric oncology patients. The ability to assess pain in children of all ages and developmental ability as well as identify and diagnose different pain types is an imperative skill, and various assessment tools are discussed. Management of pain in children is based on the World Health Organization's pain ladder, and a step-by-step approach to opioid management is provided along with case examples and common side

J. Feusner et al. (eds.), *Supportive Care in Pediatric Oncology:
A Practical Evidence-Based Approach*, Pediatric Oncology,
DOI 10.1007/978-3-662-44317-0_9, © Springer Berlin Heidelberg 2015

effects. Since neuropathic pain is a common symptom experienced by children with cancer, a separate section with descriptions of adjuvant therapies is also provided. More recently, data are emerging in support of non-pharmacologic pain management techniques, and a brief overview is discussed. Finally, oncology-specific pain topics such as vincristine-related peripheral neuropathy, osteonecrosis and post-lumbar puncture headache are addressed.

9.1 Introduction

One of the most common symptoms experienced by children with life-threatening and chronic conditions is pain. Pain in children is often underreported and undertreated (Wolfe et al. 2000). When left untreated, pain can have significant effects on children, their families and caregivers. Children with cancer who undergo aggressive treatment are more likely to experience severe pain at the end of life (Schindera et al. 2013). An effective treatment plan first requires practitioners to accurately recognize and assess pain. Frequent reevaluation of symptoms and treatment plans is equally vital. The main goal of pain management is for the child to be pain free. To accomplish this goal, it is important for practitioners to have a validated, evidence-based method of assessing pain and initiating a treatment plan. When achieving this goal is difficult, early referral to a palliative care physician or pain specialist should occur.

9.2 General Assessment

Pain is a subjective feeling and requires a detailed history from the patient and caregiver. Developmentally appropriate validated pain assessment scales (Fig. 9.1) should be used in the evaluation of pain (Twycross et al. 2009). The same assessment method should be used throughout to evaluate the effectiveness of the treatment plan. It is important in the assessment of pain that previous pain history and management are addressed as well as current medications and allergies. Additionally, contributing factors such as disease course, anxiety, age, development and temperament should be explored.

The perception of pain is directly related to a child's age and developmental level (Gaffney and Dunne 1986). Pain is identifiable by children at 18 months of age, and children can identify where they "hurt" by 4 years. In the past it was incorrectly presumed that infants do not feel as much pain as adults. Although infants' pain pathways are immature, they are fully able to transmit impulses (Fitzgerald 2000). Generally children <6 years need help describing their pain. Children >6 years can describe pain, and those between the ages of 7 to 11 often find themselves responsible for it or may recognize pain as a form of punishment (Esteve and Marquina-Aponte 2012). Adolescents are able to understand the multiple layers to pain consisting of psychological and physical causes. Adolescents often can be taught coping mechanisms due to this complex and abstract view of pain.

A complete assessment should include a thorough clinical examination. Facial expression should be noted in infancy as a behavior signaling pain (Izard et al. 1987). Pain in this age group, as well as in children with developmental delay, is typified by facial grimacing, quivering of the chin, grunting and clenching of the jaw. Other signs of pain in infants include kicking, arching, high-pitched crying and inability to be consoled (Krechel and Bildner 1995; Merkel et al. 1997). Physiological changes in heart and respiratory rate, blood pressure, and oxygen saturation can be evoked by pain but often do not indicate the level of pain in clinical encounters (Sweet and McGrath 1998).

9.3 Types of Pain

Two primary types of pain, nociceptive and neuropathic, have been described. Identification of the type of pain can be made by history and physical exam along with the input of imaging modalities. Delineating which type of pain a patient is experiencing is imperative as it guides therapy and may aid in determining an underlying etiology.

a FLACC Behavioral Pain Assessment Scale[a]

Parameter	Score		
	0	1	2
Face	No particular expression or smiling	Occasional grimace or frown, withdrawn, disinterested	Frequent to constant quivering chin, clenched jaw, distressed/panicked
Legs	Normal position, relaxed	Uneasy, restless, tense, occasional tremors	Kicking or legs drawn up, increased spasticity, constant tremors or jerking
Activity	Lying quietly, normal position, moves easily	Squirming, shifting, tense/guarded	Arched, rigid, jerking, severe agitation; head banging
Cry	No cry	Moans or whimpers, occasional complaints	Crying steadily, screams or sobs, frequent complaints; constant grunting
Consolability	Content, relaxed	Reassured by touch, hugging, or talking to; distractible	Difficult to console or comfort, resistant
Total Score (higher score indicates worse pain)			

Adapted from Merkel et al. (1997)
[a]for 2 months of age to 7 years, pre-verbal or delayed

b Wong-Baker Faces Pain Scale[a]

0	No hurt	
2	Hurts a little bit	
4	Hurts a little more	
6	Hurts even more	
8	Hurts a whole lot	
10	Hurts worst	

Adapted from Whaley and Wong (1995)
[a]4-12 years of age

c Visual Analog Scale (VAS)[a]

Score	Description
0	No pain
1	
2	
3	
4	
5	Moderate pain
6	
7	
8	
9	
10	Worst pain imaginable

Adapted from Whaley and Wong (1995)
[a] >8 years of age

Fig. 9.1 Pain assessment tools. (**a**) FLACC behavioral pain assessment scale. (**b**) Wong-Baker faces pain scale. (**c**) Visual analog scale (VAS)

9.3.1 Nociceptive Pain

Nociceptive pain is caused by past or ongoing tissue injury in the form of mechanical, thermal or chemical insults to the patient. Tissue damage activates pain receptors (nociceptors) in the skin, soft tissue, skeletal muscle, bone and certain viscera as a warning signal to the body. Signals from nociceptors travel via peripheral sensory neurons and synapse within the dorsal horn of the spinal cord. Following pathways through the brainstem and thalamus, the pain signal is then interpreted by the somatosensory cortex. This process makes up the so-called ascending pathway of pain and is the therapeutic target of opioids. The interpretation and response to pain is heavily modulated by a number of factors including a subsequent descending pathway of inhibition of pain transmission from the brainstem to dorsal horn neurons. N-Methyl-D-aspartate (NMDA) receptors at the level of the dorsal horn of the spinal cord play an important role in this pathway. As signals continue to be received from the ascending pathway, NMDA receptors are activated and decrease central inhibition of the transmission of ascending pain signals from the periphery. This positive reinforcement of the pain signal is key to the continued sensation of pain. Importantly, μ-opioid receptor activity also increases NMDA activity, playing a central role in the development of opioid tolerance and opioid refractory pain. NMDA antagonists, therefore, have been shown to reduce opioid use through reduction in tolerance and by encouraging inhibition of pain signaling via the descending pathway (Collins and Walker 2006).

Important subtypes of nociceptive pain are somatic and visceral pain. Somatic pain occurs in response to inflammation and damage to the soft tissue, muscle, skin and bone. It tends to be well localized and described as a dull, aching pain or a sharp, stabbing sensation that is worse with movement. Visceral pain is caused by direct stimulation of afferent nerves due to tumor infiltration or inflammation of some, but not all, viscera. In contrast to somatic pain, visceral pain is poorly localized and is sometimes referred to another body site. Patients often describe visceral pain as dull, achy or squeezing (Friedrichsdorf and Kang 2007). Control of either type of nociceptive pain is dependent on treatment or amelioration of the underlying cause along with use of anti-inflammatory drugs and opioids.

9.3.2 Neuropathic Pain

Neuropathic pain results from disruption of neuron signaling pathways in the peripheral, autonomic, and central nervous system and is caused by direct nervous system injury or indirect injury due to medications such as vincristine (Baron et al. 2010). Nerve injury results in inflammatory mediator signaling which increases sodium channel expression on injured and surrounding neurons. The threshold of activation of the sodium channels is lowered which triggers nociceptor activation as well. Additionally, as in nociceptive pain, continued signaling from damaged afferent peripheral nerves leads to over activation of NMDA receptors with a resultant decrease in the inhibitory tone of the descending pathway. In addition to NMDA activity, serotonin and norepinephrine also play a role in the modulation of neuropathic pain, thus underlining the importance of NMDA antagonists (i.e., ketamine) and serotonin and norepinephrine reuptake inhibitors (i.e., SNRIs such as duloxetine, venlafaxine, desvenlafaxine) in the treatment of this pain (Portenoy et al. 2005). Neuropathic pain is described as numbness and tingling, itching, burning, "pins-and-needles" sensations, and sharp, shooting pain. Neuropathic pain can also present with sensory disturbances like allodynia and temperature sensitivity, causing dramatic pain with even minor, otherwise normal stimuli (Chong and Bajwa 2003).

9.4 Pharmacologic Treatment of Pain

A summary of general principles for pain management is provided in Table 9.1. Detailed discussion and case examples are given below.

Table 9.1 General analgesic principles[a]

1. Assess pain. Pain is a subjective feeling (ask the patient or use a developmentally appropriate pain assessment scale – see Sect. 9.2)

   (a) Determine previous pain history and management, current medications, allergies

   (b) Explore contributing factors (e.g. disease course, anxiety, age, development, temperament)

2. In opioid-naïve patients, start with short-acting opioids to control acute, moderate to severe pain. Do not use long-acting opioids to control acute pain

3. When titrating or changing opiate dose, start by calculating the previous day's total opioid requirement in oral morphine equivalents (OME)

   (a) Since all opioids produce analgesia by the same mechanism, they will produce similar degrees of analgesia if provided in equianalgesic doses (see Sect. 9.4.5)

4. Determine if dose is adequate for pain control, and increase as needed (see Sect. 9.4.2)

5. Choose opioid that will be used and dose adjust for incomplete cross-tolerance if necessary (see Sect. 9.4.5)

   (a) Typically, the only reasons to change from one opioid to another are side effects or renal failure

   (b) When rotating, decrease dose by 25–50 % to correct for incomplete cross-tolerance

6. Determine route that opioid will be given. IM administration is rarely, if ever, indicated

   (a) Rectal = oral = sublingual dosing and SC = IM = IV dosing

7. Determine a dosing schedule

   (a) Use only short-acting prn doses until a sense is gained as to how much opioid is needed

   (b) Once stable daily needs are determined (and need for pain medication is expected to persist), consider giving 66–75 % of daily OME as a long-acting opioid (see Sect. 9.4.3)

   (c) For patient-controlled analgesia (PCA) dosing see Sect. 9.4.6

8. Determine breakthrough dose for acute pain not controlled by the long-acting medication (see Sect. 9.4.4)

   (a) Use same opioid for short- and long-acting when possible

   (b) Give 10–15 % of total daily long-acting dose as breakthrough dose q3h prn

9. Manage side effects as they arise (see Sect. 9.4.7)

   (a) Constipation is typically treated prophylactically

10. Determine whether co-analgesics/adjuvants and/or non-pharmacologic treatments would be beneficial (see Sects. 9.5 and 9.6)

IM intramuscular, *SC* subcutaneous, *IV* intravenous, *prn* as needed
[a]Level of evidence 1C for all recommendations per Guyatt et al. (2006); see Preface

Practitioners should utilize pain assessment tools, expectation for length of pain control required, and the patient's individual pain history to help guide decisions in pain management while continuing to reassess the patient for pain control and monitoring of side effects after initiation of pain medications.

9.4.1 World Health Organization Pain Ladder

The World Health Organization (WHO) created a three-step pain ladder as a basic approach to pain management in children with cancer (Fig. 9.2). A fourth step has also been developed for cancer pain not responding to pharmacotherapy alone and therefore requiring adjunct therapies such as interventional anesthesia. Morphine is the opioid used in the algorithm due to its ease of administration, tolerability, wide availability and well-understood side effects (Sirkia et al. 1997). Substitution with a different opioid is acceptable. The ladder is based on four major principles:

1. *By the ladder:* a stepwise approach should be taken on the escalation of analgesics depending on the severity of symptoms.

2. *By the clock:* scheduled analgesics should be given for steady state blood concentrations with appropriate as-needed (PRN) dosing.

3. *By the mouth:* the least invasive route of administration should be used that is convenient and cost-effective with effective pain control.

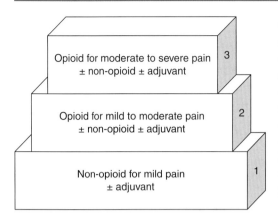

Fig. 9.2 World Health Organization three-step pain ladder

4. *By the child:* treatment plans should be individualized to the child's pain level and response to therapy.

For mild pain (step 1), a nonopioid analgesic should be primarily utilized. Ibuprofen and acetaminophen have been established for analgesia in children >3 months of age; newborn trials have found these agents to be ineffective (Berde and Sethna 2002). Although not evidence-based, nonsteroidal anti-inflammatory drugs (NSAIDs) are generally avoided in pediatric oncology patients due to reversible antiplatelet and fever-masking effects.

Step 2 in the WHO pain ladder calls for weak opioid therapy with the consideration of adjuvants such as combined opioid-NSAIDs. Step 2 has not been well characterized and calls for the use of pain medications that are controversial in pediatrics (Tremlett et al. 2010). Codeine, for example, should be avoided in children due to concerns for both efficacy and safety. Genetic variability in cytochrome P450 isoenzyme 2D6 (CYP2D6) significantly alters the ability to metabolize the drug into its active metabolite, morphine. Roughly one-third of Caucasian children have limited ability or are unable to metabolize codeine to morphine, and codeine-related deaths have been reported in children with CYP2D6 alleles associated with ultrarapid metabolism (Williams et al. 2002; Kelly et al. 2012; Anderson 2013). The latter has led to a Food and Drug Administration (FDA) black box warning which advises that

codeine is contraindicated in children after adenotonsillectomy for obstructive sleep apnea (Kuehn 2013). Additionally, medications such as tramadol have not been well studied in pediatrics, have a number of drug-drug interactions and reach a ceiling analgesic effect (Zernikow et al. 2009). Fixed combination products, such as acetaminophen/oxycodone and acetaminophen/hydrocodone, cause difficulty in dose escalation of the opioid due to dose limitations from the nonopioid component.

Step 3 in the WHO pain ladder calls for opioid therapy with consideration of an adjuvant. Several studies have demonstrated the efficacy of opioids in pain treatment. Although adjuvant therapy can be considered for the treatment of certain types of pain, a prospective non-randomized study in pediatric oncology patients demonstrated little additional analgesic benefit from the addition of nonopioids in children already receiving opioids (Zernikow et al. 2006). Further, analgesia was not improved when NSAIDs were added to a standing regimen of opioids, and the benefit of NSAIDs given for >7 days has not been established (McNicol et al. 2005). Lastly, children with cancer are at increased risk of NSAID-related bleeding as well as renal and gastrointestinal toxicity due to concurrent use of medications required for treatment of their tumors.

9.4.2 Intermittent Opioid Use

In opioid-naïve pediatric oncology patients, it is important to start with short-acting opioids to control acute, moderate to severe pain. Long-acting opioids should not be used for acute pain as they are designed to slowly release medication over a long period of time, generally 12 h. In children it is important to choose the type, preparation, dose and route of opioid such that the patient can comply with therapy. For example, intramuscular doses are avoided due to pain associated with administration and bleeding risks in patients with coagulopathy. Dosing depends on the route of administration, which in turn dictates the time to onset of medication effect. Rectal, sublingual and oral dosing are equivalent and have maximal

Table 9.2 Opioid equianalgesia conversions

Medication	Parenteral (mg)	Oral (mg)
Morphine	10	30
Oxycodone	–	20
Hydromorphone	1.5	7.5
Oxymorphone	1	10
Fentanyl	0.1[a]	–

Adapted from Friedrichsdorf and Kang (2007); McGhee et al. (2011)

[a]This dosing is not equivalent for transdermal fentanyl patches. Please refer to the specific drug information sheet from the manufacturer for fentanyl transdermal patch equivalency.

analgesic onset within 30–45 min. Subcutaneous, intramuscular and intravenous (IV) dosing are also equivalent, but the onset of action is faster, typically within 15 min (Mercadante 2012). When switching between oral and IV routes, dosing must be adjusted using a standardized equianalgesia table (Table 9.2). It is important to remind patients changing from IV to oral dosing that while the analgesic effect is expected to be similar between routes, the time to onset of analgesia is not.

Short-acting doses are given as needed until a clear sense of the total daily opioid dose required to keep the patient comfortable is established. Once stable daily needs are determined and the need for pain medication is expected to persist, long-acting doses should be considered. Unless there are contraindications such as renal failure, morphine is generally used as the first-line opioid. Initial doses should be calculated using a dose-per-kilogram basis (Table 9.3). Doses should be increased by 25–30 % for uncontrolled pain.

Case 1: Initiating Opioid Therapy
A 10-year-old, 30 kg boy presents to your outpatient clinic with a 3-month history of progressive right hip and knee pain. CT scan shows a pelvic lesion concerning for Ewing sarcoma, and now you and the family are planning an outpatient work-up of his tumor prior to starting therapy. The mother reports that he has been using five doses a day of acetaminophen for pain relief. Eric says he feels like he's being "stabbed in the leg" and rates his pain as 8 of 10 with little relief from the

acetaminophen. He has no drug allergies. They are asking if he can try something else for pain relief.

Plan
Looking at the WHO pain ladder, you decide to move up to opioids for moderate pain. Since he will be outpatient, you decide on an oral route, noting the patient prefers tablets to liquid medications. You decide to start with immediate-release morphine at a dose of 0.2–0.3 mg/kg every 3 h as needed (Table 9.3).

$$30 \text{ kg} \times 0.2 - 0.3 \text{ mg po morphine} / \text{kg}$$
$$= 6 - 9 \text{ mg po morphine}$$

You note that the smallest tablet preparation of immediate-release morphine is 15 mg, so you instruct him to take 7.5 mg (0.5 tab) every 3 h as needed and to call if it is ineffective. Of note, preparations including hydrocodone rather than oral morphine would also be reasonable in this case.

9.4.3 Long-Acting Opioids

One should consider the use of long-acting opioids when a stable daily dose of opioids is achieved and a persistent use of pain medication is expected. As described above, long-acting agents should not be used for acute pain as they slowly release medication. Long-acting opioids allow for around-the-clock analgesia and are used in combination with short acting opioids that serve to manage acute or breakthrough episodes of pain. The benefits of long-acting opioids include less use of breakthrough medication, improved sleep at night, improved comfort upon waking from sleep and less drowsiness.

When determining the amount of long-acting opioids, it is important to calculate the previous day's total opioid requirement (oral morphine equivalent or OME). Long-acting opioids should be dosed at 1/2 to 2/3 of the total OME. Slow-release morphine is used as first-line treatment and generally prescribed every 8–12 h. Doses should be reevaluated and titrated upwards if optimal pain control is not reached. This often occurs with disease progression or, less often, as a result of opioid tolerance.

Table 9.3 Pain management algorithm[a]

	Pain level	Rescue medication	Sustained medication
Step 1	Mild pain	Start rescue medication: Start a nonopioid analgesic (NSAID or acetaminophen) as needed	Consider sustained therapy: Consider a standing dose for short period of time
Step 2	Moderate pain	Start or escalate rescue medication: Acetaminophen with hydrocodone	Consider sustained therapy: Acetaminophen with hydrocodone (same dosage on scheduled basis)
Step 3	Severe pain	Start or escalate rescue medication: Morphine oral immediate-release preparation (a) Opioid naïve: 0.2–0.3 mg/kg/dose q3-4 h prn (b) Opioid exposed: increase previous dose 25–50 % for moderate pain and 50–100 % for severe pain	Start or escalate sustained medication: Morphine oral immediate-release preparation (a) Opioid naïve: 0.2–0.3 mg/kg/dose q3-4 h prn (b) Opioid exposed: total daily morphine dose divided every 3–4 h prn If meant for prolonged use, consider sustained-release morphine formulation Use of methadone or fentanyl patch should be in conjunction with palliative care or pain specialist
Step 4	Severe-persistent pain	Start or increase rescue medication: Morphine: IV, SC (a) Opioid naïve <6 months: 0.05–0.1 mg/kg/dose q3-4 h prn (b) Opioid naïve >6 months: 0.1–0.2 mg/kg/dose every 3–4 h prn (c) Opioid exposed: previous total daily oral dose converted to IV morphine equivalent and divided by frequency Consider patient-controlled analgesia (PCA) with morphine: (a) Opioid naïve: basal infusion, 0–0.02 mg/kg/h; demand dose, 0.015–0.02 mg/kg/dose; lockout interval, 5–15 min (b) Opioid exposed: basal infusion, daily dose divided by 24 h; demand dose, 50–100 % of hourly dose; lockout interval, 5–15 min	Initiate or escalate sustained medication: (a) Transition sustained medication to IV equivalent (b) Consider an infusion

NSAID nonsteroidal anti-inflammatory drug, *IV* intravenous, *SC* subcutaneous
Adapted from Klick and Hauer (2010)
[a]Level of evidence 1C for all recommendations per Guyatt et al. (2006); see Preface

Fentanyl patches and methadone are also effective as long-acting agents but are generally reserved when therapy with morphine or oxycodone has been unsuccessful or side effects have precluded their use. Equianalgesic conversions of fentanyl and methadone can be complicated and vary based on the total amount of OMEs. Methadone has unique pharmacokinetic properties that must be taken into consideration due to a long half-life requiring initially frequent dosing but later only every 12–24 h dosing. Methadone is potentially beneficial as it has less pruritus side effect and also may help treat concomitant nausea. A fentanyl patch can be a convenient way to provide pain medication delivery in the patient unable to easily take oral medications. Fentanyl and methadone should be prescribed by clinicians experienced in their use.

Case 1 (Continued) Starting Long-Acting Opioids
You see Eric 2 days later and he tells you the morphine is working well. Eric says his pain drops

from 8 of 10 to 3 of 10 within about 30 min of taking the medication, and the pain relief lasts for 3–4 h. His mother says he uses seven doses a day, but that he has excellent pain control. However, Eric does say that when he wakes up from sleeping his pain is really bad and takes some time to come back under control. Thus, his mother has been waking him up at night to give him the morphine. His mom is tired, but she tells you she's willing to do whatever it takes to keep him comfortable.

Plan

You decide that Eric would best be served with a long-acting opioid. To start, you calculate his total daily opioid requirement.

$$7.5 \, \text{mg po morphine} \times 7 \, \text{doses / day}$$
$$= 52.5 \, \text{mg po morphine per day}$$

You then determine that about 2/3 of his daily dose should be in his long-acting medication. Taking 2/3 of 52.5 mg, you decide that approximately 35 mg of morphine per day should be given in a long-acting form. Since morphine has worked so well for him, you choose sustained-release morphine as your long-acting agent. Noting that it comes in 15 mg tablets, you prescribe 15 mg by mouth twice a day, which will provide 30 mg per day in a long-acting form. You take care to advise Eric and his mother that this should be taken roughly every 12 h regardless of his pain level and that this medication will not help with breakthrough pain. He will also need a breakthrough dose; instructions for this calculation are in Sect. 9.4.4.

9.4.4 Breakthrough Dosing

Breakthrough dosing of pain medications should be used for acute pain that is not controlled by a long-acting medication. When possible, the same opioid should be used as the short- and long-acting agent. This dose should be calculated as 10–20 % of the total daily long-acting dose every 3–4 h as needed. All patients should have access to a breakthrough medication. An adult study demonstrated that up to 67 % of cancer patients with well-controlled pain have transitory episodes

of breakthrough pain requiring treatment (Bruera and Neumann 1999). Younger children with cancer tend to experience more breakthrough pain than older children (Friedrichsdorf et al. 2007).

If more than three breakthrough doses are needed in 24 h, consideration should be given to increasing the long-acting opioid dose. This should be done by calculating the daily OME from the long-acting opioid and from the total amount of breakthrough medicine required. A new long-acting dose can then be calculated using the principles listed in Sect. 9.4.3. A new, higher, breakthrough dose should be calculated as 10–20 % of the new, total daily long-acting dose.

Case 2 Calculating Breakthrough Dosing

You are taking care of a 50 kg girl with osteosarcoma of the proximal tibia. She is now 6 days post gross total resection of her tumor with a limb-sparing procedure. She has been on morphine by patient-controlled analgesia (PCA), and from a surgical standpoint, she is ready for discharge. Her morphine PCA settings have been a continuous rate of 1 mg/h with a demand dose of 1.5 mg every 15 min. She has been receiving about eight demand doses per day for the past 2 days and notes good pain control. The surgical team is asking you to determine an outpatient pain plan. She requests that you attempt to keep things in pill form.

Plan

The first step is to determine the total daily morphine requirement. Each day she receives 24 mg (1 mg/h) from her continuous rate and 12 mg (1.5 mg × 8 doses) from her demand, giving a total dose of 36 mg of IV morphine/day. Next you must decide on the oral formulation. Since morphine has worked well for her, you decide that you will use sustained-release morphine as your long-acting agent and immediate-release morphine for breakthrough.

To calculate the proper dose, you then need to convert the medication into OMEs (Table 9.2, see Sect. 9.4.5):

$$36 \, \text{mg IV morphine} \times \frac{30 \, \text{mg PO morphine}}{10 \, \text{mg IV morphine}}$$
$$= 108 \, \text{mg PO morphine}$$

The next step is to determine the amount of medication to place in long-acting form. In general, you would choose to take 2/3 of the total daily dose. Thus, 2/3 of 108 mg PO morphine is about 72 mg PO morphine. Noting that sustained-release morphine comes in 30 mg tablets given every 12 h, you decide to use 30 mg twice daily as the long-acting dose.

Next you need to calculate the breakthrough dose. Knowing that you are now going to give 60 mg per day as a long-acting dose, you can estimate the breakthrough dose at 10–20 % of the long-acting dose. This gives you a dose somewhere between 6 and 12 mg of immediate-release morphine. Recognizing that immediate-release morphine comes in 15 mg tablets, you choose a breakthrough dose of 7.5 mg.

Hence, you have settled on the following plan:
1. Sustained-release morphine 30 mg PO twice a day
2. Immediate-release morphine 7.5 mg PO every 3 h as needed for breakthrough pain

9.4.5 Opioid Rotation and Equianalgesia

When titrating or changing opiates, it is important to start by calculating the previous day's OME. All opioids produce analgesia by the same mechanism; thus, if provided in equianalgesic doses, they will produce the same degree of analgesia (Table 9.2). The most common reasons to change from one opioid to another are side effects and poor response to pain control despite appropriate titration (Drake et al. 2004). Other indications for opioid rotation include renal failure, problematic drug-drug interactions, preference or need for different route of administration or financial considerations.

When rotating opioids it is important to consider incomplete cross-tolerance. This concept takes into account that tolerance developed to one opioid does not imply complete tolerance to another. Also, the new drug may be more effective due to differences in drug bioavailability or potency (Pasero and McCaffery 2011). To account for this phenomenon, a dose reduction

by 25–50 % should occur when rotating opioids (Indelicato and Portenoy 2002). In most cases a 25 % reduction is appropriate but practitioners should use clinical judgment in determining how much of a dose reduction should occur as a result of incomplete cross-tolerance. For example, in the case of a patient who has undergone rapid increases in opioid dosing for pain subsequently deemed to be allodynia, a dose reduction of 50 % may be more appropriate.

Case 3 Opioid Switching
You are taking care of a 50 kg young man with newly diagnosed leukemia. He's been using morphine 5 mg IV every 3 h as needed for bone pain. Although he notes good pain relief, he has been itching uncontrollably. He asks you if there is anything you can do to help with his pain but keep him from itching.

Plan
This is one of the most common reasons to switch opioids. Although you could try a medication to treat the itching, changing the offending agent avoids polypharmacy. You decide that hydromorphone would be a nice alternative. To calculate a dose, you first need to determine the equianalgesic dose of hydromorphone and morphine (Table 9.2):

$$5\,\text{mg IV morphine} \times \frac{1.5\,\text{mg IV hydromorphone}}{10\,\text{mg IV morphine}}$$
$$= 0.75\,\text{mg IV hydromorphone}$$

The last step is to account for incomplete cross-tolerance. A dose reduction of 25 % would provide a dose of about 0.56 mg of IV hydromorphone. Thus, an order for 0.6 mg of IV hydromorphone every 3 h as needed for pain would be appropriate.

9.4.6 Patient-Controlled Analgesia Calculations

Patient-controlled analgesia (PCA) is indicated for use when pain is not controlled with oral medications, there is inability to take oral medications, there is possibly poor gastrointestinal absorption of pain medications, or if the child or parent has a preference for the PCA. Studies have demonstrated PCA effectiveness in postoperative pain, but PCA use is additionally effective in burns, mucositis, bone marrow transplant and sickle cell disease (Gaukroger et al. 1991; Mackie et al. 1991; Collins et al. 1996a; Dunbar et al. 1995; Trentadue et al. 1998; Walder et al. 2001). Children as young as 6 years are able to independently provide effective postoperative pain control when taught appropriate PCA use (Berde et al. 1991).

General principles and dosing of PCA are listed in Table 9.3. Opioid naïve patients should be started at low doses of medication. Lockout intervals, which represent how often a patient can push their PCA button to receive medication, should range between 5 and 15 min. Children currently receiving opioids should have their total daily OME calculated and a proportion of that dose (usually 2/3) divided over 24 h to give a continuous PCA rate. Demand (or breakthrough) doses for these patients should range from 50 to 100 % of their total hourly doses. PCA dosing plans should be frequently reassessed and titrated as necessary.

Initiation of PCA requires close monitoring of respiratory rate, oxygen saturation, blood pressure, heart rate, pain score, sedation score and nausea. Continuous pulse oximetry should be considered when PCA is started and naloxone should be available. If the child becomes somnolent, difficult to arouse, has a respiratory rate <8 or oxygen saturation <92 % with respiratory rate <12, or pinpoint pupils, administration of the opioid should be stopped and supplemental oxygen given along with naloxone. Doses can be cautiously restarted at 50 % of the original dose once the patient is alert and if they are experiencing pain. Many institutions have developed protocols for authorized agent-controlled analgesia (AACA) for children <6 years which can include either nurse-controlled or caregiver-controlled analgesia as long as the caregiver is consistently available, competent, and properly educated and the authorized agent is designated in the medical order (Wuhrman et al. 2007).

Case 4 PCA Calculations

A 15-year-old boy with acute myelogenous leukemia has developed mucositis while pancytopenic. He has been using 6 mg of IV morphine every 3 h around the clock. He tells you that the morphine has been very helpful, but his pain returns prior to the 3 h mark. He also complains that he gets somnolent immediately after the morphine dose is given. You decide that a PCA is warranted in order to give him better pain control.

Plan

The first step is to calculate his total 24 h use of morphine:

$$6 \, \text{mg of IV morphine} \times 8 \, \text{doses per day}$$
$$= 48 \, \text{mg IV morphine per day}$$

Next, you take 2/3 of that dose (48 mg × 0.67 = 32 mg) and plan for it as your continuous rate. Dividing 32 mg by 24 h gives you a continuous rate of about 1.2 mg/h. Next you must plan for your demand dose. There are a number of ways of doing this, but a good place to start would be to simply have the demand dose provide 50 % of the hourly rate with two demand doses per hour. The goal is to return the patient to comfort with a single demand dose, thus you may need to adjust this depending on his response. Finally you need to determine a lockout interval. The timing of this is patient dependent, but since the analgesic onset of action for morphine occurs within 10–15 min, this is a standard lockout interval.

Hence, you've decided on a morphine PCA with the following settings:

Morphine 1.2 mg/h plus 0.6 mg demand dose every 15 min as needed with a maximum hourly dose of 2.4 mg (bolus + 2 demand doses)

Follow-up:

The next morning the intern reports to you that the patient used 25 demand doses for a total daily dose of 43.8 mg (~1.8 mg/h). When you speak with the patient, he tells you that he is overall comfortable, but he sometimes needs two demand doses to return to comfort, especially upon waking from sleep.

Plan

In general, you'd like the patient to receive about 2/3 of his daily dose from the continuous and 1/3 from his demand, which when calculated is what he is receiving per hour ($43.8 \text{ mg} \times 0.67 = 29.3 \text{ mg}$, which divided by 24 h is 1.2 mg/h). However, his requirement for multiple doses after sleeping indicates that his continuous rate may be too low and also that he may need a higher demand dose. In such a situation, simply adjusting both continuous and demand dosing by 20–30% is a reasonable strategy, in this case increasing his basal rate to 1.4 mg/h and pushes to 0.7 mg, assuming no untoward opioid side effects as discussed below.

9.4.7 Side Effects of Opioids

Although generally well tolerated, opioids can cause adverse side effects in a minority of patients. Much of what has been studied about side effects has been investigated in adults (Cherny et al. 2001). Side effects can be managed by a reduction in the total opioid dose, but this is usually inappropriate as it would lead to ineffective pain management. Additionally, opioids can be switched to a different class (i.e., opioid rotation; see Sect. 9.4.5), which successfully manages most side effects (Drake et al. 2004). Symptomatic management of side effects is also a preferred method but adds to the medication burden. Low-dose naloxone has potential benefit in some opioid-induced side effects as described below, with the optimal dose in pediatric patients reported to be ≥ 1 μg/kg/h (Monitto et al. 2011).

9.4.7.1 Constipation

Intestinal motility is slowed by all opioids. Constipation should be anticipated and children should have one non-forced bowel movement every 1–2 days. In opioid-induced constipation, no laxative has been shown superior (Candy et al. 2011). Stool softeners such as docusate work by drawing water into the stool making it softer and thus require adequate fluid intake to be effective. Although commonly prescribed, efficacy of stool softeners as single agents in opioid-induced constipation is poor; thus, they should be used in combination with laxatives (Thomas 2008). Similar to stool softeners, fiber bulking agents draw and maintain water in stool, allowing multiple bowel movements to pass. Without adequate water intake, these agents may worsen constipation. Osmotic laxatives such as lactulose, sorbitol, magnesium citrate, and polyethylene glycol cause increased passage of stools through softening and pushing forward. Stimulant laxatives (i.e., senna and bisacodyl) increase peristalsis through stimulation of the myenteric plexus. Stimulant laxatives also increase intestinal secretions by altering fluid and electrolyte transport. Feudtner et al. (2014) have recently shown that senna therapy is more effective than other oral bowel medications for problematic opioid-induced constipation in pediatric oncology patients. Lubricant laxatives like mineral oil are primarily used for fecal impaction and work by softening fecal mass. Mineral oil, however, is generally avoided in children, especially infants and those with neurologic impairment, due to the risk of pneumonitis with aspiration (Phatak and Pashankar 2013). Rectal laxatives such as suppositories and enemas are generally used when other therapies have failed. In oncologic care, rectal agents are discouraged due to risk of infection in immunosuppressed patients.

Naloxone and methylnaltrexone are opioid antagonists which have potential benefit for reversal of opioid-induced constipation in the pediatric population. Naloxone is a nonselective opioid receptor antagonist that reverses all peripheral and central opioid mechanisms by crossing the blood-brain barrier. Oral naloxone is extensively metabolized in the liver with <2 % systemic bioavailability (Holzer 2010). Use of IV naloxone in this scenario is not appropriate as it will lead to rapid reversal of analgesia with onset of acute pain and may cause withdrawal symptoms. Methylnaltrexone is a selective, quaternary opioid antagonist that works only at peripheral μ-opioid receptors. This inability to cross the blood-brain barrier allows methylnaltrexone to treat opioid-induced constipation without interfering with analgesia. In a randomized trial, Thomas et al. (2008) showed benefit of subcutaneous methylnaltrexone in adult patients with opioid-induced constipation. One pediatric case series of 15 oncology patients has shown the potential benefit of subcutaneous methylnaltrexone in this setting at a mean dose of 0.15 mg/kg/dose (Rodrigues et al. 2013).

9.4.7.2 Nausea and Vomiting

Nausea and vomiting are rare opioid side effects in children but can occur with therapy initiation and will usually resolve within a few days. If nausea or vomiting persists, antiemetics such as ondansetron can be helpful. A detailed history is necessary to rule out constipation which can be a troublesome side effect of opioid therapy and result in significant nausea and vomiting. Low-dose naloxone has shown potential benefit in opioid-induced nausea and vomiting (Cepeda et al. 2004; Maxwell et al. 2005; Monitto et al. 2011).

9.4.7.3 Pruritus

Pruritus is a common side effect of opioid use and is the most common cause of opioid rotation in children (Drake et al. 2004). Pruritus often occurs with opioid initiation and clears within a few days. Low-dose naloxone has shown potential benefit in relieving opioid-induced pruritus (Cepeda et al. 2004; Maxwell et al. 2005; Monitto et al. 2011). If not improved with time and low-dose naloxone, opioid dose reduction can be considered. If this is unsuccessful or leads to inadequate pain management, diphenhydramine or hydroxyzine can be used. However, it is important to recognize that this is not an allergic or histamine-mediated reaction. Opioid rotation should be reserved when the above interventions have not successfully controlled pruritus and pain control is still required.

9.4.7.4 Sedation

Initiation and increase of opioid therapy may lead to a period of drowsiness that typically resolves within a few days. Persistence of sedation often is the result of renal, hepatic or CNS disease. In renal dysfunction, one of morphine's centrally acting metabolites, M6G, can accumulate. In this example, opioid rotation to an agent not renally excreted such as fentanyl is appropriate. Psychostimulants such as methylphenidate have shown benefit for their role as pain adjuncts and anti-sedatives in adult and adolescent trials but with adverse effects such as decreased appetite and tremor (Yee and Berde 1994). These medications have not been studied as an adjunct to opioid analgesia in younger children.

9.4.7.5 Confusion and Agitation

Renal and hepatic function should be checked when children become confused or agitated with opioids, and it should be ensured that correct dosing is being given. Opioid doses should be decreased or dosing intervals increased if with underlying hepatic or renal dysfunction. If confusion and agitation persist, opioid rotation should be strongly considered.

9.4.7.6 Respiratory Depression

When dosed appropriately, opioids rarely result in respiratory depression (Olkkola et al. 1988; Lynn et al. 1993). Cases of respiratory depression have primarily been seen when intravenous opioids are rapidly administered for procedures, when there is inability to excrete opioids or with concurrent use of benzodiazepines. Through its release of catecholamines, pain itself acts as a respiratory drive stimulant. Signs to evaluate for true respiratory depression include sleepiness, decreased consciousness, decreased respiratory rate and central apnea. If these symptoms are noted, an opioid antagonist such as naloxone should be administered and opioids restarted at 50 % dosing after resolution of symptoms.

9.4.7.7 Myoclonus

Patients receiving very high doses of opioids for a prolonged duration may experience myoclonus. Myoclonus typically presents as brief, involuntary muscle contractions that occur due to an accumulation of neurotoxic metabolites such as morphine-3-glucuronide (M3G). Treatment of myoclonus consists of the use of benzodiazepines such as midazolam or clonazepam or muscle relaxants such as baclofen or dantrolene (Mercadante 1998). Opioid rotation should be strongly considered.

9.4.7.8 Urinary Retention

Urinary retention can be caused by any opioid but is seen more frequently with epidural or spinal opioids, often after rapid dose escalation. Interventions to help treat urinary retention include external bladder pressure, intermittent catheterization, and bethanechol or tamsulosin to stimulate bladder contraction. However, the easiest and least invasive way to manage this is through opioid rotation. Gallo et al. (2008) have shown in adult postoperative patients treated with morphine PCA that low-dose naloxone improved urinary residuals and increased urinary frequency.

9.5 Neuropathic Pain

Neuropathic pain, as described in Sect. 9.3, is caused by damage to nociceptors and nociceptive pathways leading to abnormal pain signaling. Neuropathic pain has not been well studied in children. Characteristics that make neuropathic pain distressful include underassessment, prolonged duration and poor response to currently available treatments (Simon et al. 2012). Causes of neuropathic pain include lesions of the spinal cord, tumor-related pain that may damage tissues and nerves, and chemotherapeutic agents such as vincristine (see Sect. 9.8.1), cisplatin, and paclitaxel. Symptoms can last for months to years and can be exacerbated at the end of life (Drake et al. 2003).

Guidelines on assessment and diagnostic scales for evaluation have been designed for adults and can be used in adolescents (Haanpaa et al. 2011). Diagnosis in children is based primarily on symptom character and quality (see Sects. 9.3 and 9.8.1). A Cochrane review in adults found mixed results for the use of opioids in the treatment of neuropathic pain (Eisenberg et al. 2006). Adjuvants are typically used with opioids since an effective pain response with opioids alone may not be achieved (Chaparro et al. 2012). Adjuvant medications can cause significant side effects requiring patient and family education about these effects. Systematic evidence on the use of such adjuvant agents in pediatric oncology patients is lacking (Jacob 2004; Anghelescu et al. 2014). Additionally,

these medications can be used solely but require weeks of gradual titration. Topical agents such as capsaicin and lidocaine have shown some promise in producing analgesia in adult populations (Babbar et al. 2009; Cheville et al. 2009).

9.5.1 Calcium Channel Blockers

Calcium channel blockers such as gabapentin and pregabalin bind presynaptic voltage-gated calcium channels in the dorsal horn reducing the release of neuroexcitatory transmitters such as glutamate, noradrenaline and substance P. These agents have been the most studied in the pediatric population for neuropathic pain and inhibit the development of hyperalgesia and allodynia (Buck 2002; Vondracek et al. 2009). Doses can be titrated upwards as often as every 3 days although side effects may be limiting (see Sect. 9.8.1 for dosing). Side effects include lethargy, nausea and vomiting, dizziness, weight gain, and behavioral problems such as aggression, restlessness, and hyperactivity. Gabapentin and pregabalin are renally excreted and doses must be adjusted for renal insufficiency or failure.

9.5.2 Serotonin and Norepinephrine Reuptake Inhibitors

SNRIs inhibit serotonin and norepinephrine reuptake and have no effect on postsynaptic receptors. A few adult studies have shown improved neuropathic pain and minimal side effects with these agents (Goodyear-Smith and Halliwell 2009). Nausea is the most common reported side effect. Doses are generally titrated upwards on a weekly basis. Venlafaxine is available in an extended release form.

9.5.3 Tricyclic Antidepressants

The mechanism of action of tricyclic antidepressants (TCAs) is not well understood but appears to result from a combination of serotonin and norepinephrine presynaptic reuptake and inhibition of sodium channels. TCAs used in management of neuropathic pain include amitriptyline, imipramine, doxepin, desipramine and nortriptyline. Amitriptyline, imipramine, and doxepin are tertiary amines and cause increased levels of sedation. Other side effects include anticholinergic effects such as urinary retention, dry mouth, constipation and blurred vision. Doses should be titrated upwards weekly. TCAs are contraindicated in epileptic children because they lower the seizure threshold and in children with heart failure or cardiac conduction defects due to QTc prolongation effects.

9.6 Non-pharmacologic Treatment of Pain

The combination of pharmacologic and non-pharmacologic techniques to relieve pain and improve comfort has become increasingly recognized as complementary components in pain management (Twycross et al. 2009). Non-pharmacologic treatments address both physical and psychological aspects of pain and are often combined for improved pain control (Culbert and Olness 2010). Children with cancer often use alternative therapies in conjunction with standard pharmacologic treatments (Friedman et al. 1997). It is important to create a treatment plan that combines non-pharmacologic modalities that engage the child and compliment the child's energy level and comorbidities. Early introduction of these techniques helps them become therapeutically effective over time. Ideally all patients would utilize complementary therapies, especially when faced with chronic pain, although this is often limited by lack of resources.

9.6.1 Guided Imagery

Guided imagery uses personalized storytelling to aid children in mastering situations that provoke anxiety or fear. Parental involvement in the process is encouraged so the story can be retold during stressful treatments or procedures. Attention-distraction imagery involves teaching children to imagine a pleasant mental image during a painful experience (Turk 1978). Several studies have demonstrated the synergy of guided imagery with pharmacologic therapy in reducing pain and distress (Kuttner et al. 1988). In children undergoing bone marrow aspiration, an 18 % reduction in behavioral distress scores and 25 % reduction in self-reported pain scores has been noted with guided imagery (Jay et al. 1987). Imagery has been studied in older children and adults but has been particularly helpful in children from the age of 3–6 years where the boundaries between fantasy and reality are less concrete (Kuttner et al. 1988; Syrjala et al. 1995).

9.6.2 Biofeedback

Biofeedback is the process of converting physiologic signals such as blood pressure, pulse, muscle contractions, skin temperature and sweat response into audio or visual signals. Children are taught to observe these signals to help voluntarily control their physiologic response to pain and stress. Biofeedback is commonly used by pediatric anesthesia services for pain and anxiety management (Lin et al. 2005). Most studies demonstrating success using biofeedback have been conducted in children with chronic headache, with a 50 % symptom reduction in >2/3 of children (Blanchard and Schwarz 1988; Hermann and Blanchard 2002).

9.6.3 Acupuncture

Acupuncture is an ancient Chinese healing tradition that inserts needles into acupuncture points to balance the body's energy. Older children are more likely to prefer acupuncture as a complementary technique to manage pain (Tsao 2006). Acupuncture has been shown effective in postoperative and chronic pain, reducing cancer-related pain by 36 % at 2 months from baseline (Alimi et al. 2003). An adult study of acupuncture and chemotherapy-induced nausea and vomiting showed that over a 5 day period, a median of ten less episodes of nausea and vomiting were reported per patient in those who received acupuncture with pharmacologic therapy versus pharmacologic therapy alone (Shen et al. 2000).

9.6.4 Transcutaneous Electrical Nerve Stimulation

Transcutaneous electrical nerve stimulation (TENS) units provide electrical stimulation via electrodes to the underlying nerves near the source of maximal pain. A Cochrane review found conflicting evidence on the efficacy of TENS units in alleviating chronic low-back pain in adults (Khadilkar et al. 2008). Small pediatric studies have showed moderate success using TENS for chronic back pain in children (Van Epps et al. 2007). No studies in pediatric oncology patients have been reported.

9.6.5 Other Complementary Therapies

Several studies conducted in adults have demonstrated efficacy of other complementary therapies such as music therapy, support groups, and reiki in reducing the burden of pain and anxiety. Music therapy has been shown to increase length of life in adult hospice nursing home patients (Hilliard 2004). A 1-year prospective, randomized study demonstrated the value of support groups in reducing mood-disturbance scores, decreasing phobia and improving maladaptive responses in women with metastatic breast cancer (Spiegel et al. 1981). The use of reiki, a complementary technique using therapeutic touch, has shown improvement in quality of life rating and visual analogue scale pain rating for patients with cancer (Olson et al. 2003).

9.7 Interventional Techniques

Anesthesiologists with expertise in pain management can aid in the treatment of refractory recalcitrant pain through interventional techniques including epidural or intrathecal injections and peripheral nerve blocks. These techniques are used when there are limiting side effects of opioids, neuropathic pain that is unresponsive to rapid escalation or massive doses of opioids, and with procedural anesthesia (Collins et al. 1996b). At the end of life, rapid escalation of opioid medications is often required (Hewitt et al. 2008). Central neuraxial blocks (i.e., intrathecal or epidural blocks) and continuous peripheral nerve blocks help avoid systemic toxicity when rapid escalation of oral medications is required. Relative contraindications to central neuraxial blocks include fever, thrombocytopenia, wound at the catheter site, vertebral or spinal metastases, or fractures at the catheter site. Pain blockade via these methods has demonstrated efficacious analgesia with a moderation of opioid requirements and few side effects despite relative contraindications to catheter placement (Anghelescu et al. 2010).

9.8 Oncology-Specific Pain Issues

9.8.1 Vincristine-Related Peripheral Neuropathy

Vincristine is an effective antineoplastic agent used widely in pediatric oncology but is associated with both autonomic and sensorimotor neuropathy leading to peripheral neuropathy and neuropathic pain (Moore 2009). Symptoms of neuropathic pain due to vincristine include tingling, shooting pain, numbness, and pins-and-needles-type pain primarily in the hands, feet, and legs. Vincristine disrupts microtubular formation during mitosis and damages intraepidermal nerve fibers possibly via mitochondrial dysfunction. Longer axons tend to be most vulnerable, thus explaining the stocking glove distribution pattern of the neuropathy (Han and Smith 2013). Vincristine toxicity is significant and can lead to dose reduction and delays in therapy. In patients being treated for acute lymphoblastic leukemia (ALL), 35 % experienced at least one episode of neuropathic pain, with events clustered around periods of weekly vincristine administration (Anghelescu et al. 2011).

Gabapentin and opioid agents have been used to treat vincristine-related neuropathic pain alone or in combination. Gabapentin, in doses ranging from 10 mg/kg/day up to 50–70 mg/kg/day, was well tolerated and reduced pain scores amongst children undergoing ALL treatment (Anghelescu et al. 2011). Studies from adult patients with peripheral neuropathy from other causes have shown that coadministration of gabapentin with opioids resulted in significantly better pain control than placebo or either agent alone (Gilron et al. 2005). This synergistic effect was also observed in rat models (Matthews and Dickenson 2002).

Prior to gabapentin, TCAs were considered first-line therapy for neuropathic pain and can be considered (see Sect. 9.5.3) (Sindrup and Jensen 1999). Mouse models implicating 5-HT2A receptor involvement in neuropathic pain have led to interest in the use of SNRIs though clinical evidence in humans is lacking (Marchand et al. 2003; Thibault et al. 2008). Case reports have discussed use of pyridoxine and pyridostigmine with some effect but larger case series or trials have not been performed (Akbayram et al. 2010). Other chemotherapeutic agents linked to neuropathic pain syndromes include other vinca alkaloids (vinblastine, vinorelbine), platinum agents (cisplatin, oxaliplatin), taxanes (paclitaxel, docetaxel) and newer agents like bortezomib (Han and Smith 2013).

9.8.2 Osteonecrosis

Osteonecrosis (ON) is a painful and potentially crippling condition typified by ischemic and necrotic changes in bone. In children, ON is commonly associated with corticosteroid exposure in ALL and lymphoma but can occur independent of steroid therapy in cancers involving bone or bone marrow (Vora 2011). Additional risk factors for ON include age >10 years, obesity, Caucasian race, treatment intensity and asparaginase use (Mattano et al. 2000; Niinimaki et al. 2007; Kawedia et al. 2011). While many children treated for ALL have evidence of ON on magnetic resonance imaging (MRI), symptomatic ON incidence is <20 % (Mattano et al. 2000; Kawedia et al. 2011; Hyakuna et al. 2014).

Pain from ON ranges from mild intermittent pain to chronic debilitating pain. Analgesic treatment for ON should follow the general guidelines of the WHO pain ladder (see Sect. 9.4.1) starting with NSAIDs, if appropriate. COX2 inhibitors such as celecoxib may be preferable in patients for whom antiplatelet effects are a concern. Intermittent short-acting opioids may be sufficient for patients who cannot tolerate NSAID therapy. Patients with persistent pain requiring multiple doses of opioids per day benefit from long-acting opioids. In patients with chronic pain, methadone is an attractive option given its resistant nature to opioid tolerance. Patients who develop chronic pain from ON may best be served by a chronic pain management specialist.

Bisphosphonate therapy has been recently investigated as a method for reducing pain in patients with ON. An Australian study risk stratified a small population of children with ON and found reduction in pain amongst "severe risk" patients who received monthly IV pamidronate versus "moderate risk" patients receiving oral bisphosphonates and "mild risk" patients receiving calcium/vitamin D supplementation (Kotecha et al. 2010). A Canadian study similarly found that 14/17 (77 %) patients with symptomatic ON noted pain relief with a 3-day course of IV pamidronate given every 4 months (Leblicq et al. 2013). A study investigating zoledronic acid in children has demonstrated similar results (Padhye et al. 2013). Referral to an orthopedic surgeon experienced in ON management can be beneficial, especially for patients with significant debilitating symptoms. Surgical options which can improve functionality and reduce pain include core decompression and joint replacement. Other suggested supportive care measures for ON include physical therapy, weight loss, and treatment of vitamin D deficiency, if present (Vora 2011).

9.8.3 Post-lumbar Puncture Headache

Lumbar puncture (LP) is a common diagnostic and therapeutic procedure in pediatric oncology. Although relatively uneventful, the most common adverse effect of LP is a post-procedure headache. Typically occurring within 72 h of the procedure, symptoms of post-LP headache include throbbing pain in the bilateral occipital and frontal regions that is exacerbated by vertical position and Valsalva and palliated by lying flat. Most headaches resolve within 7 days, but some last for several weeks. The headache is thought to be caused by leakage of cerebrospinal fluid (CSF) and subsequent loss of CSF pressure. It is theorized that loss of CSF pressure leads to traction on pain-sensitive intracranial structures or an increase in cerebrovascular blood volume with resultant vasodilation, either of which could cause headache (Turnbull and Shepherd 2003). In children, the incidence of post-LP headache has been reported to be between 6 and 15 % and has been shown to occur in even young children although is much more common in adolescents (Kokki et al. 1999; Lee et al. 2007; Crock et al. 2014).

Various methods have been proposed to reduce the occurrence of post-LP headache. General guidelines suggest that LP performed with cutting needles should have the beveled edge oriented parallel to the dural fibers, which run longitudinally (Janssens et al. 2003). Post-procedure bed rest has been suggested, but not found to be helpful (Lee et al. 2007). Studies investigating the use of smaller gauge needles have not found significant differences in incidence (Ebinger et al. 2004; Crock et al. 2014). Use of an atraumatic, or "pencil-tip," needle (i.e., Whitacre), has been shown to significantly reduce the incidence of post-LP headache although one study found no difference (Kokki et al. 1999; Thomas et al. 2000; Apiliogullari et al. 2010).

When a post-LP headache occurs, various methods have been employed to treat pain not responsive to NSAIDs or opioids. Oral and IV caffeine has been most widely studied in adults and shown to reduce pain when compared to placebo (Sechzer and Abel 1978; Camann et al. 1990). It is hypothesized that caffeine causes relief by decreasing cerebrospinal pressure via cerebrovascular vasoconstriction (Janssens et al. 2003). Dosing of caffeine ranges from 300 to 500 mg in adult studies (Lee et al. 2007; Basurto Ona et al. 2011). The effectiveness of

caffeine has not been reported in pediatrics, but dosing has been suggested at 100 mg for children aged 6–10 years and 200 mg for children >10 years (McGhee et al. 2011). In studies with small sample sizes, gabapentin and the combination of caffeine and ergotamine have been shown to reduce pain measured on a visual analog scale when compared with placebo (Dogan 2006; Erol 2011). Hydration, although mentioned in supportive care for post-LP headache, has not demonstrated effectiveness when studied (Janssens et al. 2003; Lee et al. 2007). A Cochrane review concluded that there is no evidence that sumatriptans are effective (Basurto Ona et al. 2011).

Severe post-LP headache refractory to medical management can be treated with an epidural blood patch (EBP). The procedure involves obtaining access to the epidural space in the area of the previous LP. The patient's peripheral blood, obtained under sterile technique, is then inserted into the epidural space. The purpose of the procedure is to create pressure to seal the dural tear and prevent further CSF leakage (Turnbull and Shepherd 2003). Kokki and colleagues (2012) reviewed 41 cases of EBP procedures in children and found that 90 % had immediate and complete pain relief, with 85 % noting permanent relief. In pediatric oncology, blood patches should be considered cautiously given infectious risks for immunosuppressed patients and the theoretical risk of introduction of tumor cells into the CSF.

9.8.4 Mucositis Pain

Pathogenesis and management of mucositis is discussed in Chap. 11. General pain practices described here are necessary interventions for patients experiencing oral mucositis.

9.9 Summary

The large majority of pediatric oncology patients will suffer from pain at some point during their treatment course secondary to the underlying malignancy; surgical procedures including tumor resection, central venous catheter placement, lumbar puncture and bone marrow aspirate/ biopsy; and as side effects from chemotherapy including specific drug effects such as vincristine-associated neuropathy and general effects such as oral mucositis. Appropriate assessment of pain is the vital first step in appropriate pain management. Patients who are assessed as having pain should be treated according to the WHO pain ladder with the appropriate analgesic chosen based on the level of pain, expected course of pain, as well as with consideration to the individual patient's pain history. Appropriate pain management requires frequent reassessment to determine if pain control is adequate and side effects are tolerable. The pediatric oncology practitioner must also be aware of the potential for development of refractory pain or neuropathic pain not well controlled with the use of opioids. In these situations, an interdisciplinary team approach is ideal, utilizing the expertise of a pain service (if available) as well as alternative and complementary therapies to assist in treatment of the pain experience. Generally, recommendations for pain control are based on expert opinion and consensus guidelines, as firm evidence is lacking in pediatric patients.

References

Akbayram S, Akgun C, Dogan M et al (2010) Use of pyridoxine and pyridostigmine in children with vincristine-induced neuropathy. Indian J Pediatr 77:681–683

Alimi D, Rubino C, Pichard-Leandri E et al (2003) Analgesic effect of auricular acupuncture for cancer pain: a randomized, blinded, controlled trial. J Clin Oncol 21:4120–4126

Anderson BJ (2013) Is it farewell to codeine? Arch Dis Child 98:986–988

Anghelescu DL, Faughnan LG, Baker JN et al (2010) Use of epidural and peripheral nerve blocks at the end of life in children and young adults with cancer: the collaboration between a pain service and a palliative care service. Paediatr Anaesth 20:1070–1077

Anghelescu DL, Faughnan LG, Jeha S et al (2011) Neuropathic pain during treatment for childhood acute lymphoblastic leukemia. Pediatr Blood Cancer 57:1147–1153

Anghelescu DL, Faughman LG, Popenhagen MP et al (2014) Neuropathic pain referrals to a multidisciplinary pediatric cancer pain service. Pain Manag Nurs 15:126–131

Apiliogullari S, Duman A, Gok F et al (2010) Spinal needle design and size affect the incidence of postdural puncture headache in children. Paediatr Anaesth 20:177–182

Babbar S, Marier JF, Mouksassi MS et al (2009) Pharmacokinetic analysis of capsaicin after topical administration of a high-concentration capsaicin patch to patients with peripheral neuropathic pain. Ther Drug Monit 31:502–510

Baron R, Binder A, Wasner G (2010) Neuropathic pain: diagnosis, pathophysiological mechanisms, and treatment. Lancet Neurol 9:807–819

Basurto Ona X, Martinez Garcia L, Sola I et al (2011) Drug therapy for treating post-dural puncture headache. Cochrane Database Syst Rev (8):CD007887

Berde CB, Lehn BM, Yee JD et al (1991) Patient-controlled analgesia in children and adolescents: a randomized, prospective comparison with intramuscular administration of morphine for postoperative analgesia. J Pediatr 118:460–466

Berde CB, Sethna NF (2002) Analgesics for the treatment of pain in children. N Engl J Med 347:1094–1103

Blanchard E, Schwarz S (1988) Clinically significant changes in behavioral medicine. Behav Assess 10:171–188

Bruera E, Neumann CM (1999) Respective limits of palliative care and oncology in the supportive care of cancer patients. Support Care Cancer 7:321–327

Buck M (2002) Paediatric use of gabapentin. Pediatr Pharmacother 8:1–4

Camann WR, Murray RS, Mushlin PS et al (1990) Effects of oral caffeine on postdural puncture headache. A double-blind, placebo-controlled trial. Anesth Analg 70:181–184

Candy B, Jones L, Goodman ML et al (2011) Laxatives or methylnaltrexone for the management of constipation in palliative care patients. Cochrane Database Syst Rev (1):CD003448

Cepeda MS, Alvarez H, Morales O, Carr DB (2004) Addition of ultralow dose naloxone to postoperative morphine PCA: unchanged analgesia and opioid requirement but decreased incidence of opioid side effects. Pain 107:41–46

Chaparro LE, Wiffen PJ, Moore RA et al (2012) Combination pharmacotherapy for the treatment of neuropathic pain in adults. Cochrane Database Syst Rev (7):CD008943

Cherny N, Ripamonti C, Pereira J et al (2001) Strategies to manage the adverse effects of oral morphine: an evidence-based report. J Clin Oncol 19:2542–2554

Cheville AL, Sloan JA, Northfelt DW et al (2009) Use of a lidocaine patch in the management of postsurgical neuropathic pain in patients with cancer: a phase III double-blind crossover study (N01CB). Support Care Cancer 17:451–460

Chong MS, Bajwa ZH (2003) Diagnosis and treatment of neuropathic pain. J Pain Symptom Manage 25:S4–S11

Collins J, Walker S (2006) Pain: an introduction. In: Goldman A, Hain R, Liben S (eds) Oxford textbook of palliative care for children. Oxford University Press, New York

Collins JJ, Geake J, Grier HE et al (1996a) Patient-controlled analgesia for mucositis pain in children: a three-period crossover study comparing morphine and hydromorphone. J Pediatr 129:722–728

Collins JJ, Grier HE, Sethna NF et al (1996b) Regional anesthesia for pain associated with terminal pediatric malignancy. Pain 65:63–69

Crock C, Orsini F, Lee KJ et al (2014) Headache after lumbar puncture: randomised crossover trial of 22-gauge versus 25-gauge needles. Arch Dis Child 99:203–207

Culbert T, Olness K (2010) Integrative pediatrics. Oxford University Press, New York

Dogan D (2006) The effect of oral gabapentin on post-dural puncture headache. Acute Pain 8:169–173

Drake R, Frost J, Collins JJ (2003) The symptoms of dying children. J Pain Symptom Manage 26:594–603

Drake R, Longworth J, Collins JJ (2004) Opioid rotation in children with cancer. J Palliat Med 7:419–422

Dunbar PJ, Buckley P, Gavrin JR et al (1995) Use of patient-controlled analgesia for pain control for children receiving bone marrow transplant. J Pain Symptom Manage 10:604–611

Ebinger F, Kosel C, Pietz J et al (2004) Headache and backache after lumbar puncture in children and adolescents: a prospective study. Pediatrics 113:1588–1592

Eisenberg E, McNicol E, Carr DB (2006) Opioids for neuropathic pain. Cochrane Database Syst Rev (3): CD006146

Erol DD (2011) The analgesic and antiemetic efficacy of gabapentin or ergotamine/caffeine for the treatment of postdural puncture headache. Adv Med Sci 56:25–29

Esteve R, Marquina-Aponte V (2012) Children's pain perspectives. Child Care Health Dev 38:441–452

Feudtner C, Freedman J, Kang T et al (2014) Comparative effectiveness of senna to prevent problematic constipation in pediatric oncology patients receiving opioids: a multicenter study of clinically detailed administrative data. J Pain Symptom Manage 48:272–280

Fitzgerald M (2000) Development of the peripheral and spinal pain system. In: Pain in neonates, 2nd edn. Elsevier, Amsterdam

Friedman T, Slayton WB, Allen LS et al (1997) Use of alternative therapies for children with cancer. Pediatrics 100:E1

Friedrichsdorf SJ, Finney D, Bergin M et al (2007) Breakthrough pain in children with cancer. J Pain Symptom Manage 34:209–216

Friedrichsdorf SJ, Kang TI (2007) The management of pain in children with life-limiting illnesses. Pediatr Clin North Am 54:645–672

Gaffney A, Dunne EA (1986) Developmental aspects of children's definitions of pain. Pain 26:105–117

Gallo S, DuRand J, Pshon N (2008) A study of naloxone effect on urinary retention in the patient receiving morphine patient-controlled analgesia. Orthop Nurs 27:111–115

Gaukroger PB, Chapman MJ, Davey RB (1991) Pain control in paediatric burns–the use of patient-controlled analgesia. Burns 17:396–399

Gilron I, Bailey JM, Tu D et al (2005) Morphine, gabapentin, or their combination for neuropathic pain. N Engl J Med 352:1324–1334

Goodyear-Smith F, Halliwell J (2009) Anticonvulsants for neuropathic pain: gaps in the evidence. Clin J Pain 25:528–536

Guyatt G, Gutterman D, Baumann MH et al (2006) Grading strength of recommendations and quality of evidence in clinical guidelines: report from an American College of Chest Physicians Task Force. Chest 129:174–181

Haanpaa M, Attal N, Backonja M et al (2011) NeuPSIG guidelines on neuropathic pain assessment. Pain 152: 14–27

Han Y, Smith MT (2013) Pathobiology of cancer chemotherapy-induced peripheral neuropathy (CIPN). Front Pharmacol 4:156

Hermann C, Blanchard EB (2002) Biofeedback in the treatment of headache and other childhood pain. Appl Psychophysiol Biofeedback 27:143–162

Hewitt M, Goldman A, Collins GS et al (2008) Opioid use in palliative care of children and young people with cancer. J Pediatr 152:39–44

Hilliard RE (2004) A post-hoc analysis of music therapy services for residents in nursing homes receiving hospice care. J Music Ther 41:266–281

Holzer P (2010) Opioid antagonists for prevention and treatment of opioid-induced gastrointestinal effects. Curr Opin Anaesthesiol 23:616–622

Hyakuna N, Shimomura Y, Watanabe A et al (2014) Assessment of corticosteroid-induced osteonecrosis in children undergoing chemotherapy for acute lymphoblastic leukemia: a report from the Japanese Childhood Cancer and Leukemia Study Group. J Pediatr Hematol Oncol 36:22–29

Indelicato RA, Portenoy RK (2002) Opioid rotation in the management of refractory cancer pain. J Clin Oncol 20:348–352

Izard C, Hembree E, Huebner R (1987) Infants' emotion expressions to acute pain: developmental change and stability of individual differences. Dev Psychol 23:105–113

Jacob E (2004) Neuropathic pain in children with cancer. J Pediatr Nurs 21:350–357

Janssens E, Aerssens P, Alliet P et al (2003) Post-dural puncture headaches in children. A literature review. Eur J Pediatr 162:117–121

Jay SM, Elliott CH, Katz E, Siegel SE (1987) Cognitive-behavioral and pharmacologic interventions for childrens' distress during painful medical procedures. J Consult Clin Psychol 55:860–865

Kawedia JD, Kaste SC, Pei D et al (2011) Pharmacokinetic, pharmacodynamic, and pharmacogenetic determinants of osteonecrosis in children with acute lymphoblastic leukemia. Blood 117:2340–2347

Kelly LE, Rieder M, van den Anker J et al (2012) More codeine fatalities after tonsillectomy in North American children. Pediatrics 129:e1343–e1347

Khadilkar A, Odebiyi DO, Brosseau L et al (2008) Transcutaneous electrical nerve stimulation (TENS) versus placebo for chronic low-back pain. Cochrane Database Syst Rev (4):CD003008

Klick JC, Hauer J (2010) Pediatric palliative care. Curr Probl Pediatr Adolesc Health Care 40:120–151

Kokki H, Salonvaara M, Herrgard E et al (1999) Postdural puncture headache is not an age-related symptom in children: a prospective, open-randomized, parallel group study comparing a 22-gauge Quincke with a 22-gauge Whitacre needle. Paediatr Anaesth 9:429–434

Kokki M, Sjovall S, Kokki H (2012) Epidural blood patches are effective for postdural puncture headache in pediatrics–a 10-year experience. Paediatr Anaesth 22:1205–1210

Kotecha RS, Powers N, Lee SJ et al (2010) Use of bisphosphonates for the treatment of osteonecrosis as a complication of therapy for childhood acute lymphoblastic leukaemia (ALL). Pediatr Blood Cancer 54:934–940

Krechel SW, Bildner J (1995) CRIES: a new neonatal postoperative pain measurement score. Initial testing of validity and reliability. Paediatr Anaesth 5:53–61

Kuehn BM (2013) FDA: no codeine after tonsillectomy for children. JAMA 309:1100

Kuttner L, Bowman M, Teasdale M (1988) Psychological treatment of distress, pain, and anxiety for young children with cancer. J Dev Behav Pediatr 9:374–381

Leblicq C, Laverdiere C, Decarie JC et al (2013) Effectiveness of pamidronate as treatment of symptomatic osteonecrosis occurring in children treated for acute lymphoblastic leukemia. Pediatr Blood Cancer 60:741–747

Lee LC, Sennett M, Erickson JM (2007) Prevention and management of post-lumbar puncture headache in pediatric oncology patients. J Pediatr Oncol Nurs 24:200–207

Lin YC, Lee AC, Kemper KJ et al (2005) Use of complementary and alternative medicine in pediatric pain management service: a survey. Pain Med 6:452–458

Lynn AM, Nespeca MK, Opheim KE et al (1993) Respiratory effects of intravenous morphine infusions in neonates, infants, and children after cardiac surgery. Anesth Analg 77:695–701

Mackie AM, Coda BC, Hill HF (1991) Adolescents use patient-controlled analgesia effectively for relief from prolonged oropharyngeal mucositis pain. Pain 46:265–269

Marchand F, Alloui A, Pelissier T et al (2003) Evidence for an antihyperalgesic effect of venlafaxine in vincristine-induced neuropathy in rat. Brain Res 980:117–120

Mattano LA Jr, Sather HN, Trigg ME et al (2000) Osteonecrosis as a complication of treating acute lymphoblastic leukemia in children: a report from the Children's Cancer Group. J Clin Oncol 18:3262–3272

Matthews EA, Dickenson AH (2002) A combination of gabapentin and morphine mediates enhanced inhibitory effects on dorsal horn neuronal responses in a rat model of neuropathy. Anesthesiology 96:633–640

Maxwell LG, Kaufmann SC, Bitzer S et al (2005) The effects of a small-dose naloxone infusion on opioid-induced side effects and analgesia in children and adolescents treated with intravenous patient-controlled analgesia: a double-blind, prospective, randomized, controlled study. Anesth Analg 100:953–958

McGhee B, Howrie D, Vetterly C et al (2011) Pediatric drug therapy handbook & formulary, 6th edn. Lexicomp, Hudson

McNicol E, Strassels SA, Goudas L et al (2005) NSAIDS or paracetamol, alone or combined with opioids, for cancer pain. Cochrane Database Syst Rev (1):CD005180

Mercadante S (1998) Pathophysiology and treatment of opioid-related myoclonus in cancer patients. Pain 74:5–9

Mercadante S (2012) Pharmacotherapy for breakthrough cancer pain. Drugs 72:181–190

Merkel SI, Voepel-Lewis T, Shayevitz JR et al (1997) The FLACC: a behavioral scale for scoring postoperative pain in young children. Pediatr Nurs 23:293–297

Monitto C, Kost-Byerly S, White E et al (2011) The optimal dose of prophylactic intravenous naloxone in ameliorating opioid-induced side effects in children receiving intravenous patient-controlled analgesia morphine for moderate to severe pain: a dose finding study. Anesth Analg 113:834–842

Moore SW (2009) Developmental genes and cancer in children. Pediatr Blood Cancer 52:755–760

Niinimaki RA, Harila-Saari AH, Jartti AE et al (2007) High body mass index increases the risk for osteonecrosis in children with acute lymphoblastic leukemia. J Clin Oncol 25:1498–1504

Olkkola KT, Maunuksela EL, Korpela R et al (1988) Kinetics and dynamics of postoperative intravenous morphine in children. Clin Pharmacol Ther 44:128–136

Olson K, Hanson J, Michaud M (2003) A phase II trial of Reiki for the management of pain in advanced cancer patients. J Pain Symptom Manage 26:990–997

Padhye B, Dalla-Pozza L, Little DG et al (2013) Use of zoledronic acid for treatment of chemotherapy related osteonecrosis in children and adolescents: a retrospective analysis. Pediatr Blood Cancer 60:1539–1545

Pasero C, McCaffery M (2011) Pain assessment and pharmacologic management. Elsevier/Mosby, St. Louis

Phatak UP, Pashankar DS (2013) Role of polyethylene glycol in childhood constipation. Clin Pediatr (Phila) 53:927–932

Portenoy R, Forbes K, Lussier D et al (2005) Difficult pain problems: an integrated approach. In: Doyle D, Hanks G, Cherny N, Calman K (eds) Oxford textbook of palliative medicine. Oxford University Press, New York

Rodrigues A, Wong C, Mattiussi A et al (2013) Methylnaltrexone for opioid-induced constipation in pediatric oncology patients. Pediatr Blood Cancer 60:1667–1670

Schindera C, Tomlinson D, Bartels U et al (2013) Predictors of symptoms and site of death in pediatric palliative patients with cancer at end of life. Am J Hosp Palliat Care 31:548–552

Sechzer P, Abel L (1978) Post-spinal anesthesia headache treated with caffeine: evaluation with demand method. Curr Ther Res 24:307–312

Shen J, Wenger N, Glaspy J et al (2000) Electroacupuncture for control of myeloablative chemotherapy-induced emesis: a randomized controlled trial. JAMA 284:2755–2761

Simon T, Niemann CA, Hero B et al (2012) Short- and long-term outcome of patients with symptoms of spinal cord compression by neuroblastoma. Dev Med Child Neurol 54:347–352

Sindrup SH, Jensen TS (1999) Efficacy of pharmacological treatments of neuropathic pain: an update and effect related to mechanism of drug action. Pain 83:389–400

Sirkia K, Saarinen UM, Ahlgren B et al (1997) Terminal care of the child with cancer at home. Acta Paediatr 86:1125–1130

Spiegel D, Bloom JR, Yalom I (1981) Group support for patients with metastatic cancer. A randomized outcome study. Arch Gen Psychiatry 38:527–533

Sweet SD, McGrath PJ (1998) Relative importance of mothers' versus medical staffs' behavior in the prediction of infant immunization pain behavior. J Pediatr Psychol 23:249–256

Syrjala KL, Donaldson GW, Davis MW et al (1995) Relaxation and imagery and cognitive-behavioral training reduce pain during cancer treatment: a controlled clinical trial. Pain 63:189–198

Thibault K, Van Steenwinckel J, Brisorgueil MJ et al (2008) Serotonin 5-HT2A receptor involvement and Fos expression at the spinal level in vincristine-induced neuropathy in the rat. Pain 140:305–322

Thomas J (2008) Opioid-induced bowel dysfunction. J Pain Symptom Manage 35:103–113

Thomas J, Karver S, Cooney GA et al (2008) Methylnaltrexone for opioid-induced constipation in advanced illness. N Engl J Med 358:2332–2343

Thomas SR, Jamieson DR, Muir KW (2000) Randomised controlled trial of atraumatic versus standard needles for diagnostic lumbar puncture. BMJ 321:986–990

Tremlett M, Anderson BJ, Wolf A (2010) Pro-con debate: is codeine a drug that still has a useful role in pediatric practice? Paediatr Anaesth 20:183–194

Trentadue NO, Kachoyeanos MK, Lea G (1998) A comparison of two regimens of patient-controlled analgesia for children with sickle cell disease. J Pediatr Nurs 13:15–19

Tsao JC (2006) CAM for pediatric pain: what is state-of-the-research? Evid Based Complement Altern Med 3:143–144

Turk D (1978) Cognitive behavioral techniques in the management of pain. In: Foreyt J, Rathjen D (eds) Cognitive behavior therapy. Plenum Press, New York

Turnbull DK, Shepherd DB (2003) Post-dural puncture headache: pathogenesis, prevention and treatment. Br J Anaesth 91:718–729

Twycross A, Dowden S, Bruce E (2009) Managing pain in children: a clinical guide. Wiley-Blackwell, Ames

Van Epps S, Zempsky W, Schechter N et al (2007) The effects of a two-week trial of transcutaneous electrical nerve stimulation for pediatric chronic back pain. J Pain Symptom Manage 34:115–117

Vondracek P, Oslejskova H, Kepak T et al (2009) Efficacy of pregabalin in neuropathic pain in paediatric oncological patients. Eur J Paediatr Neurol 13:332–336

Vora A (2011) Management of osteonecrosis in children and young adults with acute lymphoblastic leukaemia. Br J Haematol 155:549–560

Walder B, Schafer M, Henzi I et al (2001) Efficacy and safety of patient-controlled opioid analgesia for acute postoperative pain. A quantitative systematic review. Acta Anaesthesiol Scand 45:795–804

Whaley D, Wong DL (1995) Nursing care of infants and children, 5th edn. Mosby, St. Louis

Williams DG, Patel A, Howard RF (2002) Pharmacogenetics of codeine metabolism in an urban population of children and its implications for analgesic reliability. Br J Anaesth 89:839–845

Wolfe J, Grier HE, Klar N et al (2000) Symptoms and suffering at the end of life in children with cancer. N Engl J Med 342:326–333

Wuhrman E, Cooney MF, Dunwoody CJ (2007) Authorized and unauthorized ("PCA by proxy") dosing of analgesic infusion pumps: position statement with clinical practice recommendations. Pain Manag Nurs 8:4–11

Yee JD, Berde CB (1994) Dextroamphetamine or methylphenidate as adjuvants to opioid analgesia for adolescents with cancer. J Pain Symptom Manage 9:122–125

Zernikow B, Michel E, Craig F et al (2009) Pediatric palliative care: use of opioids for the management of pain. Paediatr Drugs 11:129–151

Zernikow B, Smale H, Michel E et al (2006) Paediatric cancer pain management using the WHO analgesic ladder—results of a prospective analysis from 2265 treatment days during a quality improvement study. Eur J Pain 10:587–595

Nausea and Vomiting

10

Tiffany Chang

Contents

Abstract

Nausea and vomiting induced by antineoplastic therapy can significantly affect quality of life and continues to be a prevalent and distressing treatment-related issue faced by children with cancer and their families. Chemotherapy-induced nausea and vomiting (CINV) can result in metabolic derangements, nutritional depletion and anorexia, esophageal tears, deterioration of mental and performance status, prolonged hospitalizations, and potential poor compliance or withdrawal from anticancer treatment. Despite advances in pharmacologic and nonpharmacologic management of nausea and vomiting, prevention of CINV remains a particular issue in the pediatric population where existing guidelines are constrained by lack of robust evidence. Few studies have been carried out in children, and results obtained in adults cannot be directly applied to young children since metabolism and side effects of drugs differ. The pathophysiology of CINV, principles of antiemetic prophylaxis, emetogenicity of chemotherapy, classes of antiemetic agents, and current guidelines for prevention and treatment of CINV in children are addressed in this chapter. Specific attention is also given to nonpharmacologic strategies and approaches to anticipatory, breakthrough, and radiation-induced nausea and vomiting. This chapter provides health care providers with a summary of evidence-based information with the goal of

T. Chang, MD
Division of Hematology/Oncology,
Department of Pediatrics, Benioff Children's Hospital,
University of California-San Francisco,
505 Parnassus Avenue, San Francisco, CA 94143, USA
e-mail: changt@peds.ucsf.edu

J. Feusner et al. (eds.), *Supportive Care in Pediatric Oncology:
A Practical Evidence-Based Approach*, Pediatric Oncology,
DOI 10.1007/978-3-662-44317-0_10, © Springer Berlin Heidelberg 2015

guiding optimal emetic control in pediatric cancer patients.

10.1 Introduction

Chemotherapy-induced nausea and vomiting (CINV) are two of the most prevalent and distressing adverse effects reported among children before, during, and after chemotherapy, with frequency reports of 20–80 % noted in the literature (Rodgers et al. 2012). CINV can significantly affect quality of life, result in metabolic imbalances, malnutrition, anorexia, decline of performance and mental status, prolonged hospitalizations, and potential discontinuation of subsequent chemotherapy cycles (Laszlo 1983; Richardson et al. 1988; Mitchell 1992). This can result in suboptimal cancer therapy and reduced survival. Additionally, chronic nausea and vomiting can occur in advanced cancer patients or patients receiving radiation therapy and may be due to gastrointestinal (GI), cranial, metabolic and drug induced-problems (Schwartzberg 2006). The incidence and severity of nausea or vomiting in patients receiving chemotherapy or radiation therapy are affected by numerous factors, including type, dose and schedule of chemotherapy, target of radiation therapy (i.e., whole body, abdomen, brain), and individual patient variability based on age, gender, or prior chemotherapy (Herrstedt 2008). Compared to adult data, there are a paucity of randomized clinical trials investigating newer antiemetic agents in pediatric cancer patients. Furthermore, recognition of symptom severity continues to be an issue as parents and health care providers tend to underestimate the occurrence of delayed nausea and vomiting (Tyc et al. 1993; Small et al. 2000). Recent evidence-based guidelines have been published to provide recommendations for antiemetic prophylaxis according to the emetogenic potential of antineoplastic therapies in pediatric patients (Basch et al. 2011; Dupuis et al. 2011; Jordan et al. 2011; Dupuis et al. 2013). Progress in relieving the symptoms of CINV will require further education of oncology physicians and nurses, aggressive use of current medications, and continued development of pharmacologic and alternative therapies for children.

10.2 Chemotherapy-Induced Nausea and Vomiting (CINV)

CINV is commonly classified as acute, delayed, anticipatory, breakthrough and refractory. Although there are no standard definitions, the following are commonly used to classify the different types of CINV (Wickham 1999):

- *Acute*: Occurs within a few minutes to several hours after drug administration and commonly resolves within the first 24 h. The intensity of acute CINV typically peaks after 4–6 h.
- *Delayed*: Arises >24 h after chemotherapy administration. Delayed CINV commonly occurs following cisplatin, carboplatin, cyclophosphamide and anthracyclines. For cisplatin, emesis reaches its maximal intensity 48–72 h after administration, but can last for 1 week.
- *Anticipatory*: Usually develops in patients who have previously experienced significant CINV as a conditioned response (Morrow 1984). Symptoms occur prior to chemotherapy administration and may be triggered by stimuli such as the smells, sights and sounds of the treatment room.
- *Breakthrough*: Breakthrough CINV results despite prophylactic treatment and requires "rescue" with additional antiemetic agents (Roila et al. 2006).
- *Refractory*: Emesis that takes place in subsequent treatment cycles when antiemetic prophylaxis and rescue have failed in prior cycles.

10.2.1 Pathophysiology of Emesis

The neurophysiologic mechanisms that control nausea and vomiting are fairly well characterized. Nausea is mediated through the autonomic nervous system. Vomiting results from the stimulation of a complex reflex that is coordinated by a putative true vomiting center, which may be located in the dorsolateral reticular formation near the medullary respiratory centers. The vomiting center receives afferent input from four neuronal pathways that carry emetogenic signals: (1) the chemoreceptor trigger zone (CTZ), (2) peripheral stimuli from the gastrointestinal tract via vagus and splanchnic nerves, (3) cortical pathways in response to sensory or psychogenic stimuli, and (4) the vestibular-labyrinthine apparatus of the inner ear in response to body motion (Carpenter 1990).

The CTZ, located in the area postrema in the floor of the fourth ventricle, lacks a true blood-brain barrier (Miller and Leslie 1994). This allows the CTZ to sense fluctuations in the concentration of certain substances in the bloodstream, including chemotherapy and its metabolites. Several receptors have been identified in the CTZ including muscarinic, dopamine D_2, serotonin (5-HT$_3$), neurokinin-1 (NK$_1$) and histamine H$_1$ receptors (Dodds 1985). The CTZ may also be stimulated by posterior fossa tumors.

The emetic center (EC), located in the nucleus tractus solitarii of the brainstem, coordinates afferent pathways from the GI tract via the vagus and splanchnic nerves. Nausea may be elicited through gut irritation from medications, tumor infiltration, obstruction, distension or constipation. The EC also coordinates the efferent activities of the salivation center, abdominal muscles, respiratory center and autonomic nerves that result in vomiting (Miller and Leslie 1994). The phenomenon of anticipatory emesis suggests that inputs from the cerebral cortex may be involved. CNS or meningeal tumors, increased intracranial pressure, anxiety or uncontrolled pain can also result in cortically induced nausea and vomiting.

Current findings indicate that acute emesis following chemotherapy is initiated by the release of neurotransmitters from cells that are susceptible to the presence of toxic substances in the blood or CSF. The most critical and clinically relevant neuroreceptors involved are serotonin, dopamine and substance P. The significant advancement in antiemetic therapy came in the early 1990s when 5-HT$_3$ receptor antagonists became available (Jordan et al. 2007). Substance P, which binds to the NK$_1$ receptor, is a newer target in antiemetic therapy, and the NK$_1$ receptor antagonist aprepitant has demonstrated clinical utility in the pediatric population (Choi et al. 2010).

The exact mechanism by which chemotherapy and its metabolites induce emetic effects is unclear. Metabolites may directly stimulate the CTZ and serotonin, and other neurotransmitters may be released from intestinal enterochromaffin cells damaged by chemotherapy. Sensory neurons release substance P, and a number of NK$_1$ receptors have been identified in both the CTZ and EC. The relative contribution from these multiple pathways culminating in CINV is complex and likely accounts for the variable emetogenic profile of agents. As there is no single common pathway controlling emetic response, it is unlikely that any single agent will be able to provide complete antiemetic protection from chemotherapy.

10.2.2 Principles of Emesis Control in the Cancer Patient

The most important principle in managing CINV is the *prevention* of nausea and vomiting. The risk of CINV in patients receiving moderate to high emetogenic chemotherapy persists for at least 2–3 days after the final dose of chemotherapy, and prophylactic therapy should be given during the full period of risk (Grunberg et al. 2004). Antiemetics should be given at the minimal efficacious dose with consideration of their side effect profiles as well as the patient's prior history with specific antiemetics. Consider the use of an H$_2$ blocker or proton pump inhibitor to prevent dyspepsia, which can mimic nausea. Finally, lifestyle measures such as eating small, frequent and healthy meals may help alleviate CINV.

10.2.3 Emetogenicity of Chemotherapy

Although patient factors are important, the specific chemotherapeutic agents used are most predictive of CINV risk. Several classifications have been developed to define the emetogenicity of chemotherapy; Hesketh et al. (1997) developed a widely accepted classification system for adults that divides chemotherapy into five levels of emetogenicity based on the percentage of patients experiencing CINV following administration of each particular agent without any antiemetic prophylaxis. This classification was recently updated by Grunberg et al. (2010) and has been

Table 10.1 Acute emetic potential of antineoplastic agents in pediatric cancer patients[a]

High risk (>90% frequency of emesis in the absence of prophylaxis)

Altretamine	[b]Cytarabine 3 g/m^2/dose	Procarbazine (oral)
[b]Carboplatin	Dacarbazine	Streptozocin
Carmustine >250 mg/m^2	[b]Dactinomycin	[b]Thiotepa ≥300 mg/m^2
[b]Cisplatin	Mechlorethamine	
[b]Cyclophosphamide ≥1 g/m^2	[b]Methotrexate ≥12 g/m^2	

Moderate risk (30–90% frequency of emesis in absence of prophylaxis)

Aldesleukin >12–15 million IU/m^2	Cytarabine >200 mg to <3 g/m^2	Lomustine
Amifostin >300 mg/m^2	Daunorubicin	Melphalan >50 mg/m^2
Arsenic trioxide	[b]Doxorubicin	Methotrexate ≥250 mg to <12 g/m^2
Azacitidine	Epirubicin	Oxaliplatin >75 mg/m^2
Bendamustine	Etoposide (oral)	Temozolomide (oral)
Busulfan	Idarubicin	Vinorelbine (oral)
[b]Carmustine ≤250 mg/m^2	Ifosfamide	
[b]Clofarabine	Imatinib (oral)	
[b]Cyclophosphamide <1 g/m^2	[b]Intrathecal therapy (methotrexate, hydrocortisone and cytarabine)	
Cyclophosphamide (oral)	Irinotecan	

Low risk (10–30% frequency of emesis in the absence of prophylaxis)

Amifostine ≤300 mg/m^2	Fludarabine (oral)	Paclitaxel
Bexarotene	5-Fluorouracil	Paclitaxel-albumin
[b]Busulfan (oral)	Gemcitabine	Pemetrexed
Capecitabine	Ixabepilone	Teniposide
Cytarabine ≤200 mg/m^2	Methotrexate >50 to <250 mg/m^2	Thiotepa >300 mg/m^2
Docetaxel	Mitomycin	Vorinostat
Doxorubicin (liposomal)	Mitoxantrone	
Etoposide	Nilotinib (oral)	

Minimal risk (<10% frequency of emesis in the absence of prophylaxis)

Alemtuzumab	Erlotinib	Rituximab
Alpha interferon	Fludarabine	Sorafenib
Asparaginase (IM or IV)	Gefitinib	Sunitinib
Bevacizumab	Gemtuzumab ozogamicin	Temsirolimus
Bleomycin	Hydroxyurea (oral)	Thalidomide
Bortezomib	Lapatinib	Thioguanine (oral)
Cetuximab	Lenalidomide	Trastuzumab
Chlorambucil (oral)	Melphalan (oral low dose)	Valrubicin
Cladribine	Mercaptopurine (oral)	Vinblastine
Dasatinib	Methotrexate ≤50 mg/m^2	Vincristine
Decitabine	Nelarabine	Vinorelbine
Denileukin diftitox	Panitumumab	
Dexrazoxane	Pentostatin	

Adapted from Dupuis et al. (2011)

[a]All agents given intravenously (IV) unless stated otherwise

[b]Pediatric evidence available (per Dupuis et al. [2011])

incorporated into the National Comprehensive Cancer Network (NCCN) antiemesis guidelines. Similar to the current classification system in pediatric patients, the updated guidelines divide intravenous chemotherapeutic agents into four categories of emetogenic potential, focusing on acute emesis: (1) high emetic risk, ≥90 % of patients experiencing acute emesis; (2) moderate emetic risk, 30–90 %; (3) low emetic risk, 10–30 %; and (4) minimal emetic risk, <10 % (Table 10.1) (Dupuis et al. 2010; Grunberg et al. 2010).

Recent data suggest that the frequency and severity of delayed CINV are often underestimated and remain a significant problem for patients (Dupuis et al. 2010). In order to properly manage both acute and delayed symptoms, appropriate antiemetic prophylaxis should cover the entire duration of days that symptoms are anticipated. Furthermore, for multi-agent chemotherapy regimens, antiemetic choices should be determined based on the chemotherapeutic agent with the highest emetogenic risk.

10.2.4 Classes of Antiemetics

The basis for antiemetic therapy is the neurochemical control of vomiting. Many antiemetics act by competitively blocking receptors for these substances, thereby inhibiting stimulation of peripheral nerves at the CTZ and possibly the EC. Most drugs with proven antiemetic activity in children are categorized into five groups which are discussed individually below: (1) dopamine receptor antagonists, (2) corticosteroids, (3) 5-HT$_3$ receptor antagonists, (4) neurokinin-1 receptor (substance P) antagonists, and (5) cannabinoids. Antihistamines such as diphenhydramine which affect histaminergic receptors in the CTZ are widely utilized but have not been systematically studied. Similarly, anticholinergics, especially scopolamine, are utilized but have not been studied specifically in CINV.

10.2.4.1 Dopamine Receptor Antagonists

There are three classes of dopamine receptor antagonists effective in the prevention and treatment of CINV: phenothiazines, butyrophenones and benzamide. The most commonly used phenothiazine is prochlorperazine and has efficacy in all classes except in highly emetogenic chemotherapy (Moertel et al. 1963). A newer agent, metopimazine has been utilized with benefit in adult patients but has not been studied in children (Croom and Keating 2006; Dupuis et al. 2013). Butyrophenones, such as the antipsychotic drug haloperidol, are infrequently used in the pediatric setting secondary to their side effect profile. Of the benzamides, metoclopramide is the best studied and most widely used in children with CINV (Roila et al. 2006). Metoclopramide blocks central and peripheral D$_2$ dopaminergic receptors at low doses and exhibits weak 5-HT$_3$ inhibition at high doses. It is also known to speed gastric emptying and increase sphincter tone at the gastroesophageal junction.

Prior to the introduction of 5-HT$_3$ antagonists, a combination of high-dose metoclopramide and dexamethasone was the most effective prophylaxis for highly emetogenic chemotherapy (Moertel et al. 1963). Extrapyramidal effects including dystonia, tardive dyskinesia, and neuroleptic malignant syndrome (uncommon) may be seen with benzamides and thus they are not typically first-line agents (Terrin et al. 1984; Allen et al. 1985). If given for breakthrough CINV, high-dose metoclopramide at a dose of 1 mg/kg q4–6 h is typically administered in conjunction with diphenhydramine to decrease the risk of extrapyramidal symptoms (Marshall et al. 1989; Koseoglu et al. 1998). Pediatric guidelines recommend an initial metoclopramide dose of 1 mg/kg followed by 0.075 mg/kg PO q6 h for moderately emetogenic chemotherapy as a strong recommendation with minimal evidence (Dupuis et al. 2013).

10.2.4.2 Corticosteroids

Steroids, most commonly dexamethasone, are effective in preventing CINV when used alone or in combination with other antiemetic agents for all emetogenic classes of chemotherapy. The antiemetic mechanism of action is not fully understood, but they may inhibit prostaglandin synthesis in the brain (Weidenfeld et al. 1987). Clinically, steroids quantitatively decrease or eliminate episodes of CINV and may improve mood, though can also induce anxiety and insomnia.

Steroids should be given before chemotherapy for acute CINV and may or may not be repeated. Both dexamethasone and methylprednisolone have good efficacy in the prevention of acute CINV in children and are superior to low-dose metoclopramide and phenothiazines with few side effects with short-term use (Mehta et al. 1986). Dosages and administration schedules vary. Dexamethasone is also used orally for delayed CINV. Long-term corticosteroid use is inappropriate and may cause substantial morbidity. As previously shown with metoclopramide, numerous studies have demonstrated that dexamethasone potentiates the antiemetic properties of 5-HT$_3$-blocking agents and NK$_1$-blocking agents (Hesketh 1994; Hesketh et al. 2003; Gore et al. 2009; Choi et al. 2010). The combination of dexamethasone and ondansetron has been most studied and is recommended for first-line therapy in children receiving moderately or highly emetogenic chemotherapy; the combination of a 5-HT$_3$ antagonist with dexamethasone has been shown to be more efficacious than a 5-HT$_3$ antagonist alone (Dupuis et al. 2013). In one study, the "complete protection" rates increased from 43 % with ondansetron alone to 75 % with the combination of ondansetron and dexamethasone when given prior to high-dose cytarabine (Holdsworth et al. 2006). Dexamethasone may be particularly useful in patients who have demonstrated intolerance to other antiemetics given with high-dose chemotherapy or in patients with breakthrough, refractory or delayed CINV (Alvarez et al. 1995; Holdsworth et al. 2006).

Special considerations must be made prior to choosing corticosteroids for antiemetic therapy. Steroids cannot be given for CINV if the patient receives steroids as part of their chemotherapeutic regimen, as in leukemia or lymphoma. They are also typically avoided in patients with CNS malignancies, as dexamethasone has been shown to inhibit the influx of chemotherapy into the brain in preclinical models by "sealing" the blood-brain barrier (Straathof et al. 1998). Attention to protocol guidelines should be made prior to dexamethasone initiation particularly in hematologic and CNS malignancies but also potentially in protocols that utilize immunologic and biologic therapies.

Dexamethasone dosing for CINV is not well-studied. The most current pediatric CINV guidelines developed by the Pediatric Oncology Group of Ontario (POGO) suggest that dexamethasone should be dosed at 6 mg/m^2 IV/PO q6 h for highly emetogenic chemotherapy (Dupuis et al. 2013). For moderately emetogenic chemotherapy, dexamethasone can be dosed at 2 mg IV/PO q12 h for patients $\leq$0.6 m^2 and 4 mg q12 h for patients >0.6 m^2. If given concurrently with aprepitant, guidelines suggest reducing dexamethasone doses by half (Dupuis et al. 2013).

10.2.4.3 5-HT$_3$ Receptor Antagonists

Four serotonin receptor antagonists—ondansetron, granisetron, dolasetron and palonosetron—are available in the United States. Tropisetron is only available internationally and has not yet been approved by the Federal Drug Administration (FDA). When first approved in the early 1990s, these agents revolutionized the antiemetic prophylaxis of highly and moderately emetogenic chemotherapy, largely replacing phenothiazines and benzamides as first-line therapy due to superior efficacy and significantly fewer side effects (Grunberg et al. 2010). 5-HT$_3$ receptor antagonists are thought to prevent CINV by inhibiting serotonin, which is released from enterochromaffin cells in the gastrointestinal mucosa, from initiating afferent transmission to the CNS via vagal and spinal sympathetic nerves (Jordan et al. 2007). They may also work by blocking serotonin stimulation at the CTZ and other CNS structures. Prior to 2003, there were three FDA-approved 5-HT$_3$ receptor antagonists: ondansetron, granisetron and dolasetron. Numerous clinical trials demonstrated their clinical equivalence and showed there was no significant difference whether given orally or intravenously (Corapcioglu and Sarper 2005; Dupuis et al. 2013).

Ondansetron

Ondansetron is highly effective in controlling acute emesis induced by moderately and highly emetogenic chemotherapy in pediatric oncology patients (Carden et al. 1990; Hewitt et al. 1993). Used alone, ondansetron is superior to combination therapy with metoclopramide and dexamethasone or chlorpromazine and dexamethasone and is free of extrapyramidal and sedative side effects (Dick et al. 1995; Jimenez et al. 1997; Koseoglu et al. 1998). Ondansetron used in combination with corticosteroids has been shown superior to ondansetron monotherapy in control of CINV with highly emetogenic chemotherapy in pediatric cancer patients (Alvarez et al. 1995; Roila et al. 1998). Alvarez et al. (1995) conducted a small but significant double-blind, placebo-controlled, randomized crossover trial comparing ondansetron and dexamethasone to ondansetron and placebo in 25 children 3–8 years of age receiving highly emetogenic chemotherapy for solid tumors. Complete emetic control was achieved in 61 % receiving both ondansetron and dexamethasone versus 23 % in those treated with ondansetron alone ($p = 0.04$).

The lowest fully effective dose of ondansetron is 0.45 mg/kg/day, with a single daily dose schedule no less efficacious than a multiply divided dose schedule (Sandoval et al. 1999). Oral and intravenous (IV) drug administration has also been found statistically equivalent (White et al. 2000). White et al. (2000) conducted a double-blind, parallel-group, multicenter study comparing the efficacy and safety of IV and liquid ondansetron (both arms with oral dexamethasone) in the prevention of CINV in pediatric patients receiving moderately to highly emetogenic chemotherapy. Complete control of emesis was achieved in 89 % of patients in the IV group and 88 % of patients in the oral syrup group during the worst day of chemotherapy treatment and was well tolerated in both arms (White et al. 2000). For highly emetogenic chemotherapy, the recommended dose of ondansetron is 0.15 mg/kg 30 min prior to initiation of chemotherapy and repeated q8 h, although other regimens (such as 0.45 mg/kg as a single daily dose) have been shown equally effective (Dupuis et al. 2013). When giving multiple-daily dosing, ondansetron can potentially be spaced to q12 h for moderately emetogenic chemotherapy (Dupuis et al. 2013). A single-center retrospective chart review has reported ondansetron-loading doses of 16 mg/m^2 (maximum, 24 mg) IV, followed by two doses of 5 mg/m^2 q8 h, to be safe in infants, children and adolescents (Hasler et al. 2008).

Currently, the oral and injectable ondansetron formulations are approved for use without dosage modification in patients >4 years, including patients with renal insufficiency. Ondansetron clearance is diminished in patients with severe hepatic insufficiency; therefore, such patients should receive a single injectable or oral dose ≤8 mg. The major adverse effects include: headache, constipation or diarrhea, fatigue, dry mouth and electrocardiographic (ECG) abnormalities including QTc prolongation (Culy et al. 2001). Buyukavci et al. (2005) monitored ECGs in 22 children with acute lymphoblastic leukemia randomized to receive a single dose of either ondansetron (0.1 mg/kg) or granisetron (40 mcg/kg). The granisetron group demonstrated a significant decrease in mean heart rate at 1 and 3 h post dosing and a significant QTc prolongation at 1 h post dosing although all values eventually returned to baseline; no significant changes were seen in the ondansetron group (Buyukavci et al. 2005). Pinarli et al. (2006) randomized 38 children to either ondansetron or granisetron, and patients were monitored with a 24-h ECG post antiemetic administration. Compared to baseline, patients who received granisetron (but not ondansetron) demonstrated a significant prolongation of the QTc interval and shortening of the PR interval and QRS complex, though none of these abnormalities were clinically significant (Pinarli et al. 2006).

Granisetron

Granisetron has demonstrated efficacy in preventing and controlling CINV due to moderately to highly emetogenic chemotherapy in children and when used alone is superior to combination therapy using metoclopramide and promethazine, metoclopramide and dexamethasone, and chlorpromazine and dexamethasone (Hählen et al. 1995; Komada et al. 1999). In a small study, Hirota et al. (1993) showed no significant difference between the combination of granisetron and methylprednisolone compared with granisetron alone in pediatric oncology patients. Effective granisetron doses in children range from 20 to 40 mcg/kg/day, often administered IV once daily prior to chemotherapy or orally q12 h (Dupuis et al. 2011). In the United States, granisetron injection, transdermal patch, and oral tablets are approved for initial and repeat prophylaxis in patients receiving emetogenic chemotherapy, including high-dose cisplatin. Granisetron is pharmacologically and pharmacokinetically distinct from ondansetron; however, clinically it appears equally efficacious and safe (Gebbia et al. 1994). Current pediatric guidelines recommend granisetron at 40 mcg/kg IV as a single daily dose for moderately to highly emetogenic chemotherapy or 40 mcg/kg/dose PO q12 h for prevention of CINV from moderately emetogenic chemotherapy (Dupuis et al. 2013).

Palonosetron

A second-generation 5-HT$_3$ receptor antagonist palonosetron was FDA approved in 2003 and boasts advantages over first-generation 5-HT$_3$ receptor antagonists including a higher binding affinity to the 5-HT$_3$ receptor and longer elimination half-life (i.e., 40 h in adults versus 4–8 h for first-generation agents). Large drug company sponsored adult trials have demonstrated at least non-inferiority and potential superior control of acute emesis with single-dose palonosetron compared with single-dose ondansetron or dolasetron (Eisenberg et al. 2003; Gralla et al. 2003). Gralla et al. (2003) randomized 570 adult patients receiving moderately emetogenic chemotherapy to either 0.25 or 0.75 mg palonosetron or 32 mg ondansetron on the first day of chemotherapy and showed a significantly increased prevention of acute CINV (81 % vs. 68.8 %, $p=0.009$) for the 0.25 mg palonosetron arm compared with ondansetron. Of note, there was no significant difference in response to acute nausea comparing 0.75 mg palonosetron and 32 mg of ondansetron (Gralla et al. 2003). Eisenberg et al. (2003), on the other hand, showed only non-inferiority of both 0.25 and 0.75 mg palonosetron as compared with 100 mg of dolasetron. Although both studies showed significant improved response in delayed CINV for palonosetron compared with single-dose ondansetron as a secondary outcome measure, this conclusion is confounded by the inappropriate utilization of single-dose (with a 4–8 h half-life) ondansetron as a comparison dosing schedule for the prevention of delayed CINV (Eisenberg et al. 2003; Gralla et al. 2003). In a meta-analysis of adult studies of palonosetron in CINV, Likun et al. (2011) showed a significant benefit to 0.25 and 0.75 mg palonosetron in acute, delayed, and overall CINV prevention compared with first-generation agents although due to the methodologic concerns described above, it is difficult to conclude the superiority of palonosetron in delayed and overall control of CINV. However, Geling and Eichler (2005) have shown in a meta-analysis of adult patients that first-generation 5-HT$_3$ antagonists may not be effective in the prevention of delayed CINV no matter the dosing schedule. Palonosetron's three- to fourfold increased cost versus ondansetron must be weighed

with a need for significantly less total doses (Geling and Eichler 2005; De Leon 2006; Likun et al. 2011).

Only two studies of efficacy of palonosetron in children have been published. A randomized trial of 60 pediatric patients 2–17 years of age showed 3 mcg/kg (maximum dose 0.25 mg) and 10 mcg/kg (maximum dose 0.75 mg) of palonosetron were well tolerated and equally effective (Kadota et al. 2007). Sepulveda-Vildosola et al. (2008) conducted a randomized comparison of palonosetron (0.25 mg single dose 30 min before chemotherapy) and ondansetron (8 mg/m^2 every 8 h beginning 30 min before chemotherapy) in children 2–15 years, evaluating 50 chemotherapy courses in each arm and showing a significant reduction in emetic events and intensity of nausea during the acute phase of therapy (days 1–3) in the palonosetron group. Due to the decreased number of doses, they found that palonosetron was more inexpensive as well (Sepulveda-Vildosola et al. 2008). The study was limited by the fact that palonosetron was given as a standard dose rather than weight and age adjusted and also that determination of emesis and intensity of nausea was based on family report and therefore subject to potential inaccuracy (Sepulveda-Vildosola et al. 2008). Though palonosetron appears to be well tolerated, further research is needed to evaluate the optimal dose, cost-effectiveness and its relative efficacy in children based on the chemotherapeutic emetogenicity and in delayed CINV.

Comparison of Agents

Studies suggest that there are no major differences in efficacy or toxicity of the three first-generation 5-HT$_3$ receptor antagonists (dolasetron, granisetron and ondansetron) in the treatment of acute CINV when used at appropriate doses (Hesketh 1994). Although these agents have been shown effective for the treatment of acute CINV, they have not demonstrated efficacy in alleviating symptoms of delayed CINV in adult patients (Hickok et al. 2003; Geling and Eichler 2005). The second-generation 5-HT$_3$ receptor antagonist palonosetron has been approved for the control of delayed emesis for adult patients receiving moderately emetogenic chemotherapy, though definitive safety and efficacy has not been established in children and methodologic concerns exist in the comparison with first-generation agents for the treatment of delayed CINV.

The 5-HT$_3$-receptor antagonists remain the cornerstone of prophylaxis for both moderately and highly emetogenic chemotherapy in children although a recent Cochrane review concluded that our knowledge of effective antiemetics in children with CINV is quite incomplete (Phillips et al. 2010). Despite the advent of 5-HT$_3$ receptor antagonists, the control of acute and delayed CINV is suboptimal with highly emetogenic chemotherapeutic regimens, and there is considerable opportunity for improvement with either the addition or substitution of new agents in current regimens (Dupuis et al. 2011). Although lacking evidence, the recent pediatric guidelines suggest either ondansetron or granisetron can be given although no dose recommendation is given for granisetron and evidence is lacking to recommend doses or regimens with dolasetron or palonosetron (Dupuis et al. 2013).

10.2.4.4 Substance P Antagonists (NK$_1$ Receptor Antagonists)

NK$_1$ receptors are found in the nucleus tractus solitarii and the area postrema and are activated by substance P (Saito et al. 2003). Inhibitors of NK$_1$ receptors have demonstrated beneficial antiemetic effects and represent a new target for antiemetic therapy. Aprepitant and its prodrug fosaprepitant have been shown to prevent both acute and delayed CINV from moderately to highly emetogenic chemotherapy in adults (Hesketh et al. 2003). Current Multinational Association of Supportive Care in Cancer (MASCC), European Society of Medical Oncology (ESMO), NCCN, and American Society of Clinical Oncology (ASCO) guidelines recommend the use of aprepitant in adults receiving highly emetogenic chemotherapy or those receiving a combination of anthracycline and cyclophosphamide (Basch et al. 2011; Jordan et al. 2011; Ettinger et al. 2012). When compared to ondansetron and dexamethasone alone, the addition of aprepitant has been shown to increase the rate of complete emetic control (i.e., no acute

emesis or need for rescue medication) from 52–73 % in chemotherapy-naïve adults during a 5-day period after single-day cisplatin therapy (Hesketh et al. 2003). Subsequent randomized clinical trials in adults have demonstrated superior efficacy for the prevention of delayed CINV when aprepitant is added to a 5-HT$_3$ antagonist and dexamethasone, recently summarized in a pooled analysis by Jin et al. (2012). These results led to FDA approval of aprepitant for adults in March 2003 for highly emetogenic chemotherapy and in 2006 for moderately emetogenic chemotherapy.

Studies of aprepitant in the pediatric population have been limited to retrospective reviews and case reports with the exception of one randomized controlled trial (Gore et al. 2009; Choi et al. 2010; Bauters et al. 2013). Gore et al. (2009) conducted a randomized, double-blind, placebo-controlled multicenter phase III trial studying aprepitant in adolescent patients. In addition to ondansetron and dexamethasone, patients were randomized 2:1 to receive either aprepitant or placebo. Forty-six patients from 11 to 19 years of age participated, with overall complete response rates of 28.6 % in the aprepitant group versus 5.6 % in the control group (though not significantly different). Serious adverse events were 32.1 % in the aprepitant group versus 16.7 % in the control group (not statistically significant) and pharmacokinetic data showed increased aprepitant metabolism as compared to historical adult data (Gore et al. 2009). Further study is required to understand the efficacy, appropriate dose and side effect profile with aprepitant in pediatric patients.

In an effort to balance access to an apparently effective antiemetic with the lack of pediatric dosing and safety information, some centers are administering aprepitant to children ≥12 years of age, weighing ≥40 kg and receiving highly emetogenic chemotherapy. The usual adult dose is administered in conjunction with a 5-HT$_3$ receptor antagonist and dexamethasone for 3 days (Basch et al. 2011; Jordan et al. 2011; Ettinger et al. 2012). Based on the limited available data, pediatric guidelines recommend 125 mg of aprepitant on day 1 and 80 mg on days 2 and 3 (adult dosing) with a 5-HT$_3$ antagonist and dexamethasone for patients ≥12 years receiving highly emetogenic chemotherapy (Dupuis et al. 2013). Although variable dosing regimens have been utilized in children <40 kg and reported to be well tolerated, optimal dosing is yet to be determined in this population (Choi et al. 2010; Bauters et al. 2013; Bodge et al. 2014).

As aprepitant is a moderate inhibitor of and a substrate for CYP3A4, drug interactions are an important consideration, and, as mentioned, the dose of concomitant dexamethasone or methylprednisolone (utilized as an antiemetic) is recommended to be halved. Multiple chemotherapy agents including etoposide, ifosfamide, imatinib, irinotecan, paclitaxel, vinca alkaloids and steroids are metabolized by CYP3A4 (Shadle et al. 2004). As such, aprepitant should be avoided in patients receiving these chemotherapeutic agents because of the potential for unintended increases in the dose intensity and toxicity of these antineoplastic agents. More complete references should be consulted regarding the nature and extent of drug interactions with aprepitant, as interactions with non-chemotherapeutic agents (e.g., warfarin, phenytoin, midazolam, carbamazepine, erythromycin, ketoconazole) have been described (Shadle et al. 2004). Additional NK_1 receptor antagonists casopitant and rolapitant have been shown effective and safe in adult CINV but have not been studied in pediatric patients.

10.2.4.5 Cannabinoids

The plant *Cannabis* contains more than 60 different types of cannabinoids which have physiologic activity. There are two FDA-approved products for CINV: dronabinol (a synthetic isomer, *-trans-Δ9-tetrahydrocannabinol*) and nabilone. Cannabinoids likely exert antiemetic effects by targeting cannabinoid-1 (CB-1) and CB-2 receptors in the CNS (Abrahamov et al. 1995; Tramer et al. 2001). These agents have demonstrated modest efficacy in the prevention of acute CINV in children and are superior to low-dose metoclopramide and prochlorperazine, though with side effects which include euphoria, dizziness (i.e., postural hypotension) and hallucinations (Chan et al. 1987, Tramer et al. 2001). Dronabinol is dosed at 5 mg/m^2 q6 h prn (max 15 mg/m^2/dose) orally and is typically reserved for refractory patients. Pediatric guidelines recommend nabilone (<18 kg, 0.5 mg/dose PO twice daily; 18–30 kg, 1 mg/dose PO twice daily; >30 kg, 1 mg/dose PO three times daily) in patients for whom corticosteroids are contraindicated receiving moderately to highly emetogenic chemotherapy (Dupuis et al. 2013).

10.2.4.6 Other Antiemetic Agents
Antihistamines

Antihistamines such as diphenhydramine are commonly used as adjunctive agents in the treatment and prevention of CINV although systematic review of their potential benefit is not reported in the literature. Antihistamines theoretically impact the histaminergic receptors in the CTZ and should also be utilized in combination with metoclopramide to prevent extrapyramidal side effects. Adult and pediatric guidelines do not discuss antihistamines beyond utilization with metoclopramide (Basch et al. 2011; Jordan et al. 2011; Ettinger et al. 2012; Dupuis et al. 2013).

Benzodiazepines

Benzodiazepines such as lorazepam and midazolam have become recognized as valuable adjuncts in the prevention and treatment of anticipatory nausea and vomiting associated with chemotherapy. Benzodiazepines have not demonstrated intrinsic antiemetic activity as single agents and thus should be used with other antiemetics, primarily for the treatment of anticipatory and breakthrough CINV (Triozzi et al. 1988; Hesketh 2008; Basch et al. 2011; Jordan et al. 2011; Ettinger et al. 2012). Benzodiazepines are thought to act on higher CNS structures, the brainstem, and spinal cord, and they produce anxiolytic, sedative, and anterograde amnesic effects. Administration of lorazepam may be oral, IV or sublingual. Doses range from 0.03 to 0.05 mg/kg (max dose 2 mg) in children every 6–12 h (Van Hoff and Olszewski 1988). The adverse effects of lorazepam include sedation, visual disturbance, confusion and ataxia. Benzodiazepines as adjunct agents are not mentioned in the recent pediatric guidelines (Dupuis et al. 2013).

Olanzapine

Olanzapine nonspecifically antagonizes D_2 and $5\text{-}HT_3$ receptors and has been shown in nonrandomized adult studies to be effective in preventing acute and delayed CINV (Navari et al. 2005; Navari et al. 2007; Hesketh 2008). Adult guidelines include olanzapine as a suggested adjunct agent in patients with delayed or refractory CINV (Basch et al. 2011; Jordan et al. 2011; Ettinger et al. 2012). Pediatric data are lacking (Dupuis et al. 2013).

10.2.4.7 Alternative Therapies

Ginger

Ginger has been traditionally utilized as a treatment for upset stomach and is considered safe by the FDA. A Cochrane review of pregnant women showed limited and inconsistent results of ginger on the treatment of nausea (Matthews et al. 2014). Studies in CINV are limited and mixed. In randomized controlled adult trials, Zick et al. (2009) showed no benefit to ginger in the reduction of severity of acute or delayed CINV, while Ryan et al. (2012) found significant benefit of 0.5 and 1.0 g ginger in acute CINV when given 3 days prior to chemotherapy initiation. One randomized placebo-controlled study in pediatric patients found significant improvement in both acute and delayed CINV with the addition of ginger root powder in bone sarcoma patients receiving ondansetron and dexamethasone (Pillai et al. 2011). Further work is required to determine if ginger is a potentially beneficial adjunctive agent (Dupuis et al. 2013).

Acupressure/Acupuncture

Chinese medicine has for centuries utilized acupressure and acupuncture for the treatment of emesis induced by pregnancy and surgery (Jindal et al. 2008). Traditionally, the P6 acupuncture point above the wrist between the palmaris longus and flexor carpi radialis muscles of the forearm is targeted for prevention of nausea and vomiting. The role of acupuncture and acupressure has been studied systematically; in a pooled analysis of CINV, Ezzo et al. (2006) demonstrated mild reduction in acute emesis ($RR = 0.82$, 95 % CI 0.69, 0.99; $p = 0.04$), but no change in acute or delayed nausea severity compared with controls. A Cochrane review showed no benefit to acupuncture and limited evidence for acupressure in pregnant women with nausea (Matthews et al. 2014). Continuous pressure to the P6 acupuncture point can be administered continuously using acupressure wrist bands (Sea-Band®) (Molassiotis et al. 2008).

Studies of acupressure and acupuncture in the pediatric population are limited due to difficulties in patient accrual, particularly in younger patients who might fear this modality. One study was only able to enroll 11 patients ≥ 10 years of age in a 2-year period and demonstrated a significantly reduced need for additional antiemetics when acupressure was combined with $5\text{-}HT_3$ antagonists ($p = 0.024$) (Reindl et al. 2006). This conclusion was confounded by the fact that episodes of vomiting were not reduced ($p = 0.374$) (Reindl et al. 2006). Small sample sizes continue to be a barrier to future research, though efforts for stronger evidence-based studies are ongoing including a randomized controlled trial of acupressure to control CINV in children receiving cisplatin sponsored by the Children's Oncology Group. A validated pediatric nausea assessment tool (PeNAT) will be utilized to assess response to therapy in both acute and delayed phases (Dupuis et al. 2006).

Hypnosis and Other Therapies

Limited data are available in the literature regarding hypnosis although a meta-analysis of five pediatric studies in the prevention of CINV showed significant reduction in anticipatory CINV (Richardson et al. 2007). Benefit of hypnosis as well as other behavioral modification techniques such as cognitive-behavior therapy, guided imagery, music therapy, muscle relaxation, virtual reality and psychoeducational support have not been systematically studied (Dupuis et al. 2013).

10.2.5 Recommendations for Prevention and Treatment of CINV

The advent of new and improved pharmacologic antiemetic agents, accumulation of clinical experience, and ability to stratify chemotherapy regimens according to their emetogenicity has made it possible to construct guidelines for a logical approach to prevention and treatment of CINV in adults (Basch et al. 2011; Jordan et al. 2011; Ettinger et al. 2012). However, due to important differences in treatment intensity, drug metabolism and toxicity, adult guidelines cannot simply be extrapolated to the pediatric population. Evidence-based guidelines for antiemetic selection in children receiving chemotherapy have been developed by ASCO, ESMO, and MASCC; however, recommendations were based on few randomized controlled trials and extrapolation of adult data (Basch et al. 2011; Jordan et al. 2011; Ettinger et al. 2012). The recent Pediatric Oncology Group of Ontario guidelines represent a comprehensive systematic review of the pediatric literature and recommendations here are largely based on these guidelines (Dupuis et al. 2013).

10.2.5.1 Management of CINV

Management of CINV (Table 10.2) is based on the emetogenic potential of the chemotherapeutic regimen that each individual is undergoing as well as their previous history of CINV. For patients receiving regimens with high emetogenic risk such as cisplatin or cyclophosphamide (Table 10.1), the combination of a 5-HT$_3$ receptor antagonist, aprepitant and dexamethasone is recommended prior to chemotherapy. Aprepitant and dexamethasone are recommended to continue >24 h after chemotherapy (i.e., for 3 total days) for the prevention of delayed CINV. Close attention should be paid to potential drug interactions when considering use of aprepitant, and aprepitant cannot currently be recommended in children <12 years of age or <40 kg (Dupuis et al. 2013). If aprepitant cannot be used, patients should at minimum receive a 5-HT$_3$ receptor antagonist and dexamethasone. If aprepitant and corticosteroids are contraindicated, a 5-HT$_3$ receptor antagonist plus a cannabinoid (dronabinol or nabilone) or dopamine receptor antagonist (promethazine, metopimazine or metoclopramide with diphenhydramine) can be used although typical pediat-

ric oncology practice has utilized diphenhydramine and lorazepam prior to cannabinoids or D$_2$ antagonists. An anticholinergic such as scopolamine may also be used for adjuvant therapy especially in adolescents although data in CINV are lacking.

For patients receiving moderate emetogenic risk chemotherapy, the combination of a 5-HT$_3$ receptor antagonist and dexamethasone is recommended prior to chemotherapy. If corticosteroids are contraindicated, a 5-HT$_3$ receptor antagonist plus a cannabinoid (dronabinol or nabilone) or dopamine receptor antagonist (promethazine, metopimazine or metoclopramide with diphenhydramine) can be used although typical pediatric oncology practice has utilized diphenhydramine and lorazepam prior to cannabinoids or D$_2$ antagonists. An anticholinergic such as scopolamine may also be used for adjuvant therapy especially in adolescents. For regimens with low emetogenic risk, monotherapy with a 5-HT$_3$ receptor antagonist is recommended. For regimens with minimal emetogenic risk, no prophylaxis is recommended.

10.2.5.2 Special Considerations
Anticipatory Nausea and Vomiting
Prevention of anticipatory nausea and vomiting (Table 10.2) is achieved through the use of optimal antiemetic prophylaxis with each cycle of chemotherapy. Once symptoms have developed, benzodiazepines can be added to the prophylactic antiemetic regimen for anxiolysis. Patient expectancy of nausea and vomiting is an often underrecognized factor and alternative therapies have been shown to effectively treat anticipatory CINV especially when used in combination with antiemetics (Figueroa-Moseley et al. 2007; Richardson et al. 2007).

Breakthrough Nausea and Vomiting
Breakthrough emesis (Table 10.2) presents a difficult scenario as correction of refractory ongoing CINV is challenging to reverse. Prevention is far easier than treatment. The general principle of breakthrough treatment is to give an additional agent from a different drug class. Some patients require several agents utilizing differing mechanisms of action. Around the clock dosing is

Table 10.2 Management of chemotherapy-induced nausea and vomiting in pediatric cancer patients[a]

Emetogenic risk[b]	Drug	Dosing	Level of evidence[c]
High emetogenic risk	Corticosteroids permitted[d]: ondansetron or granisetron + dexamethasone + aprepitant[e]	Ondansetron 0.15 mg/kg/dose (max 8 mg/dose) IV/PO pretherapy and then q8 h	1B
		Granisetron 40 mcg/kg/dose IV daily	1B
	Corticosteroids contraindicated[d]: ondansetron or granisetron + breakthrough agent + aprepitant[e]	Dexamethasone 6 mg/m²/dose IV/PO q6 h; if given concurrently with aprepitant, reduce dexamethasone dose by half	1C
		Aprepitant 125 mg PO on day 1, 80 mg daily on day 2 and 3	1C
Moderate emetogenic risk	Corticosteroids permitted[d]: ondansetron or granisetron + dexamethasone	Ondansetron 0.15 mg/kg/dose (max 8 mg/dose) IV/PO pretherapy and then q8-12 h	1B
	Corticosteroids contraindicated[d]: ondansetron or granisetron + breakthrough agent	Granisetron 40 mcg/kg/dose IV daily OR 40 mcg/kg/dose PO q12 h	1B
		Dexamethasone ≤0.6 m²: 2 mg/dose IV/PO q12 h >0.6 m²: 4 mg/dose IV/PO q12 h	1C
Low emetogenic risk	Ondansetron or granisetron	Same dosing as above	1B
Minimal emetogenic risk	No routine prophylaxis		1C
Breakthrough nausea and vomiting	Ondansetron or granisetron	Same dosing as above (ordered prn if not already scheduled)	1B
	Lorazepam	0.05 mg/kg/dose IV q6 h prn (max 2 mg/dose)	2B
	Metoclopramide	1 mg/kg/dose IV pretherapy (max 10 mg/dose) then 0.075 mg/kg/dose PO q6 h; give diphenhydramine concurrently	1C
	Promethazine	0.125 mg/kg/dose IV q6 h (do not use in children <2 years of age)	2C
	Dronabinol	5 mg/m²/dose PO q6 h prn (may increase in 2.5 mg increments to max 15 mg/m²/dose)	2B
Anticipatory nausea and vomiting	Lorazepam	0.05 mg/kg/dose IV q6 h prn (max 2 mg/dose)	2B

IV intravenous, *PO* by mouth, *prn* as needed
Adapted from Ettinger et al. (2012), Dupuis et al. (2013)
[a]See text for full detail
[b]See Table 10.1 for chemotherapy emetogenicity classification
[c]Level of evidence per Guyatt et al. (2006); see Preface
[d]Corticosteroids as antiemetic generally contraindicated with treatment of brain tumors, leukemia and lymphoma
[e]Recommended for children ≥12 years old, investigate potential drug interactions prior to use

typically preferred rather than as needed dosing, particularly in children who may not know how to properly convey nausea. Typical breakthrough agents include lorazepam, diphenhydramine, scopolamine, metoclopramide (with diphenhydramine), promethazine or metopimazine, and cannabinoids. One can consider maximizing the starting dose of the 5-HT₃ antagonist or switching to an alternative 5-HT$_3$ antagonist (e.g., from ondansetron to granisetron or palonosetron). If the patient has dyspepsia, adding an H$_2$ blocker or proton pump inhibitor may be beneficial. Adequate hydration is imperative. Alternative therapies should be explored and may be of benefit. The patient should also be assessed for other non-chemotherapy-associated etiologies of nausea and vomiting such as electrolyte imbalances, GI obstruction or gastroparesis, tumor infiltration of bowel or brain, effect of total parenteral nutrition, and other potential diagnoses.

10.3 Radiation-Induced Nausea and Vomiting

Radiation-induced nausea and vomiting (Table 10.2) is seen in nearly all patients receiving total body irradiation prior to hematopoietic stem cell transplant and in >80 % of those receiving radiation to the upper abdomen (Feyer et al. 2005). Studies have demonstrated efficacy of 5-HT$_3$ receptor antagonist prophylaxis in this setting as well as superiority to metoclopramide (American Society of Health-System Pharmacists 1999). Adult guidelines recommend prophylaxis with ondansetron or granisetron prior to each radiation fraction delivered (Basch et al. 2011; Jordan et al. 2011; Ettinger et al. 2012).

10.4 Summary

Dramatic progress has been made in the prevention of CINV, especially with the introduction of the 5-HT$_3$ receptor antagonists in the early 1990s. Utilization of second-generation 5-HT$_3$ receptor antagonists such as palonosetron requires further study in children but will also likely be beneficial in the prevention of delayed CINV as compared to first-generation agents. The utility of NK$_1$ receptor antagonists is evident in the adult literature and dedicated pediatric studies are necessary to allow further improvement of CINV outcomes in children with cancer. Heightened awareness of patient symptoms, assessment and modification of risk factors, adherence to current guidelines for prophylaxis based on emetogenic risk, and the use of novel strategies such as long-acting and sublingual formulations, transdermal patches, and complimentary alternative therapies will ensure that fewer pediatric patients experience nausea and vomiting from antineoplastic therapy.

References

Abrahamov A, Abrahamov A, Mechoulam R (1995) An efficient new cannabinoid antiemetic in pediatric oncology. Life Sci 56:2097–2102

Allen JC, Gralla R, Reilly L et al (1985) Metoclopramide: dose-related toxicity and preliminary antiemetic studies in children receiving cancer chemotherapy. J Clin Oncol 3:1136–1141

Alvarez O, Freeman A, Bedros A (1995) Randomized double-blind crossover ondansetron-dexamethasone versus ondansetron-placebo study for the treatment of chemotherapy-induced nausea and vomiting in pediatric patients with malignancies. J Pediatr Hematol Oncol 17:145–150

American Society of Health-System Pharmacists (1999) ASHP therapeutic guidelines on the pharmacologic management of nausea and vomiting in adult and pediatric patients receiving chemotherapy or radiation therapy or undergoing surgery. Am J Health Syst Pharm 56:729–764

Basch E, Prestrud A, Hesketh P et al (2011) Antiemetics: American Society of Clinical Oncology clinical practice guideline update. J Clin Oncol 29:4189–4198

Bauters TG, Verlooy J, Robays H et al (2013) Emesis control by aprepitant in children and adolescents with chemotherapy. Int J Clin Pharm 35:1021–1024

Bodge M, Shillingburg A, Paul S, Biondo L (2014) Safety and efficacy of aprepitant for chemotherapy-induced nausea and vomiting in pediatric patients: a prospective, observational study. Pediatr Blood Cancer 61:1111–1113

Buyukavci M, Olgun H, Ceviz N (2005) The effects of ondansetron and granisetron on electrocardiography in children receiving chemotherapy for acute leukemia. Am J Clin Oncol 28:201–204

Carden PA, Mitchell SL, Waters SK et al (1990) Prevention of cyclophosphamide/cytarabine-induced emesis with ondansetron in children with leukemia. J Clin Oncol 8:1531–1535

Carpenter DO (1990) Neural mechanisms of emesis. Can J Physiol Pharmacol 68:230–236

Chan H, Correia J, MacLeod S (1987) Nabilone versus prochlorperazine for control of cancer chemotherapy-induced emesis in children: a double-blind, crossover trial. Pediatrics 79:946–952

Choi MR, Jiles C, Seibel NL (2010) Aprepitant use in children, adolescents, and young adults for the control of chemotherapy induced nausea and vomiting (CINV). J Pediatr Hematol Oncol 32:e268–e271

Corapcioglu F, Sarper N (2005) A prospective randomized trial of the antiemetic efficacy and cost-effectiveness of intravenous and orally disintegrating tablet of ondansetron in children with cancer. Pediatr Hematol Oncol 22:103–114

Croom KF, Keating GM (2006) Metopimazine. Am J Cancer 5:123–136

Culy CR, Bhana N, Plosker GL (2001) Ondansetron: a review of its use as an antiemetic in children. Paediatr Drugs 3:441–479

De Leon A (2006) Palonosetron (Aloxi): a second-generation 5-HT$_3$ receptor antagonist for chemotherapy-induced nausea and vomiting. Proc (Bayl Univ Med Cent) 19:413–416

Dick GS, Meller ST, Pinkerton CR (1995) Randomised comparison of ondansetron and metoclopramide plus dexamethasone for chemotherapy induced emesis. Arch Dis Child 73:243–245

Dodds LJ (1985) The control of cancer chemotherapy-induced nausea and vomiting. J Clin Hosp Pharm 10:143–166

Dupuis LL, Taddio A, Kerr EN et al (2006) Development and validation of a pediatric nausea assessment tool (PeNAT) for use by children receiving antineoplastic agents. Pharmacotherapy 26:1221–1231

Dupuis LL, Milne-Wren C, Cassidy M et al (2010) Symptom assessment in children receiving cancer therapy: the parents' perspective. Support Care Cancer 18:281–299

Dupuis LL, Boodhan S, Sung L et al (2011) Guideline for the classification of the acute emetogenic potential of antineoplastic medication in pediatric cancer patients. Pediatr Blood Cancer 57:191–198

Dupuis LL, Boodhan S, Holdsworth M et al (2013) Guideline for the prevention of acute nausea and vomiting due to antineoplastic medication in pediatric cancer patients. Pediatr Blood Cancer 60:1073–1082

Eisenberg P, Figueroa-Vadillo J, Zamora R et al (2003) Improved prevention of moderately emetogenic chemotherapy induced nausea and vomiting with palonosetron, a pharmacologically novel 5-HT3 receptor antagonist: results of a Phase III, single-dose trial versus dolasetron. Cancer 98:2473–2482

Ettinger D, Akerley W, Benson A et al (2012) National Comprehensive Cancer Network Clinical Practice Guidelines in Oncology: Antiemesis, V.1.2012 http://www.nccn.org/professionals/physician_gls/PDF/antiemesis.pdf

Ezzo J, Streitberger K, Schneider A (2006) Cochrane systematic reviews examine P6 acupuncture-point stimulation for nausea and vomiting. J Altern Complement Med 12:489–495

Feyer PC, Maranzano E, Molassiotis A (2005) Radiotherapy-induced nausea and vomiting (RINV): antiemetic guidelines. Support Care Cancer 13:122–128

Figueroa-Moseley C, Jean-Pierre P, Roscoe JA et al (2007) Behavioral interventions in treating anticipatory nausea and vomiting. J Natl Compr Canc Netw 5:44–50

Gebbia V, Cannata G, Testa A et al (1994) Ondansetron versus granisetron in the prevention of chemotherapy-induced nausea and vomiting. Results of a prospective randomized trial. Cancer 74:1945–1952

Geling O, Eichler HG (2005) Should 5-hydroxytryptamine-3 receptor antagonists be administered beyond 24 hours after chemotherapy to prevent delayed emesis? Systematic re-evaluation of clinical evidence and drug cost implications. J Clin Oncol 23:1289–1294

Gore L, Chawla SP, Petrilli AS et al (2009) Aprepitant in adolescent patients for prevention of chemotherapy-induced nausea and vomiting: a randomized, double-blind, placebo-controlled study of efficacy and tolerability. Pediatr Blood Cancer 52:242–247

Gralla R, Lichinitser M, Van Der Vegt S et al (2003) Palonosetron improves prevention of chemotherapy-induced nausea and vomiting following moderately emetogenic chemotherapy: results of a double-blind randomized phase III trial comparing single doses of palonosetron with ondansetron. Ann Oncol 14:1570–1577

Grunberg SM, Deuson RR, Mavros P et al (2004) Incidence of chemotherapy-induced nausea and emesis after modern antiemetics. Cancer 100:2261–2268

Grunberg SM, Warr D, Gralla RJ et al (2010) Evaluation of new antiemetic agents and definition of antineoplastic agent emetogenicity-state of the art. Support Care Cancer 19:S43–S47

Guyatt G, Gutterman D, Baumann MH et al (2006) Grading strength of recommendations and quality of evidence in clinical guidelines: report from an American College of Chest Physicians Task Force. Chest 129:174–181

Hählen K, Quintana E, Pinkerton CR, Cedar E (1995) A randomized comparison of intravenously administered granisetron versus chlorpromazine plus dexamethasone in the prevention of ifosfamide-induced emesis in children. J Pediatr 126:309–313

Hasler S, Hirt A, Ridolfi Luethy A et al (2008) Safety of ondansetron loading doses in children with cancer. Support Care Cancer 16:469–475

Herrstedt J (2008) Antiemetics: an update and the MASCC guidelines applied in clinical practice. Nat Clin Pract Oncol 5:32–43

Hesketh PJ (1994) Treatment of chemotherapy-induced emesis in the 1990s: impact of the 5-HT$_3$ receptor antagonists. Support Care Cancer 2:286–292

Hesketh PJ (2008) Chemotherapy-induced nausea and vomiting. N Engl J Med 358:2482–2494

Hesketh PJ, Kris MG, Grunberg SM et al (1997) Proposal for classifying the acute emetogenicity of cancer chemotherapy. J Clin Oncol 15:103–109

Hesketh PJ, Grunberg SM, Gralla RJ et al (2003) The oral neurokinin-1 antagonist aprepitant for the prevention of chemotherapy-induced nausea and vomiting: a multi-national, randomized, double-blind, placebo-controlled trial in patients receiving high-dose cisplati-he Aprepitant Protocol 052 Study Group. J Clin Oncol 21:4112–4119

Hewitt M, McQuade B, Stevens R (1993) The efficacy and safety of ondansetron in the prophylaxis of cancer-chemotherapy induced nausea and vomiting in children. Clin Oncol 5:11–14

Hickok JT, Roscoe JA, Morrow GR et al (2003) Nausea and emesis remain significant problems of chemotherapy despite prophylaxis with 5-hydroxytryptamine-3 antiemetics: a University of Rochester James P. Wilmot Cancer Center Community Clinical Oncology Program Study of 360 cancer patients treated in the community. Cancer 97:2880–2886

Hirota T, Honjo T, Kuroda R et al (1993) Antiemetic efficacy of granisetron in pediatric cancer treatment—(2). Comparison of granisetron and granisetron plus methylprednisolone as antiemetic prophylaxis. Gan To Kagaku Ryoho 20:2369–2373

Holdsworth MT, Raisch DW, Frost J (2006) Acute and delayed nausea and emesis control in pediatric oncology patients. Cancer 106:931–940

Jimenez M, Leon P, Gimeno J (1997) Comparison of chlorpromazine plus dexamethasone vs. ondansetron vs. tropisetron in the treatment of emesis induced by highly and moderately emetogenic chemotherapy in pediatric patients with malignancies. International Society of Pediatric Oncology XXIX meeting, Istanbul

Jin Y, Wu X, Guan Y et al (2012) Efficacy and safety of aprepitant in the prevention of chemotherapy-induced nausea and vomiting: a pooled analysis. Support Care Cancer 20:1815–1822

Jindal V, Ge A, Mansky P (2008) Safety and efficacy of acupuncture in children. J Pediatr Hematol Oncol 30:431–442

Jordan K, Hinke A, Grothey A et al (2007) A meta-analysis comparing the efficacy of four 5-HT3-receptor antagonists for acute chemotherapy- induced emesis. Support Care Cancer 15:1023–1033

Jordan K, Roila F, Molassiotis A et al (2011) Antiemetics in children receiving chemotherapy. MASCC/ESMO guideline update 2009. Support Care Cancer 19:S37–S42

Kadota R, Shen V, Messinger Y (2007) Safety, pharmacokinetics, and efficacy of palonosetron in pediatric patients: a multicenter, stratified, double-blind, phase 3, randomized study [abstract]. J Clin Oncol 25:9570

Komada Y, Matsuyama T, Takao A et al (1999) A randomised dose-comparison trial of granisetron in preventing emesis in children with leukemia receiving emetogenic chemotherapy. Eur J Cancer 35:1095–1101

Koseoglu V, Kurekci A, Atay A, Ozcan O (1998) Comparison of the efficacy and side-effects of ondansetron and metoclopramide-diphenhydramine administered to control nausea and vomiting in children treated with antineoplastic chemotherapy: a prospective randomized study. Eur J Pediatr 157:806–810

Laszlo J (1983) Emesis as limiting toxicity in cancer chemotherapy. In: Laszlo J (ed) Antiemetics and cancer chemotherapy. Williams & Wilkins, Baltimore, pp 1–5

Likun Z, Xiang J, Yi B et al (2011) A systematic review and meta-analysis of intravenous palonosetron in the prevention of chemotherapy-induced nausea and vomiting in adults. Oncologist 16:207–216

Marshall G, Kerr S, Vowels M et al (1989) Antiemetic therapy for chemotherapy-induced vomiting: metoclopramide, benztropine, dexamethasone, and lorazepam regimen compared with chlorpromazine. J Pediatr 115:156–160

Matthews A, Haas DM, O'Mathúna DP et al (2014) Interventions for nausea and vomiting in early pregnancy. Cochrane Database Syst Rev (3): CD007575

Mehta P, Gross S, Graham-Pole J et al (1986) Methylprednisolone for chemotherapy-induced emesis: a double-blind randomized trial in children. J Pediatr 108:774–776

Miller AD, Leslie RA (1994) The area postrema and vomiting. Front Neuroendocrinol 15:301–320

Mitchell EP (1992) Gastrointestinal toxicity of chemotherapeutic agents. Semin Oncol 19:566–579

Moertel CG, Reitemeier RJ, Gage RP (1963) A controlled clinical evaluation of antiemetic drugs. JAMA 186:116–118

Molassiotis A, Stricker C, Eaby B et al (2008) Understanding the concept of chemotherapy-related nausea: the patient experience. Eur J Cancer Care 17:444–453

Morrow GR (1984) Clinical characteristics associated with the development of anticipatory nausea and vomiting in cancer patients undergoing chemotherapy treatment. J Clin Oncol 2:1170–1176

Navari RM, Einhorn LH, Passik SD et al (2005) A phase II trial of olanzapine for the prevention of chemotherapy-induced nausea and vomiting: a Hoosier Oncology Group study. Support Care Cancer 13:529–534

Navari RM, Einhorn LH, Loehrer PJ Sr et al (2007) A phase II trial of olanzapine, dexamethasone, and palonosetron for the prevention of chemotherapy-induced nausea and vomiting: a Hoosier oncology group study. Support Care Cancer 15:1285–1291

Phillips RS, Gopaul S, Gibson F et al (2010) Antiemetic medication for prevention and treatment of chemotherapy induced nausea and vomiting in childhood. Cochrane Database Syst Rev (9):CD007786

Pillai AK, Sharma KK, Gupta YK, Bakhshi S (2011) Antiemetic effect of ginger powder versus placebo as an add-on therapy in children and young adults receiving high emetogenic chemotherapy. Pediatr Blood Cancer 56:234–238

Pinarli FG, Elii M, Dagdemir A et al (2006) Electrocardiographic findings after 5-HT3 receptor antagonists and chemotherapy in children with cancer. Pediatr Blood Cancer 47:567–571

Reindl TK, Geilen W, Hartmann R et al (2006) Acupuncture against chemotherapy-induced nausea and vomiting in pediatric oncology: interim results of a multicenter crossover study. Support Care Cancer 14:172–176

Richardson JL, Marks G, Levine A (1988) The influence of symptoms of disease and side effects of treatment on compliance with cancer therapy. J Clin Oncol 6:1746–1752

Richardson J, Smith JE, McCall G et al (2007) Hypnosis for nausea and vomiting in cancer chemotherapy: a systematic review of the research evidence. Eur J Cancer Care 16:402–412

Rodgers C, Kollar D, Taylor O et al (2012) Nausea and vomiting perspectives among children receiving moderate to highly emetogenic chemotherapy treatment. Cancer Nurs 35:203–210

Roila F, Aapro M, Stewart A (1998) Optimal selection of antiemetics in children receiving cancer chemotherapy. Support Care Cancer 6:215–220

Roila F, Hesketh PJ, Herrstedt J (2006) Prevention of chemotherapy- and radiotherapy-induced emesis: results of the 2004 Perugia International Antiemetic Consensus Conference. Ann Oncol 17:20–28

Ryan JL, Heckler CE, Roscoe JA et al (2012) Ginger (*Zingiber officinale*) reduces acute chemotherapy-induced nausea: a URCC CCOP study of 576 patients. Support Care Cancer 20:1479–1489

Saito R, Takano Y, Kamiya HO (2003) Roles of substance P and NK(1) receptor in the brainstem in the development of emesis. J Pharmacol Sci 91:87–94

Sandoval C, Corbi D, Strobino B, Ozkaynak M (1999) Randomized double-blind comparison of single high-dose ondansetron and multiple standard-dose ondansetron in chemotherapy-naive pediatric oncology patients. Cancer Invest 17:309–313

Schwartzberg L (2006) Chemotherapy-induced nausea and vomiting: state of the art in 2006. J Support Oncol 4:3–8

Sepulveda-Vildosola A, Betanzos-Cabrera Y, Lastiri G et al (2008) Palonosetron hydrochloride is an effective and safe option to prevent chemotherapy-induced nausea and vomiting in children. Arch Med Res 39:601–606

Shadle C, Lee Y, Majumdar A et al (2004) Evaluation of potential inductive effects of aprepitant on cytochrome P450 3A4 and 2C9 activity. J Clin Pharmacol 44:215–223

Small BE, Holdsworth MT, Raisch DW, Winter SS (2000) Survey ranking of emetogenic control in children receiving chemotherapy. J Pediatr Hematol Oncol 22:125–132

Straathof CS, Van Den Bent MJ, Ma J et al (1998) The effect of dexamethasone on the update of cisplatin in 9L glioma and the area of brain around tumor. J Neurooncol 37:1–8

Terrin BN, McWilliams NB, Maurer HM (1984) Side effects of metoclopramide as an antiemetic in childhood cancer chemotherapy. J Pediatr 104:138–140

Tramer M, Carrroll F, Campbell FA et al (2001) Cannabinoids for control of chemotherapy-induced nausea and vomiting: quantitative systematic review. BMJ 323:1–8

Triozzi PL, Goldstein D, Laszlo J (1988) Contributions of benzodiazepines to cancer therapy. Cancer Invest 6:103–111

Tyc V, Mulhern R, Fairclough D et al (1993) Chemotherapy induced nausea and emesis in pediatric cancer patients: external validity of child and parent emesis ratings. J Dev Behav Pediatr 14:236–241

Van Hoff J, Olszewski D (1988) Lorazepam for the control of chemotherapy-related nausea and vomiting in children. J Pediatr 113:146–149

Weidenfeld J, Lysy J, Shohami E (1987) Effect of dexamethasone on prostaglandin synthesis in various areas of the rat brain. J Neurochem 48:1351–1354

White L, Daly S, McKenna C et al (2000) A comparison of oral ondansetron syrup or intravenous ondansetron loading dose regimens given in combination with dexamethasone for the prevention of nausea and emesis in pediatric and adolescent patients receiving moderately/highly emetogenic chemotherapy. Pediatr Hematol Oncol 17:445–455

Wickham R (1999) Nausea and vomiting. In: Yarbo CH, Frogge MH, Goodman M (eds) Cancer symptom management, 2nd edn. Jones and Bartlett Publishers, Sudbury, pp 228–263

Zick SM, Ruffin MT, Lee J et al (2009) Phase II trial of encapsulated ginger as a treatment for chemotherapy-induced nausea and vomiting. Support Care Cancer 17:563–572

Oral Mouth Care and Mucositis

11

Denise Mills and Anne Marie Maloney

Contents

Abstract

Oral mucositis is one of the most common and distressing side effects of cancer therapy and results from damage to the mucosal lining of the gastrointestinal tract due to radiation therapy and chemotherapy. Mucositis is characterized by oral erythema, ulceration, and pain and is seen as a continuum from limited patches of mildly sore erythematous mucosae to diffuse areas of painful ulceration and pseudomembranes. The oncology health care team must proactively assess and manage the oral health of pediatric oncology patients before, during and after cancer therapy. This chapter describes the incidence, etiologies, and treatments of oral mucositis and summarizes general oral health care for pediatric oncology patients. Current evidence-based guidelines are reviewed in order to aid pediatric oncology practitioners on best practice for the oral health of their patients.

11.1   Introduction

Oral mucositis (OM) is one of the most common and distressing side effects of cancer therapy. Mucositis results from damage to the mucosal lining of the gastrointestinal tract due to radiation therapy and chemotherapy (Sonis et al. 2004). OM is a clinical condition characterized by erythema,

D. Mills, MN, NP (✉) • A.M. Maloney, MSN, NP
Division of Hematology/Oncology,
The Hospital for Sick Children,
555 University Avenue,
Toronto, ON M5G 1X8, Canada
e-mail: denise.mills@sickkids.ca

J. Feusner et al. (eds.), *Supportive Care in Pediatric Oncology:
A Practical Evidence-Based Approach*, Pediatric Oncology,
DOI 10.1007/978-3-662-44317-0_11, © Springer Berlin Heidelberg 2015

ulceration, and pain and is a continuum from limited patches of mildly sore erythematous mucosae to diffuse areas of painful ulceration and pseudomembranes (Scully et al. 2003). The variability in severity of OM contributes to the underreporting of its prevalence (Scully et al. 2003; Sonis 2004). It is often painful and can compromise nutrition and oral hygiene while increasing risk for local and systemic infection (Lalla et al. 2008).

OM is the most frequent, serious complication of chemotherapy and radiation therapy causing reductions in chemotherapy doses, need for nasogastric tube feedings and potentially total parenteral nutrition (TPN), and increasing hospitalizations and opioid use (Treister and Sonis 2007). OM has a significant adverse effect on the quality of life of children and adolescents (Cheng et al. 2012). Cheng et al. (2012) found that OM symptoms that were most distressing in this population included dysphagia, which led to an inability to eat or enjoy food, and trouble sleeping.

11.2   Incidence

The incidence of OM is highest in patients being treated for cancers of the head and neck. Approximately 90 % of patients with head and neck cancer develop OM, depending on the location of radiation therapy and the use of concomitant chemotherapy (Sonis et al. 2004). OM occurs in 52–80 % of all children receiving cancer treatment (Kuhn et al. 2009).

11.2.1 Risk Factors

Risk factors that dispose a patient to the development of mucositis are multifactorial and can be classified into two categories: patient-related and treatment-related (Table 11.1). Many chemotherapeutic and biotherapy agents can play a role in mucositis. The risk of OM increases when high-dose combination therapies are utilized such as in hematopoietic stem cell transplantation (HSCT) and particularly in combination with total body irradiation (TBI) (Scully et al. 2003).

Table 11.1 Therapy- and patient-related risk factors for oral mucositis

Therapy-related risk factors	
Chemotherapy and biotherapy agents	Antimetabolites
	Cytarabine
	5-fluorouracil
	Methotrexate
	Antitumor antibiotics
	Actinomycin D
	Amsacrine
	Mithramycin
	Mitomycin
	Alkylating agents
	Busulfan
	Cyclophosphamide
	Mechlorethamine
	Procarbazine
	Thiotepa
	Anthracyclines
	Daunorubicin
	Doxorubicin
	Epirubicin
	Taxanes
	Paclitaxel
	Docetaxel
	mTOR inhibitors
Hematopoietic stem cell transplant	Allogeneic > autologous transplant
Radiation therapy	Incidence and severity related to site and fractionation
Combination therapy	Chemotherapy + radiation therapy
Patient-related risk factors	
Age	Children have an increased risk of mucositis due to increased cell turnover
Genetic factors	Genes associated with chemotherapy metabolism may play an important role in increased development of mucositis
Oral health and hygiene	A comorbidity of dental or oral infection may complicate mucositis
Nutritional status	Poor nutritional status may affect increased breakdown and delayed healing
Smoking	Affects circulation and may delay healing
Previous experience	History of mucositis can predict future mucositis

Adapted from Scully et al. (2003)

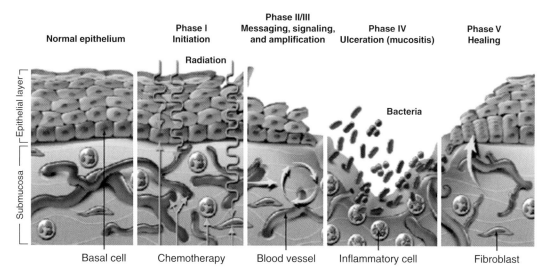

Fig. 11.1 Pathophysiology of oral mucositis (with permission from Sonis [2004])

11.2.2 Pathophysiology of Oral Mucositis

Mucositis has been described as a complex physiologic process that can be examined in five stages: initiation, primary damage response, signal amplification, ulceration, and healing (Fig. 11.1).

11.2.2.1 Initiation

The initiation stage occurs immediately following the administration of radiation or chemotherapy. In this stage, direct damage to both DNA and non-DNA occurs. This initial insult to tissues does not represent the extensive injury that characterizes the clinical presentation of mucositis. Chemotherapy agents and radiation therapy generate reactive oxygen species (ROS) that cause damage to connective tissue, DNA, and cell membranes, stimulate macrophages, and trigger a cascade of critical biologic mechanisms and molecular pathways including p53, nuclear factor kappa-B (NF-κB), and the ceramide pathway (Sonis 2004, 2011). At this point, the tissues have a normal clinical appearance.

11.2.2.2 Primary Damage Response

The primary damage response phase is an extremely active phase associated with significant inter- and intracellular signaling in connective tissue, endothelium, and the submucosa (Sonis 2011).

Activated transcription factors mediate both gene expression and the synthesis and release of biologically active mediators that impair the viability of the basal epithelium (Sonis 2007). NF-κB is thought to be the most significant transcription factor in the development of mucositis. It is responsible for regulating the expression of approximately 200 genes, many of which play a role in the pathogenesis of mucositis; specifically, it is a regulator of proinflammatory cytokines including tumor necrosis factor α (TNF-α), IL-6 and IL-1β. These proinflammatory cytokines secondarily cause damage that ultimately results in apoptosis of epithelial basal cells (Tresiter and Sonis 2007).

11.2.2.3 Signal Amplification

During signal amplification cytokine mediators generated during the primary damage response phase provide positive feedback resulting in a cascade of damaging mediators. These feedback loops reinitiate the damage response pathways. An example of this is NF-κB stimulation by TNF-α to continue its downstream activity (Sonis 2004, 2011). These feedback loops magnify the response of the initial injury by amplifying and potentiating the original biologic signals, increasing tissue injury and prolonging damage by continuing to provide signals for days after the original chemotherapeutic or radiation insult (Sonis 2007).

11.2.2.4 Ulceration

Ulceration is the phase with the most clinical significance. Ulceration develops as a consequence of the direct and indirect mechanisms noted in the previous phases that cause damage and apoptotic changes to mucosal epithelium (Sonis 2009). Mucosal integrity is lost, resulting in painful ulcers. The ulcers are covered by a pseudomembrane and are a desirable environment for secondary bacterial colonization. Neutropenic patients are at greater risk of sepsis due to the Gram-positive and Gram-negative organisms that thrive in the pseudomembrane (Sonis 2007).

11.2.2.5 Healing

In the absence of infection, healing is usually complete within 2–3 weeks. The healing phase is the least understood of the phases of mucositis but is thought to be controlled by signaling from the submucosal mesenchyme to the epithelium. Signaling controls migration, differentiation and proliferation of new tissue across the base of the ulcer (Treister and Sonis 2007).

11.2.3 Clinical Course of Oral Mucositis

On initial presentation of OM, the oral mucosa first shows erythema which then progresses to erosion and ultimately ulceration. Ulcerations are typically covered by a white fibrinous pseudomembrane. Lesions will heal approximately 2–4 weeks after the last dose of the offending chemotherapy or radiation therapy. In the case of immunosuppressed patients, resolution of OM usually coincides with granulocyte recovery (Lalla et al. 2008). Chemotherapy-induced OM is limited to nonkeratinized surfaces such as the lateral and ventral tongue, buccal mucosa, and soft palate (Lalla et al. 2008). Radiation-induced OM occurs in the radiation field with nonkeratinized tissue affected more often. Patients receiving increasing cumulative doses beyond 30 Gy will be more severely affected (Sonis 2007; Lalla et al. 2008). The clinical course of mucositis can be complicated by infection, particularly in the immunocompromised patient.

11.3 Assessment and Measurement of Oral Mucositis

Historically, mucositis measurement and assessment in pediatrics have relied on tools developed for adults (Tomlinson et al. 2009). Reliable oral assessment is essential to facilitate management strategies or implement clinical trials in mucositis prevention and treatment (Tomlinson et al. 2007, 2009). The scales currently utilized to assess pediatric OM do not address practical issues such as mechanisms for optimal visualization of the oral cavity and approaching an uncooperative child. There are also limitations to reporting subjective and functional domains in the child (Tomlinson et al. 2007).

Simple instruments such as the World Health Organization (WHO) grading system and the National Cancer Institute (NCI) Common Terminology Criteria for Adverse Events are scales that range from 0 (with no symptoms) to 4 or 5 (worst symptoms possible) (Fig. 11.2). Generally these scales are based on the ability to eat and drink combined with objective signs of mucositis. These instruments are utilized by pediatric oncology groups as part of toxicity criteria measurement. They are seen to be the most relevant scales for clinical management as a global score is achieved readily (Sonis et al. 2004). However, these simple scales may underreport mucositis if effective analgesia is administered to the patient (Sonis 2009).

The Oral Mucositis Assessment Scale (OMAS) was developed by a panel of experts to be an objective, simple, and reproducible assessment tool to be applied to multicenter clinical trials of mucositis (Sonis et al. 1999). The OMAS measures degree of ulceration, pseudomembrane formation, and mucosal erythema in specific mouth sites (Sonis et al. 1999) (Fig. 11.2). Testing has demonstrated that the OMAS is reliable and valid in adults with the only reported limitation being that patients with severe mucositis had difficulty undergoing repeated examinations (Sonis et al. 1999). Sung et al. (2007) demonstrated that the OMAS is valid in the measurement of mucositis in children ≥ 6 years of age.

a World Health Organization (WHO) Scoring Criteria for Oral Mucositis

Grade	0	1	2	3	4
Description	Normal	Soreness with or without erythema	Ulceration and erythema; patient can swallow a solid diet	Ulceration and erythema; patient cannot swallow a solid diet	Ulceration and pseudomembrane formation of such severity that alimentation is not possible

Adapted from Sonis et al. (2004a)

b National Cancer Institute Common Terminology Criteria for Adverse Events (CTCAE version 4.0)

Adverse event	Grade 1	Grade 2	Grade 3	Grade 4	Grade 5
Oral mucositis definition: a disorder characterized by inflammation of the oral mucosa	Asymptomatic or mild symptoms; intervention not indicated	Moderate pain; not interfering with oral intake; modified diet indicated	Severe pain; interfering with oral intake	Life-threatening consequences; urgent intervention indicated	Death

http://www.acrin.org/Portals/o/Administration/Regulatory/CTACE_4.02_2009-09-15_QuickReference_5x7.pdf

c Oral Mucositis Assessment Scale

Location	Ulceration/Pseudomembrane* (circle)				Erythema** (circle)		
Upper lip	0	1	2	3	0	1	2
Lower lip	0	1	2	3	0	1	2
Right cheek	0	1	2	3	0	1	2
Left cheek	0	1	2	3	0	1	2
Right ventral and lateral tongue	0	1	2	3	0	1	2
Left ventral and lateral tongue	0	1	2	3	0	1	2
Floor of mouth	0	1	2	3	0	1	2
Soft palate/fauces	0	1	2	3	0	1	2
Hard palate	0	1	2	3	0	1	2

With permission from Sonis et al. (1999)

*Ulceration/pseudomembrane:
0 = no lesion
1 = <1 cm^2
2 = 1 cm^2–3 cm^2
3 = >3 cm^2

**Erythema:
0 = none
1 = not severe
2 = severe

d Oral Assessment Guide

Category	Tools for Assessment	Methods of Measurement	Numerical and Descriptive Ratings		
			1	2	3
Voice	Auditory	Converse with patient	Normal	Deeper or raspy	Difficulty talking or painful
Swallow	Observation	Ask patient to swallow. To test gag reflex, gently place blade on back of tongue and depress	Normal swallow	Some pain on swallow	Unable to swallow
Lip	Visual/palpation	Observe and feel tissue	Smooth and pink and moist	Dry or cracked	Ulcerated or bleeding
Tongue	Visual/palpation	Feel and observe appearance of tissue	Pink and moist and papillae present	Coated or loss of papillae with a shiny appearance with or without redness	Blistered or cracked
Saliva	Tongue blade	Insert blade into mouth, touching the center of the tongue and the floor of the mouth	Watery	Thick or ropy	Absent
Mucous membrane	Visual	Observe appearance of tissue	Pink and moist	Reddened or coated (increased whiteness) without ulcerations	Ulcerations with or without bleeding
Gingiva	Tongue blade and visual	Gently press tissue with tip of blade	Pink and stippled	Edematous with or without redness	Spontaneous bleeding or bleeding with pressure
Teeth	Visual	Observe appearance of teeth	Clean and no debris	Plaque or debris in localized area (between teeth if present)	Plaque or debris generalized along gum line

Adapted from Eilers et al. (1988)

Fig. 11.2 Oral Mucositis Grading Scales. (**a**) World Health Organization scoring criteria. (**b**) National Cancer Institute Common Terminology Criteria for Adverse Events (CTCAE version 4.0). (**c**) Oral Mucositis Assessment Scale. (**d**) Oral Assessment Guide

An example of a combined scale that includes both objective and subjective experiences as well as functional dimensions is the Oral Assessment Guide (OAG) (Eilers et al. 1988). The OAG was designed primarily as a clinical tool and is useful for recording the condition of the oral cavity (Eilers et al. 1988). The OAG consists of numerical and descriptive ratings in eight categories including voice, swallowing, lips, tongue, saliva, mucous membranes, gingivae and teeth. Each descriptive category is assessed on a numeric scale from 1 to 3 with the overall oral assessment score the sum of the eight categories (Eilers et al. 1988) (Fig. 11.2). Chen et al. (2004) used the OAG to assess children with leukemia and lymphoma undergoing chemotherapy and were able to demonstrate content validity of the instrument.

Tomlinson et al. (2008a, b, c) identified four main areas of concern from the existing literature in mucositis assessment and tool development in the pediatric oncology population: (1) the challenge of oral assessment in children with relation to age and cooperation; (2) the need for proxy responses, while recognizing the challenges of reporting pain and function attributed to oral mucositis; (3) the need for an instrument that is simple, quick to complete and easy to use in almost all children; and (4) educational considerations. To address these concerns, their group developed the Children's International Mucositis Evaluation Scale (ChIMES; Fig. 11.3), an assessment instrument for both child self-report and parent proxy-report (Tomlinson et al. 2009). ChIMES assesses three main areas: (1) pain (i.e., pain assessment, amount of pain medication received), (2) function (i.e., effect on eating, drooling/pooling of saliva, effect on drinking), and (3) appearance (i.e., presence of ulcers) (Tomlinson et al. 2009). ChIMES has been shown to be understandable, with content validity and acceptability, and has been prospectively validated in a multicenter cohort of children receiving chemotherapy and after HSCT (Tomlinson et al. 2009, 2011; Jacobs et al. 2013).

11.4 Prevention and Treatment of Oral Mucositis

In recent years there has been an increase in research regarding the prevention and treatment of mucositis. However, evidence-based interventions remain limited, especially in pediatric patients. Generally, the clinical focus continues to be on palliation of the symptoms of mucositis (Eilers and Million 2011). In a Cochrane review, Clarkson et al. (2010) showed that there is limited evidence that low-level laser therapy (LLLT) may be beneficial in the treatment of OM. In a separate Cochrane analysis Worthington et al. (2011) reported that ten agents showed potential benefit in OM prophylaxis; these agents were reviewed by Eilers and Million (2011) and are summarized in Table 11.2.

11.4.1 Palifermin

Palifermin is the first targeted agent approved for the prevention of mucositis in patients receiving high-dose chemotherapy with or without radiation therapy as conditioning for HSCT. Palifermin is a recombinant form of keratinocyte growth factor-1 (KGF-1) that binds to its cognate receptor, resulting in increased cellular proliferation and mediation of epithelial cell repair (Posner and Haddad 2007). The efficacy of palifermin to reduce the incidence, duration and severity of mucosal lesions in the oral cavity has been established in adult patients undergoing autologous and allogeneic HSCT (Spielberger et al. 2004; McDonnell and Lenz 2007; Langner et al. 2008; Barasch et al. 2009). Pediatric data are quite limited. In a phase I study, Srinivasan et al. (2012) showed that palifermin was tolerated at a dose of 90 μg/kg/day with linear pharmacokinetics in children undergoing allogeneic HSCT. Lauritano et al. (2014) showed a significant reduction in duration and grade of mucositis in pediatric patients with acute lymphoblastic leukemia

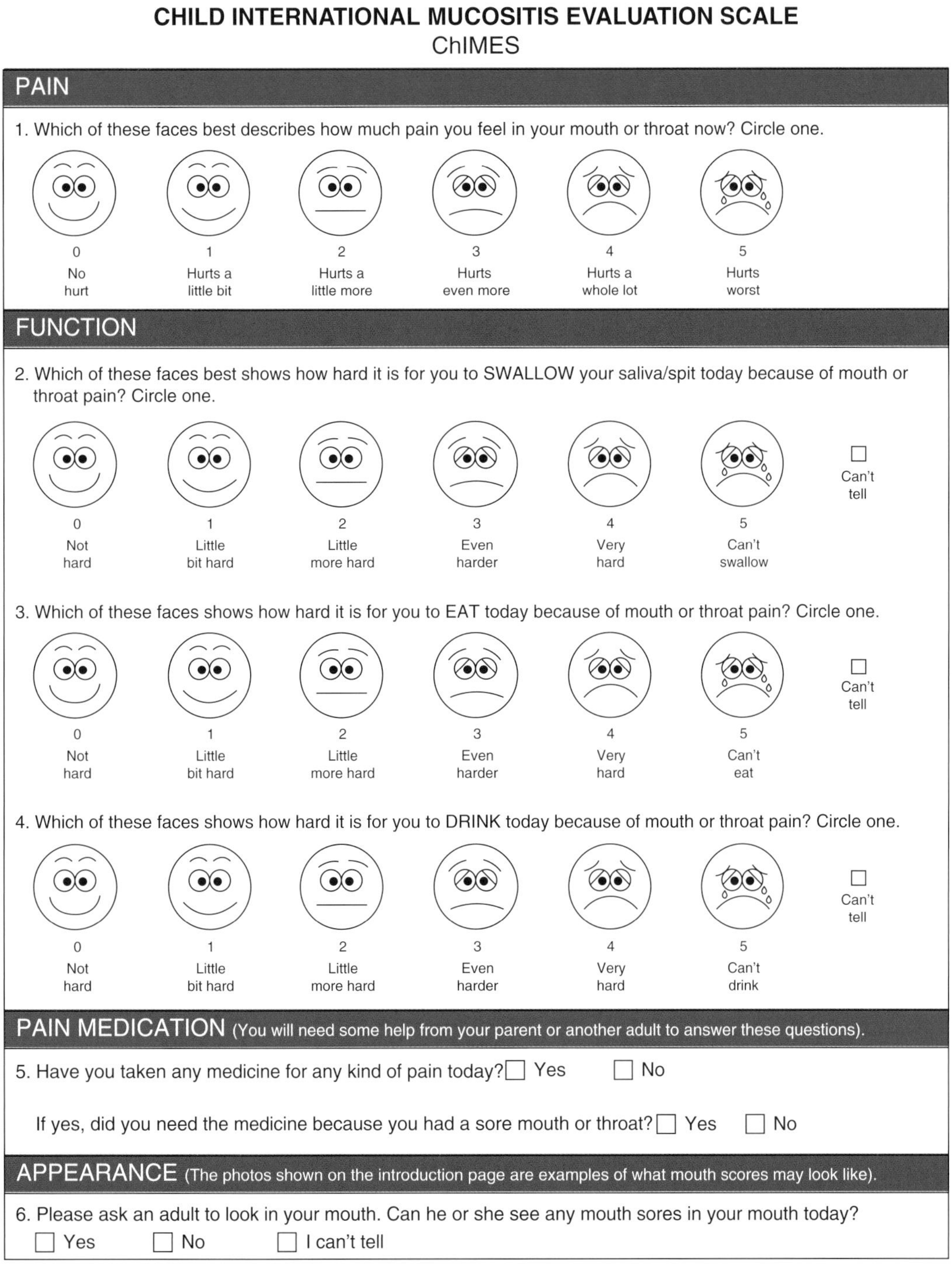

CHILD INTERNATIONAL MUCOSITIS EVALUATION SCALE
ChIMES

PAIN

1. Which of these faces best describes how much pain you feel in your mouth or throat now? Circle one.

0	1	2	3	4	5
No hurt	Hurts a little bit	Hurts a little more	Hurts even more	Hurts a whole lot	Hurts worst

FUNCTION

2. Which of these faces best shows how hard it is for you to SWALLOW your saliva/spit today because of mouth or throat pain? Circle one.

0	1	2	3	4	5	☐ Can't tell
Not hard	Little bit hard	Little more hard	Even harder	Very hard	Can't swallow	

3. Which of these faces shows how hard it is for you to EAT today because of mouth or throat pain? Circle one.

0	1	2	3	4	5	☐ Can't tell
Not hard	Little bit hard	Little more hard	Even harder	Very hard	Can't eat	

4. Which of these faces shows how hard it is for you to DRINK today because of mouth or throat pain? Circle one.

0	1	2	3	4	5	☐ Can't tell
Not hard	Little bit hard	Little more hard	Even harder	Very hard	Can't drink	

PAIN MEDICATION (You will need some help from your parent or another adult to answer these questions).

5. Have you taken any medicine for any kind of pain today? ☐ Yes   ☐ No

   If yes, did you need the medicine because you had a sore mouth or throat? ☐ Yes   ☐ No

APPEARANCE (The photos shown on the introduction page are examples of what mouth scores may look like).

6. Please ask an adult to look in your mouth. Can he or she see any mouth sores in your mouth today?
   ☐ Yes   ☐ No   ☐ I can't tell

Fig. 11.3 ChIMES tool (with permission from Tomlinson et al. [2010])

Table 11.2 Prevention and treatment of oral mucositis

Intervention	Level of support	Population studied	Grade[a]
Prevention			
Aloe Vera	Weak unreliable evidence the solution was beneficial for the prevention of moderate to severe mucositis	Head and neck cancer receiving radiotherapy	2C
Amifostine	Weak unreliable evidence from 11 low quality trials that amifostine is beneficial for the prevention of any mucositis	Combinations of head and neck cancer, other solid tumors and hematologic malignancies receiving radiotherapy, stem cell transplant, non-myeloablative chemotherapy or a combination	2C
Antibiotic (polymyxin/tobramycin/amphotericin [PTA])—lozenges/paste	Weak unreliable evidence that PTA lozenges may be beneficial for the prevention of any mucositis	Head and neck cancer receiving radiotherapy	2C
Cryotherapy	Found to be beneficial in the prevention of all the outcome categories of mucositis—any, moderate and severe mucositis	Hematologic malignancies with chemotherapy or stem cell transplantation	2B
Glutamine	Weak evidence that glutamine is beneficial for the prevention of severe mucositis	Combinations of head and neck cancer, other solid tumors and hematologic malignancies receiving radiotherapy, stem cell transplant, non-myeloablative chemotherapy or a combination	2B
Granulocyte colony-stimulating factor (G-CSF)	Weak unreliable evidence that G-CSF is effective for the prevention of severe mucositis	Combinations of head and neck cancer, other solid tumors and hematologic malignancies receiving radiotherapy, stem cell transplant, non-myeloablative chemotherapy or a combination	2C
Honey	Weak unreliable evidence with substantial heterogeneity that honey may be beneficial in the prevention of any mucositis	Head and neck cancer receiving radiotherapy	2C
Palifermin (keratinocyte growth factor)	Found beneficial for the prevention of all outcome categories of mucositis, moderate mucositis and severe mucositis	Combinations of head and neck cancer, other solid tumors and hematologic malignancies receiving radiotherapy, stem cell transplant, non-myeloablative chemotherapy or a combination	2B
Low-level laser therapy	Weak unreliable evidence that laser is beneficial for the prevention of severe mucositis	Combinations of head and neck cancer, other solid tumors and hematologic malignancies receiving radiotherapy, stem cell transplant, non-myeloablative chemotherapy or a combination	2B
Sucralfate	Evidence that sucralfate is effective in the prevention of severe mucositis, with a 33 % reduction in severe mucositis in treatment group compared to placebo	Mostly head and neck cancer receiving radiotherapy, some trials with participants with other cancer types	2B
Treatment			
Low-level laser therapy	Limited evidence that low-level laser is beneficial in reducing the severity of oral mucositis	Children with mixed cancers and adults with hematologic malignancies	2B
Patient controlled analgesia (PCA)	Unreliable evidence that less opiate is used per hour and duration of the pain is slightly reduced with PCA. No evidence that PCA is better than continuous morphine in controlling pain	Adult leukemia or lymphoma undergoing high-dose chemotherapy and total body irradiation prior to stem cell transplant	2B

Adapted from Eilers and Million (2011)

[a]Per Guyatt et al. (2006); see Preface

undergoing allogeneic HSCT while Vitale et al. (2014) showed no significant benefit in children undergoing autologous HSCT (although there was a trend toward decreased mucositis severity). Further studies are required to assess whether palifermin will be effective for other chemotherapy modalities and in the pediatric population.

11.4.2 Low-Level Laser Therapy

LLLT is an emerging therapy in the prevention and treatment of OM. LLLT is local application of a monochromatic, narrowband, coherent light source. The action of LLLT is disputed, but a cytoprotective effect before and during oxidative stress has been reported following its use. Red and infrared LLLT is believed to have an anti-inflammatory effect (Bjordal 2012). The current Multinational Association of Supportive Care in Cancer (MASCC) and International Society of Oral Oncology (ISOO) guidelines for adult patients receiving high-dose chemotherapy or chemotherapy and HSCT recommend LLLT if the institution is able to support the technology and training in LLLT (Keefe and Gibson 2007). A meta-analysis by Bensadoun and Nair (2012) reported reduced risk of OM as well as reduced duration and severity of OM with both red and infrared LLLT. Pediatric data are limited and conflicting. In a randomized, placebo-controlled trial of 21 pediatric oncology patients with chemotherapy-related OM, Kuhn et al. (2009) showed that LLLT reduced the duration of OM. This result has been supported by Abramoff et al. (2008) who similarly showed a reduction in OM frequency with LLLT as well as decreased pain and OM severity in those presenting with OM. These results conflict with Cruz et al. (2007) who showed no benefit for prevention in children with cancer in a randomized trial. As with palifermin, further data are required to support LLLT in the pediatric population given the younger age and therefore likely improved ability to heal compared to an older cohort.

11.4.3 Glutamine

Glutamine is considered a conditionally essential amino acid as stress and catabolic states lead to its depletion (Storey 2007). Theoretically, glutamine repletion may prevent damage to normal tissues such as the oral mucosa during cytotoxic therapies (Storey 2007). Adult studies showed benefit with Saforis (AES-14), an oral L-glutamine swish-and-swallow suspension, but after United States Food and Drug Administration (FDA) approval, the drug was discontinued (Posner and Haddad 2007). Studies in pediatric patients are conflicting; Anderson et al. (1998) and Aquino et al. (2005) showed benefit in pediatric patients undergoing cytotoxic therapies and HSCT, while Ware et al. (2009) showed no benefit. In the review by Storey (2007), it is concluded that studies, though promising, show an inconsistent benefit in pediatric patients and are limited by small patient numbers as well as a variety of glutamine dosages, dose intervals and administration techniques which hamper the ability to make firm conclusions about glutamine efficacy.

11.4.4 Cryotherapy

Cryotherapy has not been systematically studied in pediatric oncology patients but has shown benefit in the prevention of OM from short-acting chemotherapeutic agents such as 5-fluorouracil (5-FU) in adult patients (Posner and Haddad 2007). Administration of ice chips simply causes vasoconstriction and therefore decreased blood flow to the oral mucosa during bolus infusions of 5-FU. Benefit of this intervention on longer-acting agents is unclear although the recent Cochrane review did show potential decrement of OM incidence with prophylactic cryotherapy in adult patients (Posner and Haddad 2007; Eilers and Million 2011).

11.5 Oral Care

The purpose of basic oral care is to reduce symptoms of oral pain and bleeding related to cancer therapy and to prevent soft tissue infections that may have systemic sequelae. In addition, maintenance of good oral hygiene reduces the risk of future dental complications (Rubenstein et al. 2004). A study by Clarkson and Eden (1998) examining the dental health of children with cancer found that 43 % of patients had untreated decay and only 35 % had been seen by a dentist since diagnosis. Their study exemplified the lack of dental preventive care for pediatric oncology patients and stressed the need to continue to provide primary oral hygiene during pediatric cancer therapy (Clarkson and Eden 1998). A European multidisciplinary group, in collaboration with the United Kingdom Childhood Cancer Study Group (UKCCSG) and the Paediatric Oncology Nurses Forum (PONF), was established in 2001 principally to produce comprehensive, evidence-based guidelines on mouth care for children and adolescents being treated for cancer. The potential benefits of such guidelines include improved patient care, consistency of care, the promotion of interventions of proven benefit and a reduction in use of ineffective or potentially harmful practices (Glenny et al. 2010).

The UKCCSG-PONF Mouth Care for Children and Young People with Cancer guidelines used the agreed-upon methodology of SIGN (Scottish Intercollegiate Guidelines Network) to aid them in their development of evidence-based guidelines (Glenny et al. 2010). A consensus approach was utilized to establish the scope and basic structure of the guidelines. Three key areas were identified and covered by the guidelines: (1) dental care and basic oral hygiene, (2) methods of oral assessment, and (3) drugs and therapies (Glenny et al. 2010). The group conducted a systematic review of the literature to examine these three key areas and, where no evidence existed, a consensus opinion on best practice was determined (Glenny et al. 2010). Additionally, the American Academy of Pediatric Dentistry (AAPD) has published guidelines on the dental management of pediatric patients receiving chemotherapy, HSCT or radiation (AAPD 2013). The overarching purpose of these guidelines is to recognize that the pediatric dental professional plays an important role in the care of pediatric oncology patients. The AAPD guidelines focus on basic oral hygiene and dental care for pediatric oncology patients before, during and after cancer therapy.

The AAPD and UKCCSG-PONF guidelines make recommendations in five areas, as summarized in Table 11.3: (1) orodental care at the time of cancer diagnosis, (2) oral hygiene at diagnosis and during cancer treatment, (3) orodental care during cancer treatment, (4) orodental care after cancer therapy, and (5) prevention and treatment of xerostomia (Glenny et al. 2010).

The UKCCSG-PONF guidelines emphasize the importance of oral assessment throughout cancer treatment utilizing the discussed oral assessment tools. Frequency of oral assessment should be determined on an individual basis and should be increased if oral complications arise (Glenny et al. 2010). The AAPD describes the importance of identifying and stabilizing, or eliminating, existing and potential sources of infection or local irritants in the oral cavity. Emphasis on the education of patients and parents on the importance of oral care should occur throughout therapy as well as in regard to the potential short- and long-term effects of therapy. The AAPD further elaborates on care when the use of radiation will affect the orofacial region with the goal of reduction of radiation to healthy oral tissue through consultation with the radiation oncologist and utilization of lead-lined stents, prostheses and shields to spare structures such as the salivary glands. Patients who receive radiation therapy involving the masticatory muscles should be educated on daily oral stretching exercises to decrease the potential of trismus (AAPD 2013).

Finally, for patients that experience xerostomia, the AAPD recommends fluoride rinses and gels for the prevention of caries as well as the use of humidification for symptomatic relief.

11.6 Oral Infections

Patients experiencing OM are predisposed to infections of the oral cavity. Viral, fungal and bacterial infections may arise with incidence dependent on the use of prophylactic anti-infective regimens, oral status prior to chemotherapy, and secondary to the duration and severity of neutropenia. The most frequent documented source of sepsis in the immunocompromised cancer patient is the mouth (Allen et al. 2010). In adults, chemotherapy and radiotherapy in patients with head

Table 11.3 Summary of recommendations for oral care and hygiene for pediatric oncology patients[a]

Clinical scenario	Recommendations
Orodental care at time of cancer diagnosis	All children with an oncology diagnosis undergo a dental assessment at the time of cancer diagnosis and if possible before cancer therapy commences
	The people most suitable to undertake the initial assessment be a pediatric dentist or dental hygienist
	The possible long-term dental/orofacial effects of cancer and treatment should be discussed
	Communication and collaboration between community and cancer center dentistry should occur
	Oral hygiene advice and education should be given to patients and parents prior to starting therapy and should be provided verbally and in writing and delivered by a member of the dental team or a member of the medical team who has received appropriate training
Oral hygiene at diagnosis and during cancer treatment	Brush teeth with a fluoride toothpaste at least twice daily
	Toothbrush should be for the sole use of the patient and changed on a 3-month basis or when bristles splay. Toothbrush should be changed following an oral or respiratory infection
	For patients up to the age of 6, parents/caregivers should be educated on how to brush the child's teeth
	Oral sponges should be utilized in infants and in those unable to brush their teeth
	Use of a non-cariogenic diet should be encouraged. Education should be provided about the high cariogenic potential of dietary supplements rich in carbohydrates and oral medications rich in sucrose
Orodental care during cancer treatment	Elective dental care should not occur during periods of immunosuppression
	Close monitoring for oral mucositis and oral mucosal infection
Orodental care after cancer treatment	Review of potential long-term dental/orofacial effects of childhood cancer and treatment
	Oral health to be monitored during growth and development
	Collaboration for transfer back to routine dental provider
Treatment and prevention of xerostomia[b]	There is insufficient evidence to support the use of pharmacologic agents for the prevention of salivary gland damage and xerostomia in pediatrics
	Use of saliva stimulants (when approved for use in children), artificial saliva, sugar-free chewing gum or frequent sipping of water may aid in relief of dry mouth

Adapted from Glenny et al. (2010), American Academy of Pediatric Dentistry (2013)
[a]All recommendations are level of evidence 1C per Guyatt et al. (2006); see Preface
[b]See Chap. 13 for a detailed discussion of radiation-induced xerostomia

and neck cancer are independently and significantly associated with risk of oral fungal infection (Lalla et al. 2010).

Oropharyngeal candidiasis (i.e., thrush) is the most common oral mucosal infection in the immunocompromised patient and most often secondary to *C. albicans* (Allen et al. 2010; Lalla et al. 2010). Oral candidiasis can have multiple clinical presentations including: (1) pseudomembranous candidiasis (thrush) with whitish plaques with raised, indurated borders; (2) chronic hyperplastic candidiasis with a hyperkeratotic white patch; (3) erythematous candidiasis; and (4) angular chelitis (Lalla et al. 2010). Topical oral antifungal agents such as nystatin rinse and clotrimazole troches are often used to treat oral candidiasis although there is no evidence to support their use in neutropenic patients. (Clarkson et al. 2007; Lalla et al. 2010; Worthington et al. 2010). In a Cochrane review Clarkson et al. (2007) reported that there is strong evidence supporting the use of antifungals which are absorbed in the gastrointestinal (GI) tract (i.e., fluconazole, ketoconazole, itraconazole) in the prevention of oral candidiasis. In their review, Lalla et al. (2010) similarly reported that systemic antifungals are effective in preventing oral fungal infection. Data on treatment of fungal infection are less clear; in another Cochrane meta-analysis Worthington et al. (2010) reported there is insufficient evidence to support any particular antifungal agent although again drugs absorbed in the GI tract appear more efficacious. Both Cochrane reviews included studies which contained pediatric patients.

Viral infections differ clinically from mucositis as they are typically localized to and involve keratinized mucosa of the hard palate, gingiva, and dorsal tongue, present in crops, and may present with fever (Scully et al. 2006). Herpes simplex virus (HSV) type 1 is the most common viral pathogen isolated from mucosal lesions in immunocompromised patients and in a Cochrane review acyclovir has been found effective for both the prevention and treatment of HSV infections in adult and pediatric cancer patients (Glenny et al. 2009).

11.7   Summary

Oral mucositis is one of the most common and distressing side effects of cancer therapy occurring in >50 % of children undergoing cancer therapy. Appropriate oral care, as well as complementary patient and family education from diagnosis on the importance of oral care, is the cornerstone of prevention of mucositis and prevention of infection during periods of neutropenia. Assessment of mucositis is ideally done through the utilization of a scale validated specifically in pediatric patients. Multiple interventions have been trialled, especially in adult oncology patients, for the prevention and treatment of OM and the majority of these interventions have reported potential weak benefit or mixed results to date. Pediatric data are limited and conflicting; further studies are required to make firm recommendations on these agents in the pediatric oncology cohort.

References

Abramoff MM, Lopes NN, Lopes LA et al (2008) Low-level laser therapy in the prevention and treatment of chemotherapy-induced oral mucositis in young patients. Photomed Laser Surg 26:393–400

Allen G, Logan R, Gue S (2010) Oral manifestations of cancer treatment in children: a review of the literature. Clin J Oncol Nurs 14:481–490

American Academy of Pediatric Dentistry (2013) Guideline on dental management of pediatric patients receiving chemotherapy, hematopoietic stem cell transplantation, and/or radiation. Pediatr Dent 35:E185–E193

Anderson PM, Schroeder G, Skubitz KM (1998) Oral glutamine reduces the duration and severity of stomatitis after cytotoxic cancer chemotherapy. Cancer 83:1433–1439

Aquino VM, Harvey AR, Garvin JH et al (2005) A double-blind randomized placebo-controlled study of oral glutamine in the prevention of mucositis in children undergoing hematopoietic stem cell transplantation: a pediatric blood and marrow transplant consortium study. Bone Marrow Transplant 36:611–616

Barasch A, Epstein J, Tilashalski K (2009) Palifermin for management of treatment-induced oral mucositis in cancer patients. Biol Targets Ther 3:111–116

Bensadoun RJ, Nair RG (2012) Low-level laser therapy in the prevention and treatment of cancer therapy-induced mucositis: 2012 state of the art based on literature review and meta-analysis. Curr Opin Oncol 24:363–370

Bjordal JM (2012) Low level laser therapy (LLLT) and World Association for Laser Therapy (WALT) dosage recommendations. Photomed Laser Surg 30:61–62

Chen CF, Wang RH, Cheng SN, Chang YC (2004) Assessment of chemotherapy-induced oral complications in children with cancer. J Pediatr Oncol Nurs 21:33–39

Cheng KK, Lee V, Li CH et al (2012) Oral mucositis in pediatric and adolescent patients undergoing chemotherapy: the impact of symptoms on quality of life. Support Care Cancer 20:2335–2342

Clarkson JE, Eden OB (1998) Dental health in children with cancer. Arch Dis Child 78:560–561

Clarkson JE, Worthington HV, Eden OB (2007) Interventions for preventing oral candidiasis for patients with cancer receiving treatment. Cochrane Database Syst Rev 1:CD003807

Clarkson JE, Worthington HV, Furness S et al (2010) Interventions for treating oral mucositis for patients with cancer receiving treatment. Cochrane Database Syst Rev (4):CD001973

Cruz LB, Ribeiro AS, Rech A et al (2007) Influence of low-energy laser in the prevention of oral mucositis in children with cancer receiving chemotherapy. Pediatr Blood Cancer 48:435–440

Eilers J, Million R (2011) Clinical update: prevention and management of oral mucositis in patients with cancer. Semin Oncol Nurs 27:e1–e16

Eilers J, Berger AM, Petersen MC (1988) Development, testing, and application of the oral assessment guide. Oncol Nurs Forum 15:325–330

Glenny AM, Fernandez Mauleffinch LM, Pavitt S, Walsh T (2009) Interventions for the prevention and treatment of herpes simplex virus in patients being treated for cancer. Cochrane Database Syst Rev 1:CD006706

Glenny AM, Gibson F, Auld E (2010) The development of evidence-based guidelines on mouth care for children, teenagers and young adults treated for cancer. Eur J Cancer 46:1399–1412

Guyatt G, Gutterman D, Baumann MH et al (2006) Grading strength of recommendations and quality of evidence in clinical guidelines: report from an American College of Chest Physicians Task Force. Chest 129:174–181

Jacobs S, Baggott C, Agarwal R et al (2013) Validation of the Children's International Mucositis Evaluation Scale (ChIMES) in paediatric cancer and SCT. Br J Cancer 109:2515–2522

Keefe DM, Gibson RJ (2007) Mucosal injury from targeted anti-cancer therapy. Support Care Cancer 15:483–490

Kuhn A, Porto FA, Miraglia P, Brunetto AL (2009) Low-level infrared laser therapy in chemotherapy-induced oral mucositis: a randomized placebo-controlled trial in children. J Pediatr Hematol Oncol 31:33–37

Lalla RV, Sonis ST, Peterson DE (2008) Management of oral mucositis in patients who have cancer. Dent Clin North Am 52:61–77, viii

Lalla RV, Latortue MC, Hong CH et al (2010) A systematic review of oral fungal infections in patients receiving cancer therapy. Support Care Cancer 18:985–992

Langner S, Staber PB, Schub N et al (2008) Palifermin reduces incidence and severity of oral mucositis in allogeneic stem-cell transplant recipients. Bone Marrow Transplant 42:275–279

Lauritano D, Petruzzi M, Di Stasio D, Lucchese A (2014) Clinical effectiveness of palifermin in prevention and treatment of oral mucositis in children with acute lymphoblastic leukaemia: a case-control study. Int J Oral Sci 6:27–30

McDonnell AM, Lenz KL (2007) Palifermin: role in the prevention of chemotherapy- and radiation-induced mucositis. Ann Pharmacother 41:86–94

Posner MR, Haddad RI (2007) Novel agents for the treatment of mucositis. J Support Oncol 5:33–39

Rubenstein EB, Peterson DE, Schubert M et al (2004) Clinical practice guidelines for the prevention and treatment of cancer therapy-induced oral and gastrointestinal mucositis. Cancer 100:2026–2046

Scully C, Epstein J, Sonis S (2003) Oral mucositis: a challenging complication of radiotherapy, chemotherapy, and radiochemotherapy: part 1, pathogenesis and prophylaxis of mucositis. Head Neck 25:1057–1070

Scully C, Sonis S, Diz PD (2006) Oral mucositis. Oral Dis 12:229–241

Sonis ST (2004) A biological approach to mucositis. J Support Oncol 2:21–32

Sonis ST (2009) Mucositis: the impact, biology and therapeutic opportunities of oral mucositis. Oral Oncol 45:1015–1020

Sonis ST (2011) Oral mucositis. Anticancer Drugs 22:607–612

Sonis ST, Eilers JP, Epstein JB (1999) Validation of a new scoring system for the assessment of clinical trial research of oral mucositis induced by radiation or chemotherapy. Mucositis Study Group. Cancer 85:2103–2113

Sonis ST, Elting LS, Keefe D (2004) Perspectives on cancer therapy-induced mucosal injury: pathogenesis, measurement, epidemiology, and consequences for patients. Cancer 100:1995–2025

Sonis ST (2007) Pathobiology of oral mucositis: novel insights and opportunities. J Support Oncol 5:3–11

Spielberger R, Stiff P, Bensinger W et al (2004) Palifermin for oral mucositis after intensive therapy for hematologic cancers. N Engl J Med 351:2590–2598

Srinivasan A, Kasow KA, Cross S et al (2012) Phase I study of the tolerability and pharmacokinetics of palifermin in children undergoing allogeneic hematopoietic stem cell transplantation. Biol Blood Marrow Transplant 18:1309–1314

Storey B (2007) The role of oral glutamine in pediatric bone marrow transplant. J Pediatr Oncol Nurs 24:41–45

Sung L, Tomlinson GA, Greenberg ML et al (2007) Validation of the oral mucositis assessment scale in pediatric cancer. Pediatr Blood Cancer 49:149–153

Tomlinson D, Judd P, Hendershot E et al (2007) Measurement of oral mucositis in children: a review of the literature. Support Care Cancer 15:1251–1258

Tomlinson D, Gibson F, Treister N et al (2008a) Challenges of mucositis assessment in children: expert opinion. Eur J Oncol Nurs 12:469–475

Tomlinson D, Isitt JJ, Barron RL et al (2008b) Determining the understandability and acceptability of an oral mucositis daily questionnaire. J Pediatr Oncol Nurs 25:107–111

Tomlinson D, Judd P, Hendershot E et al (2008c) Establishing literature-based items for an oral mucositis assessment tool in children. J Pediatr Oncol Nurs 25:139–147

Tomlinson D, Gibson F, Treister N et al (2009) Understandability, content validity, and overall acceptability of the Children's International Mucositis Evaluation Scale (ChIMES): child and parent reporting. J Pediatr Hematol Oncol 31:416–423

Tomlinson D, Gibson F, Treister N et al (2010) Refinement of the Children's International Mucositis Evaluation Scale (CHiMES): child and parent perspectives on understandability, content validity and acceptability. Eur J Oncol Nurs 14:29–41

Tomlinson D, Ethier MC, Judd P et al (2011) Reliability and construct validity of the oral mucositis daily questionnaire in children with cancer. Eur J Cancer 47:383–388

Treister N, Sonis S (2007) Mucositis: biology and management. Curr Opin Otolaryngol Head Neck Surg 15:123–129

Vitale KM, Violago L, Cofnas P et al (2014) Impact of palifermin on incidence of oral mucositis and healthcare utilization in children undergoing autologous hematopoietic stem cell transplantation for malignant diseases. Pediatr Transplant 18:211–216

Ware E, Smith M, Henderson M et al (2009) The effect of high-dose enteral glutamine on the incidence and severity of mucositis in paediatric oncology patients. Eur J Clin Nutr 63:134–140

Worthington HV, Clarkson JE, Khalid T et al (2010) Interventions for treating oral candidiasis for patients with cancer receiving treatment. Cochrane Database Syst Rev 7:CD001972

Worthington HV, Clarkson JE, Bryan G et al (2011) Interventions for preventing oral mucositis for patients with cancer receiving treatment. Cochrane Database Syst Rev 4:CD000978

Nutrition

12

Elena J. Ladas and Paul C. Rogers

Contents

E.J. Ladas, PhD, RD (✉)
Division of Pediatric Hematology/Oncology/
Stem Cell Transplant,
Columbia University,
161 Ft. Washington, 7th floor,
New York, NY 10032, USA
e-mail: ejd14@cumc.columbia.edu

P.C. Rogers, MD
Division of Pediatric Hematology/Oncology/BMT,
British Columbia Children's Hospital,
Vancouver, BC, Canada

Abstract

Nutrition assessment and intervention is an important component of supportive care that is often overlooked as a part of the standards of care. The prevalence of malnutrition (i.e., undernutrition and overnutrition) has been the subject of many published papers which have found that up to 50 % of children and adolescents with cancer present with malnutrition, a prevalence that is affected by diagnosis, stage, socioeconomic status and nutritional index. Poor nutrition status has been associated with reduced survival and increased therapy-related side effects in patients with acute lymphoblastic leukemia, acute myelogenous leukemia, rhabdomyosarcoma and osteosarcoma. Current guidelines emphasize the practice of proactive nutrition therapy so as to avert the development of malnutrition, which may include the administration of enteral tube feeding. Nutrition assessment and intervention is a component of supportive care that should be offered throughout the spectrum of cancer care to optimize treatment delivery and outcomes and improve the quality of life of our patients. Here we review the evidence basis, consensus guidelines and expert opinion for the management of malnutrition in pediatric oncology.

J. Feusner et al. (eds.), *Supportive Care in Pediatric Oncology:*
A Practical Evidence-Based Approach, Pediatric Oncology,
DOI 10.1007/978-3-662-44317-0_12, © Springer Berlin Heidelberg 2015

12.1 Introduction

Nutrition-related pathologies are well described and can add to both morbidity and mortality in acute or chronic disease. Among children who are malnourished, increased infection, reduced quality of life, and poor neurodevelopmental and growth outcomes have been consistently reported in the literature (Brinksma et al. 2012). The risks associated with malnutrition are more threatening to children diagnosed with cancer and are best exemplified from epidemiologic data from low-resource countries in which children often present with overt malnutrition at diagnosis (Sala et al. 2012). After controlling for stage of disease, these studies have found that poor nutritional status correlates with reduced survival and adherence to therapy in children and adolescents (Sala et al. 2012). Remediation of malnutrition upon diagnosis in low-resource settings has been one of many strategies leading to improved survival rates for children with cancer (Antillon et al. 2013). Retrospective studies performed in high-resource countries have also found that nutritional status may affect outcomes as well as therapy-related toxicities (Lange et al. 2005; Hingorani et al. 2011; Burke et al. 2013; Orgel et al. 2014). These studies underscore the importance of directing attention and resources toward managing and, ideally, preventing malnutrition to ensure maintenance of adequate growth and development, improve well-being, and provide children with the best odds for survival.

The prevalence of malnutrition has been well documented in the medical literature; however, the degree (mild to severe) and pattern (at diagnosis or developing over the course of therapy) of poor nutrition will largely depend on the diagnosis, stage of disease, socioeconomic status and therapy intensity (Ladas et al. 2005; Brinksma et al. 2012). Malnutrition is classified as both undernutrition and overnutrition. Undernutrition is insufficient intake to support the body's requirements whereas overnutrition is excessive intake of nutrients leading to an oversupply of both macro- and micronutrients. Historically, malnutrition in children with cancer was focused on undernutrition; recent evidence suggests that

children and adolescents with cancer and concomitant overnutrition are also at risk for nutrient depletion and other related morbidities.

The severity of either undernutrition or overnutrition has been associated with the type of malignancy and degree of tumor involvement. Malnutrition frequently develops over the course of treatment due to therapy-related side effects and complications (Mosby et al. 2009). Malnutrition is most frequently seen at diagnosis in patients with advanced solid tumors such as neuroblastoma, Wilms tumor, rhabdomyosarcoma and bone sarcoma (Table 12.1) (Ladas et al. 2005). In low-resource countries, undernutrition is often associated with socioeconomic conditions that lead to delay in obtaining medical care in combination with an inadequate intake of calories and protein. During therapy, malnutrition may be exacerbated by complex interactions between the host, tumor and treatment regimen as well as concomitant psychological factors.

The importance of adequate nutritional status is best exemplified by recent studies documenting the effect of poor nutrition on therapy-related toxicities, survival and adherence to medical care. Recent studies performed in homogenous patient populations with fairly large sample sizes have addressed some of the weaknesses of earlier studies. Although most of the studies were retrospective reviews, significant relationships

Table 12.1 Risk factors for malnutrition in pediatric oncology patients

Malnutrition or evidence of cachexia present at diagnosis
Highly emetogenic chemotherapeutic regimens
Treatment regimens associated with severe GI complications such as constipation, diarrhea, loss of appetite, mucositis, enterocolitis (i.e., treatment of sarcomas, non-Hodgkin lymphoma, brain tumors)
Relapsed disease
Age <2 months
Radiation to the head and neck or abdomen
Postsurgical complications such as prolonged ileus or short gut syndrome
HSCT
Low socioeconomic status

GI gastrointestinal, *HSCT* hematopoietic stem cell transplantation

Table 12.2 Graded evidence-based recommendations for nutritional intervention in pediatric oncology patients[a]

Clinical scenario	Recommendations	Level of evidence[b]
Undernutrition	Dietary counseling	1C
	Nutritionally fortified drinks (see Table 12.4)	1C
	Medium-chain triglyceride oil	1C
	Appetite stimulants	2C
	Enteral tube feeding	1A
	Parenteral nutrition avoided when possible	1A
Severe immunosuppression	Data are lacking to recommend neutropenic or low microbial diets	2C
Overnutrition	Dietary and lifestyle counseling	1C

[a]See text for full detail
[b]Per Guyatt et al. (2006); see Preface

between nutritional status, toxicity and outcome have been reported. In one of the first studies conducted in 768 children with acute myeloid leukemia (AML), body mass index (BMI) percentile at diagnosis was associated with reduced survival (Lange et al. 2005). After controlling for age, race, leukocyte count, cytogenetics and stem cell transplantation, underweight patients had a trend toward decreased survival (HR 1.85, 95 % CI 1.19–2.87, $p = 0.06$) and were more likely to experience treatment-related mortality (HR 2.66, 95 % CI 1.38–5.11, $p = 0.03$) while overweight patients were less likely to survive (HR 1.88, 95 % CI 1.25–2.83, $p = 0.02$) and also had increased treatment-related mortality (HR 3.49, 95 % CI 1.99–6.10, $p < 0.001$) (Lange et al. 2005). In another large study of 498 pediatric osteosarcoma patients, Hingorani et al. (2011) reported an association between low BMI at the start of treatment with increased postoperative wound infection as well as significant increased risk of arterial thrombosis in children with overnutrition. A retrospective review conducted among 4,260 children with acute lymphoblastic leukemia (ALL) found a hazard ratio of 1.29 (95 % CI 1.02–1.56, $p = .04$) for relapse in those with obesity, most prominent in the preteenage and adolescent years (Butturini et al. 2007). More recently, a retrospective study exploring the effect of nutritional status at diagnosis and throughout therapy in children with high-risk ALL found that those who remained malnourished for the majority of treatment experienced increased toxicity and reduced survival

(Orgel et al. 2014). Remediation of malnutrition reduced the risk of toxicity and improved survival; similar observations have been reported in children residing in Central America (Antillon et al. 2013; Orgel et al. 2014).

Taken together, these studies consistently emphasize the importance of timely and effective nutritional interventions both for those underweight and overweight. Effective nutrition intervention appears to minimize the effects of malnutrition on therapy-related toxicity and survival. Increased attention is needed in regards to the nutritional evaluation and in management of pediatric oncology patients to scientifically evaluate nutritional interventions and monitor for improved outcomes. Here we review the evidence basis for effective measurement and management of nutritional complications and provide graded recommendations (Table 12.2).

12.2 Nutrition Assessment

Guidelines for the assessment and categorization of nutritional status, and criteria for intervention, are available to instruct the provision of nutrition therapy. Nutrition assessment should commence at diagnosis and be carried out during treatment as well as into survivorship. As in most aspects of clinical medicine, the importance of history and physical assessment cannot be underestimated. Baseline evaluation should include dietary history to ascertain the extent of caloric protein intake as well as known food aversions, allergies

Table 12.3 Components of the nutritional assessment

Basic anthropometrics	Advanced anthropometrics	Biochemical indices
Weight	Body composition assessment	Albumin
Height/length	Isotope dilution methods	Prealbumin
Head circumference (<3 years of age)	Bioelectric methods	Glucose
Weight for height/length	Absorptiometry methods (DPA and DEXA)	Lipid panel
BMI		Renal panel
Height and weight Z score		C-reactive protein
Triceps skinfold		Vitamin and trace elements
Arm circumference		
Waist circumference		

BMI body mass index, *DPA* dual-photon absorptiometry, *DEXA* dual-energy X-ray absorptiometry

and intolerance. Clinical evaluation includes appropriate anthropometric and biochemical measurements (Table 12.3).

Practically, weight is the measurement most frequently ascertained and followed. Assessments based on weight alone can be misleading, especially in the acutely ill patient when fluid balance may be disturbed, particularly by the presence of edema or mass disease. Additionally, weight may be maintained but lean body mass can be diminished. This situation may arise in the patient who is obese at the onset of treatment. BMI (calculated as weight [kg]/height squared [m^2]) is recommended for monitoring growth in children and adolescents and has to be interpreted relative to population reference data due to changes with age and differences between genders. BMI is considered a better proxy for body fat and lean body mass compared to weight alone; however, it is not without limitations, such as in those with increased muscle mass (Mosby et al. 2009). For children <2 years of age, ideal body weight (IBW) should be monitored. Mid-upper-arm circumference and triceps skinfolds provide the best estimate of lean body mass and adipose tissue and should preferably be undertaken by the same trained observer due to interobserver variability (Barr et al. 2011).

Repeat nutrition assessment during therapy is required to detect changes in nutritional status due to treatment or complications of treatment which may necessitate nutritional interventions. Assessment of hospitalized patients is usually undertaken by the dietician or nutritionist and occurs as per institutional guidelines and ideally during each admission, especially in those at high risk for nutritional depletion (Table 12.1). The

use of nutrition software to calculate protein and calories may be beneficial to the clinician. For outpatients, the maintenance of a nutritional diary of variety and quantity of foods and supplements taken is a valuable aid for the dietician to ascertain if the patient is nutritionally replete. Several methods of gathering data can be utilized; 24-h dietary recall conducted on nonsequential days or a 3–5-day food record is most optimal for dietary consultation.

Biochemical assessments need to be interpreted carefully as some proteins can also be acute-phase reactants and give spurious values. Any condition that can alter rate of protein synthesis, degradation, or excretion may alter serum protein concentration. Albumin and prealbumin are most frequently used as nutrition assessment tools, the latter of which is a better indicator of the acute state due to its shorter half-life. Biochemical laboratory assessment should include liver function, renal function, lipid panel and glucose to determine if dietary modification is required; the clinician must be cognizant that values may be altered due to cancer therapy or concurrent infection. For example, L-asparaginase inhibits liver protein synthesis and a very low-fat diet (i.e., <10 g fat/day) is often required due to asparaginase side effects. Similarly, glucose levels must be followed in patients receiving high-dose steroids such as ALL induction. Dietary intervention helps in maintaining adequate nutrition so that chemotherapy can continue at the appropriate dose and schedule and to mitigate potential side effects.

During cytotoxic therapy and with episodes of sepsis, the pediatric cancer patient undergoes a catabolic state with nutrient depletion. Decreased intake of micronutrients has been reported following chemotherapy and may be associated with therapy-related toxicity (Ladas et al. 2004). For example, reduced intake of B vitamins may be associated with the development of neuropathy; zinc, important in both immune function and mucosal integrity, has been associated with increased infection and dysgeusia (altered taste); reduced antioxidant nutrients may be associated with infection and increased hospital stay; and reduced intake of vitamin D and calcium may increase bone morbidity in children with ALL (Henkin et al. 1976; Mahajan et al. 1980; Bolze et al. 1982; Watson et al. 1983; Kennedy et al. 2004; Ozyurek et al. 2007; Youssef et al. 2008; Tylavsky et al. 2010). Thus, a thorough analysis of dietary intake should accompany anthropometric and biochemical assessments.

12.3 Nutrition Intervention

The primary goal of nutritional therapy in the pediatric oncology population is to sustain and promote normal growth and development while the patient is receiving the necessary anticancer treatments. Nutrition interventions should be proactive to prevent the development of malnutrition. If malnutrition develops, nutrition interventions should be implemented to reverse malnutrition and, secondarily, to prevent future protein-energy malnutrition. The most appropriate interventions must meet the nutritional needs of the child but be associated with the least risk. Nutrition counseling and education should be provided to the family with awareness of cultural differences in nutritional practice. The utilization of a dietitian or nutritionist to provide and support the education of healthcare staff, patient families, and patients is a crucial component of optimal nutrition care in pediatric oncology (Sacks et al. 2004). Nutritional intervention should be implemented in the following situations: (1) patients who present underweight (i.e., BMI <5th %ile or <70 % IBW); (2) patients who present overweight (i.e., BMI >95th %ile or IBW >120 %); (3) patients not meeting >80 % of their caloric requirements through oral intake during treatment; and (4) >5 % weight loss from baseline body weight.

12.3.1 Dietary Counseling

Nutrition counseling should begin with strategies to enhance dietary consumption, such as through the utilization of nutrient dense foods. Oral intake may be difficult for many children and adolescents undergoing treatment due to treatment-related toxicities such as severe nausea, vomiting, stomatitis, constipation, and diarrhea but should be offered as an initial strategy before advancing to enteral or parenteral nutrition. Nutritionally fortified drinks should be recommended for patients unable to consume food. Pediatric formulations such as Boost®, PediaSure®, and Ensure® can augment oral intake, and other formulations may be provided to ensure adequate electrolyte balance (Table 12.4). Medium-chain triglyceride (MCT) oil may complement feeding strategies by increasing total calories in a readily absorbable formulation.

Special diets, such as the neutropenic diet or low microbial diet, have been suggested for severely immunosuppressed patients such as those treated with hematopoietic stem cell transplant (HSCT) to minimize the introduction of pathogenic organisms into the gastrointestinal (GI) tract (Moody et al. 2002). Adherence to these diets is difficult and provides further restraints on dietary intake. Clinical trials performed in adults and children with cancer have found that the neutropenic diet is not associated with reduced risk of infection and does not offer an added benefit over food safety guidelines alone (Moody et al. 2006; Gardner et al. 2008). Current standards of practice should consider the

Table 12.4 Commonly used nutritional supplements

Oral	High-calorie oral	Enteral
Boost®	Boost® Plus	PediaSure® with/without fiber
Carnation® Instant Breakfast	Ensure® Plus	Jevity®
Compleat® Pediatric	PediaSure® 1.5	Nutren® 1.5/2.0
Ensure®	Resource® 2.0	Osmolite®
PediaSure® with/without fiber		Peptamen®
Nutren Junior® with/without fiber		

lack of evidence supporting a neutropenic diet as an augmentation to food safety guidelines (Table 12.5) prior to recommending it to patients at risk for severe immunosuppression.

12.3.2 Appetite Stimulants

Appetite stimulants may augment dietary intake although consistent evidence is lacking regarding efficacy and the side effect profile must be considered (Ladas et al. 2005). Both Orme et al. (2003) and Cuvelier et al. (2013) reported significant weight gain with megestrol acetate although with common severe adrenal suppression. A study of 66 evaluated pediatric oncology patients showed modest but significant weight gain with cyproheptadine hydrochloride with the main reported side effect being drowsiness (Couluris et al. 2008). Additional agents utilized include cannabinoids such as dronabinol as well as mirtazapine, a noradrenergic and serotonergic antidepressant. Systematic studies on the benefit of these agents and their comparative side effects are lacking.

12.3.3 Enteral Tube Feeding

Enteral tube feeding (TF) should be initiated when oral intake is inadequate to support growth or nutritional repletion in the child with cancer. Patients eligible for TF must have an intact GI tract. Enteral feeding has numerous advantages over total parenteral nutrition (TPN) including maintenance of GI mucosal function, cost-efficiency, and avoidance of TPN complications including bacterial infection, thrombosis, hepatic toxicity, cholestasis, and metabolic derangements (den Broeder et al. 1998; Nevin-Folino and Miller 1999). TF also offers the benefit of medication administration without oral ingestion. Despite these benefits, hesitation remains in the provision of TF in the medical community (Ladas et al. 2006). TF is often presented as a punishment for not eating. Concerns arise from patients (especially adolescents) and families due to the perceived inconvenience, discomfort and poor body image associated with the placement of a nasogastric tube. To optimize acceptance, TF

should be proposed as a positive intervention measure that is part of a comprehensive supportive care plan to aid in overall patient well-being.

Multiple studies in pediatric oncology patients have demonstrated that TF is successful in maintaining adequate nutritional status and reversing malnutrition (Aquino et al. 1995; Mathew et al. 1996; den Broeder et al. 1998; Deswarte-Wallace et al. 2001; Bakish et al. 2003; Ladas et al. 2005). Moreover, TF appears feasible and safe in patients with mucositis, severe neutropenia and thrombocytopenia. DeSwarte-Wallace et al. (2001) evaluated the use of TF in a pediatric oncology population during and after intensive oncologic treatment and demonstrated that most children tolerate TF without significant vomiting or diarrhea. The investigators concluded that TF is a safe and cost-effective intervention in pediatric patients receiving dose-intensive chemotherapy. Pietsch et al. (1999) evaluated TF in children receiving intensive chemotherapy ($n=14$) or HSCT ($n=3$) and found TF was well tolerated with minimal complications, including risk of emesis and tube dislodgment, at a substantial cost saving compared to TPN. Finally, 32 children with solid tumors were administered TF during the most intensive phase of therapy; TF was well tolerated and improved weight among the patients (Den et al. 2000). An association between TF and reduction in non-leukopenic infection was also observed ($p=.009$) (Den et al. 2000). Taken together these small studies lend support to the benefits of TF on nutritional status and possibly therapy-related toxicities.

Depending on the tolerability of TF and amount of oral intake, TF can commence as bolus feeds, nocturnal continuous feeds, nocturnal continuous feeds with bolus feeds during the day or as continuous drip-feeds. The clinical aim of TF is to supply the required nutrient intake of both macro- and micronutrients as described in the Dietary Reference Intakes (DRIs) (Otten et al. 2006). The DRIs are designed to guide health professionals in determining the dietary needs of each individual patient; recommendations by age and gender are available at the United States Department of Agriculture website (http://fnic.nal.usda.gov/dietary-guidance/dietary-reference-intakes/dri-tables).

Table 12.5 Food safety practices[a]

Food shopping

   1. Check expiration dates on food and do not buy or use if the food is out of date.

   2. Do not purchase ready-to-eat food from bulk food bins (i.e., breads, nuts, dried fruit, candies).

   3. Avoid all food in cans that are swollen, dented or damaged.

   4. Avoid produce that is bruised or damaged.

   5. Bag fresh fruits and vegetables separately from meat, poultry and seafood products.

Food storage

   1. Store perishable fresh fruits and vegetables (i.e. cucumbers, tomatoes) in a clean refrigerator at a temperature of 40 °F or below.

   2. Refrigerate all produce that is purchased pre-cut or peeled.

   3. Beef should be refrigerated at 40 °F and used within two days. Beef can be frozen at 0 °F and used within 6 months of the purchase date.

Food preparation

   1. Wash hands with water and soap for 20 s before and after any food preparation.

   2. Wash fruits or vegetables under running water even if you are going to peel them. Do not use soap, bleach or commercial produce washes to clean fruit.

   3. Dry produce with a clean cloth towel or paper towel. This will reduce the spread of bacteria. Do not wash meat, poultry or eggs.

   4. Defrost all meats in the refrigerator. Do not defrost at room temperature.

   5. Food-preparation surfaces must be cleaned first. Wash surfaces thoroughly with soap and water and thoroughly dry. As an extra precaution, you can use a solution of one tablespoon unscented, liquid chlorine bleach in one gallon of water to sanitize washed surfaces and utensils.

   6. Wash cutting boards, dishes, utensils and counter tops with hot, soapy water after preparing each food item and before you go on to the next item.

Cooking

   1. Cook foods immediately after thawing.

   2. All raw foods such as meats, poultry and entrees should be cooked until they are well-done. Beef should be cooked to 160 °F, depending on the cut. Chicken should be cooked to an internal temperature of 165 °F. Cold foods should be stored <40 °F, hot foods kept >140 °F. A home thermometer may help.

Storage of cooked foods

   1. Store leftovers within 2 h. By dividing leftovers into several clean, shallow containers, you'll allow them to chill faster. Discard leftovers that were kept at room temperature for greater than 2 h.

   2. Perishable foods (fruits, vegetables, meat, dairy) should be put into the fridge or freezer within 2 h. In the summer months, cut this time down to 1 h.

   3. Do not use leftovers prior to reheating to >165 °F before serving.

Baby food/infant formula

   1. Never put baby food in the refrigerator if the baby doesn't finish it. Do not feed your baby directly from the jar of baby food. Instead, put a small serving of food on a clean dish and refrigerate the remaining food in the jar. If the baby needs more food, use a clean spoon to serve another portion. Throw away any food in the dish that's not eaten. If you do feed a baby from a jar, always discard any remaining food.

   2. Prepare safe water for preparing formula. Bring tap water to a roiling boil and boil it for 1 min. If you use bottled water, follow this same process. Cool the water to body temperature before mixing formula.

   3. Sterilize bottles and nipples before first use. After that, wash them by hand or in a dishwasher.

   4. Formula can become contaminated during preparation, and bacteria can multiply quickly if formula is improperly stored. Prepare formula in smaller quantities on an as-needed basis to greatly reduce the possibility of contamination. Always follow the label instructions for mixing formula.

Additional information may be found at www.foodsafety.gov.

[a]Select recommendations from the United States Federal Drug Administration's Clean, Separate, Cook and Chill.

Considerations in determining the type of formula, volume of feeds, and schedule should include the patient's oral intake, sleep patterns, lifestyle, food allergies/intolerances, and GI conditions that affect dietary intake. Continuous feeding schedules are generally better tolerated than intermittent bolus feeds. Nocturnal continuous feeds allow the patient to attempt normal feeding during the day while ensuring the necessary proportion of nutrients are being delivered via TF. Daytime continuous feeds may be initiated on days when children are unable to consume significant oral intake. TF allows the family flexibility with the child's feeding schedule while continuing to support oromotor developmental skills and a more normal lifestyle. Continuous feeds are the preferred schedule in patients at high risk for nausea and vomiting, constipation, or diarrhea. If frequent vomiting continues to occur with continuous TF, post-pyloric feedings may help improve tolerance (Sacks et al. 2004; Ladas et al. 2005).

The choice of formula will depend on the clinical condition of the patient. In most cases, a standard milk-based formula with or without fiber may be used to initiate TF (Table 12.4). Unflavored formulas have a lower osmolarity than flavored products, are better tolerated and should preferentially be used for TF. In patients with lactose intolerance, a soy-based or lactose-free formula should be used. Elemental formulas are ideal for patients with GI inflammation or malabsorption. Modification of the chosen formula may be necessary in patients with underlying GI problems if with intolerance to the current formula, persistent constipation or diarrhea, or stomach pain. Continuous TF should be initiated with a full-strength formula at 1–2 mL/kg/h and increased by 1–2 mL/kg/h as tolerated until the goal rate is achieved (Sacks et al. 2004; Ladas et al. 2005). Elevating the head of the bed to >30° during and after TF and using prokinetic medications such as metoclopramide, erythromycin or cisapride (not available in the United States) may assist with reducing high gastric residuals caused by delayed gastric emptying and therefore promote digestion (Sacks et al. 2004). Feeding tubes should be flushed before and after feeds or the administration of any medication. A solution composed of a Viokase™ enzyme tablet, a 325 mg sodium bicarbonate tablet, and 5 mL of warm water

can be utilized to help unclog the tube by inserting the 5 mL solution, clamping the tube for 15–30 min and then flushing with 20–30 mL of warm water (Sacks et al. 2004). Utilization of acidic beverages such as Coca-Cola or cranberry juice has been utilized but may precipitate the caseinate in formula and should not be used. Reevaluation of nutritional status and feeding methods for the individual patient should be undertaken if feeding problems persist and growth is not observed.

Side effects associated with TF include diarrhea, constipation, abdominal pain and aspiration. Although empirically thought to increase the risk of infection or mucosal bleeding, feeding tube insertion has been shown safe during periods of mucositis (Deswarte-Wallace et al. 2001). Whether TF is tolerated with severe mucositis involving much of the GI tract is unclear. Vomiting may occur but is not a contraindication to tube reinsertion; passing the tube beyond the pyloric valve into the duodenum may prevent recurrence. Diarrhea can develop secondary to hyperosmolar feeds, lactose intolerance or refeeding syndrome. Refeeding syndrome can occur in the severely malnourished patient who is started on feeds at too rapid a rate and consists of diarrhea, vomiting and a variety of metabolic disturbances.

Criteria for placement of a percutaneous endoscopic gastrostomy (PEG) include dysphagia, risk of aspiration, intractable vomiting, esophageal strictures, cancer of the head and neck, radiation to the head, neck or chest, or anticipated long-term need for nutritional support. Adequate GI function is necessary for PEG insertion (Sacks et al. 2004; Ladas et al. 2005). Infection at the local insertion site can occur and careful hygiene is required.

12.3.4 Parenteral Nutrition

Parenteral nutrition (PN) is significantly more expensive and offers no clear advantages over enteral feeding for those patients with an intact gut. PN is required when all attempts for sufficient enteral feeding have failed or are contraindicated. Neutropenic enterocolitis, bowel obstruction and a nonfunctional GI system are indications for PN. The utility of PN has been best demonstrated in HSCT recipients who have prolonged gut damage due to the chemotherapeutic preparative regimen, graft-versus-host disease or infection (Muscaritoli et al. 2002). In many HSCT centers, PN is commenced either during the preparative conditioning regimen or shortly thereafter as routine care without consideration for enteral feeds, although studies have shown that enteral feeding is safe and feasible in patients undergoing HSCT (Sefcick et al. 2001; Garofolo 2012). When PN is required, an effort should still be made to maintain some enteral feeding (unless contraindicated), to help preserve gut integrity and function. PN is associated with mechanical complications such as increased risk of thrombosis or occlusion of the central venous catheter, infection, and GI complications including hepatic toxicity, cholestasis, and metabolic abnormalities including fluid and electrolyte imbalance, hyperglycemia, and metabolic acidosis (Christensen et al. 1993; Quigley et al. 1993; Lenssen et al. 1998; Mirtallo et al. 2004). Refeeding syndrome can also occur in the severely malnourished patient on PN. The interaction between PN and the pharmacokinetics and pharmacodynamics of other necessary medications remains unclear. It is important that all potential drug interactions be considered when prescribing PN in addition to determining which drugs can be concurrently administered in the lumen infusing PN.

Short-term (i.e., 2–3 week) PN is rarely beneficial and should only be considered in those temporally unable to tolerate enteral feeds. A central venous device is required for prolonged PN to avoid damage to peripheral veins by high-solute PN solution. In determining PN requirements, the clinician should calculate the required fluids, calories, protein, fat, carbohydrates, vitamins and trace elements (ASPEN Board of Directors and the Clinical Guidelines Task Force 2002; National Academy of Sciences and Institute of Medicine 2002). The majority of institutions have strict guidelines for the prescribing and monitoring of PN, and close clinical and biochemical monitoring is necessary to prevent and anticipate complications (Mirtallo et al. 2004).

PN should be altered or discontinued in patients experiencing significant hepatic dysfunction, cholestasis, severe hyperglycemia or other significant metabolic complications. For patients on TPN, the transition back to enteral feeding requires careful weaning dependent on GI function. A rapid transition may result in abdominal pain, diarrhea and sometimes hypoglycemia. Prolonged PN has been associated with suppressed appetite and difficulty resuming adequate oral feeding (Charuhas et al. 1997). The decision to implement and wean PN should be undertaken with the advice from a registered dietician or a dedicated PN team. PN should not be the routine or first option for nutritional intervention in pediatric oncology patients.

12.4 Nutrition and Survivorship

Survivors of childhood cancer are at increased risk for many nutrition-related conditions including obesity, metabolic syndrome, heart disease, osteopenia/osteoporosis and mechanical issues such as reduced salivary function which can make eating difficult (Hudson et al. 2003; Oeffinger and Hudson 2004; Meacham et al. 2005). Due to these risks, pediatric oncologists must provide nutritional counseling and promote healthy behaviors after the completion of therapy to prevent long-term complications of poor nutrition and a sedentary lifestyle.

Not unlike the general population, surveys of childhood cancer survivors have found that most do not meet recommended dietary guidelines for cancer prevention or heart disease and lack a general understanding of what constitutes a healthy diet and lifestyle. How this potentially impacts the risk of secondary malignancy is unknown. In a survey of 380 childhood cancer survivors, 79 % did not meet the guidelines for fruit and vegetable consumption, 84 % obtained >30 % of their calories from fat and only 48 % were meeting exercise guidelines (Demark-Wahnefried et al. 2005). Robien et al. (2008) similarly found that childhood ALL survivors did not adhere to healthy dietary guidelines. Again, not unlike the general population, childhood cancer survivors reported being too tired (57 %), too busy (53 %), finding higher fat foods more visually appealing (58 %), and consuming high-fat foods in their social interactions (50 %) the primary reasons for an unhealthy diet (Arroyave et al. 2008).

Practitioners must explore creative means for imparting beneficial dietary and behavioral interventions for patients beyond the intensive phases of therapy. A small, prospective study evaluating 13 children between 4 and 10 years of age during

Table 12.6 Internet resources for reliable nutrition information

American Institute for Cancer Research	www.aicr.org
National Cancer Institute	www.cancer.gov/cancertopics/prevention/energybalance
American Society for Cancer Research	www.cancer.org/healthy/eathealthygetactive/ acsguidelinesonnutritionphysicalactivityforcancerprevention/ acs-guidelines-on-nutrition-and-physical-activity-for-cancer-prevention-summary

ALL maintenance therapy explored the feasibility of a 12-month home-based nutrition and exercise intervention program, and although the study led to improvement in the frequency of physical activity ($p = 0.05$), no difference in dietary behaviors was observed (Moyer-Mileur et al. 2009). Due to lack of resources, effective dietary and lifestyle interventions remain a poorly studied area and emphasize the importance of ongoing education; the involvement of family, peers, schools and healthcare providers; and the need for continued care of childhood cancer survivors. The American Institute for Cancer Research (www.aicr.org) has published nutrition guidelines focused on cancer prevention and are available for medical providers to review with patients. Ideally, dietary counseling should be performed by a registered dietician so that strategies for behavior modification may be discussed with the individual and their families. Additionally, the influence on dietary choices by gender, ethnicity, age and socioeconomic status should be included when discussing behavior modification programs. The use of lifestyle education programs has been found to be successful in promoting long-term behavior change among adult survivors of cancer (Mosher et al. 2013). The effectiveness of such programs in childhood cancer survivors is unknown. Until additional research is available, current clinical practice should incorporate all aspects of lifestyle intervention and provide the opportunity for survivors to receive continual access to nutrition information specifically designed for cancer survivors (Table 12.6).

12.5 Summary

Nutrition assessment and intervention are critical components of a pediatric oncology supportive care program, both during cancer therapy and after the completion of therapy. The inclusion of nutrition therapy promotes normal growth and development over the course of cancer therapy, may improve quality of life, and prevents therapy-related toxicities and decreased survival as has been shown in patients that are under- and over-nourished. Nutritional assessment and intervention should be proactive and start at diagnosis and must continue well beyond the completion of antineoplastic therapy. Although a clear evidence basis is lacking for many recommendations, there are general indications for nutritional support during cancer therapy including the use of nutritional supplements, appetite stimulants, enteral tube feeding and parenteral nutrition.

References

Antillon F, Rossi E, Molina AL et al (2013) Nutritional status of children during treatment for acute lymphoblastic leukemia in Guatemala. Pediatr Blood Cancer 60:911–915

Aquino VM, Smyrl CB, Hagg R et al (1995) Enteral nutritional support by gastrostomy tube in children with cancer. J Pediatr 127:58–62

Arroyave WD, Clipp EC, Miller PE et al (2008) Childhood cancer survivors' perceived barriers to improving exercise and dietary behaviors. Oncol Nurs Forum 35:121–130

ASPEN Board of Directors and the Clinical Guidelines Task Force (2002) Guidelines for the use of parenteral and enteral nutrition in adult and pediatric patients. JPEN J Parenter Enteral Nutr 26:1SA–138SA

Bakish J, Hargrave D, Tariq N et al (2003) Evaluation of dietetic intervention in children with medulloblastoma or supratentorial primitive neuroectodermal tumors. Cancer 98:1014–1020

Barr R, Collins L, Nayiager T et al (2011) Nutritional status at diagnosis in children with cancer. 2. An assessment by arm anthropometry. J Pediatr Hematol Oncol 33:e101–e104

Bolze MS, Fosmire GJ, Stryker JA et al (1982) Taste acuity, plasma zinc levels, and weight loss during radiotherapy: a study of relationships. Radiology 144:163–169

Brinksma A, Huizinga G, Sulkers E et al (2012) Malnutrition in childhood cancer patients: a review on its prevalence and possible causes. Crit Rev Oncol Hematol 83:249–275

Burke M, Lyden ER, Meza JL et al (2013) Does body mass index at diagnosis or weight change during therapy predict toxicity or survival in intermediate risk rhabdomyosarcoma? A report from Children's Oncology Group Soft Tissue Sarcoma Committee. Pediatr Blood Cancer 60:748–753

Butturini AM, Dorey FJ, Lange BJ et al (2007) Obesity and outcome in pediatric acute lymphoblastic leukemia. J Clin Oncol 25:2063–2069

Charuhas PM, Fosberg KL, Bruemmer B et al (1997) A double-blind randomized trial comparing outpatient parenteral nutrition with intravenous hydration: effect on resumption of oral intake after marrow transplantation. JPEN J Parenter Enteral Nutr 21:157–161

Christensen ML, Hancock ML, Gattuso J et al (1993) Parenteral nutrition associated with increased infection rate in children with cancer. Cancer 72:2732–2738

Couluris M, Mayer JL, Freyer DR et al (2008) The effect of cyproheptadine hydrochloride (Periactin®) and megestrol acetate (Megace®) on weight in children with cancer/treatment-related cachexia. J Pediatr Hematol Oncol 30:791–797

Cuvelier GD, Baker TJ, Peddie EF et al (2013) A randomized, double-blind, placebo-controlled clinical trial of megestrol acetate as an appetite stimulant in children with weight loss due to cancer and/or cancer therapy. Pediatr Blood Cancer 61:672–679

Demark-Wahnefried W, Werner C, Clipp EC et al (2005) Survivors of childhood cancer and their guardians. Cancer 103:2171–2180

den Broeder E, Lippens RJ, van't Hof MA et al (1998) Effects of naso-gastric tube feeding on the nutritional status of children with cancer. Eur J Clin Nutr 52:494–500

den Broeder E, Lippens RJ, van't Hof MA et al (2000) Association between the change in nutritional status in response to tube feeding and the occurrence of infections in children with a solid tumor. Pediatr Hematol Oncol 17:567–575

Deswarte-Wallace J, Firouzbakhsh S, Finklestein JZ (2001) Using research to change practice: enteral feedings for pediatric oncology patients. J Pediatr Oncol Nurs 18:217–223

Gardner A, Mattiuzzi G, Faderl S et al (2008) Randomized comparison of cooked and noncooked diets in patients undergoing remission induction therapy for acute myeloid leukemia. J Clin Oncol 26:5684–5688

Garofolo A (2012) Enteral nutrition during bone marrow transplantation in patients with pediatric cancer: a prospective cohort study. Sao Paulo Med J 130:159–166

Guyatt G, Gutterman D, Baumann MH et al (2006) Grading strength of recommendations and quality of evidence in clinical guidelines: report from an American College of Chest Physicians Task Force. Chest 129:174–181

Henkin RI, Schecter PJ, Friedewald WT et al (1976) A double blind study of the effects of zinc sulfate on taste and smell dysfunction. Am J Med Sci 272:285–299

Hingorani P, Seidel K, Krailo M et al (2011) Body mass index (BMI) at diagnosis is associated with surgical wound complications in patients with localized osteosarcoma: a report from the Children's Oncology Group. Pediatr Blood Cancer 57:939–942

Hudson MM, Mertens AC, Yasui Y et al (2003) Health status of adult long-term survivors of childhood cancer: a report from the Childhood Cancer Survivor Study. JAMA 290:1583–1592

Kennedy D, Tucker K, Ladas EJ et al (2004) Low antioxidant vitamin intakes are associated with increases in adverse effects of chemotherapy in children with acute lymphoblastic leukemia. Am J Clin Nutr 79:1029–1036

Ladas EJ, Jacobson JS, Kennedy DD et al (2004) Antioxidants and cancer therapy: a systematic review. J Clin Oncol 22:517–528

Ladas EJ, Sacks N, Meacham L et al (2005) A multidisciplinary review of nutrition considerations in the pediatric oncology population: a perspective from Children's Oncology Group. Nutr Clin Pract 20:377–393

Ladas EJ, Sacks N, Brophy P, Rodgers PC (2006) Standards of nutritional care in pediatric oncology: results from a nationwide survey on the standards of practice in pediatric oncology. A Children's Oncology Group Study. Pediatr Blood Cancer 46:339–344

Lange BJ, Gerbing RB, Feusner J et al (2005) Mortality in overweight and underweight children with acute myeloid leukemia. JAMA 293:203–211

Lenssen P, Bruemmer BA, Bowden RA et al (1998) Intravenous lipid dose and incidence of bacteremia and fungemia in patients undergoing bone marrow transplantation. Am J Clin Nutr 67:927–933

Mahajan SK, Prasad AS, Lambujon J et al (1980) Improvement of uremic hypogeusia by zinc: a double-blind study. Am J Clin Nutr 33:1517–1521

Mathew P, Bowman L, Williams R et al (1996) Complications and effectiveness of gastrostomy feedings in pediatric cancer patients. J Pediatr Hematol Oncol 18:81–85

Meacham LR, Gurney JG, Mertens AC et al (2005) Body mass index in long-term adult survivors of childhood cancer: a report of the Childhood Cancer Survivor Study. Cancer 103:1730–1739

Mirtallo J, Canada T, Johnson D et al (2004) Safe practices for parenteral nutrition. JPEN J Parenter Enteral Nutr 28:S39–S70

Moody K, Charlson ME, Finlay J (2002) The neutropenic diet: what's the evidence? J Pediatr Hematol Oncol 24:717–721

Moody K, Finlay J, Mancuso C, Charlson M (2006) Feasibility and safety of a pilot randomized trial of infection rate: neutropenic diet versus standard food safety guidelines. J Pediatr Hematol Oncol 28:126–133

Mosby TT, Barr RD, Pencharz PB (2009) Nutritional assessment of children with cancer. J Pediatr Oncol Nurs 26:186–197

Mosher CE, Lipkus I, Sloane R et al (2013) Long-term outcomes of the FRESH START trial: exploring the role of self-efficacy in cancer survivors' maintenance of dietary practices and physical activity. Psychooncology 22:876–885

Moyer-Mileur LJ, Ransdell L, Bruggers CS (2009) Fitness of children with standard-risk acute lymphoblastic leukemia during maintenance therapy: response to a home-based exercise and nutrition program. J Pediatr Hematol Oncol 31:259–266

Muscaritoli M, Grieco G, Capria S et al (2002) Nutritional and metabolic support in patients undergoing bone marrow transplantation. Am J Clin Nutr 75:183–190

National Academy of Sciences and Institute of Medicine (2002) Dietary reference intakes for energy, carbohydrate, fiber, fat, fatty acids, cholesterol, protein, and amino acids (macronutrients). National Academy Press, Washington, D.C

Nevin-Folino N, Miller M (1999) Enteral nutrition. In: Samour PQ, Helm KK, Lang CE (eds) Handbook of pediatric nutrition. Aspen Publishers, Gaithersburg

Oeffinger KC, Hudson MM (2004) Long-term complications following childhood and adolescent cancer: foundations for providing risk-based health care for survivors. CA Cancer J Clin 54:208–236

Orgel E, Sposto R, Malvar J et al (2014) Impact on survival and toxicity by duration of weight extremes during treatment for pediatric acute lymphoblastic leukemia: a report from the Children's Oncology Group. J Clin Oncol 32:1331–1337

Orme LM, Bond JD, Humphrey MS et al (2003) Megestrol acetate in pediatric oncology patients may lead to severe, symptomatic adrenal suppression. Cancer 98: 397–405

Otten JJ, Hellwig Pitzi J, Meyers LD (2006) Dietary reference intakes: the essential guide to nutrient requirements. National Academy Press, Washington, D.C

Ozyurek H, Turker H, Akbalik M et al (2007) Pyridoxine and pyridostigmine treatment in vincristine-induced neuropathy. Pediatr Hematol Oncol 24:447–452

Pietsch JB, Ford C, Whitlock JA (1999) Nasogastric tube feedings in children with high-risk cancer: a pilot study. J Pediatr Hematol Oncol 21:111–114

Quigley EM, Marsh MN, Shaffer JL, Markin RS (1993) Hepatobiliary complications of total parenteral nutrition. Gastroenterology 104:286–301

Robien K, Ness KK, Klesges LM et al (2008) Poor adherence to dietary guidelines among adult survivors of childhood acute lymphoblastic leukemia. J Pediatr Hematol Oncol 30:815–822

Sacks N, Ringwald-Smith K, Hale G (2004) Nutritional support. In: Altman A (ed) Supportive care of children with cancer. The Johns Hopkins University Press, Baltimore

Sala A, Rossi E, Antillon F et al (2012) Nutritional status at diagnosis is related to clinical outcomes in children and adolescents with cancer: a perspective from Central America. Eur J Cancer 48:243–252

Sefcick A, Anderton D, Byrne JL et al (2001) Nasojejunal feeding in allogeneic bone marrow transplant recipients: results of a pilot study. Bone Marrow Transplant 28:1135–1139

Tylavsky FA, Smith K, Surprise H et al (2010) Nutritional intake of long-term survivors of childhood acute lymphoblastic leukemia: evidence for bone health interventional opportunities. Pediatr Blood Cancer 55:1362–1369

Watson AR, Stuart A, Wells FE et al (1983) Zinc supplementation and its effect on taste acuity in children with chronic renal failure. Hum Nutr Clin Nutr 37:219–225

Youssef S, Hachem R, Chemaly RF et al (2008) The role of vitamin B6 in the prevention of haematological toxic effects of linezolid in patients with cancer. J Antimicrob Chemother 61:421–424

Management of Acute Radiation Side Effects

13

Jong H. Chung, Anurag K. Agrawal, and Patrick S. Swift

Contents

J.H. Chung, MD
Division of Pediatric Hematology/Oncology,
University of California-Davis Children's Hospital,
Sacramento, CA, USA

A.K. Agrawal, MD (✉)
Department of Hematology/Oncology,
Childrens Hospital and Research Center Oakland,
747 52nd Street, Oakland, CA 94609, USA
e-mail: aagrawal@mail.cho.org

P.S. Swift, MD
Professor of Radiation Oncology,
Stanford University School of Medicine,
Stanford Cancer Center, Stanford, CA, USA

Abstract

Potential complications from radiation therapy requiring supportive care measures include acute, subacute (also called early delayed), and chronic (late delayed) entities and are directly related to the site of radiation, subsequent dose, and volume of tissue exposed. Here we specifically concentrate on acute and, to a lesser extent, subacute issues. Data in children, especially of a prospective nature, are quite limited, and therefore we rely on extrapolation of data from adult studies which may or may not include pediatric patients. Studies on simple and widely utilized historical treatment strategies are often lacking; therefore, reference to clinical practice guidelines is made where possible. Radiation toxicity is examined in a site- and dose-dependent fashion with a discussion of supportive care evidence to date and recommendations on evidence-based treatment guidelines, where available.

J. Feusner et al. (eds.), *Supportive Care in Pediatric Oncology:
A Practical Evidence-Based Approach*, Pediatric Oncology,
DOI 10.1007/978-3-662-44317-0_13, © Springer Berlin Heidelberg 2015

13.1 Introduction

Potential complications from radiation therapy (RT) requiring supportive care measures include acute, subacute (also called early delayed), and chronic (late delayed) entities and are directly related to the site of RT, subsequent dose, and volume of tissue exposed (Keime-Guibert et al. 1998; New 2001; Rinne et al. 2012). Here we will specifically concentrate on acute and, to a lesser extent, subacute issues such as somnolence and xerostomia. With increasing survival from pediatric cancer diagnoses, the practitioner must be cognizant of late effects of RT, especially risk of secondary malignancy; these topics are beyond the scope of this review. RT leads to direct DNA damage, and thus those cells which are rapidly dividing (i.e., skin, orogastrointestinal mucosa, hematopoietic cells) are most likely to face acute toxicity (Chopra and Bogart 2009). Such acute toxicity will often resolve with supportive care measures alone, unlike chronic etiologies which may never completely repair. Data in children, especially of a prospective nature, are quite limited, and therefore we will rely on extrapolation of data from adult studies which may or may not include pediatric patients. Studies on simple and widely utilized historical treatment strategies may be lacking in some cases; therefore, recommendations will be provided based on consensus statements in addition to evidence-based guidelines.

The increasing use of intensity-modulated radiation therapy (IMRT) and stereotactic fractionated radiation therapy (SFRT) allows the radiation oncologist to limit toxicities seen previously with external beam radiation therapy (EBRT) (Salvo et al. 2010; McQuestion 2011). The Radiation Therapy Oncology Group (RTOG) provides a grading system for both acute and late radiation morbidity which will provide a basis for our recommendations (Cox et al. 1995). In many cases these grading criteria are parallel to that provided in the National Cancer Institute's Common Terminology Criteria for Adverse Events (CTCAE) (Trotti et al. 2003). Of note, per the RTOG scoring criteria, acute toxicity is limited to the first 90 days after the commencement of RT; generally though, acute toxicity is defined as side effects during RT and early-delayed toxic-

ity can be up to 6 months postirradiation (Soussain et al. 2009). RT toxicity will be examined in a site- and dose-dependent fashion with a discussion of supportive care evidence to date and recommendations on evidence-based treatment guidelines, where available (Table 13.1).

13.2 Hematologic Toxicity

In a retrospective cohort of adult patients, MacManus et al. (1997) showed the most significant risk factors for neutropenia and thrombocytopenia were concurrent use of myelosuppressive chemotherapy as well as increasing percentage of marrow irradiated. They specifically describe that the odds ratio for myelosuppression increases for each additional 20 % of marrow irradiated. Children, unlike adults, have functional bone marrow in the appendicular skeleton, although the axial skeleton is most prominent with the pelvis and vertebrae serving the largest roles (Mauch et al. 1995). Pediatric protocols generally recommend treatment interruption for ANC between $0.3–0.5 \times 10^9$/L and platelet counts between $25–50 \times 10^9$/L.

13.2.1 Management of Neutropenia

The use of myeloid colony-stimulating factors (CSFs), specifically filgrastim (granulocyte colony-stimulating factor; G-CSF), pegfilgrastim, and granulocyte-macrophage colony-stimulating factor (GM-CSF), in the management of neutropenia during RT, whether resulting from radiation, concurrent chemotherapy, or both, is controversial. The 2006 American Society of Clinical Oncology (ASCO) guidelines for the use of CSFs make no specific recommendation with regard to pediatric patients receiving RT (Smith et al. 2006). The only specific mention of radiotherapy in these guidelines is a caution with concomitant use of CSFs, chemotherapy, and radiotherapy to the mediastinum due to a single adult trial in lung cancer patients which showed a highly significant increase in severe thrombocytopenia and pulmonary toxic deaths in the cohort receiving GM-CSF (Bunn et al. 1995). By contrast, the European Society for Medical Oncology (ESMO) released guidelines in

Table 13.1 Summary of management strategies and level of evidence for common acute and subacute pediatric radiation-induced toxicities[a]

Organ	RT side effect	Treatment	Level of evidence[b]
Hematologic	Neutropenia	Consider G-CSF (see Chap. 15 for more detail)	1C
	Thrombocytopenia	Platelet transfusion	1C
	Anemia	Red blood cell transfusion; erythropoietin (EPO)-stimulating agents should not be utilized	1C
Skin	Dermatitis	Lotion, topical steroid 0.1 % mometasone furoate to prevent/treat irritation/pruritus; other treatments or no therapy may be equally efficacious	2C
	Moist desquamation	Hydrocolloid/hydrogel dressings for comfort	2C
	Ulceration/necrosis	Referral to wound care specialist	1C
CNS	Somnolence syndrome	Dexamethasone 4 mg/m^2/day until improvement in symptoms	1C
Head and neck	Oral mucositis	Pain management with morphine PCA, fluid and nutritional assessment; benzydamine, LLLT, and palifermin not yet recommended (see Chap. 11 for more detail)	1C
	Xerostomia	IMRT for salivary gland sparing; oral mucosal lubricants/salivary substitutes; consider pilocarpine, acupuncture	1C
Gastrointestinal	Esophagitis	Supportive care with nutritional assessment and H$_2$ blocker or PPI for GER; consider promotility agent, rule out infectious etiologies	1C
	Nausea/vomiting	Supportive care with nutritional assessment; 5-HT$_3$ receptor antagonist±dexamethasone (see Chap. 10 for more detail)	1C
	GI mucositis	Bowel care and nutritional assessment; loperamide for diarrhea; atropine or octreotide for refractory cases; *Lactobacillus* spp. or sulfasalazine not yet recommended	1C
Lung	Pneumonitis	Antitussive; prednisone 1–2 mg/kg/day	2C
Bladder	Cystitis	Anesthetic agents (e.g., pyridium) and antispasmodics (e.g., oxybutynin); copious bladder irrigation for hemorrhagic cystitis, consider HBO or intravesical therapy	1C

RT radiation therapy, *GCSF* granulocyte colony-stimulating factor, *CNS* central nervous system, *PCA* patient-controlled analgesia, *LLLT* low-level laser therapy, *IMRT* intensity-modulated radiation therapy, *PPI* proton pump inhibitor, *GER* gastroesophageal reflux, *GI* gastrointestinal, *HBO* hyperbaric oxygen
[a]See text for full detail
[b]Per Guyatt et al. (2006); see Preface

2009 recommending primary prophylaxis with CSFs in high-risk situations including ANC $<1.5 \times 10^9$/L due to radiotherapy of >20 % of the bone marrow (Crawford et al. 2009).

Small adult studies have shown a decrease in RT treatment interruption secondary to neutropenia with the use of G-CSF; yet, what effect, if any, this had on local control and outcome are unclear (MacManus et al. 1993, 1995; Fyles et al. 1998a; Su et al. 2006; Kalaghchi et al. 2010). Larger meta-analyses on the use of G-CSF after chemotherapeutic regimens and hematopoietic stem cell transplant (HSCT) have failed to show an improvement in overall survival and transplant-related mortality

(Dekker et al. 2006; Sung et al. 2007a; Center for International Blood and Marrow Transplant Research et al. 2009). A potential benefit in morbidity from radiation-induced neutropenia is unclear although no study has shown any significant risk or toxicity with the use of CSFs beyond bone pain and local reactions. Similarly, there are no data in regard to the timing of CSF delivery; for instance, CSFs could be used as primary prophylaxis to prevent the development of neutropenia in high-risk cases or secondarily to treat neutropenia once it has occurred. Current pediatric treatment protocols suggest the use of CSFs in both such cases. See Chap. 15 for more detail on CSF usage.

13.2.2 Management of Thrombocytopenia

Platelet transfusion remains the mainstay of treatment for radiation-induced thrombocytopenia. Guidelines are lacking in both the adult and pediatric literature as to what the appropriate threshold for platelet transfusion should be and thus transfusion criteria are variable between pediatric institutions, clinicians, and chemotherapeutic protocols (Wong et al. 2005). Clinicians should take into account potential risk factors which will help aid in the determination of an appropriate platelet threshold. For instance, fever, minor bleeding, coagulopathy and mucositis are potential clinical complaints which might increase the platelet transfusion threshold from 10×10^9/L to $20–50 \times 10^9$/L though evidence-based data are lacking. From a radiation standpoint, radiation fields with a high degree of marrow involvement such as a pelvic or craniospinal field or those fields potentiating the risk of mucositis should also increase platelet transfusion thresholds from 10×10^9/L to $30–50 \times 10^9$/L though evidence-based data are lacking. Close monitoring and clinical judgment are warranted.

Thrombopoietin receptor agonists (TPO-RAs) including eltrombopag and romiplostim have recently been approved in adults for multiple indications including chemotherapy-induced thrombocytopenia (Bussel et al. 2006). As yet, very limited data are available on their efficacy for chemotherapy-induced thrombocytopenia and no pediatric data are available (Basciano and Bussel 2012). It is unclear if TPO-RAs will prove beneficial after chemotherapy- and secondarily after RT-induced thrombocytopenia. Additionally, concerns remain in regard to the safety of these agents specifically in pediatric patients due to reports of thrombocytosis, thrombosis, tumor/leukemia cell growth and bone marrow fibrosis (Kuter 2007; Gernsheimer 2008; Basciano and Bussel 2012).

13.2.3 Management of Anemia

Hypoxia in solid tumors, especially head and neck, uterine cervix, and bladder cancers, and possibly soft tissue sarcomas, has been shown to be an important component in the decreased effectiveness of RT to promote tumor cell death (Dische et al. 1983; Overgaard and Horsman 1996; Fyles et al. 1998b; Brizel et al. 1999; Vaupel et al. 2001; Dunst et al. 2003; Pinel et al. 2003; Harrison and Blackwell 2004; Nordsmark and Overgaard 2004; Nordsmark et al. 2005; Overgaard 2007). Causes for tumor hypoxia are multifactorial and include abnormalities in tumor microvasculature, increased diffusion distances and underlying anemia (Vaupel et al. 2001; Vaupel and Harrison 2004). In normal cells, tissue hypoxia eventually leads to cell death while tumor cells have adapted cellular pathways, such as by upregulation of hypoxia-inducible factor 1 (HIF1), to allow for survival and growth in such conditions (Harris 2002; Dewhirst et al. 2008). Tumor hypoxia has independently been shown to be a poor prognostic factor representing an aggressive phenotype (Brizel et al. 1999; Harris 2002; Harrison and Blackwell 2004; Vaupel and Harrison 2004; Nordsmark et al. 2005; Vaupel 2008).

Determining what role underlying anemia has in tumor tissue hypoxia is as yet to be fully understood. Brizel et al. (1999) showed that even in non-anemic patients, 50 % of tumors were still poorly oxygenated. Studies in patients with head and neck and uterine cervix cancers undergoing radiation therapy have shown that patient outcomes are worse with underlying anemia (Grogan et al. 1999; Thomas 2001; Dunst et al. 2003; Prosnitz et al. 2005; Hoff et al. 2011). Yet, it is not well understood whether anemia causes poor outcomes secondary to the ineffectiveness of therapy or, plausibly, is a marker of tumor aggressiveness and the severity of the underlying disease (Harrison and Blackwell 2004; Prosnitz et al. 2005; Hoff et al. 2011). Effectiveness of transfusion was mixed with Grogan et al. (1999) and Thomas (2001) showing that transfusion could overcome negative pretreatment and average weekly nadir hemoglobin during radiotherapy for cervical cancer, while Hoff et al. (2011) showed no improvement in outcomes based on transfusion for patients with head and neck cancers. Nordsmark et al. (2005) showed that tumor hypoxia, independent of hemoglobin concentration, was singularly associated with poor outcomes in adult patients with head and neck cancers.

Multiple xenograft studies have shown a potential benefit with the use of erythropoietin (EPO)-stimulating agents (ESAs) to increase tumor radiosensitivity and potentially improve patient outcomes (Pinel et al. 2003; Stüben et al. 2003; Ning et al. 2005). Yet, clinical studies with uterine cervix and head and neck cancers and a recent Cochrane review of adult patients with head and neck cancers have failed to show a benefit in outcome with ESAs concurrent with RT (Thomas et al. 2008; Hoskin et al. 2009; Lambin et al. 2009). Additionally, meta-analyses of ESA usage in adult patients are troubling due to increased risk of thromboembolism and possible increased mortality (Bohlius et al. 2006; Bennett et al. 2008). Pediatric data are lacking. Recently updated American Society of Hematology (ASH) and ASCO guidelines by Rizzo et al. (2010) recommend ESAs with caution for adult patients with chemotherapy-induced anemia and hemoglobin (hgb) <10 g/dL. No mention is made of ESA usage for treatment of radiation-induced anemia. Pediatric consensus guidelines by the French National Cancer Institute recommend avoiding systematic administration of ESAs in pediatric cancer patients with anemia (Marec-Berard et al. 2009).

Without any pediatric data, it is difficult to imply what potential benefit transfusion may impart to solid tumor patients, such as patients with soft tissue sarcomas, undergoing radiotherapy. Patients with leukemia, lymphoma and germ cell tumors will likely not benefit due to the inherent radiosensitivity of such tumor types. Additionally, it is unclear what level of hemoglobin would be optimal for radiosensitization. In the adult head and neck cancer studies, hgb <13 g/dL was prognostic although again transfusion did not prove useful in altering outcomes (Dunst et al. 2003; Prosnitz et al. 2005). The cervical cancer studies, on the other hand, showed benefit of transfusion, keeping the hgb ≥12 g/dL (Grogan et al. 1999; Thomas 2001). Survey of

pediatric oncologists' blood transfusion practice with concurrent radiotherapy showed a bimodal distribution, with 47 % of respondents transfusing for hgb >9 g/dL (Wong et al. 2005). This again underscores the lack of clear evidence-based guidelines to provide for a more uniform treatment strategy, with data to date not supporting transfusion.

13.3 Central Nervous System Complications

Risk factors for radiation-induced brain and spinal injury include higher total radiation dose, increased dose fractions (e.g., >180–200 cGy/dose), extended radiation field volume and concomitant usage of central nervous system (CNS) toxic drugs such as intrathecal methotrexate (New 2001; Butler et al. 2006; Chopra and Bogart 2009; Rinne et al. 2012). The developed brain is able to tolerate high total RT doses with a 5 % chance of radiation necrosis with daily fractionated doses to a total effective dose of 120 Gy (Lawrence et al. 2010). In comparison, the adult brain stem and spinal cord can tolerate effective doses of 54 Gy (Kirkpatrick et al. 2010; Mayo et al. 2010). Maximum standard of care doses are generally below these threshold levels.

Acute neurologic complications include paresthesias, seizures, encephalopathy, myelopathy, paralysis and coma and are most likely secondary to underlying brain and spinal pathology and the resulting alteration in the blood-brain barrier and tumor edema (and potential mass effect) which occurs with RT (Keime-Guibert et al. 1998; Chopra and Bogart 2009; Soussain et al. 2009; Rinne et al. 2012). Management of these symptoms may require hospitalization as well as medications such as anticonvulsants and steroids (e.g., dexamethasone) to reduce symptomatic edema. Unlike adults, radiation fatigue has not been reported in pediatric patients and is likely quite rare in this population. Methylphenidate can be used to treat fatigue as in adults if present (Butler et al. 2006). Somnolence syndrome, a subacute toxicity, has been reported in pediatric patients undergoing CNS irradiation (Sect. 13.3.1).

Late complications include cerebral edema, radionecrosis, leukoencephalopathy, neuroendocrine dysfunction, neurocognitive delay and secondary development of brain tumors; a discussion of these is beyond the scope of this chapter (Keime-Guibert et al. 1998; Butler et al. 2006; Chopra and Bogart 2009; Soussain et al. 2009; Rinne et al. 2012).

13.3.1 Somnolence Syndrome

Somnolence syndrome was first described in 1929 in children receiving scalp irradiation for the treatment of ringworm and has since become associated with prophylactic cranial irradiation in children with acute lymphoblastic leukemia (ALL) (Freeman et al. 1973). Freeman et al. (1973) noted that 39 % of ALL patients developed pronounced symptoms including lethargy, excessive sleeping (up to 20 h per day), anorexia, headache, irritability, fever, nausea and vomiting and transient cognitive dysfunction. An additional 39 % had mild symptoms. All patients received 24 Gy cranial irradiation (spinal irradiation ranged from 10 to 24 Gy) and there was no difference in frequency in somnolence between those children that received concomitant intrathecal methotrexate versus those who received RT alone. Mean onset of symptoms was 38 days after the completion of RT with symptoms resolving spontaneously without neurologic sequelae in a median of 18.5 days. Electroencephalogram done in a small subset of patients showed rhythmic slowing which improved with resolution of symptoms. Somnolence syndrome has also been reported after total body irradiation (TBI) with HSCT and in adult patients with primary brain tumors (Miyahara et al. 2000; Powell et al. 2011).

Follow-up studies have confirmed the findings of Freeman et al. (1973), showing a frequency of symptoms ranging from 58–71 % of patients (Parker et al. 1978; Ch'ien et al. 1980; Littman et al. 1984; Vern and Salvi 2009). Berg et al. (1983) performed neuropsychological testing on 48 children with ALL 1.5 and 3.75 years after somnolence syndrome and found no significant difference in cognitive function compared to 31 children with ALL who had not experienced somnolence after

RT. Littman et al. (1984) compared the daily fractionated dose of RT, giving 100 and 180 cGy to a total dose of 18 Gy, and found the same rate of somnolence syndrome in both groups.

Symptoms of somnolence syndrome are thought due to demyelination injury of oligodendrocytes (Butler et al. 2006; Rinne et al. 2012). Two studies have looked at prophylactic administration of steroids during RT. Mandell et al. (1989) showed a 3 % incidence of symptoms in patients receiving daily prednisone ≥ 15 mg/m^2 and Uzal et al. (1998) reported an incidence of 17.6 % in patients receiving 4 mg/m^2 of daily dexamethasone (there was no significant difference between studies due to small patient numbers). Current pediatric ALL protocols do not recommend prophylactic steroids during RT secondary to the lack of large multicenter prospective trials. Steroid treatment at the onset of symptoms has also shown benefit in reducing the duration of illness (Butler et al. 2006; Kelsey and Marks 2006; Rinne et al. 2012).

13.3.2 Lhermitte's Sign

Lhermitte's sign is a transient spinal radiation myelopathy which occurs after cervical irradiation and presents with electric-like sensations in the spine and extremities with neck flexion thought to be secondary to transient demyelination of the cord (Keime-Guibert et al. 1998; Chopra and Bogart 2009; Soussain et al. 2009). It has not been specifically reported in pediatrics but could presumably occur with a spinal tumor, especially in adolescent patients considering their increased vulnerability to spinal cord injury with radiation or intrathecal chemotherapy (Bleyer et al. 2009). Spontaneous clinical improvement occurs in months (Chopra and Bogart 2009; Soussain et al. 2009).

13.4 Skin Complications

Acute radiation skin changes are seen in up to 85–95 % of adult patients undergoing RT (though may be decreased in incidence with IMRT) and typically occur several days to weeks after commencement of RT and after multifractionated doses totaling >20 Gy (Archambeau et al. 1995; Chopra and Bogart 2009; Salvo et al. 2010; Feight et al. 2011). Dose tolerance in normal skin is 45 Gy with increasing symptoms with greater cumulative RT doses and concomitant chemotherapy (Archambeau et al. 1995). Fluorouracil and epidermal growth factor receptor inhibitors such as cetuximab have been reported to worsen radiation dermatitis in adult patients (Archambeau et al. 1995; Budach et al. 2007). Concurrent chemotherapy with radiosensitizers such as dactinomycin and doxorubicin may play a role in the severity of radiation dermatitis in pediatric patients but has not been characterized in part due to the scheduling of these agents around RT (Archambeau et al. 1995; Krasin et al. 2009). Areas most affected are those containing skin folds such as the axillae, groin and inframammary folds (Feight et al. 2011). The earliest skin changes are pruritus, mild erythema, anhydrosis, and dry desquamation progressing to tender erythema, edema, and moist desquamation and, in severe cases, ulceration and necrosis. Data on incidence of dermatitis in children are lacking. Radiation recall, which can be precipitated by multiple agents and can occur days to years after RT, most often presents as low-grade dermatitis in a previously irradiated region although more severe reactions can also occur (Burris and Hurtig 2010).

Although there are a large number of adult studies which have reported on prevention and management of acute radiation dermatitis, many have small patient numbers with conflicting results. Pediatric data are almost completely lacking with only one reported study with 45 patients (Merchant et al. 2007). Multiple systematic reviews have been conducted though which are a useful guide from which to give direction (Bolderston et al. 2006; Kedge 2009; Kumar et al. 2010; Salvo et al. 2010; Feight et al. 2011; McQuestion 2011; Chan et al. 2012; Wong et al. 2013). General management recommendations include the use of loose fitting clothing, prevention of scratching or other abrasive activities, protection from the sun with hats and sunscreen,

avoidance of temperature extremes, avoidance of cornstarch or baby powder especially to skin folds, use of an electric razor rather than a straight blade, use of non-aluminum-based deodorant on intact skin, avoidance of cosmetic products in the treatment field, avoidance of swimming in lakes or chlorinated pools, and use of gentle, non-perfumed soaps and lotions (Feight et al. 2011; McQuestion 2011). Although initially thought that washing of skin and hair in the radiation field would lead to increased toxicity, multiple studies have shown this to be safe (Bolderston et al. 2006; Kumar et al. 2010; Salvo et al. 2010; Feight et al. 2011; McQuestion 2011; Chan et al. 2012; Wong et al. 2013). It is vital though that the irradiated areas be dry at the immediate time of treatment to prevent increasing the RT dose to the skin surface (Bernier et al. 2008).

Multiple topical agents for the prevention and treatment of radiation dermatitis have been studied including aloe vera, steroid creams, trolamine (Biafine®), calendula (marigold extract), hyaluronic acid (Xclair®), sucralfate, silver sulfadiazine, 3M™ Cavilon™ no-sting barrier film, and petroleum-based ointment (Aquaphor), among other more obscure substances (Salvo et al. 2010; Feight et al. 2011; McQuestion 2011; Wong et al. 2013). Certain agents such as aloe vera, sucralfate, and trolamine are clearly without benefit, while others such as calendula, Aquaphor, hyaluronic acid, steroid creams, and silver sulfadiazine are lacking in evidence (Kumar et al. 2010; Salvo et al. 2010; Feight et al. 2011; Wong et al. 2013). Benefit of silymarin (milk thistle extract) has also been reported in a nonrandomized trial (Becker-Schiebe et al. 2011). Due to the lack of consistent and well-powered results, recommendations from the systematic reviews are variable with Salvo et al. (2010) and Chan et al. (2012) favoring no topical agent, McQuestion (2011) and Feight et al. (2011) endorsing calendula and hyaluronic acid, Bolderston et al. (2006) supporting topical steroids, Kumar et al. (2010) favoring calendula, Cavilon™, and topical steroids, and Wong et al. (2013) sanctioning topical steroids and silver sulfadiazine. All agree that larger, prospective, better designed studies are required to answer the many remaining questions about efficacy. Finally, the majority of studies address prevention of symptoms, and thus there is even less evidence to support topical therapy as treatment for radiation dermatitis (Salvo et al. 2010; Wong et al. 2013).

Prophylactic oral agents including zinc, proteolytic enzymes (Wobe-Mugos E), pentoxifylline, and sucralfate and dressings for management of moist desquamation such as hydrogels and hydrocolloids (e.g., DuoDERM®, Spenco 2nd Skin®, Intrasite™), silver leaf, moisture vapor permeable (Tegaderm™), soft silicone (Mepilex®), GM-CSF impregnated, gentian violet, and more obscure dressings are also discussed in the systematic reviews (Kedge 2009; Kumar et al. 2010; Salvo et al. 2010; Feight et al. 2011; McQuestion 2011; Wong et al. 2013). As with the topical agents, poor study design and lack of power limit conclusions that can be made on any of these agents (Kedge 2009; Kumar et al. 2010; Salvo et al. 2010; Feight et al. 2011; McQuestion 2011; Wong et al. 2013). Kedge (2009) notes in her review of hydrogels and hydrocolloid dressings that although improved healing may not occur with these agents, patient comfort may be an important benefit in some cases.

13.5 Head and Neck Complications

Radiotherapy to the head and neck can lead to complications in multiple different structures including the oral mucosa, salivary glands, bone, masticatory musculature, dentition, middle and outer ear, larynx, pharynx, and upper esophagus. The most common side effects with RT to the oral mucosa and salivary glands include mucositis, taste loss, parotitis/sialadenitis, xerostomia, trismus, and osteoradionecrosis (Kielbassa et al. 2006). Mucositis and taste loss are transitory, while xerostomia can be a long-term complication although conformal radiation therapy and proper planning have been shown to reduce this risk (Kielbassa et al. 2006; Jensen et al. 2010a). Head and neck cancer patients receiving RT must also be monitored for oropharyngeal candidiasis (Bensadoun et al. 2011). Serous otitis media and

externa, laryngeal edema, dysphagia, and pharyngeal dysfunction can all occur. Tooth decay, sensorineural hearing loss, osteonecrosis, and bone growth arrest are long-term effects that must be considered but are beyond the scope of this chapter.

13.5.1 Oral Mucositis

Mucositis is a common and debilitating complication of chemoradiation occurring several days to weeks after RT initiation which can lead to treatment interruption, dose-limiting toxicity, and decreased patient quality of life and is most likely to occur in patients receiving high-dose radiation for head and neck cancers (e.g., 60–70 Gy), with 85 % of adult patients clinically affected (Sonis et al. 2004; Peterson et al. 2011). Incidence is dependent on the underlying therapeutic regimen with combination chemoradiation to the head and neck being a more likely culprit as well as total body irradiation (TBI) with HSCT (Sonis et al. 2004; Peterson et al. 2011). Incidence in children has not been widely reported but is likely similar to that for adults (Allen et al. 2010; Qutob et al. 2013b). Multiple scoring systems have been utilized in the literature, and only some have been validated for children (Sonis et al. 2004; Sung et al. 2007b; Tomlinson et al. 2007).

Due to the large number of adult trials reporting on management of oral mucositis, multiple clinical practice guidelines and systematic reviews from ASCO, ESMO, MASCC/ International Society of Oral Oncology (ISOO), and the Cochrane Collaboration are available in the literature to help guide management (Keefe et al. 2007; Hensley et al. 2009; Clarkson et al. 2010; Peterson et al. 2011; Worthington et al. 2011; Gibson et al. 2013). Pediatric data are limited to small studies with variable treatment designs and therefore extrapolation from adult studies is required (Allen et al. 2010; Qutob et al. 2013b). Treatment of radiation-induced oral mucositis is similar to chemotherapy-induced mucositis; the interested reader should refer to Chap. 11 for a more detailed review of mucositis treatment guidelines.

Prior to the initiation of chemoradiation, the pediatric patient should have an oral exam to determine what, if any, treatments are required to help prevent the development of mucositis and to ensure there is no interference with the radiation field (Otmani 2007; Barbería et al. 2008; Qutob et al. 2013a). If possible, cavities should be filled and fixed appliances in the radiation field removed 7–10 days before the initiation of therapy (Barbería et al. 2008). Families and patients should be advised in regard to the importance of maintaining oral hygiene including regular tooth and tongue brushing with a soft brush and fluoridated toothpaste (in children ≥18 months) and regular mouth washing (Qutob et al. 2013b). A standardized multidisciplinary hospital oral care protocol has been shown beneficial, as well as bland rinses such as saline or sodium bicarbonate; chlorhexidine has not been proven helpful (Keefe et al. 2007; Peterson et al. 2011; McGuire et al. 2013). Nutritional status should be monitored and those at risk for malnutrition (>5 % weight loss from baseline) should be started on total parenteral nutrition (TPN) if with orogastrointestinal mucositis or have percutaneous endoscopic gastrostomy (PEG) placement if with a head and neck tumor (Ladas et al. 2005). Additionally, hydration status in patients with severe mucositis must be monitored with intravenous fluids given if required.

Multiple well-studied agents in adult patients receiving RT have not been shown beneficial including cryotherapy (i.e., ice chips, oral cooling), antimicrobial lozenges, misoprostol mouthwash, amifostine, glutamine, and pilocarpine for the prevention of oral mucositis and oral sucralfate for treatment of mucositis (Keefe et al. 2007; Hensley et al. 2009; Gibson et al. 2013; Jensen et al. 2013; Nicolatou-Galitis et al. 2013; Peterson et al. 2013; Saunders et al. 2013; Yarom et al. 2013). Therapies that have shown potential benefit include prophylactic zinc, morphine mouth rinse, doxepin rinse, morphine patient-controlled analgesia (PCA), use of midline radiation blocks (with EBRT, not utilized with IMRT), benzydamine (locally acting nonsteroidal anti-inflammatory), low-level laser therapy (LLLT), and palifermin (keratinocyte growth factor-1

[KGF-1]) (Keefe et al. 2007; Hensley et al. 2009; Clarkson et al. 2010; Peterson et al. 2011; Gibson et al. 2013; Migliorati et al. 2013; Nicolatou-Galitis et al. 2013a; Raber-Durlacher et al. 2013; Saunders et al. 2013; Yarom et al. 2013). The strongest evidence in the adult literature exists for benzydamine, LLLT and palifermin. Of note, benzydamine has not been approved by the United States Food and Drug Administration.

LLLT is recommended in adult patients receiving HSCT with or without TBI and head and neck patients undergoing RT (Peterson et al. 2011; Migliorati et al. 2013). A pilot study of LLLT in children showed potential benefit in the prevention of chemotherapy-induced mucositis (Abramoff et al. 2008). Palifermin, 60 mcg/kg/day, for 3 days prior to conditioning and 3 days posttransplantation for autologous (and possibly allogeneic) HSCT with TBI has shown benefit in adult patients (Keefe et al. 2007; Hensley et al. 2009; Raber-Durlacher et al. 2013). Recent studies in adult head and neck cancer patients are promising in reducing the severity and duration of mucositis symptoms although without improvement in event-free and overall survival (Le et al. 2011; Henke et al. 2011). Data on palifermin usage in the pediatric population are significantly limited. Srinivasan et al. (2012) recently reported on a phase I dose-finding study in 12 children receiving myeloablative HSCT and found that 90 mcg/kg/day was tolerated with skin rash being the most common side effect; mucositis was seen in only 25 % of the cohort but without a comparative control group. See Chap. 11 for a full discussion regarding oral mucositis and mouth care.

13.5.2 Dysgeusia

Patients undergoing radiation for head and neck tumors are at risk for altered taste due to direct radiation effect on the fungiform papillae and taste buds (Otmani 2007). Taste loss can precede mucositis with histologic signs of degeneration and atrophy occurring after 10 Gy, with taste loss increasing exponentially with higher cumulative RT doses, and with bitter and acid flavors being most affected (Kielbassa et al. 2006). Pediatric patients may develop anorexia due to dysgeusia and therefore nutritional status must be monitored closely. Zinc and amifostine for prophylaxis or treatment of dysgeusia in adult patients have not consistently shown benefit and are not recommended (Hovan et al. 2010). Dysgeusia usually returns to normal weeks to months after the completion of RT though in a small subsegment of patients may persist.

13.5.3 Xerostomia

A reduction in salivary function is most commonly seen with head and neck RT and has also been noted post-HSCT with and without TBI (Jensen et al. 2010a). In a systematic review by Jensen et al. (2010a), xerostomia prevalence remained >70 % from the time of development to >2 years post conventional RT. Pediatric data are limited; it appears the risk of chronic xerostomia is low although has been described after both head and neck RT and TBI conditioning with HSCT (Jensen et al. 2010a). Xerostomia risk is dose related, with minimal risk at mean doses of 10–15 Gy to the parotid gland and a decrease in glandular function >75 % with mean doses >40 Gy (Deasy et al. 2010). Xerostomia risk has been reported to be significantly reduced with sparing of one parotid or even, potentially, one submandibular gland, with IMRT although in the review by Jensen et al. (2010a) prevalence of xerostomia after IMRT was similar to that noted with conventional RT at all time points due to variation in technique and ability to spare the parotid and submandibular glands (Saarilahti et al. 2006).

Multiple potential management strategies exist in the adult literature and have most recently been systematically reviewed by Jensen et al. (2010b) as part of MASCC/ISOO. Recommendations include the use of IMRT with salivary gland sparing when oncologically feasible, muscarinic agonist stimulation (pilocarpine over newer and less well-studied agents cevimeline and bethanechol) after RT completion (but not during RT), oral mucosal lubricants/salivary substitutes, salivary gland transfer in strictly selected cases, and acupuncture to stimulate salivary gland secretion

(Jensen et al. 2010b). Agents that are not recommended include amifostine (as opposed to the 2008 ASCO guidelines by Hensley et al. [2009]), gustatory and masticatory stimulation (sugar-free lozenges, acidic candy, chewing gum), and hyperbaric oxygen (HBO) therapy (Jensen et al. 2010b). Pediatric data on such interventions are extremely limited.

13.5.4 Ear Complications

Depending on the extent of the radiation field and cumulative dose, patients have been reported to acutely develop serous otitis media and externa in addition to radiation dermatitis of the external ear and ear canal. Otitis media occurs in conjunction with mucosal edema leading to tinnitus and high-frequency hearing loss in rare cases requiring myringotomy tubes (Chopra and Bogart 2009). Excessive earwax buildup has also been noted after the completion of RT (Chopra and Bogart 2009). Patients may require decongestants and oral antibiotics for serous otitis media, otic antibiotic drops for otitis externa, and carbamide peroxide ear drops for wax buildup. Corticosteroid drops can be utilized for radiation dermatitis in the external ear canal. Audiometric testing should be done on clinically symptomatic patients. Sensorineural deafness, a late effect of RT, is dose dependent and permanent, occurring at >50 Gy and synergistic with platinum chemotherapy (Huang et al. 2002). Tissue protection with IMRT has significantly reduced the risk of this complication (Huang et al. 2002).

13.5.5 Laryngeal Complications

Radiation to the oropharynx can lead to laryngeal edema as well as reduced laryngeal closure resulting in aspiration, especially at doses >50 Gy although risk has been decreased with the use of IMRT (Chopra and Bogart 2009; Rancati et al. 2010). Patients should be monitored closely and treated symptomatically with antitussives, pain medication, and steroids to reduce edema. RT treatment interruption may be necessary depending on the underlying cause of the edema and the severity. ENT evaluation and hospitalization may be required for more complicated cases. Adolescent patients should be advised against smoking during and after RT as it has been reported to lead to persistent hoarseness in adults with glottic tumors (Chopra and Bogart 2009).

13.6 Gastrointestinal Complications

The stomach and small bowel are often incidentally irradiated when treating upper GI tract, inferior lung, retroperitoneal, and pelvic tumors. Acute gastrointestinal RT-induced side effects include nausea, vomiting, and anorexia immediately after treatment as well as dysphagia, esophagitis, dyspepsia, ulceration, bleeding, enteritis (GI mucositis manifesting as cramping, diarrhea, and malabsorption), and proctitis within the first few weeks of therapy (Kavanagh et al. 2010; Michalski et al. 2010). Late small bowel obstruction due to RT-induced fibrosis and secondary adhesions as well as chronic dyspepsia, ulceration, diarrhea, fistula, perforation, bleeding, strictures, and chronic radiation proctitis must be considered but are beyond the scope of this chapter. RT dose-volume constraints for the stomach and small bowel are difficult to determine as partial volume irradiation is usually undertaken; ≥45 Gy for the whole stomach and for partial small bowel <195 mL are thresholds that have been published for adult patients (Kavanagh et al. 2010).

13.6.1 Dysphagia and Esophagitis

Radiation to the oropharynx can lead to pharyngeal edema as well as dysphagia while RT to the thorax can lead to esophagitis. Adult patients receiving chemoradiation or hyperfractionated RT have been noted to have a 15–25 % risk of severe acute esophagitis with symptoms peaking 4–8 weeks after the commencement of RT (Werner-Wasik et al. 2010). Of note, esophageal infections such as oroesophageal (OE) candidiasis

or herpes simplex esophagitis can lead to similar symptoms and must be ruled out; additionally, preexisting gastroesophageal reflux (GER) can worsen esophagitis and should be treated (Werner-Wasik et al. 2010). If infection is a concern, patients should undergo diagnostic endoscopy unless the level of symptoms contradicts such a procedure; in such cases empiric therapy (e.g., fluconazole) for OE candidiasis may be required. Radiation doses >40–50 Gy in adults have been shown to correlate with increased risk of acute esophagitis (Werner-Wasik et al. 2010). Data in the pediatric population are lacking.

Amifostine has shown some potential benefit in non-small cell lung cancer patients, but the reports are inconsistent, and recommendation for its use is also not uniform (Keefe et al. 2007; Hensley et al. 2009; Peterson et al. 2011). No other agent has been well studied; oral sucralfate has been utilized, but data are conflicting, and it is not recommended in consensus guidelines for RT-induced esophagitis (Bradley and Movsas 2004). General treatment strategies include treatment of underlying GER with an H_2 blocker or proton pump inhibitor, ruling out and treating infectious etiologies for esophagitis, and prescribing viscous lidocaine and analgesics for pain. Promotility agents such as metoclopramide can also be tried. Patients should be advised to avoid acidic and spicy foods as well as alcohol and coffee. Nutritional status should be closely monitored, and patients at risk for malnutrition should receive oral supplementation, nasogastric feeds, PEG placement (if with a head and neck tumor), or TPN, depending on the underlying clinical situation; see Chap. 12 for more details. Pediatric patients with a history of chemoradiation-induced esophagitis are at risk for esophageal stricture and should be monitored for this potential late complication (Mahboubi and Silber 1997).

13.6.2 Nausea, Vomiting and Anorexia

Radiation-induced nausea and vomiting (RINV) has been reported to occur in 50–80 % of adult patients dependent on the radiation field, RT dose, and use of concurrent chemotherapy (Feyer et al. 2011). MASCC/ISOO and ASCO have created clinical practice guidelines for antiemetics with RINV and have devised an RT emetogenic risk stratification, with high risk in those receiving TBI, moderate risk with RT to the upper abdomen, low risk for cranial, craniospinal, head and neck, lower thorax, and pelvic RT, and minimal risk with extremity and breast RT (Basch et al. 2011; Feyer et al. 2011). Emetic prophylaxis should be per the chemotherapy-related antiemetic schedule unless the risk of emesis is higher with RT (Basch et al. 2011; Feyer et al. 2011). Pediatric guidelines for RINV are lacking. Chap. 10 has a more extensive discussion of antiemetics in relation to chemotherapy-induced nausea and vomiting in children.

MASCC/ISOO and ASCO guidelines both recommend prophylaxis with a 5-HT$_3$ receptor antagonist in the high- and moderate-risk groups with prophylactic dexamethasone in the high-risk group and optional dexamethasone in the moderate-risk group. MASCC/ISOO guidelines recommend prophylaxis or rescue with a 5-HT$_3$ receptor antagonist in the low-risk group while ASCO guidelines recommend no prophylaxis in this cohort. Finally, both guidelines advise rescue only with either a 5-HT$_3$ receptor antagonist or dopamine antagonist in the minimal-risk group (Basch et al. 2011; Feyer et al. 2011). ASCO guidelines recommend a 5-HT$_3$ receptor antagonist prior to each fraction with 5 days of dexamethasone; MASCC/ISOO guidelines make no particular recommendation in regard to duration of prophylaxis (Basch et al. 2011; Feyer et al. 2011). Gastric protection should be considered with repeated or prolonged dexamethasone therapy.

13.6.3 Enteritis

Abdominopelvic radiation can cause acute injury to the small bowel mucosa leading to enteritis (GI mucositis) with cramping, diarrhea, and malabsorptive symptoms, potentially exacerbated by concomitant chemotherapy administration (Chopra and Bogart 2009). Basic bowel care

is recommended including maintenance of adequate hydration and consideration for possible lactose intolerance and bacterial pathogens (Keefe et al. 2007; Peterson et al. 2011). Symptoms of radiation-induced enteritis have traditionally been managed with moderate bowel rest, such as institution of a low-residue, low-fat and low-lactose diet. For severe diarrhea, antimotility agents such as loperamide or atropine may be utilized. Due to the risk of bacterial pathogens, treatable causes such as *Clostridium difficile* should be ruled out. A recent systematic review by MASCC/ISOO suggests the prophylactic use of probiotics with *Lactobacillus* spp. and sulfasalazine, 500 mg twice daily, to prevent RT-induced enteritis for adult patients with pelvic tumors (Gibson et al. 2013). The recommendation for sulfasalazine is specifically for patients receiving pelvic EBRT. Additionally the guidelines recommend octreotide in patients after HSCT with chemotherapy conditioning that fail loperamide for control of diarrhea (Gibson et al. 2013). Patients undergoing RT are not included in this recommendation. Agents that have not shown benefit and should not be utilized include amifostine, 5-ASA and related compounds, and sucralfate (Peterson et al. 2011; Gibson et al. 2013). Pediatric data are lacking.

13.6.4 Proctitis

Adult patients receiving radiation for anal cancer are at risk for the development of radiation proctitis which is usually self-limited and leads to softer or diarrhea-like stools, pain, a sense of rectal distension with cramping, urgency, increased frequency, and rarely bleeding (Chopra and Bogart 2009; Michalski et al. 2010). A potential example in pediatric patients could be perineal sarcoma; evidence is lacking. RT doses to the rectum >45 Gy increase the risk for proctitis (Michalski et al. 2010). Recent guidelines by MASCC/ISOO and ESMO suggest the use of IV/intrarectal amifostine prior to RT as well as HBO and sucralfate enemas for the treatment of proctitis and recommend against misoprostol suppositories (Peterson et al. 2011; Gibson et al. 2013).

13.7 Major Organ Inflammation

Acute and long-term toxicity to organs within the radiation field is directly related to RT dose, fractionation, concomitant chemotherapy and any underlying morbidities. The lungs and kidneys are particularly sensitive to RT and the kidneys specifically are the dose-limiting organ with TBI (Dawson et al. 2010). Acute organ toxicity is often poorly defined in the pediatric population, but the practitioner must be cognizant of this potential complication which is often a risk factor for the development of chronic complaints.

13.7.1 Pneumonitis

Lung tissue is extremely sensitive to radiation with histologic effects seen in all patients, even those receiving only a few hundred cGy (McDonald et al. 1995). The risk of long-term damage is increased with fractionated lung irradiation >20 Gy (Marks et al. 2010). Chemotherapeutic agents including bleomycin, methotrexate, alkylating agents, dactinomycin, anthracyclines and vinca alkaloids can synergistically add to lung injury (McDonald et al. 1995; Abid et al. 2001). Pathologic exudative changes, directly related to the dose and volume of lung tissue irradiated, can lead to acute radiation pneumonitis which can be followed by healing over weeks to months. Late lung injury with chronic pneumonitis, fibrosis and bronchiolitis obliterans can also result (McDonald et al. 1995; Abid et al. 2001). Pneumonitis is usually seen 1–3 months after completion of RT although can be seen more acutely, with 5–15 % incidence in adult patients receiving mediastinal EBRT for lung and breast cancer and lymphoma; recent data show a decreased risk with IMRT (McDonald et al. 1995; Marks et al. 2010). Data on acute incidence of radiation pneumonitis in pediatric patients are lacking. Weiner et al. (2006) noted in a small cohort of pediatric patients who received whole lung irradiation (median 12 Gy) that the majority had long-term reductions in total lung capacity and diffusion capacity although most had also received doxorubicin.

Common symptoms of acute radiation pneumonitis include cough, dyspnea, low-grade fever, and pleuritic chest pain, with minimal physical signs although moist rales and pleural friction rub have been noted (McDonald et al. 1995; Abid et al. 2001). Early chest radiograph findings include diffuse haziness with interstitial markings or ground-glass opacification in the radiation field; the chest radiograph may also be normal (McDonald et al. 1995; Abid et al. 2001). Computed tomography is a more sensitive test for the diagnosis of acute radiation pneumonitis (McDonald et al. 1995). Acute radiation pneumonitis is a risk factor for the development of chronic changes and patients should be followed clinically and with serial pulmonary function testing. Treatment for acute radiation pneumonitis is empirical; steroids at a dose of 1–2 mg/kg/day for several weeks followed by a slow taper have been shown beneficial although randomized controlled trial data are lacking (Abid et al. 2001). Other potential etiologies including infection, pulmonary embolism, and tumor recurrence should be considered and ruled out (Chopra and Bogart 2009).

13.7.2 Pericarditis

Acute pericarditis is an unlikely toxicity, especially with conformal RT, but can be seen with RT to a substantial volume of the entire heart such as in patients with Hodgkin lymphoma (Chopra and Bogart 2009; Gagliardi et al. 2010). Treatment includes utilization of diuretics and cardiac inotropic support as needed. Synergistic acute risk with anthracycline therapy has not been defined. Long-term effects including coronary artery disease, cardiomyopathy, valvular damage, dysrhythmias and cardiac fibrosis are more likely with whole heart doses >30 Gy (Gagliardi et al. 2010).

13.7.3 Hepatitis

RT-induced liver disease in adults is split between classic and nonclassic presentations

(Pan et al. 2010). Classic RT-induced liver toxicity presents with anicteric hepatomegaly and ascites, with onset usually occurring months after the completion of RT although it can occur more rapidly (Chopra and Bogart 2009; Pan et al. 2010). Elevated alkaline phosphatase >2× the upper limit of normal (ULN) is a commonly reported finding; pathologic findings are similar to veno-occlusive disease/sinusoidal obstructive syndrome (VOD/SOS) (Lawrence et al. 1995; Chopra and Bogart 2009; Pan et al. 2010). Nonclassic presentations are usually seen in the setting of hepatocellular carcinoma with elevated liver transaminases >5× ULN (Pan et al. 2010). Other potential signs of liver toxicity include thrombocytopenia and coagulopathy.

Cumulative radiation doses to the liver should be <28–32 Gy to decrease the risk of liver toxicity (Pan et al. 2010). Concurrent hepatic disease, secondary to hepatitis B, hepatitis C or the underlying malignancy, is a potential risk factor for RT-induced hepatitis (Pan et al. 2010). Synergistic risk secondary to concomitant chemotherapy is likely but poorly defined. Infectious etiologies, metastases, and drug-induced hepatitis must be considered and ruled out (Chopra and Bogart 2009). Treatment includes diuretics as needed. The use of steroids and anticoagulants has been suggested; since the underlying pathology is similar to VOD/SOS, an analogous treatment strategy could be considered although this is not evidence-based. Liver failure is often irreversible in adult patients (Pan et al. 2010). Pediatric data are lacking. The presence of focal nodular hyperplasia has been noted as a late effect after liver RT (Bouyn et al. 2003).

13.7.4 Nephropathy

Acute RT-induced kidney injury is usually subclinical with signs and symptoms such as decreased glomerular filtration rate and proteinuria occurring in the subacute time period (Dawson et al. 2010). Chronic injury occurs with a long latency and the development of hypertension, elevated creatinine and renal failure, although the risk in the pediatric population

receiving multimodal chemoradiotherapy appears low (Dawson et al. 2010; Bölling et al. 2011). Acute injury can rarely present with a hemolytic-uremic type syndrome or an increased creatinine, with the total RT dose to the kidney being the most important risk factor (Dawson et al. 2010). Data on incidence in children are lacking. In their review, Dawson et al. (2010) recommend a mean kidney dose of <10 Gy with TBI and <18 Gy with bilateral partial kidney irradiation. Although multiple factors can influence kidney function after HSCT, in their review of 92 children after TBI and HSCT, Gerstein et al. (2009) found a very low incidence of persistent renal dysfunction with cumulative fractionated RT doses <12 Gy. Treatment may include low-protein diet, fluid and salt restriction, use of antihypertensives and diuretics as needed, treatment of anemia, and, if necessary, dialysis (Cassady 1995).

13.7.5 Cystitis

RT to the bladder and urethra can acutely lead to urinary frequency, urgency and dysuria; incontinence is rarely seen in the acute period (Marks et al. 1995; Chopra and Bogart 2009). The mechanism for acute symptoms is unclear; smooth muscle edema as well as inflammation and injury to the epithelial cell layer are proposed mechanisms (Marks et al. 1995). Bladder toxicity is unlikely to occur with cumulative fractionated RT doses <40–50 Gy (Viswanathan et al. 2010). Concurrent chemotherapy, especially with cyclophosphamide, ifosfamide or busulfan, is an additional potential risk factor (Payne et al. 2013). Anesthetic agents (e.g., pyridium) and antispasmodics (e.g., oxybutynin) can be used symptomatically (Chopra and Bogart 2009). Pediatric data on acute RT-induced cystitis are lacking but is a potential complication in the treatment of pelvic tumors. Urinary tract infections should be considered and ruled out (Chopra and Bogart 2009). Hematuria is an unlikely early complication but should be treated with two-way Foley catheter insertion for copious bladder irrigation. Patients who are refractory to such therapy may benefit from HBO or intravesical therapy (Payne et al. 2013).

13.8 Summary

Radiation-induced toxicity is a real possibility that is likely underrecognized in the pediatric population. The pediatric oncologist must be aware of potential RT-induced complications based on the radiation field, RT dose, fractionation, concurrent chemotherapy and potential underlying patient morbidities. A multidisciplinary approach is often required to plan for and treat any potential complications. Although evidence-based prevention and treatment strategies are generally lacking in the pediatric literature, the adult literature, through both evidence and consensus guidelines, provides an excellent resource from which to extrapolate reasonable management plans.

References

Abid SY, Malhotra V, Perry MC (2001) Radiation-induced and chemotherapy-induced pulmonary injury. Curr Opin Oncol 13:242–248

Abramoff MM, Lopes NN, Lopes LA et al (2008) Low-level laser therapy in the prevention and treatment of chemotherapy-induced oral mucositis in young patients. Photomed Laser Surg 26:393–400

Allen G, Logan R, Gue S (2010) Oral manifestations of cancer treatment in children: a review of the literature. Clin J Oncol Nurs 14:481–490

Archambeau JO, Pezner R, Wasserman T (1995) Pathophysiology of irradiated skin and breast. Int J Radiat Oncol Biol Phys 31:1171–1185

Barbería E, Hernandez C, Miralles V et al (2008) Paediatric patients receiving oncology therapy: review of the literature and management guidelines. Eur J Paediatr Dent 9:188–194

Basch E, Prestrud AA, Hesketh PJ et al (2011) Antiemetics: American Society of Clinical Oncology clinical practice guideline update. J Clin Oncol 29:4189–4198

Basciano PA, Bussel JB (2012) Thrombopoietin-receptor agonists. Curr Opin Hematol 19:392–398

Becker-Schiebe M, Mengs U, Schaefer M et al (2011) Topical use of a silymarin-based preparation to prevent radiodermatitis. Strahlenther Onkol 187:485–491

Bennett CL, Silver SM, Djulbegovic B et al (2008) Venous thromboembolism and mortality associated with recombinant erythropoietin and darbopoietin administration for the treatment of cancer-associated anemia. JAMA 299:914–924

Bensadoun RJ, Patton LL, Lalla RV et al (2011) Oropharyngeal candidiasis in head and neck cancer patients treated with radiation: update 2011. Support Care Cancer 19:737–744

Berg RA, Ch'ien LT, Lancaster W et al (1983) Neuropsychological sequelae of postradiation somnolence syndrome. J Dev Behav Pediatr 4:103–107

Bernier J, Bonner J, Vermorken JB et al (2008) Consensus guidelines for the management of radiation dermatitis and coexisting acne-like rash in patients receiving radiotherapy plus EGFR inhibitors for the treatment of squamous cell carcinoma of the head and neck. Ann Oncol 19:142–149

Bleyer A, Choi M, Wang SJ et al (2009) Increased vulnerability of the spinal cord to radiation or intrathecal chemotherapy during adolescence: a report from the Children's Oncology Group. Pediatr Blood Cancer 53:1205–1210

Bohlius J, Wilson J, Seidenfeld J et al (2006) Recombinant human erythropoietins and cancer patients: updated meta-analysis of 57 studies including 9353 patients. J Natl Cancer Inst 98:708–714

Bolderston A, Lloyd NS, Wong RK et al (2006) The prevention and management of acute skin reactions related to radiation therapy: a systematic review and practice guidelines. Support Care Cancer 14:802–817

Bölling T, Ernst I, Pape H et al (2011) Dose-volume analysis of radiation nephropathy in children: preliminary report of the risk consortium. Int J Radiat Oncol Biol Phys 80:840–844

Bouyn CI, Leclere J, Raimondo G et al (2003) Hepatic focal nodular hyperplasia in children previously treated for a solid tumor. Incidence, risk factors, and outcome. Cancer 97:3107–3113

Bradley J, Movsas B (2004) Radiation esophagitis: predictive factors and preventive strategies. Semin Radiat Oncol 14:280–286

Brizel DM, Dodge RK, Clough RW et al (1999) Oxygenation of head and neck cancer: changes during radiotherapy and impact on treatment outcome. Radiother Oncol 53:113–117

Budach W, Bölke E, Homey B (2007) Severe cutaneous reaction during radiation therapy with concurrent cetuximab. N Engl J Med 357:514–515

Bunn PA Jr, Crowley J, Kelly K et al (1995) Chemoradiotherapy with or without granulocyte-macrophage colony stimulating factor in the treatment of limited-stage small-cell lung cancer: a prospective phase III randomized study of the Southwest Oncology Group. J Clin Oncol 13:1632–1641

Burris HA 3rd, Hurtig J (2010) Radiation recall with anticancer agents. Oncologist 15:1227–1237

Bussel JB, Kuter DJ, George JN et al (2006) AMG 531, a thrombopoiesis-stimulating protein for chronic ITP. N Engl J Med 355:1672–1681

Butler JM, Rapp SR, Shaw EG (2006) Managing the cognitive effects of brain tumor radiation therapy. Curr Treat Options Oncol 7:517–523

Cassady JR (1995) Clinical radiation nephropathy. Int J Radiat Oncol Biol Phys 31:1249–1256

Center for International Blood and Marrow Transplant Research (CIBMTR), National Marrow Donor Program (NMDP), European Blood and Marrow Transplant Group (EBMT) et al (2009) Guidelines for preventing infectious complications among hematopoietic cell transplant recipients: a global perspective. Bone Marrow Transplant 44:453–558

Ch'ien LT, Aur RJ, Stanger S et al (1980) Long-term neurological implications of somnolence syndrome in children with acute lymphocytic leukemia. Ann Neurol 8:273–277

Chan RJ, Larsen E, Chan P (2012) Re-examining the evidence in radiation dermatitis management literature: an overview and a critical appraisal of systematic reviews. Int J Radiat Oncol Biol Phys 84:e357–e362

Chang EL, Allen P, Wu C et al (2002) Acute toxicity and treatment interruption related to electron and photon craniospinal irradiation in pediatric patients treated at the University of Texas M. D. Anderson Cancer Center. Int J Radiat Oncol Biol Phys 52:1008–1016

Chopra RR, Bogart JA (2009) Radiation therapy-related toxicity (including pneumonitis and fibrosis). Emerg Med Clin North Am 27:293–310

Clarkson JE, Worthington HV, Furness S et al (2010) Interventions for treating oral mucositis for patients with cancer receiving treatment. Cochrane Database Syst Rev (8):CD001973

Cox JD, Stetz J, Pajak TF (1995) Toxicity criteria of the Radiation Therapy Oncology Group (RTOG) and the European Organization for Research and Treatment of Cancer (EORTC). Int J Radiat Oncol Biol Phys 31:1341–1346

Crawford J, Caserta C, Roila F et al (2009) Hematopoietic growth factors: ESMO recommendations for the applications. Ann Oncol 20:162–165

Dawson LA, Kavanagh BD, Paulino AC et al (2010) Radiation-associated kidney injury. Int J Radiat Oncol Biol Phys 76:S108–S115

Deasy JO, Moiseenko V, Marks L et al (2010) Radiotherapy dose-volume effects on salivary gland function. Int J Radiat Oncol Biol Phys 76:S58–S63

Dekker A, Bulley S, Beyene J et al (2006) Meta-analysis of randomized controlled trials of prophylactic granulocyte colony-stimulating factor and granulocyte-macrophage colony-stimulating factor after autologous and allogeneic stem cell transplantation. J Clin Oncol 24:5207–5215

Dewhirst MW, Cao Y, Moeller B (2008) Cycling hypoxia and free radicals regulate angiogenesis and radiotherapy response. Nat Rev Cancer 8:425–437

Dische S, Anderson PJ, Sealy R et al (1983) Carcinoma of the cervix–anaemia, radiotherapy and hyperbaric oxygen. Br J Radiol 56:251–255

Dunst J, Kuhnt T, Strauss HG et al (2003) Anemia in cervical cancers: impact on survival, patterns of relapse, and association with hypoxia and angiogenesis. Int J Radiat Oncol Biol Phys 56:778–787

Feight D, Baney T, Bruce S et al (2011) Putting evidence into practice: evidence-based interventions for radiation dermatitis. Clin J Oncol Nurs 15:481–492

Feyer PC, Maranzano E, Molassiotis A et al (2011) Radiotherapy-induced nausea and vomiting (RINV): MASCC/ESMO guideline for antiemetics in radiotherapy: update 2009. Support Care Cancer 19:S5–S14

Freeman JE, Johnston PG, Voke JM (1973) Somnolence after prophylactic cranial irradiation in children with acute lymphoblastic leukaemia. Br Med J 4:523–525

Fyles AW, Manchul L, Levin W et al (1998a) Effect of filgrastim (G-CSF) during chemotherapy and abdomino-pelvic radiation therapy in patients with ovarian carcinoma. Int J Radiat Oncol Biol Phys 41:843–847

Fyles AW, Milosevic M, Wong R et al (1998b) Oxygenation predicts radiation response and survival in patients with cervix cancer. Radiother Oncol 48:149–156

Gagliardi G, Constine LS, Moiseenko V et al (2010) Radiation dose-volume effects in the heart. Int J Radiat Oncol Biol Phys 76:S77–S85

Gernsheimer T (2008) The pathophysiology of ITP revisited: ineffective thrombopoiesis and the emerging role of thrombopoietin receptor agonists in the management of chronic immune thrombocytopenic purpura. Hematol Am Soc Hematol Educ Program:219–226

Gerstein J, Meyer A, Sykora KW et al (2009) Long-term renal toxicity in children following fractionated total-body irradiation (TBI) before allogeneic stem cell transplantation (SCT). Strahlenther Onkol 185:751–755

Gibson RJ, Keefe DM, Lalla RV et al (2013) Systematic review of agents for the management of gastrointestinal mucositis in cancer patients. Support Care Cancer 21:313–326

Grogan M, Thomas GM, Melamed I et al (1999) The importance of hemoglobin levels during radiotherapy for carcinoma of the cervix. Cancer 86:1528–1536

Guyatt G, Gutterman D, Baumann MH et al (2006) Grading strength of recommendations and quality of evidence in clinical guidelines: report from an American College of Chest Physicians Task Force. Chest 129:174–181

Harris AL (2002) Hypoxia—a key regulatory factor in tumour growth. Nat Rev Cancer 2:38–47

Harrison L, Blackwell K (2004) Hypoxia and anemia: factors in decreased sensitivity to radiation therapy and chemotherapy? Oncologist 9:31–40

Henke M, Alfonsi M, Foa P et al (2011) Palifermin decreases severe oral mucositis of patients undergoing postoperative radiochemotherapy for head and neck cancer: a randomized, placebo-controlled trial. J Clin Oncol 29:2815–2820

Hensley ML, Hagerty KL, Kewalramani T et al (2009) American Society of Clinical Oncology 2008 clinical practice guideline update: use of chemotherapy and radiation therapy protectants. J Clin Oncol 27:127–145

Hoff CM, Hansen HS, Overgaard M et al (2011a) The importance of haemoglobin level and effect of transfusion in HNSCC patients treated with radiotherapy—results from the randomized DAHANCA 5 study. Radiother Oncol 98:28–33

Hoff CM, Lassen P, Eriksen JG et al (2011b) Does transfusion improve the outcome for HNSCC patients treated with radiotherapy?—results from the randomized DAHANCA 5 and 7 trials. Acta Oncol 50:1006–1014

Hoskin PJ, Robinson M, Slevin N et al (2009) Effect of epoetin alfa on survival and cancer treatment-related anemia and fatigue in patients receiving radical radiotherapy with curative intent for head and neck cancer. J Clin Oncol 27:5751–5756

Hovan AJ, Williams PM, Stevenson-Moore P et al (2010) A systematic review of dysgeusia induced by cancer therapies. Support Care Cancer 18:1081–1087

Huang E, Teh BS, Strother DR et al (2002) Intensity-modulated radiation therapy for pediatric medulloblastoma: early report on the reduction of ototoxicity. Int J Radiat Oncol Biol Phys 52:599–605

Jensen SB, Pedersen AM, Vissink A et al (2010a) A systematic review of salivary gland hypofunction and xerostomia induced by cancer therapies: prevalence, severity and impact on quality of life. Support Care Cancer 18:1039–1060

Jensen SB, Pedersen AM, Vissink A et al (2010b) A systematic review of salivary gland hypofunction and xerostomia induced by cancer therapies: management strategies and economic impact. Support Care Cancer 18:1061–1079

Jensen SB, Jarvis V, Zadik Y et al (2013) Systematic review of miscellaneous agents for the management of oral mucositis in cancer patients. Support Care Cancer 21:3223–3232

Kalaghchi B, Kazemian A, Hassanloo J et al (2010) Granulocyte colony stimulating factor for prevention of craniospinal radiation treatment interruption among central nervous system tumor patients. Asian Pac J Cancer Prev 11:1499–1502

Kavanagh BD, Pan CC, Dawson LA et al (2010) Radiation dose-volume effects in the stomach and small bowel. Int J Radiat Oncol Biol Phys 76:S101–S107

Kedge EM (2009) A systematic review to investigate the effectiveness and acceptability of interventions for moist desquamation in radiotherapy patients. Radiography 15:247–257

Keefe DM, Schubert MM, Elting LS et al (2007) Updated clinical practice guidelines for the prevention and treatment of mucositis. Cancer 109:820–831

Keime-Guibert F, Napolitano M, Delattre JY (1998) Neurological complications of radiotherapy and chemotherapy. J Neurol 245:695–708

Kelsey CR, Marks LB (2006) Somnolence syndrome after focal radiation therapy to the pineal region: case report and review of the literature. J Neurooncol 78:153–156

Kielbassa AM, Hinkelbein W, Hellwig E et al (2006) Radiation-related damage to dentition. Lancet Oncol 7:326–335

Kirkpatrick JP, van der Kogel AJ, Schultheiss TE (2010) Radiation dose-volume effects in the spinal cord. Int J Radiat Oncol Biol Phys 76:S42–S49

Krasin MJ, Hoth KA, Hua C et al (2009) Incidence and correlates of radiation dermatitis in children and adolescents receiving radiation therapy for the treatment of paediatric sarcomas. Clin Oncol 21:781–785

Kumar S, Juresic E, Barton M et al (2010) Management of skin toxicity during radiation therapy: a review of the evidence. J Med Imaging Radiat Oncol 54:264–279

Kuter DJ (2007) New thrombopoietic growth factors. Blood 109:4607–4616

Ladas EJ, Sacks N, Meacham L et al (2005) A multidisciplinary review of nutrition considerations in the pediatric oncology population: a perspective from Children's Oncology Group. Nutr Clin Pract 20:377–393

Lambin P, Ramaekers BL, van Mastrigt GA et al (2009) Erythropoietin as an adjuvant treatment with (chemo) radiation therapy for head and neck cancer. Cochrane Database Sys Rev (8):CD006158

Lawrence TS, Robertson JM, Anscher MS et al (1995) Hepatic toxicity resulting from cancer treatment. Int J Radiat Oncol Biol Phys 31:1237–1248

Lawrence YR, Li XA, el Naqa I et al (2010) Radiation dose-volume effects in the brain. Int J Radiat Oncol Biol Phys 76:S20–S27

Le QT, Kim HE, Schneider CJ et al (2011) Palifermin reduces severe mucositis in definitive chemoradiotherapy of locally advanced head and neck cancer: a randomized, placebo-controlled study. J Clin Oncol 29:2808–2814

Littman P, Rosenstock J, Gale G et al (1984) The somnolence syndrome in leukemic children following reduced daily dose fractions of cranial radiation. Int J Radiat Oncol Biol Phys 10:1851–1853

MacManus MP, Clarke J, McCormick D et al (1993) Use of recombinant granulocyte-colony stimulating factor to treat neutropenia occurring during craniospinal irradiation. Int J Radiat Oncol Biol Phys 26:845–850

MacManus MP, McCormick D, Trimble A et al (1995) Value of granulocyte colony stimulating factor in radiotherapy induced neutropenia: clinical and laboratory studies. Eur J Cancer 31A:302–307

MacManus M, Lamborn K, Khan W et al (1997) Radiotherapy-associated neutropenia and thrombocytopenia: analysis of risk factors and development of a predictive model. Blood 89:2303–2310

Mahboubi S, Silber JH (1997) Radiation-induced esophageal strictures in children with cancer. Eur Radiol 7:119–122

Mandell LR, Walker RW, Steinherz P et al (1989) Reduced incidence of the somnolence syndrome in leukemic children with steroid coverage during prophylactic cranial radiation therapy. Cancer 63:1975–1978

Marec-Berard P, Chastagner P, Kassab-Chahmi D et al (2009) 2007 standards, options, and recommendations: use of erythropoiesis-stimulating agents (ESA: epoetin alfa, epoetin beta, and darbopoietin) for the management of anemia in children with cancer. Pediatr Blood Cancer 53:7–12

Marks LB, Carroll PR, Dugan TC et al (1995) The response of the urinary bladder, urethra, and ureter to radiation and chemotherapy. Int J Radiat Oncol Biol Phys 31:1257–1280

Marks LB, Bentzen SM, Deasy JO et al (2010) Radiation dose-volume effects in the lung. Int J Radiat Oncol Biol Phys 76:S70–S76

Mauch P, Constine L, Greenberger J et al (1995) Hematopoietic stem cell compartment: acute and late effects of radiation therapy and chemotherapy. Int J Radiat Oncol Biol Phys 31:1319–1339

Mayo C, Yorke E, Merchant TE (2010) Radiation associated brainstem injury. Int J Radiat Oncol Biol Phys 76:S36–S41

McDonald S, Rubin P, Phillips TL et al (1995) Injury to the lung from cancer therapy: clinical syndromes, measurable endpoints, and potential scoring systems. Int J Radiat Oncol Biol Phys 31:1187–1203

McGuire DB, Fulton JS, Park J et al (2013) Systematic review of basic oral care for the management of oral mucositis in cancer patients. Support Care Cancer 21:3165–3177

McQuestion M (2011) Evidence-based skin care management in radiation therapy: clinical update. Semin Oncol Nurs 27:e1–e17

Merchant TE, Bosley C, Smith J et al (2007) A phase III trial comparing an anionic phospholipid-based cream and aloe vera-based gel in the prevention of radiation dermatitis in pediatric patients. Radiat Oncol 2:45

Michalski JM, Gay H, Jackson A et al (2010) Radiation dose-volume effects in radiation-induced rectal injury. Int J Radiat Oncol Biol Phys 26:S123–S129

Migliorati C, Hewson I, Lalla RV et al (2013) Systematic review of laser and other light therapy for the management of oral mucositis in cancer patients. Support Care Cancer 21:333–341

Miyahara M, Azuma E, Hirayama M et al (2000) Somnolence syndrome in a child following 1200-cGy total body irradiation in an unrelated bone marrow transplantation. Pediatr Hematol Oncol 17:489–495

New P (2001) Radiation injury to the nervous system. Curr Opin Neurol 14:725–734

Nicolatou-Galitis O, Sarri T, Bowen J et al (2013a) Systematic review of anti-inflammatory agents for the management of oral mucositis in cancer patients. Support Care Cancer 21:3179–3189

Nicolatou-Galitis O, Sarri T, Bowen J et al (2013b) Systematic review of amifostine for the management of oral mucositis in cancer patients. Support Care Cancer 21:357–364

Ning S, Hartley C, Molineux G et al (2005) Darbepoietin alfa potentiates the efficacy of radiation therapy in mice with corrected or uncorrected anemia. Cancer Res 65:284–290

Nordsmark M, Overgaard J (2004) Tumor hypoxia is independent of hemoglobin and prognostic for loco-regional tumor control after primary radiotherapy in advanced head and neck cancer. Acta Oncol 43:396–403

Nordsmark M, Bentzen SM, Rudat V et al (2005) Prognostic value of tumor oxygenation in 397 head and neck tumors after primary radiation therapy. An international multi-center study. Radiother Oncol 77:18–24

Otmani N (2007) Oral and maxillofacial side effects of radiation therapy on children. J Can Dent Assoc 73:257–261

Overgaard J (2007) Hypoxic radiosensitization: adored and ignored. J Clin Oncol 25:4066–4074

Overgaard J, Horsman MR (1996) Modification of hypoxia-induced radioresistance in tumors by the use of oxygen and sensitizers. Semin Radiat Oncol 6:10–21

Pan CC, Kavanagh BD, Dawson LA et al (2010) Radiation-associated liver injury. Int J Radiat Oncol Biol Phys 76:S94–S100

Parker D, Malpas JS, Sandland R et al (1978) Outlook following "somnolence syndrome" after prophylactic cranial irradiation. Br Med J 1:554

Payne H, Adamson A, Bahl A et al (2013) Chemical- and radiation-induced haemorrhagic cystitis: current treatments and challenges. BJU Int 112:885–897

Peterson DE, Bensadoun RJ, Rolla F et al (2011) Management of oral and gastrointestinal mucositis: ESMO Clinical Practice Guidelines. Ann Oncol 22:vi78–vi84

Peterson DE, Öhrn K, Bowen J et al (2013) Systematic review of oral cryotherapy for management of oral mucositis caused by cancer therapy. Support Care Cancer 21:327–332

Pinel S, Barberi-Heyob M, Cohen-Jonathan E et al (2004) Erythropoietin-induced reduction of hypoxia before and during fractionated irradiation contributes to improvement of radioresponse in human glioma xenografts. Int J Radiat Oncol Biol Phys 59:250–259

Powell C, Guerrero D, Sardell S et al (2011) Somnolence syndrome in patients receiving radical radiotherapy for primary brain tumors: a prospective study. Radiother Oncol 100:131–136

Prosnitz RG, Yao B, Farrell CL et al (2005) Pretreatment anemia is correlated with the reduced effectiveness of radiation and concurrent chemotherapy in advanced head and neck cancer. Int J Radiat Oncol Biol Phys 61:1087–1095

Qutob AF, Allen G, Gue S et al (2013a) Implementation of a hospital oral care protocol and recording of oral mucositis in children receiving cancer treatment. Support Care Cancer 21:1113–1120

Qutob AF, Gue S, Revesz T et al (2013b) Prevention of oral mucositis in children receiving cancer therapy: a systematic review and evidence-based analysis. Oral Oncol 49:102–107

Raber-Durlacher JE, von Bültzingslöwen I, Logan RM et al (2013) Systematic review of cytokines and growth factors for the management of oral mucositis in cancer patients. Support Care Cancer 21:343–355

Rancati T, Schwarz M, Allen AM et al (2010) Radiation dose-volume effects in the larynx and pharynx. Int J Radiat Oncol Biol Phys 76:S64–S69

Rinne ML, Lee EQ, Wen PY (2012) Central nervous system complications of cancer therapy. J Support Oncol 10:133–141

Rizzo JD, Brouwers M, Hurley P et al (2010) American Society of Hematology/American Society of Clinical

Oncology clinical practice guideline update on the use of epoetin and darbepoetin in adult patients with cancer. Blood 116:4045–4059

Saarilahti K, Kouri M, Collan J et al (2006) Sparing of the submandibular glands by intensity modulated radiotherapy treatment of head and neck cancer. Radiother Oncol 78:270–275

Salvo N, Barnes E, van Draanen J et al (2010) Prophylaxis and management of acute radiation-induced skin reactions: a systematic review of the literature. Curr Oncol 17:94–112

Saunders DP, Epstein JB, Elad S et al (2013) Systematic review of antimicrobials mucosal coating agents, anesthetics, and analgesics for the management of oral mucositis in cancer patients. Support Care Cancer 21:3191–3207

Smith T, Khatcheressian J, Lyman G et al (2006) 2006 update of recommendations for the use of white blood cell growth factors: an evidence-based clinical practice guideline. J Clin Oncol 24:3187–3205

Sonis ST, Elting LS, Keefe D et al (2004) Perspective on cancer therapy-induced mucosal injury: pathogenesis, measurement, epidemiology, and consequences for patients. Cancer 100:1995–2025

Soussain C, Ricard D, Fike JR et al (2009) CNS complications of radiotherapy and chemotherapy. Lancet 374:1639–1651

Srinivasan A, Kasow KA, Cross S et al (2012) Phase I study of the tolerability and pharmacokinetics of palifermin in children undergoing allogeneic hematopoietic stem cell transplantation. Biol Blood Marrow Transplant 18:1309–1314

Stüben G, Thews O, Pöttgen C et al (2003) Impact of anemia prevention by recombinant human erythropoietin on the sensitivity of xenografted glioblastomas to fractionated irradiation. Strahlenther Onkol 179:620–625

Su YB, Vickers AJ, Zelefsky MJ et al (2006) Double-blind, placebo-controlled, randomized trial of granulocyte-colony stimulating factor during postoperative radiotherapy for squamous head and neck cancer. Cancer J 12:182–188

Sung L, Nathan PC, Alibhai SM et al (2007a) Meta-analysis: effect of prophylactic hematopoietic colony-stimulating factors on mortality and outcomes of infection. Ann Intern Med 147:400–411

Sung L, Tomlinson GA, Greenberg ML et al (2007b) Validation of the oral mucositis assessment scale in pediatric cancer. Pediatr Blood Cancer 49:149–153

Thomas G (2001) The effect of hemoglobin level on radiotherapy outcomes: the Canadian experience. Semin Oncol 28:60–65

Thomas G, Ali S, Hoebers FJ et al (2008) Phase III trial to evaluate the efficacy of maintaining hemoglobin levels above 12.0 g/dL with erythropoietin vs above 10.0 g/dL without erythropoietin in anemic patients receiving concurrent radiation and cisplatin for cervical cancer. Gynecol Oncol 108:317–325

Tomlinson D, Judd P, Hendershot E et al (2007) Measurement of oral mucositis in children: a review of the literature. Support Care Cancer 15:1251–1258

Trotti A, Colevas AD, Setser A et al (2003) CTCAE v3.0: development of a comprehensive grading system for the adverse effects of cancer treatment. Semin Radiat Oncol 13:176–181

Uzal D, Özyar E, Hayran M et al (1998) Reduced incidence of the somnolence syndrome after prophylactic cranial irradiation in children with acute lymphoblastic leukemia. Radiother Oncol 48:29–32

Vaupel P (2008) Hypoxia and aggressive tumor phenotype: implications for therapy and prognosis. Oncologist 13:21–26

Vaupel P, Harrison L (2004) Tumor hypoxia: causative factors, compensatory mechanisms, and cellular response. Oncologist 9:4–9

Vaupel P, Thews O, Hoeckel M (2001) Treatment resistance of solid tumors: role of hypoxia and anemia. Med Oncol 18:243–259

Vern TZ, Salvi S (2009) Somnolence syndrome and fever in pediatric patients with cranial irradiation. J Pediatr Hematol Oncol 31:118–120

Viswanathan AN, Yorke ED, Marks LB et al (2010) Radiation dose-volume effects of the urinary bladder. Int J Radiat Oncol Biol Phys 76:S116–S122

Weiner DJ, Maity A, Carlson CA et al (2006) Pulmonary function abnormalities in children treated with whole lung irradiation. Pediatr Blood Cancer 46:222–227

Werner-Wasik M, Yorke E, Deasy J et al (2010) Radiation dose-volume effects in the esophagus. Int J Radiat Oncol Biol Phys 76:S86–S93

Wong EC, Perez-Albuerne E, Moscow JA et al (2005) Transfusion management strategies: a survey of practicing pediatric hematology/oncology specialists. Pediatr Blood Cancer 44:119–127

Wong RK, Bensadoun RJ, Boers-Doets CB et al (2013) Clinical practice guidelines for the prevention and treatment of acute and late radiation reactions from the MASCC Skin Toxicity Study Group. Support Care Cancer 21:2933–2948

Worthington HV, Clarkson JE, Bryan G et al (2011) Interventions for preventing oral mucositis for patients with cancer receiving treatment. Cochrane Database Syst Rev (4):CD000978

Yarom N, Ariyawardana A, Hovan A et al (2013) Systematic review of natural agents for the management of oral mucositis in cancer patients. Support Care Cancer 21:3209–3221

Prevention of Infection

14

Brian T. Fisher, Christopher C. Dvorak,
and Sarah Alexander

Contents

B.T. Fisher, DO, MSCE, MPH (✉)
Pediatrics, Division of Infectious Diseases,
Children's Hospital of Philadelphia,
34th Street and Civic Center Boulevard,
CHOP North Room 1515,
Philadelphia, PA 19104, USA
e-mail: fisherbria@email.chop.edu

C.C. Dvorak, MD
Pediatric Stem Cell Transplantation,
Benioff Children's Hospital,
University of California-San Francisco,
San Francisco, CA, USA

S. Alexander, MD
Pediatric Hematology/Oncology,
Hospital for Sick Children,
Toronto, ON, Canada

Abstract

Significant advances in chemotherapy protocols for the treatment of many childhood cancers have resulted in improved survival rates; however, opportunistic infections continue to plague this vulnerable population, especially with concomitant increased therapeutic intensity. Empiric antibiotic and antifungal therapy in patients with suspected infection have helped limit the effect of such infections although infection persists as a leading cause of treatment-related mortality.

J. Feusner et al. (eds.), *Supportive Care in Pediatric Oncology:*
A Practical Evidence-Based Approach, Pediatric Oncology,
DOI 10.1007/978-3-662-44317-0_14, © Springer Berlin Heidelberg 2015

Preventative interventions represent an opportunity to reduce the incidence of infection and thus reduce mortality. The pediatric evidence for specific preventative measures to reduce bacterial, fungal and viral infections is reviewed. Areas for future research to improve knowledge regarding infection prevention in children with malignancy are also identified.

14.1   Introduction

The use of increasingly complex treatment regimens including intensive chemotherapy, radiation therapy and surgical interventions place patients at risk for infection due to altered anatomical barriers, impairment of various arms of innate and adaptive immunity, and worsening in their nutritional status (Lehrnbecher et al. 1997). Together, these negative sequelae of cancer therapy translate into a significant risk for infection. Early reports of acute leukemia cohorts suggested that 70 % of mortality was attributable to infection (Hersh et al. 1965; Hughes 1971). Soon after these reports, adult and pediatric studies suggested the benefit of empiric antibiotic and antifungal therapy in the setting of febrile neutropenia (FN) (Schimpff et al. 1971; Pizzo et al. 1979, 1982). While empiric antimicrobial therapy has become standard of care in FN (see Chap. 1), contemporary epidemiology studies still identify infection as the major contributing cause of treatment-related mortality in children receiving myelosuppressive chemotherapy (Creutzig et al. 2004; Sung et al. 2007; Freifeld et al. 2011).

In recent years, strategies for the management of infection in pediatric cancer patients have been broadened from a reactionary approach to a more proactive one utilizing preventative measures. Preventing the development of infection may prove more successful than attempting to clear a pathogen in an immunocompromised patient. This chapter will focus on current and potential future preventative therapeutic options for bacterial and fungal infections and discuss both pediatric and adult data. In addition, options for

suppression of latent viral infection and postexposure chemoprophylaxis with antiviral therapy will be explored. Discussion of prevention of infection through vaccination is discussed in detail in Chap. 16. Consideration of the prevention or suppression of other important infections such as tuberculosis or parasitic illnesses is important in communities where such infections are more prominent; however, such a discussion is outside the scope of this chapter. At the conclusion of each section, tables of graded recommendations (Tables 14.1, 14.5 and 14.7) are included for ease of reference. Finally, the chapter concludes with a discussion on hospital-based infection control practices which can reduce hospital-acquired communicable diseases in these vulnerable patients.

14.2   Prevention of Bacterial Infection

Bacterial infection is the leading cause of treatment-related morbidity and mortality in pediatric oncology patients. Evaluation and treatment of suspected or proven bacterial infection is a core component of care in children receiving myelosuppressive chemotherapy and is discussed extensively in Chap. 1. Strategies to prevent such infection, including both pharmacologic and non-pharmacologic approaches, are not as well established; data to support prophylactic measures, as well as gaps in our current knowledge, are the focus of this section.

14.2.1 Risk Stratification

As discussed in Chap. 1, the child with cancer may have multiple risk factors for serious bacterial infection including a central venous catheter, interruption of normal mucosal surfaces secondary to mucositis, surgical wounds and altered anatomy from tumor masses. Certain cancer predisposition syndromes may contribute to increased risk of infection. For example, children with Down syndrome and acute lymphoblastic leukemia (ALL) have a higher rate of infectious complications than those with ALL alone (Rabin et al. 2012). The factor most strongly associated with risk of serious bacterial infection is chemotherapy-related neutropenia; patients receiving the most intensive myelosuppressive regimens are at the highest risk. For example, 39–50 % of children treated on Children's Cancer Group protocol 2961 for acute myelogenous leukemia (AML) had Gram-positive infections and 18–28 % had Gram-negative sterile site infections during the three phases of therapy (Sung et al. 2007). Treatment-related mortality from bacterial infection in children with AML is consistently 3–4 % across cooperative group studies over the last several decades (Woods et al. 1996; Riley et al. 1999; Creutzig et al. 2004; Sung et al. 2007, 2009). Similarly, children with relapsed ALL receiving intensive chemotherapy have high rates of infectious morbidity and mortality related to bacterial infection (Abshire et al. 2000; Lawson et al. 2000; Thomson et al. 2004; Raetz et al. 2008; Locatelli et al. 2009).

14.2.2 Antimicrobial Approaches

14.2.2.1 Adult Data

Antibacterial prophylaxis for afebrile patients receiving myelosuppressive chemotherapy is widely adopted in adult oncology practice based on data from trials preformed over the last 30 years with more than 100 published studies evaluating various antibiotic regimens. Two large contemporary studies in adult solid tumor, lymphoma and leukemia patients compared levofloxacin to placebo using a double-blind, randomized, controlled design (Bucaneve et al. 2005, Cullen et al. 2005). Although neither study was able to show a significantly decreased rate of death in the levofloxacin arm, both studies showed that prophylaxis significantly decreased episodes of fever, clinically documented infection and hospitalization. In solid tumor and lymphoma patients, Cullen et al. (2005) reported a 34.2 % rate of infection with levofloxacin compared to 41.5 % in the placebo arm (RR 0.82, 95 % CI 0.73–0.94, $p=0.004$) while Bucaneve et al. (2005) reported 22 % infection rate in the levofloxacin arm versus

39 % with placebo (absolute risk difference –0.17, 95 % CI –0.24 to –0.10) in patients with leukemia, lymphoma and solid tumors.

Meta-analysis of randomized controlled trials has shown that prophylaxis has an impact on incidence of infection and, more important, is associated with a decreased risk of death (Gafter-Gvili et al. 2012). All-cause mortality was reduced in patients receiving prophylaxis (RR 0.66, 95 % CI 0.55–0.79), with the number of patients needed to treat to prevent death from any cause being 34 (95 % CI 26–56). The most substantial effect was found in studies that used fluoroquinolones (FQs) as prophylaxis with the greatest benefit in those at the highest risk.

14.2.2.2 Pediatric Data

Data regarding the utility of bacterial prophylaxis in neutropenic children are very limited. Early studies using trimethoprim-sulfamethoxazole, erythromycin, and amoxicillin-clavulanate were hampered by difficulties with patient accrual and compliance with oral therapies (Pizzo et al. 1983; van Eys et al. 1987; Castagnola et al. 2003). Studies which have documented benefit are limited by small patient numbers at single institutions. For instance, a single arm pilot trial of ciprofloxacin prophylaxis in children receiving a reinduction block of therapy for ALL showed a decreased incidence of hospitalization, bacteremia and intensive care unit admissions compared to historical controls (Yousef et al. 2004). Specifically, hospitalization was 90 % in the controls versus 58 % in the study group ($p<0.001$), the overall rate of proven bacteremia was 22 % in the controls versus 9 % in the ciprofloxacin group ($p=0.028$), and there were no Gram-negative bacteremias in this group as compared to 7.7 % in the controls ($p<0.001$) (Yousef et al. 2004).

Similarly, a retrospective study in pediatric AML patients of prophylactic cefepime, or prophylactic vancomycin with ciprofloxacin or a cephalosporin, showed decreased rates of septicemia and hospital days compared to historical controls while patients who received only an oral cephalosporin as prophylaxis had no significant decrement in bacterial sepsis or hospital days compared with controls (Kurt et al. 2008).

A recent survey by the Children's Oncology Group (COG) of institutional standards for supportive care during AML trial AAML0531 found that antibacterial prophylaxis significantly reduced Gram-positive sterile site infection (incidence rate ratio [IRR] 0.71, 95 % CI 0.57–0.90, $p=0.004$) with a trend toward reducing all bacterial infection (IRR 0.85, 95 % CI 0.72–1.01, $p=0.058$) (Sung et al. 2013).

14.2.3 Risks of Prophylaxis

The main concern when considering prophylactic antibiotics is the potential development of bacterial resistance. Any exposure to antibiotics increases the risk of colonization and possible subsequent infection with resistant pathogens. Resistance can be acquired by selection of previously undetectable but present bacteria or de novo in a previously susceptible organism. Resistant pathogens can be transmitted from patient to patient. Studies performed in the 1980s in patients with leukemia and in those undergoing hematopoietic stem cell transplant (HSCT) documented that surveillance stool cultures could often detect pathogens preceding the development of bacteremia (Schimpff et al. 1972; Tancrede and Andremont 1985; Wingard et al. 1986). Patients identified as having a resistant organism in their stool were much more likely to have a subsequent infection with a resistant pathogen. Systematic studies evaluating the impact of FQ prophylaxis on the bacterial resistance profiles from sterile site cultures in oncology patients are limited. As anticipated with any broad antibacterial use, centers with extensive use of FQs have documented increased rates of clinically relevant FQ-resistant pathogens (Razonable et al. 2002; Kern et al. 2005; Prabhu et al. 2005). The two large contemporary double-blind studies of levofloxacin prophylaxis, which combined included 2,325 patients, did not note increased rates of resistant organisms from sterile site cultures; however, the studies were not powered to detect this outcome (Bucaneve et al. 2005; Cullen et al. 2005). Specifically, Bucaneve et al. (2005) noted 3 % of patients in the levofloxacin

group had FQ-resistant Gram-negative bacilli as compared to 1 % in the placebo group (absolute risk difference 2 %, 95 % CI –0.4 % to 3 %, $p=0.10$) while Cullen et al. (2005) did not routinely test for FQ sensitivity.

The use of antibacterial prophylaxis also has potential risk for other infectious complications. Exposure to FQs in adult oncology patients has been associated with increased incidence of *Clostridium difficile*-associated diarrhea (CDAD) (von Baum et al. 2006). Rates of CDAD in hospitalized pediatric patients remain significantly lower than their adult counterparts although has increased in the last decade (Kim et al. 2008a). Additionally, there is theoretical concern that antibacterial prophylaxis may increase the rate of invasive fungal infection (IFI) though the data available do not support this concern (Gafter-Gvili et al. 2012).

FQs are the class of antibiotic most intensively investigated for antibacterial prophylaxis in adult oncology patients; in meta-analysis, FQs are the agents associated with the greatest benefit (Gafter-Gvili et al. 2012). As a class their safety profile is similar to other antibiotics with unique toxicities including rare but consistent association with tendonitis and tendon rupture (with those >60 years of age and receiving concomitant steroids at greatest risk), as well as possible association with retinal detachment (Owens and Ambrose 2005; Etminan et al. 2012). Concern regarding potential FQ toxicity in children arose from early preclinical data that associated FQ exposure to articular cartilage damage in young animals although there is now significant literature describing the safety in children (Hampel et al. 1997; Jick 1997; Redmond 1997; Bradley et al. 2007; Schaad 2007, Noel et al. 2008). Toxicity analysis in more than 2,500 pediatric patients reported that levofloxacin exposure was associated with an increased rate (3.4 % vs. 1.8 %, $p=0.025$) of musculoskeletal complaints (primarily arthralgia) at 12 months postexposure though the quality of symptoms was not different in the exposed and unexposed groups (Noel et al. 2007). Some concern remains that the results were biased by the open-label study design. Currently only ciprofloxacin is approved in the

United States for limited indications in those <18 years of age by the Food and Drug Administration (FDA).

14.2.4 Guidelines and Current Usage of Antibacterial Prophylaxis

The Infectious Diseases Society of America (IDSA) guidelines recommend the use of FQ prophylaxis in high-risk adult patients, with high-risk being defined as anticipated prolonged and profound neutropenia (i.e., absolute neutrophil count [ANC] $\leq 0.1 \times 10^9$/L for >7 days) (Freifeld et al. 2011). Similarly, the National Comprehensive Cancer Network (NCCN) guidelines recommend FQ prophylaxis in patients whose infection risk is considered to be intermediate- or high-risk (i.e., neutropenia >7 days) (NCCN 2008). The paucity of data in children have precluded the generation of pediatric-specific recommendations and these guidelines do not address the use of prophylaxis in pediatric patients. Thus, survey data for pediatric AML patients show that only approximately 13 % receive routine antibacterial prophylaxis in North American settings (Lehrnbecher et al. 2009; Sung et al. 2013).

14.2.5 Central Venous Catheter-Related Interventions

Central venous catheters (CVCs) are a common site of infection in pediatric oncology patients and prophylactic methods including CVC care plans, lock therapy as well as chlorhexidine cleansing are reviewed briefly here. See Chap. 17 for a more detail review of CVC care.

14.2.5.1 Protocols for Line Placement and Care

Revised guidelines for the prevention of infection with intravascular catheters have been recently published (O'Grady et al. 2011). The strategies recommended include systems for training those involved in the placement and care of catheters, the use of maximal sterile barrier precautions at the time of line placement and using a >0.5 % chlorhexidine skin solution with alcohol for local antisepsis. The guidelines emphasize the quality assurance and safety aspects of standardized "bundles" of central line care and systems for evaluation of compliance with institutional standards.

14.2.5.2 Antibiotic and Ethanol Locks

Antibiotic and ethanol lock therapy involves using an antimicrobial agent to fill the lumen of the central venous catheter in an attempt to prevent line-related bacterial infections. A number of studies have shown efficacy for various antimicrobial agents used as lock therapy, including studies in children with cancer (Henrickson et al. 2000). A meta-analysis of randomized controlled studies comparing vancomycin/heparin lock versus heparin alone, which included five studies in children with cancer, showed a benefit to the use of antibiotic lock in prevention of infection (Safdar and Maki 2006). As with any antibacterial prophylactic strategy, use of the agent raises concerns for emergence of resistance which has been documented in a study of gentamicin central catheter locks (Landry et al. 2010).

Ethanol locks have a potential advantage by not creating antimicrobial resistance. Studies of ethanol locks have varied in the ethanol concentrations and luminal dwell times as well as other concurrent catheter care strategies (Majetschak et al. 1999). Several studies have been performed in children receiving home parenteral nutrition; meta-analysis of four retrospective studies in this patient group suggested that ethanol lock therapy decreased the rate of central line-related infections by 81 % (Oliveira et al. 2012). Rarely, occlusion of the central line and catheter-related clots have been described with the use of ethanol locks. Data in children with cancer are lacking (Wolf et al. 2013).

14.2.5.3 Chlorhexidine Cleansing

Chlorhexidine gluconate (CHG) is a bactericidal antiseptic agent that causes membrane disruption. A cloth product with 2 % CHG (Sage Products, Inc., Cary, IL) was approved by the FDA in 2005

Table 14.1 Graded recommendations for interventions to prevent bacterial infections in children with cancer

Recommendation	Grade			Comments	Reference
	Data from studies of non-oncology patients[a]	Data from studies of adult oncology patients[a]	Data from studies of pediatric oncology patients[a]		
Antibacterial prophylaxis with a fluoroquinolone should be considered for pediatric patients with expected durations of prolonged and profound neutropenia	Not applicable	1A	0	Recommended for high-risk adult oncology patients; insufficient data in children to formulate a recommendation	Gafter-Gvili et al. (2012)
Antibiotic or ethanol locks should be considered for prevention of central line-related bacteremia	1B	1B	0	Specifics of antibiotic and ethanol lock therapies have varied across studies; insufficient data in children with cancer to formulate a recommendation	Majetschak et al. (1999); Henrickson et al. (2000); Safdar and Maki (2006); Oliveira et al. (2012); Wolf et al. (2013)
Chlorhexidine bathing should be considered for the prevention of central line-related bacteremia	1B	0	0	Insufficient data in oncology patients to formulate a recommendation	Bleasdale et al. (2007); Popovich et al. (2009)

[a]Level of evidence per Guyatt et al. (2006); see Preface

for preoperative skin cleansing. Studies of this product in adult intensive care patients have shown a significant decrease in central line infections and acquisition of multidrug-resistant pathogens (Bleasdale et al. 2007; Climo et al. 2009; Popovich et al. 2009). No data are available utilizing this strategy in children with cancer.

14.2.6 Future Directions

Data to evaluate the efficacy and potential toxicity of various strategies for the prevention of serious bacterial infection in pediatric oncology are urgently needed. Use of prophylactic antimicrobial agents needs to be evaluated for efficacy as well as safety in terms of potential short- and longer-term impact on the evolution of bacterial resistance. Studies of levofloxacin prophylaxis (ACCL0934) and CHG cleansing (ACCL1034) in children receiving intensive therapy for cancer are underway. Such research will be critical in understanding the potential

merit of various preventative strategies with the ultimate goal of decreasing the burden of bacterial infection and resultant morbidity and mortality in children with cancer. Current recommendations and evidence-based grading for prevention of bacterial infection are summarized in Table 14.1.

14.3 Prevention of Fungal Infections

Children undergoing treatment for cancer are also at increased risk of developing an IFI secondary to breakdown in natural barriers (e.g., indwelling catheter, mucositis), defects in cell-mediated immunity (i.e., lymphopenia from corticosteroids and other anti-T-cell cytotoxic agents), and deficient numbers of phagocytes (due to myelosuppressive chemotherapy) (Lehrnbecher et al. 1997). Having a single defect in the host defense system is often insufficient for development of an opportunistic IFI, but, with multiple defects, IFI begins to emerge as a significant problem. The data on IFI development and potential prevention in immunocompromised hosts derive primarily from adult studies. However, children differ from adults in the types of IFI they develop and in their metabolism of antifungal agents. For example, invasive infections caused by *Candida parapsilosis* are more common, and *Candida glabrata* rarer, in children as compared to adults, and invasive aspergillosis (IA) can be more difficult to diagnose in children due to different radiologic findings (Malani et al. 2001, Burgos et al. 2008). Thus, extrapolating clinical decisions from adult trials may be problematic. Once IFI develops, even with the advent of newer antifungal agents, treatment success rates are suboptimal, especially for mold infections. For example, Burgos et al. (2008) found that 53 % of children diagnosed with IA died; therefore, prevention of IFI in pediatric oncology patients is likely most important in improving morbidity and mortality.

14.3.1 Risk Stratification

Based on retrospective reports, as well as toxicity data collected during therapeutic trials, several groups of pediatric patients are at high risk of developing an IFI: patients undergoing HSCT (especially from an alternative allogeneic donor), patients receiving chemotherapy for AML or relapsed ALL and patients with severe aplastic anemia (SAA) (Zaoutis et al. 2006; Burgos et al. 2008). In children being treated for AML, several studies have demonstrated a high incidence (i.e., up to 29 %) of IFI, both in newly diagnosed and relapsed patients (Table 14.2) (Groll et al. 1999; Rosen et al. 2005; Sung et al. 2007, 2009). The high rate of mold infection and secondary morbidity and mortality suggest this group of patients may benefit from anti-mold prophylaxis. Conversely, studies of ALL patients (Table 14.2) suggest that only those with relapsed disease have a high enough incidence of IFI to justify routine prophylaxis (Groll et al. 1999; Leahey et al. 2000; Rosen et al. 2005; Afzal et al. 2009). From a biologic standpoint, patients with relapsed ALL will have generally received years of lympholytic chemotherapy during which time they could have theoretically become colonized with fungal spores which are more likely to become invasive when treated with more aggressive myelosuppressive chemotherapy for their relapsed disease. The risk of IFI in newly diagnosed ALL and solid tumor patients is not high enough to justify routine use of prophylactic antifungals (Rosen et al. 2005; Afzal et al. 2009). A pediatric meta-analysis came to

Table 14.2 Incidence of invasive fungal infection (IFI) in pediatric oncology patients

Study design	# of patients	Disease/procedure	Prophylaxis agent	IFI incidence	Reference
Prospective (CCG 2961)	492	New AML	None[a]	14–23 % per phase	Sung et al. (2007)
Prospective (CCG 2891)	335	New AML	Nonabsorbable[a]	10–27 % per phase	Sung et al. (2009)
Prospective	18	New AML	Fluconazole or nonabsorbable antifungal agent	29 %	Groll et al. (1999)
	7	Relapsed AML		28 %	
	97	New ALL		2 %	
	35	Relapsed ALL		9 %	
Retrospective	261	ALL	None	10 %	Rosen et al. (2005)
	117	AML		9 %	
Retrospective	425	New ALL	None	1 %	Afzal et al. (2009)
Prospective (CHP-540)	21	Relapsed ALL	Fluconazole	19 %	Leahey et al. (2000)

CHP-540 Children's Hospital of Philadelphia Trial 540, *CCG* Children's Cancer Group, *AML* acute myelogenous leukemia, *ALL* acute lymphoblastic leukemia
Adapted from Dvorak et al. (2012)
[a]Some patients may have received systemic antifungals

similar conclusions, recommending antifungal prophylaxis in patients with AML/MDS (myelodysplastic syndrome) but not in those with other malignancies even if with anticipated neutropenia >7 days (Science et al. 2014).

14.3.2 Approaches to Antifungal Prophylaxis

Whether antifungal prophylaxis is beneficial in high-risk pediatric cohorts remains controversial due to a lack of sufficient data. Robenshtok et al. (2007) performed a meta-analysis of 64 antifungal prophylaxis trials and demonstrated in patients with acute leukemia that the risk of IFI development was lower with antifungal prophylaxis, yet did not result in a statistical improvement in all-cause mortality. Only 5 of the 64 analyzed trials included pediatric patients making it difficult to generalize to the pediatric oncology cohort. Additionally, data were not collected on potential altered morbidity with IFI prophylaxis such as decreased hospital days or need for intensive care.

Several published randomized prospective trials comparing antifungal agents have included pediatric patients, although rarely younger than 12 years of age, and pediatric patients have generally not been separately analyzed (Table 14.3) (Goodman et al. 1992; Slavin et al. 1995; van Burik et al. 2004; Cornely et al. 2007; Wingard et al. 2010). Therefore, conclusions about the optimal prophylactic agent in pediatric oncology patients are based almost exclusively upon extrapolation from adult data. Currently, the most commonly recommended agent for antifungal prophylaxis in high-risk children is fluconazole although this recommendation is based on two older placebo-controlled trials performed in patients >12 years older of age undergoing autologous or allogeneic HSCT (Goodman et al. 1992; Slavin et al. 1995).

Although it reduced the risk of IFI relative to placebo, fluconazole lacks activity against *Aspergillus* spp., which is the second most common cause of IFI in these patients. Given this lack of anti-mold activity, several trials have compared it to mold-active agents in hopes of further decreasing rates of IFI. The first of these trials compared fluconazole to low-dose conventional deoxycholate amphotericin B deoxycholate (D-AMB); however, D-AMB did not show improvement over fluconazole and resulted in a higher adverse event rate (Wolff et al. 2000). With the advent of liposomal amphotericin B (L-AMB), there was renewed interest in prophylaxis with an amphotericin B product, and several trials, including one in children, have evaluated L-AMB (often given only three times per week) for antifungal prophylaxis in HSCT and acute leukemia patients (Kelsey et al. 1999; Mattiuzzi et al. 2003; Penack et al. 2006; Roman et al. 2008). Again, like D-AMB, L-AMB has not been shown superior to fluconazole and typically demonstrates increased side effects.

Extended-spectrum azoles such as itraconazole, voriconazole and posaconazole do possess anti-*Aspergillus* activity (Ashley et al. 2006). Several trials of itraconazole versus fluconazole have been performed and although a meta-analysis showed significantly less IFI, increased side effects, greater drug interactions and poor tolerability have led to itraconazole being abandoned in pediatric patients (Marr et al. 2004; Vardakas et al. 2005). The results of a multicenter, double-blind trial showed that voriconazole was not superior to fluconazole in the prevention of IFI, though the safety profile was similar (Wingard et al. 2010). Given the broader spectrum of activity with voriconazole, this result was surprising, but may have been due to an incomplete understanding of the complex pharmacokinetics of voriconazole and subsequent underdosing. Posaconazole is a triazole with broad coverage of most fungi, including zygomycetes (Ashley et al. 2006). In a randomized, blinded, multicenter trial of AML/MDS patients ≥ 13 years of age with neutropenia, posaconazole prophylaxis was superior to fluconazole or itraconazole in the prevention of IFI (absolute risk reduction -6 %; 95 % CI, -9.7 % to -2.5 %, $p < 0.001$), but was also associated with an increased risk of serious adverse events (6 % vs. 2 %, $p = 0.01$) (Cornely et al. 2007).

Table 14.3 Selected antifungal prophylaxis trials

Prophylaxis	Design	# of patients (# pediatric)	Disease/procedure	Control outcome[a]	Intervention outcome[a]	Reference
Fluconazole	DB, PC, MC	356 (?)[b]	Auto- and allo-HSCT	16 % at 50 days (placebo)	3 % at 50 days	Goodman et al. (1992)
Fluconazole	DB, PC, SC	300 (?)[b]	Auto- and allo-HSCT	18 % at 75 days (placebo)	7 % at 75 days	Slavin et al. (1995)
Amphotericin B	OL, MC	355 (0)	Auto- and allo-HCT	9 % (fluconazole)	14 %	Wolff et al. (2000)
L-AMB	OL Pilot	57 (57)	Allo-HSCT	NA	0 % at 100 days[a]	Roman et al. (2008)
Itraconazole	OL, SC	304 (5)[b]	Allo-HSCT	15 % (fluconazole)	7 %	Marr et al. (2004)
Voriconazole	DB, MC	600 (51)	Allo-HSCT	11 % (fluconazole) at 6 months	7 % at 6 months	Wingard et al. (2010)
Posaconazole	OL, MC	602 (?)[b]	AML/MDS	11 % (fluconazole or itraconazole) at 100 days	5 % at 100 days	Cornely et al. (2007)
Micafungin	DB, MC	882 (84)	Auto- and allo-HSCT	1.6 % (fluconazole) at 70 days	2.4 % at 70 days	van Burik et al. (2004)
Caspofungin	OL, SC	200 (0)	AML/MDS	6 % (itraconazole)	6 %	Mattiuzzi et al. (2006)
Caspofungin	Retrospective	123 (0)	Auto- and allo-HSCT	NA	7.3 % at 100 days	Chou et al. (2007)

DB double-blind, *PC* placebo-controlled, *MC* multicenter, *Auto* autologous, *Allo* allogeneic, *OL* open-label, *SC* single-center, *L-AMB* liposomal amphotericin B, *NA* not applicable, *AML* acute myelogenous leukemia, *MDS* myelodysplastic syndrome

With permission from Dvorak et al. (2012)

[a]Incidence of probable or proven fungal infection

[b]Only patients >12 years of age were eligible

The echinocandins (i.e., caspofungin, micafungin, anidulafungin) are a novel class of antifungals that target (1,3)-β-ᴅ-glucan synthase and thus interrupt biosynthesis of the glucan polymers that make up fungal cell walls. Because mammalian cells do not possess cell walls, echinocandin administration to patients has resulted in minimal toxicity. Echinocandins possess fungicidal activity against *Candida* spp. (including *Candida krusei* and *Candida glabrata*, which possess significant degrees of fluconazole resistance) and *Pneumocystis jiroveci*, as well as fungistatic activity against *Aspergillus* spp. (Ashley et al. 2006). However, they have limited efficacy against *Candida parapsilosis*. The echinocandins may be superior to fluconazole or amphotericin B for treatment of invasive candidiasis which, when combined with their anti-*Aspergillus* activity and excellent safety profile, makes them an attractive option for antifungal prophylaxis (Mora-Duarte et al. 2002; Reboli et al. 2007). In a prophylactic trial, micafungin demonstrated reduced need for empiric antifungal therapy and an improved safety profile compared to fluconazole (van Burik et al. 2004). However, the number of pediatric subjects enrolled was small ($n=84$), and a reduction in the incidence of proven or probable IFI was not demonstrated. The lack of impact on IFI may have been because the incidence of breakthrough IFI in both groups was very low, likely due to the inclusion of low-risk patients (46 % autologous HSCT recipients) and very few patients undergoing umbilical cord blood transplant (UCBT; $n=30$). Caspofungin has been shown to be at least equivalent to itraconazole in the setting of antifungal prophylaxis for adults with AML/MDS with few adverse events (Mattiuzzi et al. 2006; Chou et al. 2007). Similarly, a randomized, blinded, multicenter study of pediatric patients with persistent febrile neutropenia found comparable tolerability, safety and efficacy between caspofungin and L-AMB (Maertens et al. 2010).

14.3.3 Guideline Recommendations for Antifungal Prophylaxis

Most antifungal prophylaxis guidelines are focused on adults with hematologic malignancies or those undergoing HSCT. The IDSA guidelines recommend patients undergoing allogeneic HSCT or intensive remission induction or salvage-induction chemotherapy for acute leukemia to receive anti-*Candida* agents, with all four azoles, micafungin, and caspofungin as acceptable choices (Freifeld et al. 2011). In patients ≥13 years of age undergoing intensive chemotherapy for AML or MDS, *Aspergillus*-directed prophylaxis with posaconazole should be considered (Freifeld et al. 2011). Conversely, anti-*Aspergillus* agents have not been shown to be beneficial in HSCT recipients unless there is a prior history of IA, anticipated neutropenia (i.e., ANC $<0.5 \times 10^9$/L) for >2 weeks or a prolonged period of neutropenia pre-HSCT (Freifeld et al. 2011). The European Conference on Infections in Leukemia (ECIL) guidelines are also focused on adult patients undergoing induction chemotherapy or allogeneic HSCT (Maertens et al. 2011). For patients with leukemia, the ECIL guidelines consider posaconazole as having the strongest supportive evidence, with aerosolized L-AMB combined with fluconazole, fluconazole alone, itraconazole and low-dose amphotericin B all having lesser support (Maertens et al. 2011). North American pediatric guidelines strongly recommend fluconazole at a dose of 6–12 mg/kg/day (maximum 400 mg/day) for children with AML/MDS and suggest that posaconazole 200 mg three times daily is an alternative in children ≥13 years of age in settings with a high local incidence of mold infection (Science et al. 2014). In contrast, pediatric ECIL guidelines suggest either posaconazole in children ≥13 years or itraconazole in those >2 years as a recommendation with moderate evidence in patients with high-risk ALL, AML or relapsed leukemia (Groll et al. 2014).

14.3.4 Limitations of Current Options for Antifungal Prophylaxis

The current options for antifungal prophylaxis all have certain limitations: fluconazole is generally well tolerated, but has a limited spectrum of activity that does not include invasive molds; itraconazole is poorly tolerated due to gastrointestinal side effects; voriconazole, though an attractive option in children >12 years of age (age of most trial data), has questionable standard dosing regimens and multiple drug interactions; posaconazole lacks pharmacokinetic data in children <13 years of age, lacks an intravenous formulation, has unreliable absorption in the setting of limited oral intake, and shares many of the same enzymatic pathways and therefore drug interactions as voriconazole; and finally, echinocandins are expensive and lack an available oral formulation.

For voriconazole in particular, relatively well-established dosing regimens exist for children and adults although recent studies have questioned these standard dosing regimens and have instead proposed dosing based on serum drug levels although the optimal serum voriconazole level is still uncertain (Smith et al. 2006; Trifilio et al. 2007). Part of this variability may be due to allelic polymorphisms of the gene encoding CYP2C19, which can result in an increase or decrease in voriconazole metabolism (Pascual et al. 2008). In children the situation is further complicated by linear kinetics; the optimal dose may be 7 mg/kg twice daily for children from 2 to 12 years of age, while in children <2 years of age it may be as high as 8.5 mg/kg twice daily (Karlsson et al. 2009; Neely et al. 2010; Shima et al. 2010). Even more recent data has led to a proposed maintenance dose of 8 mg/kg twice daily for all children <12 years of age and for those 12–14 years of age weighing <50 kg (Friberg et al. 2012). Currently there is no universally accepted approach to dosing or monitoring of serum levels. Voriconazole also has significant drug interactions with commonly used agents in pediatric oncology patients: voriconazole is a substrate of CYP2CP (major), 2C19 (major), and 3A4 (minor) and an inhibitor of 2C9 (moderate), 2C19 (weak), and 3A4 (moderate) (Cronin and Chandrasekar 2010). Proton pump inhibitors increase voriconazole levels, while voriconazole increases serum levels and toxicity of corticosteroids, vincristine, imatinib, bortezomib, irinotecan and many other medications (Cronin and Chandrasekar 2010).

14.3.5 Risks of Prophylaxis

In addition to direct toxicities (such as renal or hepatic) and medication interactions (especially with azoles), utilization of an antifungal agent can induce selective pressure and lead to the development of resistant organisms. Resistance of various *Candida* spp. to fluconazole is a well-known phenomenon and recently echinocandin resistance has also been noted (Pfaller et al. 2012). There is also concern that more widespread usage of prophylactic voriconazole has led to more cases of Mucorales infection (Trifilio et al. 2007). Theoretically this may be due to competitive inhibition such that Mucorales will not invade if *Aspergillus* spp. are present, but with voriconazole inhibition of *Aspergillus*, the less common Mucorales will find an opportunity to invade. In vitro data also suggest that voriconazole directly increases the virulence of zygomycetes (Lamaris et al. 2009).

14.3.6 Biomarkers

The European Organisation for Research and Treatment of Cancer and Mycoses Study Group (EORTC/MSG) has established guidelines to standardize the definitions of proven, probable and possible IFI (De Pauw et al. 2008). However, in practice, the diagnosis of IFI is often difficult because of the lack of specific symptoms and the invasiveness of standard diagnostic tests. Significant attention has been focused on developing noninvasive assays such as galactomannan (GMN) and $(1,3)$-β-D-glucan (BDG) to diagnose IFI and as discussed in Chap. 1. GMN is a polysaccharide cell wall component that is released by *Aspergillus* during growth and BDG is a cell wall polymer found in all fungi except *Cryptococcus* spp. and zygomycetes. Although commercially available kits for detection of both GMN and BDG are approved by the FDA for adults, the role of GMN in diagnosing IFI in the pediatric population remains undefined and data on BDG testing in pediatric patients are extremely limited (Steinbach et al. 2007). Until further research on these and other noninvasive tests is performed, the potential for early diagnosis of IFI in pediatric oncology patients remains elusive.

Table 14.4 Genetic risk factors for development of invasive fungal infection (IFI) following allogeneic hematopoietic stem cell transplant (HSCT)

Infection	Gene	Source	# of HSCTs	Hypothetical mechanism	Reference
IA	TLR1 and TLR6	Host	127	Decreased recognition by phagocytes	Kesh et al. (2005)
IA	IL-10 promoter	Host	105	Less production of IL-10	Seo et al. (2005)
IA	Plasminogen	Host	236	Increased tissue damage and invasion	Zaas et al. (2008)
IA	TLR4	Donor	366	Decreased recognition by phagocytes	Bochud et al. (2008)
IA	Chemokine ligand 10	Donor	139	Less response to IFN-γ, so less Th1 cells	Mezger et al. (2008)
IA	Dectin-1	Both	205	Less production of IFN-γ and IL-10	Cunha et al. (2010)
IFI	MBL	Donor	106	Decreased complement fixation	Granell et al. (2006)
IFI	MASP2	Host	106	Decreased complement fixation	Granell et al. (2006)

IA invasive aspergillosis, *TLR* toll-like receptor, *IL* interleukin, *IFN* interferon, *Th1* T-helper 1, *MBL* mannan-binding lectin, *MASP2 MBL*-associated serine protease
With permission from Dvorak et al. (2012)

14.3.7 Future Directions

The profound lack of data for this patient population have led to a clinical situation where there is no clear agent of choice for patients at high risk of developing an IFI. Because of this, in April 2011 the COG initiated a randomized open-label trial of caspofungin compared to fluconazole to prevent IFI in children undergoing chemotherapy for AML. As noted previously, a number of therapy-induced alterations in host defense have been identified as risk factors for IFI. However, there is also considerable emerging evidence that a genetic component exists in the susceptibility and outcome of IFI for immunocompromised populations. In allogeneic HSCT recipients, several polymorphisms in both host and donor genes appear to significantly predispose patients to IFI (Table 14.4) (Kesh et al. 2005; Seo et al. 2005; Granell et al. 2006; Bochud et al. 2008; Mezger et al. 2008; Zaas et al. 2008; Cunha et al. 2010). Future investigation will likely uncover additional polymorphisms that place immunocompromised hosts at increased risk of IFI. As more details on genetic risk factors emerge and are validated, personalized risk stratification will be improved beyond the current system that only utilizes traditional IFI risk factors. Furthermore, although all such studies to date have been performed in allogeneic HSCT patients, biologically it is rea-

sonable to assume that these polymorphisms will also play a role in the development of IFI during treatment of AML, relapsed ALL, SAA and, potentially, even lower-risk diseases. Current recommendations and evidence grading for prevention of IFI are summarized in Table 14.5.

14.4 Prevention of *Pneumocystis jiroveci* Pneumonia (PCP)

Previously referred to as *Pneumocystis carinii*, the distinct yeastlike fungal species that infects humans is now known as *Pneumocystis jiroveci*, with the classic abbreviation PCP used to refer to pneumocystis pneumonia.

14.4.1 Risk Stratification

Because PCP prophylaxis has been broadly applied in pediatric oncology patients for over 25 years, it is difficult to firmly ascertain the risk factors for PCP infection in the setting of modern chemotherapeutic regimens. Older data suggest that the intensity of chemotherapy, concomitant use of corticosteroids with other chemotherapeutic agents, and possibly craniospinal irradiation were risk factors for PCP infection (Chusid and Heyrman 1978; Harris et al. 1980). Newer data show that children <2 years of

Table 14.5 Graded recommendations for interventions to prevent fungal infections in pediatric oncology patients

	Grade			
	Data from studies of adult or adolescent patients[a]	Data from studies of or including pediatric patients[a]	Comments	References
Antifungal prophylaxis should generally not be utilized for patients with newly diagnosed ALL	0	0		None
Antifungal prophylaxis with fluconazole should be considered for patients undergoing reinduction for relapsed ALL	0	0[b]		None
Antifungal prophylaxis with a minimum of fluconazole can be considered for patients undergoing chemotherapy for AML although pediatric evidence is mixed	1A	1B[b]	Antifungal prophylaxis with an echinocandin or posaconazole can also be considered; there is no accepted dose of posaconazole for children <13 years of age	Mattiuzzi et al. (2006); Cornely et al. (2007); Robenshtok et al. (2007); Lehrnbecher et al. (2009); Sung et al. (2013); Science et al. (2014)
Antifungal prophylaxis should generally not be utilized for patients with solid tumors	0	2B		Science et al. (2014)

ALL acute lymphoblastic leukemia, *AML* acute myelogenous leukemia
[a]Level of evidence per Guyatt et al. (2006); see Preface
[b]Area in urgent need of further investigation

age and, especially, infant HSCT recipients are at highest risk for PCP infection (Kim et al. 2008b).

14.4.2 Approaches to PCP Prophylaxis

PCP reactivation or infection is generally thought preventable in patients with cancer with administration of classical prophylaxis with trimethoprim-sulfamethoxazole (TMP-SMX). However, in the setting of alternative prophylaxis agents or TMP-SMX noncompliance, episodes of PCP do still occur beginning about 2 months following initiation of chemotherapy and continuing through recovery of T-cell functional immunity. TMP acts by interfering with dihydrofolate reductase, inhibiting synthesis of tetrahydrofolic acid and thus nucleic acid synthesis. TMP-SMX administration in conjunction with antifolates for ALL treatment can lead to marrow suppression and may require lowering of chemotherapy doses (Levinsen et al.

2012). The necessary amount of TMP-SMX required to prevent PCP has not been well studied, and a variety of dosing regimens exist, with 2 or 3 days per week administration being the most common (Agrawal et al. 2011). Generally, TMP-SMX is continued for at least 3 months following chemotherapy, though this recommendation is not evidence-based as studies have shown a variable rate of T-cell recovery after chemotherapeutic regimens, potentially dependent on patient age and chemotherapeutic intensity (Mackall et al. 1995; Azuma et al. 1998; Mazur et al. 2006).

In addition to possible bone marrow suppression, many patients have allergies or other reactions to TMP-SMX that induce clinicians to prematurely discontinue its use. However, the optimal second-line prophylactic agent is not well defined and all options appear to be potentially less effective than TMP-SMX. Agents that have been used include oral dapsone, intravenous or inhaled pentamidine and oral atovaquone. Dapsone is inexpensive but has a high incidence of adverse events, especially in patients with glucose-6-phosphate dehydrogenase (G6PD) deficiency (Sangiolo et al. 2005). Intravenous pentamidine every 4 weeks has also been used, though inadequate protection has been noted in children <2 years of age and in those undergoing HSCT, who may require more frequent dosing (Kim et al. 2008b). Aerosolized pentamidine is generally well tolerated other than occasional bronchospasm, but its effectiveness has been questioned and it requires a compliant patient, generally 6 years of age and older (Vasconcelles et al. 2000). Atovaquone is also well tolerated, but absorption can be limited in patients not eating diets containing fatty foods. In vitro, the echinocandin class of antifungal agents appears to have some activity against the cyst form of *P. jiroveci*. To date, no study has evaluated an echinocandin as a solitary prophylactic agent; however, a few case reports have described their potential utility in combination with TMP-SMX for the treatment of PCP (Annaloro et al. 2006; Beltz et al. 2006).

14.4.3 Summary of the Recommendations from Guidelines for PCP Prophylaxis

Perhaps because PCP prophylaxis is near-universal and of little controversy, the IDSA does not have guidelines for PCP prophylaxis in patients receiving chemotherapy. The joint guidelines of the American Society for Blood and Marrow Transplantion (ASBMT), IDSA and others list TMP-SMX as first choice, with dapsone, atovaquone and both forms of pentamidine as acceptable alternatives in pediatric HSCT patients (Tomblyn et al. 2009).

14.4.4 Future Directions

Although questions remain regarding the dosing schedule and toxicities of TMP-SMX as well as the optimal second-line agents, the relative rarity of PCP infection today (except in the setting of medication noncompliance) makes the performance of future prospective trials a daunting endeavor, as the power required to show differ-

ences in outcome would require enormous numbers of patients. In this unique infection, large retrospective analyses may be the only way to obtain useful information on how to standardize approaches to optimal PCP prophylaxis.

14.5 Prevention of Viral Infections

Although significant questions are yet to be answered, the foundation for preventing bacterial and fungal infections has been established. This foundation includes a logical approach of stratifying patients by risk of infection and then instituting prophylactic therapy for high-risk patients. For many reasons, this preventative model cannot be easily adapted to viral pathogens. First, children with cancer are at risk of infection from a wide variety of viruses with various modes of transmission including from close contacts and the surrounding environment or from reactivation within the patient. Second, establishing risk strata that can be generically applied to all viral infections is extremely challenging; host factors, such as prolonged lymphopenia in a well-appearing child with ALL that increases the risk for certain viral infections, are not traditionally considered risk factors and the course of infection can be extremely variable from benign in one immunosuppressed patient to fatal in another. Third, there are limited effective antiviral therapeutic options that can be employed in a prophylactic manner; the few antiviral options that do exist often have activity against specific viruses, thus limiting their impact as broad-spectrum prophylactic options.

Therefore, in order to effectively prevent viral infections, a more comprehensive approach that targets the patient, close contacts of the patient and the patient's environment is necessary. Despite these challenges some important strategies have been developed including preexposure prophylaxis (i.e., vaccination), postexposure passive prophylaxis (i.e., immunoglobulin), chemoprophylaxis, suppressive therapy (i.e., prevention of viral reactivation), hospital infection control practices and anticipatory guidance to be applied in the home or school setting. Here, suppressive therapy, chemoprophylaxis and hospital infection

Table 14.6 Postexposure chemoprophylaxis regimens for influenza in immunocompromised children

Prophylaxis regimen	Comment

First-line therapy options:
  Oseltamivir:
    3–11 months: 3 mg/kg/dose once daily
    1–12 years:
      ≤15 kg: 30 mg once daily
      >15 kg to ≤23 kg: 45 mg once daily
      >23 kg to ≤40 kg: 60 mg once daily
      >40 kg: 75 mg once daily
    >12 years: 75 mg once daily
  Zanamivir:
    ≥5 years: two inhalations (10 mg) once daily
	Therapy to be started within 48 h of exposure and continued for 10 days; seasonal and regional resistance patterns may dictate variation in therapeutic choices; exposed patients who have not received their yearly influenza vaccine should also be administered with the inactivated influenza vaccine

control are discussed while active and passive prophylaxis is discussed in Chap. 16.

14.5.1 Postexposure Chemoprophylaxis

Every viral infection has an incubation period which establishes a window of time during which preventative efforts, if available, may be enacted to avert progression to symptomatic infection. Currently, chemoprophylaxis is routinely employed for influenza exposure. Randomized trials have established the efficacy of antiviral prophylaxis in immunocompetent healthy household contacts of a person with influenza (Hayden et al. 2000; Welliver et al. 2001). Although similar data do not exist for immunocompromised individuals exposed to influenza, it is reasonable to extrapolate the aforementioned studies to support postexposure antiviral prophylaxis in such cases. Based on these data the Advisory Committee on Immunization Practices (ACIP) currently recommends administration of an antiviral regimen after face-to-face exposure with an influenza-infected person. The antiviral therapy should be initiated within 48 h of exposure for optimal benefit and continued for 10 days (Fiore et al. 2011). Neuraminidase inhibitors (i.e., oseltamivir, zanamivir) are typically first-line antiviral prophylactic agents; however, seasonal and regional resistance patterns may vary yearly, necessitating awareness of annual resistance characteristics (Table 14.6).

14.5.2 Suppressive Therapy

Daily suppressive antiviral therapy is an option for preventing some herpesviruses from reactivating during periods of immunosuppression. Given the available antiviral agents, predominant interest regards suppressive therapy for cytomegalovirus (CMV), herpes simplex virus (HSV) and varicella-zoster virus (VZV). Prophylaxis against each of these herpesviruses is primarily discussed in relationship to allogeneic HSCT recipients where the potential for viral reactivation secondary to patient or donor seropositivity is significant.

CMV reactivation disease has been reported in children receiving chemotherapy for malignancy; however, there are no comprehensive data to support a recommendation for universal prophylaxis or preemptive therapy in this patient population (Licciardello et al. 2011). Data from HSCT populations report the efficacy of ganciclovir in preventing CMV reactivation although comparison of prophylaxis to preemptive therapy (i.e., started if a patient becomes positive for CMV on surveillance testing) showed no difference in the rate of progression to CMV disease or death (Goodrich et al. 1993; Winston et al. 1993; Boeckh et al. 1996). Additionally, concern remains in regard to the significant myelosuppression caused by ganciclovir.

Although the mortality risk of HSV reactivation is not as significant as CMV, the high rate of HSV reactivation in adult HSCT recipients and oncology patients prompted early investigations into the benefits of suppressive therapy. Multiple controlled trials in adult seropositive allogeneic HSCT and malignancy patients have revealed the benefits of acyclovir prophylaxis leading to a consensus among various published guidelines of endorsing acyclovir suppressive therapy in these adult populations (Saral et al. 1981, 1983; Anderson et al. 1984; Sullivan et al. 2001; Styczynski et al. 2009; Tomblyn et al. 2009). Unfortunately, there are limited pediatric-specific data to guide decisions on HSV prophylaxis in children. For children receiving chemotherapy for malignancy, it has not been recommended to routinely administer acyclovir prophylaxis but instead to monitor for evidence of breakthrough infection (Licciardello et al. 2011). There are no recommendations to guide therapeutic decisions for pediatric cancer patients suffering from recurrent HSV reactivation. In this scenario it is reasonable to consider acyclovir or valacyclovir suppressive therapy for the period of time that the patient is immunosuppressed. The clinician must balance the benefit of reducing morbidity from HSV reactivation with the side effects of daily suppressive therapy.

Beyond vaccination and passive immunoprophylaxis (see Chap. 16), suppressive therapy with acyclovir has also been explored and found effective to prevent VZV infections, mainly in adult and pediatric HSCT recipients (Boeckh et al. 2006).

No data are available in regard to high-risk pediatric oncology populations.

14.5.3 Future Directions

The available diagnostic modalities to identify viruses far surpass knowledge on preventing acquisition and suppressing reactivation of these viral pathogens in pediatric oncology patients. There remain a paucity of antiviral options for a number of viral pathogens. Even when a reasonable antiviral option exists, there often are limited pediatric-specific data to guide recommendations for prophylactic or preemptive approaches. Efforts to discover improved preventative or suppressive interventions, either through antiviral medications or passive immune therapies, are necessary. As these novel therapeutic interventions become clinically utilized, it is important that pediatric-specific trials be designed so that continued extrapolation from predominantly adult data is no longer required. Recommendations and their evidence basis for suppression of viral infection are summarized in Table 14.7.

Table 14.7 Graded recommendations for chemoprophylaxis for the prevention or suppression of viral infections in pediatric oncology patients

Recommendation	Grade		Comments	Reference
	Data from studies of adult oncology patients[a]	Data from studies of pediatric oncology patients[a]		
Postexposure influenza antiviral prophylaxis should be administered after face-to-face contact with an influenza-infected person	0	0	Recommendation by ACIP based on RCTs in immunocompetent exposed household contacts	Hayden et al. (2000); Welliver et al. (2001)
No data to support either a prophylactic or preemptive approach for CMV reactivation in high-risk pediatric oncology patients	1B	Pediatric patients included in the adult trials	Published guidelines support either a prophylactic or preemptive approach	
Suppressive therapy for patients with a history of HSV can be considered in children with leukemia	1B	Few pediatric patients included in the adult trials	No definitive evidence that daily suppressive therapy is superior in children compared to initiating therapy at the time of breakthrough HSV infection	Saral et al. (1981); Saral et al. (1983); Anderson et al. (1984)

ACIP Advisory Committee on Immunization Practices, *RCT* randomized controlled trial, *CMV* cytomegalovirus, *HSV* herpes simplex virus
[a]Level of evidence per Guyatt et al. (2006); see Preface

14.6 Infection Control Practices

As evidenced by the preceding sections, much of the focus for infection prevention has been on interventions (i.e., antimicrobial prophylaxis, suppressive therapy) aimed at reducing the incidence of specific pathogens. Although these specific interventions are vital in reducing the impact of infection in pediatric oncology patients, such strategies can only account for a minority of pathogens that patients are exposed to in the hospital and community. Therefore, infection control practices should be considered paramount in these vulnerable patients. This section highlights various hospital-based interventions that should be employed to reduce exposures to infectious pathogens. Community- and home-based infection control practices are also important but are outside the scope of this chapter.

14.6.1 Hand Hygiene

Healthcare worker (HCW) compliance with hand hygiene is arguably the most important practice for reducing patient exposures to infectious pathogens. The Centers for Disease Control and Prevention (CDC) and the World Health Organization (WHO) have each endorsed protocols for appropriate hand hygiene (Boyce et al. 2002; WHO 2009). Despite the known benefits of hand hygiene, HCW compliance on oncology wards has been reported to be <60 % (Siegel and Korniewicz 2007). Given recent national focus on hand hygiene compliance, this rate has likely improved; however, anything less than 100 % compliance should be considered unacceptable.

14.6.2 Mandatory Vaccination

Vaccination of family members is an important practice in creating a cocoon of protection against certain vaccine-preventable diseases for immunocompromised patients. HCWs should consider themselves "family members" to inpatients and should be motivated to help establish this cocoon of protection in the hospital setting. Unfortunately, despite the personal benefits of vaccination and potential for some vaccines such as influenza to extend protection to vulnerable patients, HCW compliance with vaccination has been traditionally poor (Feemster et al. 2011). Although mandatory HCW influenza vaccination has been debated, recent data on mandating influenza vaccine for all hospital staff employees support this as an appropriate action plan (Helms and Polgreen 2008; Isaacs and Leask 2008; Feemster et al. 2011).

In addition to influenza, it has been well documented that children with malignancy have a reduction in their humoral and cellular immunities to pertussis during chemotherapy and up to 18 months after chemotherapy completion (Cheng et al. 2010). The recent epidemic increase in cases of pertussis in the United States amplifies the potential for pertussis infection in children with malignancy (Cherry 2012). Because immunity to pertussis after childhood and adolescent vaccination wanes, booster vaccination in adults is necessary and specifically recommended in healthcare personnel (ACIP 2012; Klein et al. 2012). Similar to influenza vaccine, mandatory vaccination of HCWs against pertussis has been successfully employed at a university hospital and should be considered by all medical institutions to extend protection to the vulnerable pediatric oncology population (Weber et al. 2012).

14.6.3 Hospital Isolation Practices

Appropriate isolation of patients diagnosed with a communicable infection or with symptoms consistent with such infection is also pivotal in reducing transmission between patients. A general guideline for isolation precautions has been published by the Healthcare Infection Control Practices Advisory Committee sponsored by the CDC (Siegel et al. 2007). Although this document does not dictate specific isolation practices for each infectious organism, it does serve as a foundation for hospitals to establish their own infection control protocols. Additionally, the guideline briefly discusses isolation practices in immunocompromised patients. In many instances, the application of infection control policies can be consistent across immunocompetent and immunocompromised patient populations. However, in certain circumstances, adapting isolation precautions to children with malignancy or HSCT recipients can be challenging. In 2000, a collaborative effort between the CDC, IDSA and ASBMT resulted in a guideline for infection control practices in HSCT recipients, with a majority of the recommendations based on expert opinion or committee consensus, not specific to pediatric patients, and not focused on patients undergoing chemotherapy for malignancy (CDC et al. 2000). Updated guidelines are warranted so gaps in knowledge can be effectively identified and further investigated. In the meantime, local oncologists are encouraged to interact with their hospital infection control teams in applying isolation guidelines that are most appropriate for their patient populations.

14.6.4 Visitor Screening Policies

In addition to isolation of hospitalized patients with infectious pathogens, visitors should be considered a potential reservoir for infectious organisms, especially in hospital units caring for high-risk patients (Siegel et al. 2007). The aforementioned HSCT-specific infection control guidelines recommend visitors with symptomatic infectious illnesses be restricted from entering the HSCT unit, and a similar approach is reasonable for the oncology ward (Sullivan et al. 2001). In order to identify visitors with such illnesses, hospitals should establish formal visitor screening protocols; however, there is limited evidence to guide the most effective mechanism for such screening. Some hospitals have used passive programs including signs to communicate symptoms of infections to visiting family members and friends, while other hospitals have employed more active surveillance programs that include screening questions administered to visitors prior to hospital entry (Siegel et al. 2007). The effectiveness of either strategy has not been well delineated in the medical literature. While an active surveillance approach would seemingly be more effective, the implementation of such a practice requires trained hospital personnel to be consistently available for screening of all visitors.

Future investigations are necessary to determine an effective visitor screening policy that is feasible to implement.

14.6.5 Work Restriction

Patient visitors are not the only source of community-acquired pathogens. HCWs represent an additional important reservoir from which patients can be exposed to communicable diseases. A survey of HCWs found that 86 % of hospital personnel with a recent upper respiratory infection admitted to providing care after their symptoms had started (LaVela et al. 2007). This misguided dedication to patient care can place pediatric oncology patients at risk for significant morbidity. Guidelines exist that recommend institutions to restrict HCWs with viral upper respiratory symptoms from attending clinical duties for high-risk patients (Bolyard et al. 1998). While it is unlikely that HCWs will restrict themselves, institutions should enact policies that prevent HCWs with such symptoms from coming to work.

14.6.6 Cytomegalovirus (CMV) Status of Transfused Blood Products

Transfusion of platelets or packed red blood cells represents a source for transmission of CMV infection via latent virus in white blood cells that are in the transfusion product (Ziemann et al. 2007). The potential for transmission is of particular concern in CMV-seronegative children presenting for allogeneic HSCT as reactivation of CMV during the posttransplant period can be devastating (Bueno et al. 2002). No data in regard to CMV infection in high-risk pediatric oncology patients are available in the literature. In HSCT patients, transfusion of leukocyte-reduced blood products has been shown to be as safe as transfusion from a CMV-seronegative donor and should be considered standard of care (Bowden et al. 1995; Thiele et al. 2011). See Chap. 2 for a more detailed discussion of this topic.

14.7 Summary

Infection remains a significant contributor to both morbidity and mortality in children with cancer. Because of the difficulty in treating some infections in the setting of a compromised immune system, the importance of safe and effective preventative strategies is paramount. Knowledge from studies performed in adult oncology patients can be informative. However, issues unique to children such as the types of cancer, therapeutic regimens employed, immune system ontogeny, as well as age-related drug metabolism and toxicities underlie the need for pediatric-specific data. A number of studies are underway which will fill some of the current gaps in knowledge. It is anticipated that research into the prevention of infection in children with cancer will ultimately have a significant impact on reducing the burden of disease and improving disease suppression.

References

Abshire TC, Pollock BH, Billett AL et al (2000) Weekly polyethylene glycol conjugated L-asparaginase compared with biweekly dosing produces superior induction remission rates in childhood relapsed acute lymphoblastic leukemia: a Pediatric Oncology Group Study. Blood 96:1709–1715

Advisory Committee on Immunization Practices (2012) Recommended adult immunization schedule: United States. Ann Intern Med 156:211–217

Afzal S, Ethier MC, Dupuis LL et al (2009) Risk factors for infection-related outcomes during induction therapy for childhood acute lymphoblastic leukemia. Pediatr Infect Dis J 28:1064–1068

Agrawal A, Chang P, Feusner J (2011) Twice weekly Pneumocystis jiroveci pneumonia prophylaxis with trimethoprim-sulfamethoxazole in pediatric patients with acute lymphoblastic leukemia. J Pediatr Hematol Oncol 33:e1–e4

Anderson H, Scarffe JH, Sutton RN et al (1984) Oral acyclovir prophylaxis against herpes simplex virus in non-Hodgkin lymphoma and acute lymphoblastic leukaemia patients receiving remission induction chemotherapy. A randomised double blind, placebo controlled trial. Br J Cancer 50:45–49

Annaloro C, Della Volpe A, Usardi P et al (2006) Caspofungin treatment of Pneumocystis pneumonia during conditioning for bone marrow transplantation. Eur J Clin Microbiol Infect Dis 25:52–54

Ashley ES, Lewis R, Lewis JS et al (2006) Pharmacology of systemic antifungal agents. Clin Infect Dis 43:28–39

Azuma E, Nagai M, Qi J et al (1998) CD4+ T-lymphocytopenia in long-term survivors following intensive chemotherapy in childhood cancers. Med Pediatr Oncol 30:40–45

Beltz K, Kramm C, Laws H et al (2006) Combined trimethoprim and caspofungin treatment for severe Pneumocystis jiroveci pneumonia in a five year old boy with acute lymphoblastic leukemia. Klin Padiatr 218:177–179

Bleasdale SC, Trick WE, Gonzalez IM et al (2007) Effectiveness of chlorhexidine bathing to reduce catheter-associated bloodstream infections in medical intensive care unit patients. Arch Intern Med 167:2073–2079

Bochud P-Y, Chien JW, Marr KA et al (2008) Toll-like receptor 4 polymorphisms and aspergillosis in stem-cell transplantation. N Engl J Med 359:1766–1777

Boeckh M, Gooley TA, Myerson D et al (1996) Cytomegalovirus pp 65 antigenemia-guided early treatment with ganciclovir versus ganciclovir at engraftment after allogeneic marrow transplantation: a randomized double-blind study. Blood 88: 4063–4071

Boeckh M, Kim HW, Flowers ME et al (2006) Long-term acyclovir for prevention of varicella zoster virus disease after allogeneic hematopoietic cell transplantation—a randomized double-blind placebo-controlled study. Blood 107:1800–1805

Bolyard EA, Tablan OC, Williams WW et al (1998) Guideline for infection control in healthcare personnel, 1998. Hospital Infection Control Practices Advisory Committee. Infect Control Hosp Epidemiol 19:407–463

Bowden RA, Slichter SJ, Sayers M et al (1995) A comparison of filtered leukocyte-reduced and cytomegalovirus (CMV) seronegative blood products for the prevention of transfusion-associated CMV infection after marrow transplant. Blood 86:3598–3603

Boyce JM, Pittet D (2002) Guideline for hand hygiene in health-care settings. Recommendations of the Healthcare Infection Control Practices Advisory Committee and the HICPAC/SHEA/APIC/IDSA Hand Hygiene Task Force. Soceity for Healthcare Epidemiology of America/Association for Professionals in Infection Control/Infectious Disease Society of America. MMWR Recomm Rep 51:1–45

Bradley JS, Arguedas A, Blumer JL et al (2007) Comparative study of levofloxacin in the treatment of children with community-acquired pneumonia. Pediatr Infect Dis J 26:868–878

Bucaneve G, Micozzi A, Menichetti F et al (2005) Levofloxacin to prevent bacterial infection in patients with cancer and neutropenia. N Engl J Med 353: 977–987

Bueno J, Ramil C, Green M (2002) Current management strategies for the prevention and treatment of cytomegalovirus infection in pediatric transplant recipients. Paediatr Drugs 4:279–290

Burgos A, Zaoutis TE, Dvorak CC et al (2008) Pediatric invasive aspergillosis: a multicenter retrospective analysis of contemporary cases. Pediatrics 121: e1286–e1294

Castagnola E, Boni L, Giacchino M et al (2003) A multicenter, randomized, double blind placebo-controlled trial of amoxicillin/clavulanate for the prophylaxis of fever and infection in neutropenic children with cancer. Pediatr Infect Dis J 22:359–365

Centers for Disease Control and Prevention, Infectious Disease Society of America, American Society of Blood and Marrow Transplantation (2000) Guidelines for preventing opportunistic infections among hematopoietic stem cell transplant recipients. MMWR Recomm Rep 49(1–125):CE1–CE7

Cheng FW, Leung TF, Chan PK et al (2010) Recovery of humoral and cellular immunities to vaccine-preventable infectious diseases in pediatric oncology patients. Pediatr Hematol Oncol 27:195–204

Cherry JD (2012) Epidemic pertussis in 2012–the resurgence of a vaccine-preventable disease. N Engl J Med 367:785–787

Chou L, Lewis R, Ippoliti C et al (2007) Caspofungin as primary antifungal prophylaxis in stem cell transplant recipients. Pharmacotherapy 27:1644–1650

Chusid MJ, Heyrman KA (1978) An outbreak of Pneumocystis carinii pneumonia at a pediatric hospital. Pediatrics 62:1031–1035

Climo MW, Sepkowitz KA, Zuccotti G et al (2009) The effect of daily bathing with chlorhexidine on the acquisition of methicillin-resistant Staphylococcus aureus, vancomycin-resistant Enterococcus, and healthcare-associated bloodstream infections: results of a quasi-experimental multicenter trial. Crit Care Med 37:1858–1865

Cornely OA, Maertens J, Winston DJ et al (2007) Posaconazole vs. fluconazole or itraconazole prophylaxis in patients with neutropenia. N Engl J Med 356:348–359

Creutzig U, Zimmermann M, Reinhardt D et al (2004) Early deaths and treatment-related mortality in children undergoing therapy for acute myeloid leukemia: analysis of the multicenter clinical trials AML-BFM 93 and AML-BFM 98. J Clin Oncol 22:4384–4393

Cronin S, Chandrasekar P (2010) Safety of triazole antifungal drugs in patients with cancer. J Antimicrob Chemother 65:410–416

Cullen M, Steven N, Billingham L et al (2005) Antibacterial prophylaxis after chemotherapy for solid tumors and lymphomas. N Engl J Med 353:988–998

Cunha C, Di Ianni M, Bozza S et al (2010) Dectin-1 Y238X polymorphism associates with susceptibility to invasive aspergillosis in hematopoietic transplantation through impairment of both recipient- and donor-dependent mechanisms of antifungal immunity. Blood 116:5394–5402

De Pauw B, Walsh T, Donnelly J et al (2008) Revised definitions of invasive fungal disease from the European Organization for Research and Treatment of Cancer/ Invasive Fungal Infections Cooperative Group and the National Institute of Allergy and Infectious Diseases Mycoses Study Group (EORTC/MSG) Consensus Group. Clin Infect Dis 46:1813–1821

Dvorak CC, Fisher BT, Sung L et al (2012) Antifungal prophylaxis in pediatric hematology/oncology: new choices and new data. Pediatr Blood Cancer 59:21–26

Etminan M, Forooghian F, Brophy JM et al (2012) Oral fluoroquinolones and the risk of retinal detachment. JAMA 307:1414–1419

Feemster KA, Prasad P, Smith MJ et al (2011) Employee designation and health care worker support of an influenza vaccine mandate at a large pediatric tertiary care hospital. Vaccine 29:1762–1769

Fiore AE, Fry A, Shay D et al (2011) Antiviral agents for the treatment and chemoprophylaxis of influenza – recommendations of the Advisory Committee on Immunization Practices (ACIP). MMWR Recomm Rep 60:1–24

Freifeld A, Bow E, Sepkowitz K et al (2011) Clinical practice guideline for the use of antimicrobial agents in neutropenic patients with cancer: 2010 Update by the Infectious Diseases Society of America. Clin Infect Dis 52:427–431

Friberg L, Ravva P, Karlsson M et al (2012) Integrated population pharmacokinetics of voriconazole in children, adolescents, and adults. Antimicrob Agents Chemother 56:3032–3042

Gafter-Gvili A, Fraser A, Paul M et al (2012) Antibiotic prophylaxis for bacterial infections in afebrile neutropenic patients following chemotherapy. Cochrane Database Syst Rev 1, CD004386

Goodman J, Winston D, Greenfield R et al (1992) A controlled trial of fluconazole to prevent fungal infections in patients undergoing bone marrow transplantation. N Engl J Med 326:845–851

Goodrich JM, Bowden RA, Fisher L et al (1993) Ganciclovir prophylaxis to prevent cytomegalovirus disease after allogeneic marrow transplant. Ann Intern Med 118:173–178

Granell M, Urbano-Ispizua A, Suarez B et al (2006) Mannan-binding lectin pathway deficiencies and invasive fungal infections following allogeneic stem cell transplantation. Exp Hematol 34:1435–1441

Groll A, Kurz M, Schneider W et al (1999) Five-year-survey of invasive aspergillosis in a paediatric cancer centre. Epidemiology, management and long-term survival. Mycoses 42:431–442

Groll AH, Castagnola E, Cesaro S et al (2014) Fourth European Conference on Infections in Leukaemia (ECIL-4): guidelines for diagnosis, prevention, and treatment of invasive fungal diseases in paediatric patients with cancer or allogeneic haemopoietic stem-cell transplantation. Lancet Oncol 15:e327–e340

Guyatt G, Gutterman D, Baumann MH et al (2006) Grading strength of recommendations and quality of evidence in clinical guidelines: report from an American College of Chest Physicians Task Force. Chest 129:174–181

Hampel B, Hullmann R, Schmidt H (1997) Ciprofloxacin in pediatrics: worldwide clinical experience based on compassionate use–safety report. Pediatr Infect Dis J 16:127–129; discussion 60–62

Harris R, McCallister J, Allen S et al (1980) Prevention of pneumocystis pneumonia. Use of continuous sulfamethoxazole-trimethroprim therapy. Am J Dis Child 134:35–38

Hayden FG, Gubareva LV, Monto AS et al (2000) Inhaled zanamivir for the prevention of influenza in families. Zanamivir Family Study Group. N Engl J Med 343:1282–1289

Helms CM, Polgreen PM (2008) Should influenza immunisation be mandatory for healthcare workers? Yes. BMJ 337:a2142

Henrickson KJ, Hoover SM, Kuhn SM et al (2000) Prevention of central venous catheter–related infections and thrombotic events in immunocompromised children by the use of vancomycin/ciprofloxacin/heparin flush solution: a randomized, multicenter, double-blind trial. J Clin Oncol 18:1269–1278

Hersh EM, Bodey GP, Nies BA et al (1965) Causes of death in acute leukemia: a ten-year study of 414 patients from 1954–1963. JAMA 193:105–109

Hughes WT (1971) Fatal infections in childhood leukemia. Am J Dis Child 122:283–287

Isaacs D, Leask J (2008) Should influenza immunisation be mandatory for healthcare workers? No. BMJ 337:a2140

Jick S (1997) Ciprofloxacin safety in a pediatric population. Pediatr Infect Dis J 16:130–133; discussion 3–4, 60–62

Karlsson M, Lutsar I, Milligan P (2009) Population pharmacokinetic analysis of voriconazole plasma concentration data from pediatric studies. Antimicrob Agents Chemother 53:935–944

Kelsey S, Goldman J, McCann S et al (1999) Liposomal amphotericin (AmBisome) in the prophylaxis of fungal infections in neutropenic patients: a randomised, double-blind, placebo-controlled study. Bone Marrow Transplant 23:163–168

Kern WV, Klose K, Jellen-Ritter AS et al (2005) Fluoroquinolone resistance of Escherichia coli at a cancer center: epidemiologic evolution and effects of discontinuing prophylactic fluoroquinolone use in neutropenic patients with leukemia. Eur J Clin Microbiol Infect Dis 24:111–118

Kesh S, Mensah N, Peterlongo P et al (2005) TLR1 and TLR6 polymorphisms are associated with susceptibility to invasive aspergillosis after allogeneic stem cell transplantation. Ann N Y Acad Sci 1062:95–103

Kim J, Smathers SA, Prasad P et al (2008a) Epidemiological features of Clostridium difficile-associated disease among inpatients at children's hospitals in the United States, 2001–2006. Pediatrics 122:1266–1270

Kim S, Dabb A, Glenn D et al (2008b) Intravenous pentamidine is effective as second line Pneumocystis pneumonia prophylaxis in pediatric oncology patients. Pediatr Blood Cancer 50:779–783

Klein NP, Bartlett J, Rowhani-Rahbar A et al (2012) Waning protection after fifth dose of acellular pertussis vaccine in children. N Engl J Med 367:1012–1019

Kurt B, Flynn P, Shenep JL et al (2008) Prophylactic antibiotics reduce morbidity due to septicemia during intensive treatment for pediatric acute myeloid leukemia. Cancer 113:376–382

Lamaris GA, Ben-Ami R, Lewis RE et al (2009) Increased virulence of zygomycetes organisms following exposure to voriconazole: a study involving fly and murine models of zygomycosis. J Infect Dis 199:1399–1406

Landry DL, Gobielle SL, Haessler SD et al (2010) Emergence of gentamicin-resistant bacteremia in hemodialysis patients receiving gentamicin lock catheter prophylaxis. Clin J Am Soc Nephrol 5:1799–1804

LaVela S, Goldstein B, Smith B et al (2007) Working with symptoms of a respiratory infection: staff who care for high-risk individuals. Am J Infect Control 35:448–454

Lawson SE, Harrison G, Richards S et al (2000) The UK experience in treating relapsed childhood acute lymphoblastic leukaemia: a report on the medical research council UKALLR1 study. Br J Haematol 108:531–543

Leahey AM, Bunin NJ, Belasco JB et al (2000) Novel multiagent chemotherapy for bone marrow relapse of pediatric acute lymphoblastic leukemia. Med Pediatr Oncol 34:313–318

Lehrnbecher T, Foster C, Vázquez N et al (1997) Therapy-induced alterations in host defense in children receiving therapy for cancer. J Pediatr Hematol Oncol 19:399–417

Lehrnbecher T, Ethier MC, Zaoutis T et al (2009) International variations in infection supportive care practices for paediatric patients with acute myeloid leukaemia. Br J Haematol 147:125–128

Levinsen M, Shabaneh D, Bohnstedt C et al (2012) Pneumocystis jiroveci pneumonia prophylaxis during maintenance therapy influences methotrexate/6-mercaptopurine dosing but not event-free survival for childhood acute lymphoblastic leukemia. Eur J Haematol 88:78–86

Licciardello M, Pegoraro A, Cesaro S (2011) Prophylaxis and therapy of viral infections in pediatric patients treated for malignancy. Pediatr Rep 3:e5

Locatelli F, Testi AM, Bernardo ME et al (2009) Clofarabine, cyclophosphamide and etoposide as single-course re-induction therapy for children with refractory/multiple relapsed acute lymphoblastic leukaemia. Br J Haematol 147:371–378

Mackall CL, Fleisher TA, Brown MR et al (1995) Age, thymopoiesis, and CD4+ T lymphocyte regeneration after intensive chemotherapy. N Engl J Med 332:143–149

Maertens J, Madero L, Reilly A et al (2010) A randomized, double-blind, multicenter study of caspofungin versus liposomal amphotericin B for empiric antifungal therapy in pediatric patients with persistent fever and neutropenia. Pediatr Infect Dis J 29:415–420

Maertens J, Marchetti O, Herbrecht R et al (2011) European guidelines for antifungal management in leukemia and hematopoietic stem cell transplant recipients: summary of the ECIL 3–2009 update. Bone Marrow Transplant 46:709–718

Majetschak M, Flohe S, Obertacke U et al (1999) Relation of a TNF gene polymorphism to severe sepsis in trauma patients. Ann Surg 230:207–214

Malani P, Bradley S, Little R et al (2001) Trends in species causing fungaemia in a tertiary care medical centre over 12 years. Mycoses 44:446–449

Marr KA, Crippa F, Leisenring W et al (2004) Itraconazole versus fluconazole for prevention of fungal infections in patients receiving allogeneic stem cell transplants. Blood 103:1527–1533

Mattiuzzi G, Estey E, Raad I et al (2003) Liposomal amphotericin B versus the combination of fluconazole and itraconazole as prophylaxis for invasive fungal infections during induction chemotherapy for patients with acute myelogenous leukemia and myelodysplastic syndrome. Cancer 97:450–456

Mattiuzzi G, Alvarado G, Giles F et al (2006) Open-label, randomized comparison of itraconazole versus caspofungin for prophylaxis in patients with hematologic malignancies. Antimicrob Agents Chemother 50:143–147

Mazur B, Szczepański T, Karpe J et al (2006) Decreased numbers of CD4+ T lymphocytes in peripheral blood after treatment of childhood acute lymphoblastic leukemia. Leuk Res 30:33–36

Mezger M, Steffens M, Beyer M et al (2008) Polymorphisms in the chemokine (C-X-C motif) ligand 10 are associated with invasive aspergillosis after allogeneic stem-cell transplantation and influence CXCL10 expression in monocyte-derived dendritic cells. Blood 111:534–536

Mora-Duarte J, Betts R, Rotstein C et al (2002) Comparison of caspofungin and amphotericin B for invasive candidiasis. N Engl J Med 347:2020–2029

National Comprehensive Cancer Network (2008) Practice guidelines in oncology. Prevention and treatment of cancer related infections. www.nccn.org

Neely M, Rushing T, Kovacs A et al (2010) Voriconazole pharmacokinetics and pharmacodynamics in children. Clin Infect Dis 50:27–36

Noel GJ, Bradley JS, Kauffman RE et al (2007) Comparative safety profile of levofloxacin in 2523 children with a focus on four specific musculoskeletal disorders. Pediatr Infect Dis J 26:879–891

Noel GJ, Blumer JL, Pichichero ME et al (2008) A randomized comparative study of levofloxacin versus amoxicillin/clavulanate for treatment of infants and young children with recurrent or persistent acute otitis media. Pediatr Infect Dis J 27:483–489

O'Grady NP, Alexander M, Burns LA et al (2011) Guidelines for the prevention of intravascular catheter-related infections. Clin Infect Dis 52:e162–e193

Oliveira C, Nasr A, Brindle M et al (2012) Ethanol locks to prevent catheter-related bloodstream infections in parenteral nutrition: a meta-analysis. Pediatrics 129:318–329

Owens RC Jr, Ambrose PG (2005) Antimicrobial safety: focus on fluoroquinolones. Clin Infect Dis 41:S144–S157

Pascual A, Calandra T, Bolay S et al (2008) Voriconazole therapeutic drug monitoring in patients with invasive mycoses improves efficacy and safety outcomes. Clin Infect Dis 46:201–211

Penack O, Schwartz S, Martus P et al (2006) Low-dose liposomal amphotericin B in the prevention of invasive fungal infections in patients with prolonged neutropenia: results from a randomized, single-center trial. Ann Oncol 17:1306–1312

Pfaller M, Castanheira M, Lockhart S et al (2012) Frequency of decreased susceptibility and resistance to echinocandins among fluconazole-resistant bloodstream isolates of Candida glabrata. J Clin Microbiol 50:1199–1203

Pizzo PA, Robichaud KJ, Gill FA et al (1979) Duration of empiric antibiotic therapy in granulocytopenic patients with cancer. Am J Med 67:194–200

Pizzo PA, Robichaud KJ, Gill FA et al (1982) Empiric antibiotic and antifungal therapy for cancer patients with prolonged fever and granulocytopenia. Am J Med 72:101–111

Pizzo PA, Robichaud KJ, Edwards BK et al (1983) Oral antibiotic prophylaxis in patients with cancer: a double-blind randomized placebo-controlled trial. J Pediatr 102:125–133

Popovich KJ, Hota B, Hayes R et al (2009) Effectiveness of routine patient cleansing with chlorhexidine gluconate for infection prevention in the medical intensive care unit. Infect Control Hosp Epidemiol 30:959–963

Prabhu RM, Piper KE, Litzow MR et al (2005) Emergence of quinolone resistance among viridans group streptococci isolated from the oropharynx of neutropenic peripheral blood stem cell transplant patients receiving quinolone antimicrobial prophylaxis. Eur J Clin Microbiol Infect Dis 24:832–838

Rabin KR, Smith J, Kozinetz CA (2012) Myelosuppression and infectious complications in children with Down syndrome and acute lymphoblastic leukemia. Pediatr Blood Cancer 58:633–635

Raetz EA, Borowitz MJ, Devidas M et al (2008) Reinduction platform for children with first marrow relapse of acute lymphoblastic Leukemia: A Children's Oncology Group Study[corrected]. J Clin Oncol 26:3971–3978

Razonable RR, Litzow MR, Khaliq Y et al (2002) Bacteremia due to viridans group Streptococci with diminished susceptibility to Levofloxacin among neutropenic patients receiving levofloxacin prophylaxis. Clin Infect Dis 34:1469–1474

Reboli A, Rotstein C, Pappas P et al (2007) Anidulafungin versus fluconazole for invasive candidiasis. N Engl J Med 356:2472–2482

Redmond AO (1997) Risk-benefit experience of ciprofloxacin use in pediatric patients in the United Kingdom. Pediatr Infect Dis J 16:147–149; discussion 60–62

Riley LC, Hann IM, Wheatley K et al (1999) Treatment-related deaths during induction and first remission of acute myeloid leukaemia in children treated on the Tenth Medical Research Council acute myeloid leukaemia trial (MRC AML10). The MCR Childhood Leukaemia Working Party. Br J Haematol 106:436–444

Robenshtok E, Gafter-Gvili A, Goldberg E et al (2007) Antifungal prophylaxis in cancer patients after chemotherapy or hematopoietic stem-cell transplantation:

systematic review and meta-analysis. J Clin Oncol 25:5471–5489

Roman E, Osunkwo I, Militano O et al (2008) Liposomal amphotericin B prophylaxis of invasive mold infections in children post allogeneic stem cell transplantation. Pediatr Blood Cancer 50:325–330

Rosen G, Nielsen K, Glenn S et al (2005) Invasive fungal infections in pediatric oncology patients: 11-year experience at a single institution. J Pediatr Hematol Oncol 27:135–140

Safdar N, Maki DG (2006) Use of vancomycin-containing lock or flush solutions for prevention of bloodstream infection associated with central venous access devices: a meta-analysis of prospective, randomized trials. Clin Infect Dis 43:474–484

Sangiolo D, Storer B, Nash R et al (2005) Toxicity and efficacy of daily dapsone as Pneumocystis jiroveci prophylaxis after hematopoietic stem cell transplantation: a case–control study. Biol Blood Marrow Transplant 11:521–529

Saral R, Burns WH, Laskin OL et al (1981) Acyclovir prophylaxis of herpes-simplex-virus infections. N Engl J Med 305:63–67

Saral R, Ambinder RF, Burns WH et al (1983) Acyclovir prophylaxis against herpes simplex virus infection in patients with leukemia. A randomized, double-blind, placebo-controlled study. Ann Intern Med 99:773–776

Schaad UB (2007) Will fluoroquinolones ever be recommended for common infections in children? Pediatr Infect Dis J 26:865–867

Schimpff S, Satterlee W, Young VM et al (1971) Empiric therapy with carbenicillin and gentamicin for febrile patients with cancer and granulocytopenia. N Engl J Med 284:1061–1065

Schimpff SC, Young VM, Greene WH et al (1972) Origin of infection in acute nonlymphocytic leukemia. Significance of hospital acquisition of potential pathogens. Ann Intern Med 77:707–714

Science M, Robinson PD, MacDonald T et al (2014) Guideline for primary antifungal prophylaxis for pediatric patients with cancer or hematopoietic stem cell transplant recipients. Pediatr Blood Cancer 61:393–400

Seo K, Kim D, Sohn S et al (2005) Protective role of interleukin-10 promoter gene polymorphism in the pathogenesis of invasive pulmonary aspergillosis after allogeneic stem cell transplantation. Bone Marrow Transplant 36:1089–1095

Shima H, Miharu M, Osumi T et al (2010) Differences in voriconazole trough plasma concentrations per oral dosages between children younger and older than 3 years of age. Pediatr Blood Cancer 54:1050–1052

Siegel JD, Rhinehart E, Jackson M et al (2007) 2007 guideline for isolation precautions: preventing transmission of infectious agents in health care settings. Am J Infect Control 35:S65–S164

Siegel JH, Korniewicz DM (2007) Keeping patients safe: an interventional hand hygiene study at an oncology center. Clin J Oncol Nurs 11:643–646

Slavin M, Osborne B, Adams R et al (1995) Efficacy and safety of fluconazole prophylaxis for fungal infections after marrow transplantation–a prospective, randomized, double-blind study. J Infect Dis 171:1545–1552

Smith J, Safdar N, Knasinski V et al (2006) Voriconazole therapeutic drug monitoring. Antimicrob Agents Chemother 50:1570–1572

Steinbach W, Addison R, McLaughlin L et al (2007) Prospective Aspergillus galactomannan antigen testing in pediatric hematopoietic stem cell transplant recipients. Pediatr Infect Dis J 26:558–564

Styczynski J, Reusser P, Einsele H et al (2009) Management of HSV, VZV and EBV infections in patients with hematological malignancies and after SCT: guidelines from the Second European Conference on Infections in Leukemia. Bone Marrow Transplant 43:757–770

Sullivan KM, Dykewicz CA, Longworth DL et al (2001) Preventing opportunistic infections after hematopoietic stem cell transplantation: the Centers for Disease Control and Prevention, Infectious Diseases Society of America, and American Society for Blood and Marrow Transplantation Practice Guidelines and beyond. Hematology Am Soc Hematol Educ Program 392–421

Sung L, Lange BJ, Gerbing RB et al (2007) Microbiologically documented infections and infection-related mortality in children with acute myeloid leukemia. Blood 110:3532–3539

Sung L, Gamis A, Alonzo TA et al (2009) Infections and association with different intensity of chemotherapy in children with acute myeloid leukemia. Cancer 115:1100–1108

Sung L, Aplenc R, Alonzo TA et al (2013) Effectiveness of supportive care measures to reduce infections in pediatric AML: a report from the Children's Oncology Group. Blood 121:3573–3577

Tancrede CH, Andremont AO (1985) Bacterial translocation and gram-negative bacteremia in patients with hematological malignancies. J Infect Dis 152:99–103

Thiele T, Kruger W, Zimmermann K et al (2011) Transmission of cytomegalovirus (CMV) infection by leukoreduced blood products not tested for CMV antibodies: a single-center prospective study in high-risk patients undergoing allogeneic hematopoietic stem cell transplantation (CME). Transfusion 51:2620–2626

Thomson B, Park JR, Felgenhauer J et al (2004) Toxicity and efficacy of intensive chemotherapy for children with acute lymphoblastic leukemia (ALL) after first bone marrow or extramedullary relapse. Pediatr Blood Cancer 43:571–579

Tomblyn M, Chiller T, Einsele H et al (2009a) Guidelines for preventing infectious complications among hematopoietic cell transplant recipients: a global perspective. Preface. Bone Marrow Transplant 44:453–455

Tomblyn M, Chiller T, Einsele H et al (2009b) Guidelines for preventing infectious complications among hematopoietic cell transplant recipients: a global perspective. Biol Blood Marrow Transplant 15:1143–1238

Trifilio S, Singhal S, Williams S et al (2007) Breakthrough fungal infections after allogeneic hematopoietic stem cell transplantation in patients on prophylactic voriconazole. Bone Marrow Transplant 40:451–456 van Burik J, Ratanatharathorn V, Stepan D et al (2004) Micafungin versus fluconazole for prophylaxis against invasive fungal infections during neutropenia in patients undergoing hematopoietic stem cell transplantation. Clin Infect Dis 39:1407–1416

van Eys J, Berry DM, Crist W et al (1987) Effect of trimethoprim/sulfamethoxazole prophylaxis on outcome of childhood lymphocytic leukemia. A Pediatric Oncology Group Study. Cancer 59:19–23

Vardakas K, Michalopoulos A, Falagas M (2005) Fluconazole versus itraconazole for antifungal prophylaxis in neutropenic patients with haematological malignancies: a meta-analysis of randomised-controlled trials. Br J Haematol 131:22–28

Vasconcelles M, Bernardo M, King C et al (2000) Aerosolized pentamidine as pneumocystis prophylaxis after bone marrow transplantation is inferior to other regimens and is associated with decreased survival and an increased risk of other infections. Biol Blood Marrow Transplant 6:35–43

von Baum H, Sigge A, Bommer M et al (2006) Moxifloxacin prophylaxis in neutropenic patients. J Antimicrob Chemother 58:891–894

Weber DJ, Consoli SA, Sickbert-Bennett E et al (2012) Assessment of a mandatory tetanus, diphtheria, and pertussis vaccination requirement on vaccine uptake over time. Infect Control Hosp Epidemiol 33:81–83

Welliver R, Monto AS, Carewicz O et al (2001) Effectiveness of oseltamivir in preventing influenza in household contacts: a randomized controlled trial. JAMA 285:748–754

Wingard JR, Dick J, Charache P et al (1986) Antibiotic-resistant bacteria in surveillance stool cultures of patients with prolonged neutropenia. Antimicrob Agents Chemother 30:435–439

Wingard JR, Carter SL, Walsh TJ et al (2010) Randomized double-blind trial of fluconazole versus voriconazole for prevention of invasive fungal infection (IFI) after allogeneic hematopoietic cell transplantation. Blood 116:5111–5118

Winston D, Ho W, Bartoni K et al (1993) Ganciclovir prophylaxis of cytomegalovirus infection and disease in allogeneic bone marrow transplant recipients. Results of a placebo-controlled, double-blind trial. Ann Intern Med 118:179–184

Wolf J, Shenep JL, Clifford V et al (2013) Ethanol lock therapy in pediatric hematology and oncology. Pediatr Blood Cancer 60:18–25

Wolff S, Fay J, Stevens D et al (2000) Fluconazole vs low-dose amphotericin B for the prevention of fungal infections in patients undergoing bone marrow transplantation: a study of the North American Marrow Transplant Group. Bone Marrow Transplant 25:853–859

Woods WG, Kobrinsky N, Buckley JD et al (1996) Timed-sequential induction therapy improves postremission outcome in acute myeloid leukemia: a report from the Children's Cancer Group. Blood 87:4979–4989

World Health Organization (2009) WHO guidelines on hand hygiene in health care. World Health Organization, Geneva

Yousef AA, Fryer CJ, Chedid FD et al (2004) A pilot study of prophylactic ciprofloxacin during delayed intensification in children with acute lymphoblastic leukemia. Pediatr Blood Cancer 43:637–643

Zaas A, Liao G, Chien J et al (2008) Plasminogen alleles influence susceptibility to invasive aspergillosis. PLoS Genet 4:e1000101

Zaoutis TE, Heydon K, Chu JH et al (2006) Epidemiology, outcomes, and costs of invasive aspergillosis in immunocompromised children in the United States, 2000. Pediatrics 117:e711–e716

Ziemann M, Krueger S, Maier AB et al (2007) High prevalence of cytomegalovirus DNA in plasma samples of blood donors in connection with seroconversion. Transfusion 47:1972–1983

Hematopoietic Growth Factors

15

Anurag K. Agrawal and Jeffrey D. Hord

Contents

Abstract

Several recombinant human hematopoietic growth factors are approved and in clinical use but not all are approved for use in children with cancer. Here we review the evidence-based guidelines for neutrophil stimulating factors granulocyte colony-stimulating factor (G-CSF) and granulocyte-macrophage colony-stimulating factor (GM-CSF) as well as evidence regarding erythropoietins and platelet growth factors interleukin-11 (IL-11) and thrombopoietin (TPO)-receptor agonists. Among these hematopoietic growth factors, only G-CSF and GM-CSF are approved in children with cancer; we review the evidence regarding their use in different clinical scenarios as well as the appropriate timing and dose of therapy. Evidence regarding the current status of the other hematopoietic cytokines in regard to pediatric oncology patients is also reviewed.

A.K. Agrawal, MD
Department of Hematology/Oncology,
Children's Hospital and Research Center Oakland,
Oakland, CA, USA

J.D. Hord, MD (✉)
Pediatric Hematology/Oncology,
Children's Hospital Medical Center of Akron,
One Perkins Square,
Akron, OH 44308, USA
e-mail: jhord@chmca.org

15.1 Introduction

Several recombinant human hematopoietic growth factors are approved and in clinical use but not all are approved for use in children with cancer. Here we review the evidence-based guidelines for neutrophil stimulating factors granulocyte colony-stimulating factor (G-CSF) and granulocyte-macrophage colony-stimulating factor

J. Feusner et al. (eds.), *Supportive Care in Pediatric Oncology:
A Practical Evidence-Based Approach*, Pediatric Oncology,
DOI 10.1007/978-3-662-44317-0_15, © Springer Berlin Heidelberg 2015

(GM-CSF) as well as evidence regarding erythro-poietins and platelet growth factors interleukin-11 (IL-11) and thrombopoietin (TPO)-receptor agonists. Among these hematopoietic growth factors, only G-CSF and GM-CSF are approved in children with cancer; we review the evidence regarding their use in different clinical scenarios as well as the appropriate timing and dose of therapy. Evidence regarding the current status of the other hematopoietic cytokines in regard to pediatric oncology patients is also reviewed.

Multiple excellent reviews of hematopoietic growth factors as well as consensus statements by the American Society of Clinical Oncology (ASCO), American Society of Hematology (ASH) and European Society for Medical Oncology (ESMO) are additionally available in the literature although the ASCO, ASH and ESMO consensus statements are mainly for adult patients (Schaison et al. 1998; Feusner and Hastings 2002; Lehrnbecher and Welte 2002; Smith et al. 2006; Kuter 2007; Rizzo et al. 2010; Schrijvers et al. 2010). The following guidelines should be considered a general framework that must be refined as additional data become available. When no specific recommendations for the use of hematopoietic growth factors exist within a study protocol or the patient is not enrolled in a study, the following graded guidelines may prove useful (Table 15.1).

Table 15.1 Graded recommendations for the utilization of hematopoietic growth factors[a]

Clinical scenario	Recommendation	Level of evidence[b]
Treatment of myelosuppression after chemotherapy (primary prophylaxis)	Consider if risk of neutropenia is ≥20 % or if patient had neutropenia with previous course of chemotherapy	1B
Prevention of febrile neutropenia to avoid delay or dose reduction in subsequent chemotherapy (secondary prophylaxis)	Can be considered in cases where delay or dose reduction is shown to be harmful in treatment outcome	2C
Treatment of neutropenia to prevent infection or with known infection	G-CSF should be given in patients with high-risk neutropenia (i.e., pneumonia, hypotension, multiorgan dysfunction, fungal infection, neutropenia >28 days, bacterial sepsis, age <12 months)	1C
Treatment of myelosuppression with radiation therapy	Can be considered without concomitant chemotherapy and if radiation is not to the mediastinum	1C
Utilization of G-CSF versus GM-CSF for neutropenia	G-CSF should be utilized for neutropenia due to increased efficacy and decreased side effects	1B
Utilization of filgrastim (G-CSF) versus pegfilgrastim	Likely equal efficacy; data are lacking in pediatric patients to routinely recommend pegfilgrastim	2C
Dose of G-CSF to use for neutropenia	Recommended 5 mcg/kg/day; alternative day schedules may be adequate but have not been studied	1A
Route of administration for G-CSF	Subcutaneous is the preferred route	2B
Timing of G-CSF after chemotherapy	Can be started 1–5 days after completion of chemotherapy; data are lacking to distinguish efficacy between starting 1 or 5 days after chemotherapy completion	1B
Timing of G-CSF discontinuation	Stop when post-nadir (i.e., >7–10 days after chemo initiation and ANC >$0.5–1.0 \times 10^9$/L); stop ≥24 h before next chemotherapy cycle	1B
Utilization of EPO for chemotherapy-induced anemia	Can be considered only if there is contraindication to red blood cell transfusion	1C
Utilization of IL-11 for chemotherapy-induced thrombocytopenia	Significant side effects; lack of evidence to recommend	1A
TPO-receptor antagonists for chemotherapy-induced thrombocytopenia	Data are lacking to recommend	1B

[a]See text for full detail
[b]Level of evidence per Guyatt et al. (2006); see Preface

15.2 Granulocyte Colony-Stimulating Factors

Colony-stimulating factors (CSFs) can be non-lineage specific such as IL-3, IL-6, IL-11 and stem cell factor or be restricted to a single lineage such as G-CSF (filgrastim) with neutrophils. Serum levels of CSFs are low unless stimulated by infection or by a reduction in terminally differentiated cells (Lieschke and Burgess 1992). CSF concentration may then be altered by both changes in production and rates of clearance; high neutrophil levels increase CSF clearance (Layton et al. 1989). Normal G-CSF levels are approximately 25 pg/mL with levels ≥1,000 pg/mL seen in response to severe infection (Kawakami et al. 1990). GM-CSF (sargramostim) was the first cytokine approved by the United States Food and Drug Administration (FDA) for stimulation of myelopoiesis in the posttransplant setting and has activity on multiple cell lineages including monocytes and neutrophils. GM-CSF was subsequently followed by G-CSF for both chemotherapy-induced neutropenia and in the posttransplant setting. A longer lasting pegylated form of G-CSF, pegfilgrastim, is FDA approved in adults for stimulation of granulopoiesis after myelosuppressive chemotherapy in nonmyeloid malignancies but is yet to be approved in pediatric patients (Holmes et al. 2002). Limited studies are available on the use of pegfilgrastim in pediatric oncology but it appears effective with a similar side effect profile to G-CSF in solid tumor patients (Wendelin et al. 2005; te Poele et al. 2005; André et al. 2007; Borinstein et al. 2009; Fox et al. 2009; Milano-Bausset et al. 2009; Spunt et al. 2010).

15.2.1 Clinical Usage of Myeloid Growth Factors

Utilization of myeloid CSFs has been reported for the following clinical situations: (1) treatment of myelosuppression after chemotherapy (primary prophylaxis), (2) prevention of febrile neutropenia and delay or dose reduction in subsequent chemotherapy delivery (secondary prophylaxis), (3) treatment of neutropenia to prevent infection,

and (4) treatment of infection with neutropenia. Pediatric guidelines are lacking although reviews and meta-analyses have been published (Lehrnbecher and Welte 2002; Sung et al. 2004; Wittman et al. 2006). Although established for adult oncology patients, guidelines by ASCO, ESMO and the European Organisation for Research and Treatment of Cancer (EORTC) can be generalized to pediatric patients as pediatric data alone are inconclusive (Smith et al. 2006; ESMO 2007; Aapro et al. 2011). Generally, the three sets of adult guidelines are similar, recommending CSFs in patients who are: (1) expected to have a ≥20 % risk of chemotherapy-induced neutropenia, (2) have previously suffered chemotherapy-induced febrile neutropenia and delay or dose reduction in chemotherapy delivery which may affect treatment outcome, and (3) as supportive treatment in patients with high-risk febrile neutropenia, variably defined as >7–10 days of neutropenia with uncontrolled primary disease, hypotension, profound neutropenia (i.e., ANC $<0.1 \times 10^9$/L), sepsis, pneumonia or fungal infection (Smith et al. 2006; ESMO 2007; Aapro et al. 2011).

15.2.1.1 Treatment of Myelosuppression with Chemotherapy Delivery

As stated, adult ASCO, ESMO and EORTC guidelines support the use of CSFs in patients with ≥20 % risk of neutropenia or in patients who have suffered neutropenia in previous courses of chemotherapy. Meta-analyses in pediatric patients by Sung et al. (2004) and Wittman et al. (2006) similarly support this recommendation in pediatric patients. Both found a significant reduction in febrile neutropenia, length of hospital stay and documented infection with prophylactic G-CSF although there was no benefit in infection-related mortality (Sung et al. 2004; Wittman et al. 2006). A meta-analysis by Sasse et al. (2005) in the use of CSFs in pediatric acute lymphoblastic leukemia (ALL) patients similarly found shorter hospital stays and fewer infections with prophylactic CSF use although there was no reduction in duration of neutropenia and no useful information on survival. Sung et al. (2013)

recently analyzed G-CSF prophylaxis in pediatric acute myelogenous leukemia (AML) patients treated on the AAML0531 Children's Oncology Group (COG) study and found a significant reduction in bacterial infection; this contrasts with Lehrnbecher et al. (2007) who reported that although G-CSF significantly reduced time of neutropenia in the AML-BFM 98 trial, there was no decrement in episodes of febrile neutropenia, documented infections, infection-related mortality or 5-year event-free survival. A meta-analysis of AML patients similarly found no benefit of CSF prophylaxis in the prevention of infection (Gurion et al. 2012).

15.2.1.2 Prevention of Febrile Neutropenia, Delay in Chemotherapy Delivery, or Dose Reduction

Adult guidelines recommend consideration for CSFs in patients in which delay in chemotherapy delivery or dose reduction is known to be potentially harmful in treatment outcome (Smith et al. 2006; ESMO 2007; Aapro et al. 2011). Early phase I and II studies in adult patients have shown that reduction in chemotherapy delay can be achieved with G-CSF and GM-CSF (Antman et al. 1988; Bronchud et al. 1989). Pediatric data are unclear although the recently published improved survival in localized Ewing sarcoma patients who received compressed every 2-week therapy with G-CSF support as compared to the standard every 3-week arm implies there are situations in which G-CSF may be beneficial (Womer et al. 2012). Further data are required to make more generalized pediatric recommendations. As a corollary, G-CSF has been analyzed as a method to increase dose intensity since chemotherapeutic effect is directly related to the dose delivered (Bonadonna and Valagussa 1981; Kwak et al. 1990). Multiple pediatric studies have evaluated increased dose intensity with G-CSF support, and although these studies have shown the safety of this method, benefit on outcome has not been delineated (Woods et al. 1993; Kushner et al. 1994; White et al. 1994; Jones et al. 1995; Kushner et al. 1995; Michon et al. 1998; Fernandez et al. 2000; Kushner et al. 2000;

Michel et al. 2000; Saarinen-Pihkala et al. 2000; Alonzo et al. 2002). In the meta-analysis by Sasse et al. (2005) in pediatric ALL patients, CSF usage had no effect on chemotherapy delays.

15.2.1.3 Treatment of Febrile Neutropenia

As described, adult consensus guidelines recommend utilization of CSFs in patients with high-risk neutropenia which is variably defined as neutropenia for >7–10 days, profound neutropenia with ANC $<0.1 \times 10^9$/L, as well as clinical situations including pneumonia, hypotension, sepsis syndrome with multiorgan failure, uncontrolled primary disease and invasive fungal infection (Smith et al. 2006; ESMO 2007; Aapro et al. 2011). In a meta-analysis of randomized controlled trials, Clark et al. (2005) found that the use of CSFs in established febrile neutropenia reduced hospital stay and neutrophil recovery with potential marginal effect on infection-related mortality; no subgroup analysis on patients defined as high-risk could be performed. Limited data exist in pediatric patients: three randomized prospective trials have shown shortened median hospital stays, days of antibiotic use, cost of treatment and a reduction in duration of the febrile neutropenic episode (Riikonen et al. 1994; Mitchell et al. 1997; Ozkaynak et al. 2005). Pediatric consensus guidelines suggest similar parameters for utilization of CSFs in febrile neutropenia as adult guidelines, recommending usage in patients with pneumonia, hypotension, multiorgan dysfunction and fungal infection as well as, potentially, prolonged neutropenia (i.e., >28 days), bacterial sepsis and age <12 months (Schaison et al. 1998; Lehrnbecher and Welte 2002). Although no pediatric study has demonstrated that CSF usage impacts infection-related mortality, reduction in hospital stay and therefore cost are reasonable parameters to support CSF utilization, especially in the high-risk patient.

15.2.1.4 Treatment of Myelosuppression with Radiation Therapy

Adult guidelines recommend avoidance of CSFs during concomitant radiation therapy to the mediastinum due to a noted increased risk of mortality (Smith et al. 2006; ESMO 2007). The ASCO guidelines also warn against the use of CSFs when chemotherapy and radiation therapy are being administered jointly (Smith et al. 2006). No pediatric data are available to make recommendations for these clinical scenarios. The 2002 pediatric guidelines by Lehrnbecher and Welte recommend against G-CSF usage with concomitant chemotherapy and radiation therapy while no mention is made of utilization with radiation therapy alone.

15.2.2 Optimal Administration of Colony-Stimulating Factors

The optimal CSF formulation in pediatric oncology patients as well as the best dosing schedule, route of administration and timing of administration must all be considered when administering CSFs.

15.2.2.1 Comparison of Granulocyte Colony-Stimulating Factor and Granulocyte-Macrophage Colony-Stimulating Factor

GM-CSF is not FDA approved for treating chemotherapy-induced myelosuppression or febrile neutropenia. A meta-analysis of G-CSF and GM-CSF trials for this purpose in adult oncology patients reported a significantly increased rate of fever in patients receiving GM-CSF, a lack of head to head trials between GM-CSF and G-CSF, and GM-CSF being ineffective in reducing febrile neutropenia compared with placebo (Dubois et al. 2004). EORTC adult guidelines recommend filgrastim, pegfilgrastim or lenograstim (not FDA approved) with equipotency; ESMO recommends either filgrastim or pegfilgrastim; and ASCO gives consideration for filgrastim, pegfilgrastim and GM-CSF while cautioning that there is no long-term data with pegfilgrastim and no significant comparative studies between G-CSF and GM-CSF (Smith et al. 2006; ESMO 2007; Aapro et al. 2011). Pediatric data are lacking. Lydaki et al. (1995) randomized a small cohort of pediatric oncology patients to

G-CSF or GM-CSF and found a significant delay in neutrophil recovery in those treated with GM-CSF although this had no bearing on antibiotic usage or mean hospital stay.

15.2.2.2 Optimal Dosing

Adult guidelines recommend dosing of 5 mcg/kg of filgrastim, 100 mcg/kg of pegfilgrastim (max 6 mg) and 250 mcg/m^2 of sargramostim (Smith et al. 2006; ESMO 2007; Aapro et al. 2011). Few pediatric studies are available. Cairo et al. (2001) compared 5 and 10 mcg/kg of G-CSF starting 24 h after intensive chemotherapy for 123 pediatric patients with relapsed or refractory solid tumors and found no significant difference in time to ANC $\geq 1.0 \times 10^9$/L, incidence of infection, febrile days, incidence of hospitalization or overall survival. A small pediatric study comparing 100 mcg/m^2 vs. 250 mcg/m^2 of GM-CSF showed that duration of neutropenia was significantly shortened in the 250 mcg/m^2 arm with a trend toward decreased duration of febrile neutropenia and no noted difference in side effects (Kubota et al. 1995).

15.2.2.3 Route of Administration

Although package inserts for CSFs consider intravenous and subcutaneous administration to be equipotent, adult data have found that 2–4 times dosing is required to achieve equivalent effect when either G-CSF or GM-CSF is given intravenous as compared to subcutaneous (Eguchi et al. 1990; Kaneko et al. 1991; Stute et al. 1995; Honkoop et al. 1996). Adult guidelines all suggest subcutaneous administration for CSFs (Smith et al. 2006; ESMO 2007; Aapro et al. 2011). No pediatric data are available and no mention of route of administration is made in pediatric guidelines (Schaison et al. 1998; Lehrnbecher and Welte 2002). In the pediatric clinical setting, intravenous G-CSF is often used when the patient is admitted while subcutaneous dosing is given when at home with no dose adjustment.

15.2.2.4 Optimal Timing

Pediatric guidelines suggest initiation of CSFs 1–5 days after completion of chemotherapy while adult guidelines suggest 24–72 h (Schaison et al. 1998; Lehrnbecher and Welte 2002; Smith et al. 2006; ESMO 2007; Aapro et al. 2011). Limited adult and pediatric data have both shown that delay in CSF initiation does not lead to significant difference in mean duration of neutropenia, number of hospital days on parenteral antibiotics or number of febrile neutropenic episodes (Ciernik et al. 1999; Hägglund et al. 1999; Lee et al. 1999; Rahiala et al. 1999; Hofmann et al. 2002). Optimal timing for stoppage of CSFs is also poorly studied. Both pediatric and adult guidelines recommend continuing CSFs through the neutrophil nadir, approximately 7–10 days after chemotherapy (Aapro et al. 2011). The ideal ANC threshold for discontinuation of CSFs is unknown with guidelines recommending ANC $>0.5–5 \times 10^9$/L as a potential stopping point (Schaison et al. 1998; Lehrnbecher and Welte 2002; Smith et al. 2006). ESMO guidelines suggest a sufficient and stable recovery with no ANC threshold, although they do state the historical practice of continuing until ANC $>10 \times 10^9$/L is unnecessary (ESMO 2007). The necessity of a daily dosing schedule (i.e., versus every other day or other potential schedules) has not been well studied in the literature and alternative schedules may potentially be equally efficacious at a reduced cost (Djulbegovic et al. 2005). CSFs should be discontinued at least 24 h prior to the initiation of the subsequent chemotherapy cycle due to risk for enhanced myelosuppression by destruction of CSF-stimulated precursors by cell-cycle-specific chemotherapy (Meropol et al. 1992).

15.3 Erythropoietin

Erythropoietin (EPO) is a sialoglycoprotein produced primarily in the cortical region of the kidneys. EPO stimulates the proliferation and terminal differentiation of erythroid precursors in the bone marrow and is specifically stimulated by hypoxic conditions (Krantz 1991; Jelkmann 1992). In addition to effects on proliferation and differentiation, EPO has been shown to modulate apoptosis and increase erythrocyte survival time (Masuda et al. 1999). Additional studies have shown that EPO stimulates the proliferation and migration of endothelial cells in vitro and stimulates the expression of other angiogenic growth factors including vascular endothelial growth factor (VEGF) and placental growth factor (Batra et al. 2003). Recombinant human erythropoietin (rhEPO) was first approved in 1989 for the treatment of anemia associated with chronic kidney disease and subsequently approved for the treatment of chemotherapy-induced anemia in patients with nonmyeloid malignancies. A second EPO-stimulating agent (ESA), darbepoetin alfa, which has a 2–3-fold half-life compared with rhEPO, is also approved by the FDA for adult patients (Zamboni and Stewart 2002). Darbepoetin has undergone a phase I trial in pediatric patients with chemotherapy-induced anemia but is not approved in this population (Blumer et al. 2007).

Multiple adult randomized controlled trials have shown that ESAs increase hemoglobin, reduce red blood cell transfusion requirements and improve quality of life in patients with chemotherapy- or radiation therapy-associated anemia (Bokemeyer 2004; Bohlius et al. 2006). Very limited data exist for pediatric oncology patients and has most recently been summarized by Shankar (2008) (Porter et al. 1996; Csáki et al. 1998; Büyükpamukçu et al 2002; Wagner et al. 2004; Yilmaz et al. 2004; Razzouk et al. 2006; Abdelrazik and Fouda 2007; Çorapcioglu et al. 2008; Durmaz et al. 2011). These studies are generally with small cohorts of patients with a mixture of different pediatric malignancies and utilize variable doses, dose schedules, and routes of administration for rhEPO. The studies all show increased hemoglobin and decreased transfusion requirement as compared to controls. Quality of life data are limited, with only a subset of patients in the largest study showing significant improvement (Razzouk et al. 2006). Data of effect on overall survival between the two groups are not ascertainable due to the small cohorts studied and was only reported in two studies (Wagner et al. 2004; Durmaz et al. 2011).

Two adult trials of rhEPO in breast and head and neck cancer reported in 2003 were concerning for increased mortality rates and increased disease recurrence in the rhEPO treatment arm as compared to controls (Henke et al. 2003; Leyland-Jones 2003). Since that time, multiple meta-analyses have shown that survival may be worsened by utilization of ESAs, possibly secondary to an increased risk of thromboembolic events which may be related to a high hemoglobin goal with rhEPO therapy (Bohlius et al. 2006; Bennett et al. 2008; Bohlius et al. 2009, 2010; Glasby et al. 2010). No pediatric study has reported any case of venous thromboembolism secondary to rhEPO. Concern has also been raised due to the promotion of angiogenic growth factors and expression of antiapoptotic genes by EPO and potential effect on tumor cell growth (Batra et al. 2003; Yasuda et al. 2003). Batra et al. (2003) additionally reported the presence of EPO receptors and expression of EPO on pediatric tumor cells including neuroblastoma, Ewing sarcoma, Wilms tumor, rhabdomyosarcoma, hepatoblastoma, medulloblastoma, ependymoma and astrocytoma. Sartelet et al. (2007) similarly reported increased EPO-R expression on neuroblastoma cell lines, although in vitro they were unable to show increased tumor cell proliferation with exogenous EPO. No study has shown an in vivo effect of ESAs on tumor proliferation and in a recent review Aapro et al. (2012) conclude that current clinical and preclinical data have not shown that ESAs have an effect on disease progression.

Updated 2010 ASH/ASCO guidelines as well as the 2010 ESMO guidelines on the use of ESAs in adult oncology patients recommend a careful weighing of the risks and potential benefits of ESA therapy in patients with hemoglobin <10 g/dL and nonmyeloid malignancies (Rizzo et al. 2010; Schrijvers et al. 2010). Concerns remain in regard to the stimulation of the leukemic clone and therefore ESAs are not recommended in leukemia, especially acute myelogenous leukemia (Takeshita et al. 2000). The combined guidelines recommend that ESAs should be used only in patients currently undergoing chemotherapy and should be used cautiously in patients undergoing therapy with curative intent and in those with risk for thromboembolism (Rizzo et al. 2010;

Schrijvers et al. 2010). Additionally, patients should be monitored and treated for other etiologies of anemia such as iron deficiency and also monitored to ensure that hemoglobin does not increase over 12 g/dL (Glaspy and Cavill 1999; Rizzo et al. 2010; Schrijvers et al. 2010). With the paucity of reported data, similar such guidelines are unavailable in the pediatric literature. For pediatric patients, the French National Cancer Institute concluded that: (1) systematic administration of ESAs is not recommended in pediatric cancer patients with anemia, (2) ESAs can be considered on a case-by-case basis in those patients with a contraindication to red blood cell transfusion, and (3) intravenous ESA use is the preferred method of administration (Marec-Berard et al. 2009). From the adult oncology literature it is unclear if there is potency difference between subcutaneous and intravenous rhEPO administration although studies in adult hemodialysis patients have shown that subcutaneous injection is approximately 30 % more effective (Kaufman et al. 1998; Galliford et al. 2005; Vercaigne et al. 2005). In his editorial response to the French guidelines, Feusner (2009) concurs that evidence is lacking to support ESA use in pediatric oncology patients as their benefit in quality of life and cost-effectiveness in this patient population as well as their potential risks in regard to tumor progression, overall survival and thromboembolism are unclear.

15.4 Platelet Growth Factors

Platelet transfusion remains the only method for treatment of clinically significant thrombocytopenia in pediatric oncology patients. Multiple growth factors have in vitro stimulatory effects on platelet production, but only IL-11, stem cell factor and thrombopoietin (TPO) have shown in vivo benefit (Broudy et al. 1995; Kuter et al. 1999; Kaushansky 2005; Bhatia et al. 2007; Zeuner et al. 2007). Only IL-11 is approved for chemotherapy-induced thrombocytopenia and only in adult patients. TPO-receptor antagonists have been approved for the treatment of adult immune thrombocytopenic purpura (ITP) but as yet have not been found effective for the treatment of chemotherapy-induced thrombocytopenia. Multiple additional agents including IL-1, IL-3, IL-6 and GM-CSF have been attempted and found ineffective, to have unacceptable toxicity or lead to antibody development (O'Shaughnessy et al. 1996; Jones et al. 1999; Miller et al. 1999; Demetri 2001; Farese et al. 2001; Vadhan-Raj et al. 2005).

15.4.1 Interleukin-11

Interleukin-11 stimulates megakaryocyte maturation in addition to effects on bone, chondrocytes, neurons, adipocytes as well as gastrointestinal and bronchial epithelium (Musashi et al. 1991; Teramura et al. 1992; Orazi et al. 1996; Du and Williams 1997). Studies in adult solid tumor patients have shown benefit in platelet count and subsequent need for platelet transfusion with no benefit in patients with AML and no benefit in overall survival (Gordon et al. 1996; Tepler et al. 1996; Isaacs et al. 1997; Vredenburgh et al. 1998; Giles et al. 2005; Cripe et al. 2006; Usuki et al. 2007). Only one study has been conducted in pediatric patients. Cairo et al. (2004) reported on 47 patients with solid tumors who received IL-11 after ifosfamide, carboplatin and etoposide chemotherapy. The study compared results to historic controls and found a decreased median time to platelet recovery and need for platelet transfusion although there were significant noted side effects including the development of IL-11 antibodies, papilledema, periosteal bone changes, cardiomegaly, edema and tachycardia (Cairo et al. 2004).

15.4.2 Thrombopoietin Receptor Agonists

TPO is the primary regulator of megakaryopoiesis and has shown both in vitro and in vivo effects with increase in platelet counts in 5–14 days in normal bone marrow (Kaushansky et al. 1994; Kuter et al. 1994; Kaushansky 1998). Although the original recombinant products, recombinant human TPO and recombinant human megakaryo-

cyte growth and development factor, were shown to increase platelet counts, both were discontinued due to development of platelet-neutralizing antibodies (Li et al. 2001; Basser et al. 2002). Prior to discontinuation, both agents had shown benefits in children and adults with solid tumors with a trend toward decreased platelet transfusion and level of thrombocytopenia; benefit on survival was not reported and important side effects included risk for thromboembolism and dose-dependent thrombocytosis (Basser et al. 1997; Fanucchi et al. 1997; Basser et al. 2000; Vadhan-Raj et al. 2000, 2003; Angiolillo et al. 2005; Muskowitz et al. 2007).

Second-generation TPO-receptor antagonists, notably TPO peptide mimetic romiplostim and non-peptide mimetic eltrombopag, have shown dose-dependent increases in platelet count without the development of neutralizing antibodies and both drugs have been FDA approved for the treatment of ITP in adult patients (Bussel et al. 2006; Andemariam et al. 2007; Bussel et al. 2007; Jenkins et al. 2007; Kuter et al. 2008; Bussel et al. 2009). Two small, randomized, placebo-controlled studies in pediatric patients with ITP have similarly shown benefit with no significant short-term side effects (Bussel et al. 2011; Elafy et al. 2011). No study has been published using second-generation TPO-receptor antagonists in chemotherapy-induced thrombocytopenia (Andemariam et al. 2007). Although longer-term treatment in adult ITP patients has been shown safe, further study on the long-term effect of these agents in pediatric patients, especially in regard to the potential for thrombosis, tumor or leukemic cell growth, development of neutralizing antibodies and increased bone marrow reticulin or collagen deposition, is warranted (Kuter 2007; Gernsheimer 2008; Kuter et al. 2013).

15.5 Summary

Although several recombinant human hematopoietic growth factors are approved and in clinical use for adult patients, only G-CSF and GM-CSF are approved in children with cancer. Pediatric oncology patients have been shown to benefit from CSF usage if there is ≥20 % risk of neutropenia or if neutropenia has occurred with previous courses of chemotherapy. Similarly there is a benefit to CSF utilization in high-risk febrile neutropenia by decreasing the days of neutropenia and the total length of hospitalization although there has been no proven benefit in overall survival. Similarly there is potential benefit of CSFs in dose-intensity regimens such as compressed Ewing sarcoma therapy by preventing delay in chemotherapy delivery. Utilization of erythropoietin is not recommended but may be considered in the patient with a contraindication to red blood cell transfusion. Platelet growth factors should not be utilized in pediatric patients with chemotherapy-induced thrombocytopenia.

References

Aapro MS, Bohlius J, Cameron DA et al (2011) 2010 Update of EORTC Guidelines for the use of granulocyte-colony stimulating factor to reduce the incidence of chemotherapy-induced febrile neutropenia in adult patients with lymphoproliferative disorders and solid tumors. Eur J Cancer 47:8–32

Aapro M, Jeklmann W, Constantinescu SN, Leyland-Jones B (2012) Effects of erythropoietin receptors and erythropoiesis-stimulating agents on disease progression in cancer. Br J Cancer 106:1249–1258

Abdelrazik N, Fouda M (2007) Once weekly recombinant human erythropoietin treatment for cancer-induced anemia in children with acute lymphoblastic leukemia receiving maintenance chemotherapy: a randomized case-controlled study. Hematology 12:533–541

Alonzo TA, Kobrinsky NL, Aledo A et al (2002) Impact of granulocyte colony-stimulating factor use during induction for acute myelogenous leukemia in children: a report from the Children's Cancer Group. J Pediatr Hematol Oncol 24:627–635

Andemariam B, Psaila B, Bussel JB (2007) Novel thrombopoietic agents. Hematology Am Soc Hematol Educ Program 106–113

André N, Kababri ME, Bertrand P et al (2007) Safety and efficacy of pegfilgrastim in children with cancer receiving myelosuppressive chemotherapy. Anticancer Drugs 18:277–281

Angiolillo AL, Davenport V, Bonilla MA et al (2005) A phase I clinical, pharmacologic, and biologic study of thrombopoietin and granulocyte colony-stimulating factor in children receiving ifosfamide, carboplatin, and etoposide chemotherapy for recurrent or refractory solid tumors: a Children's Oncology Group experience. Clin Cancer Res 11:2644–2650

Antman KS, Griffin JD, Elias A et al (1988) Effect of recombinant human granulocyte-macrophage colony-stimulating factor on chemotherapy-induced myelosuppression. N Engl J Med 319:593–598

Basser RL, Rasko JE, Clarke K et al (1997) Randomized, blinded, placebo-controlled phase I trial of pegylated recombinant human megakaryocyte growth and development factor with filgrastim after dose-intensive chemotherapy in patients with advanced cancer. Blood 89:3118–3128

Basser RL, Underhill C, Davis I et al (2000) Enhancement on platelet recovery after myelosuppressive chemotherapy by recombinant human megakaryocyte growth and development factor in patients with advanced cancer. J Clin Oncol 18:2852–2861

Basser RL, O'Flaherty E, Green M et al (2002) Development of pancytopenia with neutralizing antibodies to thrombopoietin after multicycle chemotherapy supported by megakaryocyte growth and development factor. Blood 99:2599–2602

Batra S, Perelman N, Luck LR et al (2003) Pediatric tumor cells express erythropoietin and a functional erythropoietin receptor that promotes angiogenesis and tumor cell survival. Lab Invest 83:1477–1487

Bennett CL, Silver SM, Djulbegovic B et al (2008) Venous thromboembolism and mortality associated with recombinant erythropoietin and darbepoetin administration for the treatment of cancer-associated anemia. JAMA 299:914–924

Bhatia M, Davenport V, Cairo MS (2007) The role of interleukins-11 to prevent chemotherapy-induced thrombocytopenia in patients with solid tumors, lymphoma, acute myeloid leukemia and bone marrow failure syndromes. Leuk Lymphoma 48:9–15

Blumer J, Berg S, Adamson PC et al (2007) Pharmacokinetic evaluation of darbepoetin alfa for the treatment of pediatric patients with chemotherapy-induced anemia. Pediatr Blood Cancer 49:687–693

Bohlius J, Wilson J, Seidenfeld J et al (2006) Recombinant human erythropoietins and cancer patients: updated meta-analysis of 57 studies including 9353 patients. J Natl Cancer Inst 98:708–714

Bohlius J, Schmidlin K, Brillant C et al (2009) Recombinant human erythropoiesis-stimulating agents and mortality in patients with cancer: a meta-analysis of randomized trials. Lancet 373:1532–1542

Bohlius J, Schmidlin K, Brillant C et al (2010) Erythropoietin or darbepoetin for patients with cancer—meta-analysis based on individual patient data. Cochrane Database Syst Rev (3):CD007303

Bokemeyer C (2004) EORTC guidelines for the use of erythropoietic proteins in anaemic patients with cancer. Eur J Cancer 40:2201–2216

Bonadonna G, Valagussa P (1981) Dose-response effect of adjuvant chemotherapy in breast cancer. N Engl J Med 304:10–15

Borinstein SC, Pollard J, Winter L, Hawkins DS (2009) Pegfilgrastim for prevention of chemotherapy-associated neutropenia in pediatric patients with solid tumors. Pediatr Blood Cancer 53:375–378

Bronchud MH, Howell A, Crowther D et al (1989) The use of granulocyte colony-stimulating factor to increase the intensity of treatment with doxorubicin in patients with advanced breast and ovarian cancer. Br J Cancer 60:121–125

Broudy VC, Lin NL, Kaushansky K (1995) Thrombopoietin (c-mpl ligand) acts synergistically with erythropoietin, stem cell factor, and interleukin-11 to enhance murine megakaryocyte colony growth and increases mega-karyocyte ploidy in vitro. Blood 85:1719–1726

Bussel JB, Kuter DJ, George JN et al (2006) AMG 531, a thrombopoiesis-stimulating protein for chronic ITP. N Engl J Med 355:1672–1681

Bussel JB, Cheng G, Saleh MN et al (2007) Eltrombopag for the treatment of chronic idiopathic thrombocytope-nic purpura. N Engl J Med 357:2237–2247

Bussel JB, Kuter DJ, Pullarkat V et al (2009) Safety and efficacy of long-term treatment with romiplostim in thrombocytopenic patients with chronic ITP. Blood 113:2161–2171

Bussel JB, Buchanan GR, Nugent DJ et al (2011) A ran-domized, double-blind study of romiplostim to deter-mine its safety and efficacy in children with immune thrombocytopenia. Blood 118:28–36

Büyükpamukçu M, Varan A, Kutluk T et al (2002) Is epo-etin alfa a treatment option for chemotherapy-related anemia in children? Med Pediatr Oncol 39:455–458

Cairo MS, Shen V, Krailo MD et al (2001) Prospective randomized trial between two doses of granulocyte colony-stimulating factor after ifosfamide, carbopla-tin, and etoposide in children with recurrent or refrac-tory solid tumors: a children's cancer group report. J Pediatr Hematol Oncol 23:30–38

Cairo MS, Davenport V, Bessmertny O et al (2004) Phase I/II dose escalation study of recombinant human inter-leukin-11 following ifosfamide, carboplatin and eto-poside in children, adolescents and young adults with solid tumours or lymphoma: a clinical, haematological and biological study. Br J Haematol 128:49–58

Ciernik IF, Schanz U, Gmür J (1999) Delaying treatment with granulocyte colony-stimulating factor after allo-geneic bone marrow transplantation for hematological malignancies: a prospective randomized trial. Bone Marrow Transplant 24:147–151

Clark OA, Lyman GH, Castro AA et al (2005) Colony-stimulating factors for chemotherapy-induced febrile neutropenia: a meta-analysis of randomized controlled trials. J Clin Oncol 23:4198–4214

Çorapçioglu F, Aksu G, Basar E et al (2008) Recombinant human erythropoietin beta therapy: an effective strat-egy to reduce transfusion requirement in children receiving anticancer therapy. Pediatr Hematol Oncol 25:509–521

Cripe LD, Rader K, Tallman MS et al (2006) Phase II trial of subcutaneous recombinant human interleukin 11 with subcutaneous recombinant human granulocyte-macrophage colony stimulating factor in patients with acute myeloid leukemia (AML) receiving high-dose cytarabine during induction: ECOG 3997. Leuk Res 30:823–827

Csáki C, Ferencz T, Schuler D et al (1998) Recombinant human erythropoietin in the prevention of chemotherapy-induced anaemia in children with malignant solid tumors. Eur J Cancer 34:364–367

Demetri GD (2001) Targeted approaches for the treatment of thrombocytopenia. Oncologist 6:15–23

Djulbegovic B, Frohlich A, Bennett CL (2005) Acting on imperfect evidence: how much regret are we ready to accept? J Clin Oncol 23:6822–6825

Du X, Williams DA (1997) Interleukin-11: review of molecular, cell biology, and clinical use. Blood 89:3897–3908

Dubois RW, Pinto LA, Bernal M et al (2004) Benefits of GM-CSF versus placebo or G-CSF in reducing chemotherapy-induced complications: a systematic review of the literature. Support Care Cancer 2:34–41

Durmaz O, Demirkaya M, Sevinir B (2011) Recombinant human erythropoietin β: the effect of weekly dosing on anemia, quality of life, and long-term outcomes in pediatric cancer patients. Pediatr Hematol Oncol 28:461–468

Eguchi K, Shinkai T, Sasaki Y et al (1990) Subcutaneous administration of recombinant human granulocyte colony-stimulating factor (KRN8601) in intensive chemotherapy in patients with advanced lung cancer. Jpn J Cancer Res 81:1168–1174

Elafy MS, Abdelmaksoud AA, Eltonbary KY (2011) Romiplostim in children with chronic refractory ITP: randomized placebo controlled study. Ann Hematol 90:1341–1344

ESMO Guidelines Working Group, Greil R, Psenak O (2007) Hematopoietic growth factors: ESMO recom-mendations for the application. Ann Oncol 18:ii89–ii91

Fanucchi M, Glapsy J, Crawford J et al (1997) Effects of polyethylene glycol-conjugated recombinant human megakaryocyte growth and development factor on platelet counts after chemotherapy for lung cancer. N Engl J Med 336:404–409

Farese AM, Smith WG, Giri JG et al (2001) Promegapoietin-1a, an engineered chimeric IL-3 and Mpl-L receptor agonist, stimulates hematopoietic recovery in conventional and abbreviated schedules following radiation-induced myelosuppression in non-human primates. Stem Cells 19:329–338

Fernandez MC, Krailo MD, Gerbing RR et al (2000) A phase I dose escalation of combination chemotherapy with granulocyte-macrophage-colony stimulating factor in patients with neuroblastoma. Cancer 88:2838–2844

Feusner J (2009) Guidelines for Epo use in children with cancer. Pediatr Blood Cancer 53:308–309

Feusner J, Hastings C (2002) Recombinant human eryth-ropoietin in pediatric oncology: a review. Med Pediatr Oncol 39:463–468

Fox E, Widemann BC, Hawkins DS et al (2009) Randomized trial and pharmacokinetic study of pegfil-grastim versus filgrastim after dose-intensive chemo-therapy in young adults and children with sarcomas. Clin Cancer Res 15:7361–7367

Galliford JW, Malasana R, Farrington K (2005) Switching from subcutaneous to intravenous erythropoietin α in haemodialysis patients requires a major dose increase. Nephrol Dial Transplant 20:1956–1962

Gernsheimer T (2008) The pathophysiology of ITP revisited: ineffective thrombopoiesis and the emerging role of thrombopoietin receptor agonists in the management of chronic immune thrombocytopenic purpura. Hematology Am Soc Hematol Educ Program 219–226

Giles FJ, Kantarjian HM, Cortes JE et al (2005) Adaptive randomized study of idarubicin and cytarabine alone or with interleukin-11 as induction therapy in patients aged 50 or above with acute myeloid leukemia or high-risk myelodysplastic syndromes. Leuk Res 29:649–652

Glasby J, Crawford J, Vansteenkiste J et al (2010) Erythropoiesis-stimulating agents in oncology: a study-level meta-analysis of survival and other safety outcomes. Br J Cancer 102:301–315

Glaspy J, Cavill I (1999) Role of iron in optimizing responses of anemic cancer patients to erythropoietin. Oncology 13:461–473; discussion 477–478, 483–488

Gordon MS, McCaskill-Stevens WJ, Battiato LA et al (1996) A phase I trial of recombinant human interleukin-11 (neumega rhIL-11 growth factor) in women with breast cancer receiving chemotherapy. Blood 87:3615–3624

Gurion R, Belnik-Plitman Y, Gafter-Gvili A et al (2012) Colony-stimulating factors for prevention and treatment of infectious complications in patients with acute myelogenous leukemia. Cochrane Database Syst Rev (6):CD008238

Guyatt G, Gutterman D, Baumann MH et al (2006) Grading strength of recommendations and quality of evidence in clinical guidelines: report from an American College of Chest Physicians Task Force. Chest 129:174–181

Hägglund H, Ringdén O, Oman S et al (1999) A prospective randomized trial of Filgrastim (r-metHuG-CSF) given at different times after unrelated bone marrow transplantation. Bone Marrow Transplant 24:831–836

Henke M, Laszig R, Rübe C et al (2003) Erythropoietin to treat head and neck cancer patients with anaemia undergoing radiotherapy: randomised, double-blind, placebo-controlled trial. Lancet 362:1255–1260

Hofmann WK, Seipelt G, Langerhan S et al (2002) Prospective randomized trial to evaluate two delayed granulocyte colony stimulating factor administration schedules after high-dose cytarabine therapy in adult patients with acute lymphoblastic leukemia. Ann Hematol 81:570–574

Holmes FA, O'Shaughnessy JA, Vukelja S et al (2002) Blinded, randomized, multicenter study to evaluate single administration pegfilgrastim once per cycle versus daily filgrastim as an adjunct to chemotherapy in patients with high-risk stage II or stage III/IV breast cancer. J Clin Oncol 20:727–731

Honkoop AH, Hoekman K, Wagstaff J et al (1996) Continuous infusion or subcutaneous injection of granulocyte-macrophage colony-stimulating factor: increased efficacy and reduced toxicity when given subcutaneously. Br J Cancer 74:1132–1136

Isaacs C, Robert NJ, Bailey FA et al (1997) Randomized placebo-controlled study of recombinant human interleukin-11 to prevent chemotherapy-induced thrombocytopenia in patients with breast cancer receiving dose-intensive cyclophosphamide and doxorubicin. J Clin Oncol 15:3368–3377

Jelkmann W (1992) Erythropoietin: structure, control of production, and function. Physiol Rev 72:449–489

Jenkins JM, Williams D, Deng Y et al (2007) Phase I clinical study of eltrombopag, an oral, nonpeptide thrombopoietin receptor agonist. Blood 109:4739–4741

Jones CA, Shaw PJ, Stevens MM (1995) Use of granulocyte colony stimulating factor to reduce the toxicity of super-VAC chemotherapy in advanced solid tumours in childhood. Med Pediatr Oncol 25:84–89

Jones SE, Khandelwal P, McIntyre K et al (1999) Randomized, double-blind, placebo-controlled trial to evaluate the hematopoietic growth factor PIXY321 after moderate-dose fluorouracil, doxorubicin, and cyclophosphamide in stage II and III breast cancer. J Clin Oncol 17:3025–3032

Kaneko T, Takaku F, Ogawa M (1991) Outline of clinical studies on recombinant human granulocyte colony stimulating factor (KRN 8601) in Japan. Tokai J Exp Clin Med 16:51–61

Kaufman JS, Reda DJ, Fye CL et al (1998) Subcutaneous compared with intravenous epoetin in patients receiving hemodialysis. Department of Veterans Affairs Cooperative Study Group on Erythropoietin in Hemodialysis Patients. N Engl J Med 339:578–583

Kaushansky K (1998) Thrombopoietin. N Engl J Med 339:746–754

Kaushansky K (2005) The molecular mechanisms that control thrombopoiesis. J Clin Invest 115:3339–3347

Kaushansky K, Lok K, Holly RD et al (1994) Promotion of megakaryocyte progenitor expansion and differentiation by the c-Mpl ligand thrombopoietin. Nature 369:568–571

Kawakami M, Tsutsumi M, Kumakawa T et al (1990) Levels of serum granulocyte colony-stimulating factor in patients with infections. Blood 76:1962–1964

Krantz SB (1991) Erythropoietin. Blood 77:419–434

Kubota M, Akiyama Y, Mikawa H, Tsutsui T (1995) Comparative effect of 100 versus 250 micrograms/m^2/day of G-CSF in pediatric patients with neutropenia induced by chemotherapy. Pediatr Hematol Oncol 12:393–397

Kushner BH, LaQuaglia MP, Bonilla MA et al (1994) Highly effective induction therapy for stage 4 neuroblastoma in children over 1 year of age. J Clin Oncol 12:2607–2613

Kushner BH, Meyers PA, Gerald WL et al (1995) Very-high-dose short-term chemotherapy for poor-risk peripheral primitive neuroectodermal tumors, including Ewing's sarcoma, in children and young adults. J Clin Oncol 13:2796–2804

Kushner BH, Heller G, Kramer K et al (2000) Granulocyte-colony stimulating factor and multiple cycles of strongly myelosuppressive alkylator-based combination chemotherapy in children with neuroblastoma. Cancer 89:2122–2130

Kuter DJ (2007) New thrombopoietic growth factors. Blood 109:4607–4616

Kuter DJ, Beeler DL, Rosenberg RD (1994) The purification of megapoietin: a physiological regulator of megakaryocyte growth and platelet production. Proc Natl Acad Sci U S A 91:11104–11108

Kuter DJ, Cebon J, Harker LA et al (1999) Platelet growth factors: potential impact on transfusion medicine. Transfusion 39:321–332

Kuter DJ, Bussel JB, Lyons RM et al (2008) Efficacy of romiplostim in patients with chronic immune thrombocytopenia purpura: a double-blind randomized controlled trial. Lancet 371:395–403

Kuter DJ, Bussel JB, Newland A et al (2013) Long-term treatment with romiplostim in patients with chronic immune thrombocytopenia: safety and efficacy. Br J Haematol 161:411–423

Kwak LW, Halpern J, Olshen RA et al (1990) Prognostic significance of actual dose intensity in diffuse large-cell lymphoma: results of a tree-structured survival analysis. J Clin Oncol 8:963–977

Layton JE, Hockman H, Sheridan WP et al (1989) Evidence for a novel in vivo control mechanism of granulopoiesis: mature cell-related control of a regulatory growth factor. Blood 74:1303–1307

Lee KH, Lee JH, Choi SJ et al (1999) Randomized comparison of two different schedules of granulocyte colony-stimulating factor administration after allogeneic bone marrow transplantation. Bone Marrow Transplant 24:591–599

Lehrnbecher T, Welte K (2002) Haematopoietic growth factors in children with neutropenia. Br J Haematol 116:28–56

Lehrnbecher T, Zimmermann M, Reinhardt D et al (2007) Prophylactic human granulocyte colony-stimulating factor after induction therapy in pediatric acute myeloid leukemia. Blood 109:936–943

Leyland-Jones B (2003) Breast cancer trial with erythropoietin terminated unexpectedly. Lancet Oncol 4:459–460

Li J, Yang C, Xia Y et al (2001) Thrombocytopenia caused by the development of antibodies to thrombopoietin. Blood 98:3241–3248

Lieschke GJ, Burgess AW (1992) Granulocyte colony-stimulating factor and granulocyte-macrophage colony-stimulating factor (1). N Engl J Med 327:28–35

Lydaki E, Bolonaki E, Staikaki E et al (1995) Efficacy of recombinant human granulocyte colony-stimulating factor and recombinant human granulocyte-macrophage colony-stimulating factor in neutropenic children with malignancies. Pediatr Hematol Oncol 12:551–558

Marec-Berard P, Chastagner P, Kassab-Chahmi D et al (2009) 2007 Standards, Options, and Recommendations: use of erythropoiesis-stimulating agents (ESA: epoetin alfa, epoetin beta, and darbepoetin) for the management of anemia in children with cancer. Pediatr Blood Cancer 53:7–12

Masuda S, Nagao M, Sasaki R (1999) Erythropoietic, neurotrophic, and angiogenic functions of erythropoietin and regulation of erythropoietin production. Int J Hematol 70:1–6

Meropol NJ, Miller LL, Korn EL et al (1992) Severe myelosuppression resulting from concurrent administration of granulocyte colony-stimulating factor and cytotoxic chemotherapy. J Natl Cancer Inst 84:1201–1203

Michel G, Landman-Parker J, Auclerc MF et al (2000) Use of recombinant human granulocyte colony-stimulating factor to increase chemotherapy dose-intensity: a randomized trial in very high-risk childhood acute lymphoblastic leukemia. J Clin Oncol 18:1517–1524

Michon JM, Hartmann O, Bouffet E et al (1998) An open-label, multicentre, randomised phase 2 study of recombinant human granulocyte colony-stimulating factor (filgrastim) as an adjunct to combination chemotherapy in paediatric patients with metastatic neuroblastoma. Eur J Cancer 34:1063–1069

Milano-Bausset E, Gaudart J, Rome A et al (2009) Retrospective comparison of neutropenia in children with Ewing sarcoma treated with chemotherapy and granulocyte colony-stimulating factor (G-CSF) or pegylated G-CSF. Clin Ther 31:2388–2395

Miller LL, Korn EL, Stevens DS et al (1999) Abrogation of the hematological and biological activities of the interleukin-3/granulocyte-macrophage colony-stimulating factor fusion protein PIXY321 by neutralizing anti-PIXY321 antibodies in cancer patients receiving high-dose carboplatin. Blood 93:3250–3258

Mitchell PL, Morland B, Stevens MC et al (1997) Granulocyte colony-stimulating factor in established febrile neutropenia: a randomized study of pediatric patients. J Clin Oncol 15:1163–1170

Musashi M, Yang YC, Paul SR et al (1991) Direct and synergistic effects of interleukin 11 on murine hemopoiesis in culture. Proc Natl Acad Sci U S A 88:765–769

Muskowitz CH, Hamlin PA, Gabrilove J et al (2007) Maintaining the dose intensity of ICE chemotherapy with a thrombopoietic agent, PEG-rHuMGDF, may confer a survival advantage in relapsed and refractory aggressive non-Hodgkin lymphoma. Ann Oncol 18:1842–1850

O'Shaughnessy JA, Tolcher A, Riseberg D et al (1996) Prospective, randomized trial of 5-fluorouracil, leucovorin, doxorubicin, and cyclophosphamide chemotherapy in combination with the interleukin-3/granulocyte-macrophage colony-stimulating factor (GM-CSF) fusion protein (PIXY321) versus GM-CSF in patients with advanced breast cancer. Blood 87:2205–2211

Orazi A, Copper RJ, Tong J et al (1996) Effects of recombinant human interleukin-11 (Neumega rhIL-11 growth factor) on megakaryocytopoiesis in human bone marrow. Exp Hematol 24:1289–1297

Ozkaynak MF, Krailo M, Chen Z et al (2005) Randomized comparison of antibiotics with and without granulocyte colony-stimulating factor in children with chemotherapy-induced febrile neutropenia: a report from the Children's Oncology Group. Pediatr Blood Cancer 45:274–280

Porter JC, Leahey A, Polise K et al (1996) Recombinant human erythropoietin reduces the need for erythrocyte and platelet transfusions in pediatric patients with sarcoma: a randomized, double-blind, placebo-controlled trial. J Pediatr 129:656–660

Rahiala J, Perkkio M, Riikonen P (1999) Prospective and randomized comparison of early versus delayed prophylactic administration of granulocyte colony-stimulating factor (filgrastim) in children with cancer. Med Pediatr Oncol 32:326–330

Razzouk BI, Hord JD, Hockenberry M et al (2006) Double-blind, placebo-controlled study of quality of life, hematologic end points, and safety of weekly epoetin alfa in children with cancer receiving myelosuppressive chemotherapy. J Clin Oncol 24:3583–3589

Riikonen P, Saarinen UM, Mäkipernaa A et al (1994) Recombinant human granulocyte-macrophage colony-stimulating factor in the treatment of febrile neutropenia: a double blind placebo-controlled study in children. Pediatr Infect Dis J 13:197–202

Rizzo JD, Brouwers M, Hurley P et al (2010) American Society of Clinical Oncology/American Society of Hematology clinical practice guideline update on the use of epoetin and darbepoetin in adult patients with cancer. J Clin Oncol 28:4996–5010

Saarinen-Pihkala UM, Lanning M, Perkkiö M et al (2000) Granulocyte-macrophage colony-stimulating factor support in therapy of high-risk acute lymphoblastic leukemia in children. Med Pediatr Oncol 34: 319–327

Sartelet H, Fabre M, Castaing M et al (2007) Expression of erythropoietin and its receptor in neuroblastomas. Cancer 110:1096–1105

Sasse EC, Sasse AD, Brandalise SR et al (2005) Colony-stimulating factors for prevention of myelosuppressive therapy-induced febrile neutropenia in children with acute lymphoblastic leukaemia. Cochrane Database Syst Rev (3):CD004139

Schaison G, Eden OB, Henze G et al (1998) Recommendations on the use of colony-stimulating factors in children: conclusions of a European panel. Eur J Pediatr 157:955–966

Schrijvers D, De Samblanx H, Roila F, ESMO Guidelines Working Group (2010) Erythropoiesis-stimulating agents in the treatment of anaemia in cancer patients: ESMO Clinical Practice Guidelines for use. Ann Oncol 21:v244–v247

Shankar AG (2008) The role of recombinant erythropoietin in childhood cancer. Oncologist 13:157–166

Smith TJ, Khatcheressian J, Lyman GH et al (2006) 2006 update of recommendation for the use of white blood cell growth factors: an evidence–based clinical practice guideline. J Clin Oncol 24:3187–3205

Spunt SL, Irving H, Frost J et al (2010) Phase II, randomized, open-label study of pegfilgrastim-supported VDC/IE chemotherapy in pediatric sarcoma patients. J Clin Oncol 28:1329–1336

Stute N, Furman WL, Schell M et al (1995) Pharmacokinetics of recombinant human granulocyte-macrophage colony-stimulating factor in children after intravenous and subcutaneous administration. J Pharm Sci 84:824–828

Sung L, Nathan PC, Lange B et al (2004) Prophylactic granulocyte colony-stimulating factor and granulocyte-macrophage colony-stimulating factor decrease febrile neutropenia after chemotherapy in children with cancer: a meta-analysis of randomized controlled trials. J Clin Oncol 22:3350–3356

Sung L, Aplenc R, Alonzo TA et al (2013) Effectiveness of supportive care measures to reduce infections in pediatric AML: a report from the Children's Oncology Group. Blood 121:3573–3577

Takeshita A, Shinjo K, Higuchi M et al (2000) Quantitative expression of erythropoietin receptor (EPO-R) on acute leukaemia cells: relationships between the amount of EPO-R and CD phenotypes, in vitro proliferative response, the amount of other cytokine receptors and clinical prognosis. Japan Adult Leukaemia Study Group. Br J Haematol 108:55–63

te Poele E, Kamps W, Tamminga R et al (2005) Pegfilgrastim in pediatric cancer patients. J Pediatr Hematol Oncol 27:627–629

Tepler I, Elias L, Smith JW et al (1996) A randomized placebo-controlled trial of recombinant human interleukin-11 in cancer patients with severe thrombocytopenia due to chemotherapy. Blood 87:3607–3614

Teramura M, Kobayashi S, Hoshino S et al (1992) Interleukin-11 enhances human megakaryocytopoiesis in vitro. Blood 79:327–331

Usuki K, Urabe A, Ikeda Y et al (2007) A multicenter randomized, double-blind, placebo-controlled late-phase II/III study of recombinant human interleukin 11 in acute myelogenous leukemia. Int J Hematol 85:59–69

Vadhan-Raj S, Verschraegen CF, Bueso-Ramos C et al (2000) Recombinant human thrombopoietin attenuates carboplatin-induced severe thrombocytopenia and the need for platelet transfusions in patients with gynecologic cancer. Ann Intern Med 132:364–368

Vadhan-Raj S, Patel S, Bueso-Ramos C et al (2003) Importance of predosing of recombinant human thrombopoietin to reduce chemotherapy-induced early thrombocytopenia. J Clin Oncol 21:3158–3167

Vadhan-Raj S, Cohen V, Bueso-Ramos C (2005) Thrombopoietic growth factors and cytokines. Curr Hematol Rep 4:137–144

Vercaigne LM, Collins DM, Penner SB (2005) Conversion from subcutaneous to intravenous erythropoietin in a hemodialysis population. J Clin Pharmacol 45:895–900

Vredenburgh JJ, Hussein A, Fisher D et al (1998) A randomized trial of recombinant human interleukin-11 following autologous bone marrow transplantation with peripheral blood progenitor cell support in patients with breast cancer. Biol Blood Marrow Transplant 4:134–141

Wagner L, Billups CA, Furman WL et al (2004) Combined use of erythropoietin and granulocyte colony-stimulating factor does not decrease blood transfusion requirements during induction therapy for high-risk neuroblastoma: a randomized controlled trial. J Clin Oncol 22:1886–1893

Wendelin G, Lackner H, Schwinger W et al (2005) Once-per-cycle pegfilgrastim versus daily filgrastim in pediatric patients with Ewing Sarcoma. J Pediatr Hematol Oncol 27:449–451

White L, McCowage G, Kannourakis G et al (1994) Dose-intensive cyclophosphamide with etoposide and vincristine for pediatric solid tumors: a phase I/II pilot study by the Australia and New Zealand Childhood Cancer Study Group. J Clin Oncol 12: 522–531

Wittman B, Horan J, Lyman G (2006) Prophylactic colony-stimulating factors in children receiving myelosuppressive chemotherapy: a meta-analysis of randomized controlled trials. Cancer Treat Rev 32: 289–303

Womer RB, West DC, Krailo MD et al (2012) Randomized controlled trial of interval-compressed chemotherapy for the treatment of localized Ewing sarcoma: a report from the Children's Oncology Group. J Clin Oncol 30:4148–4154

Woods WG, Kobirnsky N, Buckley J et al (1993) Intensively timed induction therapy followed by autologous or allogeneic bone marrow transplantation for children with acute myeloid leukemia or myelodysplastic syndrome: a Children's Cancer Group pilot study. J Clin Oncol 11:1448–1457

Yasuda Y, Fujita Y, Matsuo T et al (2003) Erythropoietin regulates tumour growth of human malignancies. Carcinogenesis 24:1021–1029

Yilmaz D, Çetingül N, Kantar M et al (2004) A single institutional experience: is epoetin alpha effective in anemic children with cancer? Pediatr Hematol Oncol 21:1–8

Zamboni WC, Stewart CE (2002) An overview of the pharmacokinetic disposition of darbepoetin alfa. Pharmacotherapy 22:133S–140S

Zeuner A, Signore M, Martinetti D et al (2007) Chemotherapy-induced thrombocytopenia derives from the selective death of megakaryocyte progenitors and can be rescued by stem cell factor. Cancer Res 67:4767–4773

Immunization Practice in Pediatric Oncology

16

Anurag K. Agrawal

Contents

A.K. Agrawal, MD
Department of Hematology/Oncology,
Children's Hospital and Research Center Oakland,
747 52nd Street, Oakland, CA 94609, USA
e-mail: aagrawal@mail.cho.org

Abstract

The need for vaccination before, during and after chemotherapeutic regimens remains an area of controversy due to the lack of evidence-based guidelines. Although multiple consensus statements and guidelines are available in regard to the timing and necessity of (re)vaccination, these recommendations are variable, leading to significant differences in clinical practice. In this chapter we review the literature in regard to immune status prior to chemotherapy initiation, during chemotherapy and data on immune recovery after completion of therapy for pediatric patients with malignancy. This serves as background for the available evidence on immunization practice prior to, during and after chemotherapy completion. Population-based risk assessment is also a key component of (re)vaccination guidelines; therefore, we review the evidence for active immunization in settings of high disease prevalence. Finally, we review passive and active immunization practice after exposure to disease and vaccination of household contacts.

J. Feusner et al. (eds.), *Supportive Care in Pediatric Oncology:*
A Practical Evidence-Based Approach, Pediatric Oncology,
DOI 10.1007/978-3-662-44317-0_16, © Springer Berlin Heidelberg 2015

16.1 Introduction

The need for vaccination before, during and after chemotherapeutic regimens remains an area of controversy due to the lack of evidence-based guidelines. Although multiple consensus statements and guidelines are available in regard to the timing and necessity of (re)vaccination these recommendations are variable, leading to significant differences in clinical practice (Centers for Disease Control and Prevention 1993; Sung et al. 2001; Royal College of Paediatrics and Child Health 2002; Allen 2007; Esposito et al. 2010a; Ruggiero et al. 2011). Crawford et al. (2010) showed that 39 % of childhood cancer survivors in Australia had no booster vaccinations; they theorize that lack of evidence leads to variability in practice. This was in contrast to a survey in the United Kingdom where stated compliance with reimmunization was 94.3 % (Bate et al. 2010a). No report of practice in the United States can be found in the medical literature.

Although Fioredda et al. argued in 2005 that antibody deficiency to vaccine-preventable diseases was not significantly different in children after chemotherapy as compared to healthy controls, multiple other studies have shown the development of antibody deficiency after commencement of chemotherapy with no resolution over time following the completion of therapy (van der Does-van den Berg et al. 1981; Smith et al. 1995; Feldman et al. 1998; von der Hardt et al. 2000; Nilsson et al. 2002; Reinhardt et al. 2003; Ek et al. 2004; Zignol et al. 2004; Brodtman et al. 2005; Ek et al. 2006; Cheng et al. 2009; Lehrnbecher et al. 2009; Zengin and Sarper 2009; Alavi et al. 2010; Cheng et al. 2010; Paulides et al. 2011; Kwon et al. 2012; Patel et al. 2012; Van Tilburg et al. 2012). A review of such studies was most recently conducted by Esposito et al. (2010a) and van Tilburg et al. (2006). Only two additional studies could be found corroborating the data by Fioredda et al. (Ercan et al. 2005; El-Din et al. 2012).

In this chapter we review the literature in regard to immune status prior to chemotherapy initiation, during chemotherapy, and data on immune recovery after completion of therapy for pediatric patients with malignancy. This serves as background for the available evidence

on immunization practice prior to, during and after chemotherapy completion (Table 16.1). Population-based risk assessment is also a key component of (re)vaccination guidelines; therefore, we review the evidence for active immunization in settings of high disease prevalence. Finally, we review passive and active immunization practice after exposure to disease and vaccination of household contacts.

16.2 Immune Status Prior to Chemotherapy Initiation

Immune status is normal in most cases prior to the commencement of chemotherapeutic regimens except, potentially, in hematologic malignancies that affect lymphocyte and granulocyte number and function and lymphomas which affect peripheral T- and B-lymphocytes.

Nilsson et al. (2002) quantified bone marrow plasma cells in a small number of pediatric acute lymphoblastic leukemia (ALL) patients at diagnosis and found the percentage was significantly decreased compared to healthy controls. In most studies, antibody levels to vaccine-preventable diseases are similar to a healthy population at diagnosis although van Tilburg et al. (2012) showed that children with ALL had tetanus antibody levels statistically lower than a healthy group (Feldman et al. 1998; Reinhardt et al. 2003; Ercan et al. 2005; Zengin and Sarper 2009; Alavi et al. 2010). Data on immune deficiency at diagnosis in lymphoma patients are lacking in the pediatric literature. Studies in adult lymphoma patients have shown lower baseline immunoglobulin levels and decreased lymphocyte stimulation to phytohemagglutinin and concanavalin A compared to controls (Fuks et al. 1976; Biggar et al. 2009).

16.3 Immune Status During Chemotherapy

The decline in immune status with chemotherapy initiation is due to medication effect rather than the underlying malignancy. Moritz et al. (2001) studied T-cell regenerative capacity after ALL induction chemotherapy and found that patients

Table 16.1 Immunization recommendations with chemotherapeutic regimens[a]

	Prior to chemotherapy[b]	During chemotherapy[c]	After chemotherapy completion[c, d]
Diphtheria-tetanus-acellular pertussis		Continuation of primary series during lower-intensity phases of therapy (i.e., ALL in maintenance)	Continuation of primary series; booster 3–6 months after therapy completion in those that finished primary series
Haemophilus influenzae type b		Continuation of primary series during lower-intensity phases of therapy (i.e., ALL in maintenance)	Continuation of primary series; booster 3–6 months after therapy completion in those that finished primary series and <5 years of age
Inactivated poliovirus		Continuation of primary series during lower-intensity phases of therapy (i.e., ALL in maintenance)	Continuation of primary series; booster 3–6 months after therapy completion in those that finished primary series
Pneumococcus		Continuation of primary series during lower-intensity phases of therapy (i.e., ALL in maintenance)	Continuation of primary series; booster 3–6 months after therapy completion in those that finished primary series and <5 years of age
Hepatitis B	Consider starting immunization series in high-risk settings in seronegative[a]	Continuation of primary series during lower-intensity phases of therapy (i.e., ALL in maintenance)	Continuation of primary series; booster 3–6 months after therapy completion in those that finished primary series
Measles-mumps-rubella			Continuation of primary series; booster 3–6 months after therapy completion in those that finished primary series[e]
Varicella		Consider vaccination during lower-intensity phases of therapy (i.e., ALL in maintenance) in high-risk settings[a]	Continuation of primary series; booster 3–6 months after therapy completion in those that finished primary series
Meningococcus			Booster dose for those previously vaccinated; otherwise per routine schedule
Inactivated influenza	Consider if high seasonal incidence	Annually for children ≥6 months of age	Annually for children ≥6 months of age

ALL acute lymphoblastic leukemia
[a]See text for details
[b]Level of evidence 2C per Guyatt et al. (2006); see Preface
[c]Level of evidence 1C per Guyatt et al. (2006); see Preface
[d]Can consider postvaccination titers in less immunogenic vaccines, specifically hepatitis B and varicella
[e]Washout period required after blood products and immunoglobulin therapy; see text for details

were able to regenerate T-cell subsets at this time point. They concluded that the long-lasting T-cell dysfunction seen after the completion of therapy is due to chemotherapy rather than the underlying disease process itself. At least in number, B-lymphocytes are more affected than T-lymphocytes and NK cells during therapy. Studies of children with ALL have found decreased total lymphocyte counts, lymphocyte subsets and immunoglobulin levels as compared to controls with statistically decreased levels in those treated with more intensive protocols compared to standard risk and reduced-intensity groups and with improvement in levels, especially IgG, occurring in the maintenance phase of therapy (Caver et al. 1998; Kostaridou et al. 2004; Luczynski et al. 2004; El-Chennawi et al. 2008; Eyrich et al. 2009; Van Tilburg et al. 2012).

Seroprotection to vaccine-preventable diseases declines significantly during chemotherapy, both for patients with hematologic malignancies and in those with solid tumors (Feldman et al. 1998; Reinhardt et al. 2003; Ek et al. 2004; Zignol et al. 2004; Ek et al. 2006; Zengin and Sarper 2009; Alavi et al. 2010; Kwon et al. 2012; van Tilburg et al. 2012). Comparing ALL regimens with different levels of intensity, van Tilburg et al. (2012) found that antibody levels to diphtheria, tetanus and *Bordetella pertussis* declined sharply during induction and high-dose methotrexate treatment in both groups with this decline continuing at a slower rate through therapy. Decrease in total IgG did not correlate with the level of antibody to vaccine-preventable diseases. By the end of chemotherapy, 90 % of the 41 children had lower levels of antibody compared to population-based norms. Only decline in diphtheria antibody showed a significant difference between the standard and reduced-intensity ALL regimens. On univariate analysis, Zignol et al. (2004) showed that loss of antibody protection correlated with younger patient age, while Paulides et al. (2011) showed the same on multivariate analysis.

16.4 Immune Recovery After Chemotherapy Completion

The pace of immune recovery after the completion of chemotherapy remains poorly quantified and is multifactorial, being related to the underlying malignancy, treatment intensity and age of the patient. Kovacs et al. (2008) analyzed 88

children 1 year after the completion of chemotherapy for malignancies and found that 19 % of leukemia patients and 9 % of solid tumor patients had decrement in at least one immunoglobulin level ($p < 0.001$ in the leukemia patients). At least one marker of cellular immunity was decreased in 42 % of leukemia patients and 29 % of solid tumor patients. Mustafa et al. (1998) similarly found that 1 year after therapy completion, 35 of the 43 studied patients maintained some immunologic abnormality. Patients had rapid normalization of B-lymphocyte numbers while CD4+ T-lymphocytes lagged and lymphocyte stimulation remained low in a subset of patients 9–12 months after therapy completion. IgG levels normalized rapidly while IgA and IgM were slower to recover. The number of abnormalities at 1 year correlated statistically with patient age; the younger the patient the more abnormalities at this time point. Type of malignancy and duration of therapy were not relevant factors in their study. Other studies have similarly shown the rapid pace of recovery for IgG, with IgA being restored more slowly and IgM remaining low for years after therapy completion (de Vaan et al. 1982; Abrahamsson et al. 1995). Azuma et al. (1998) and Mazur et al. (2006) also found that a subset of patients retained low CD4+ counts. This contrasts with others who have shown that immunoglobulin levels and mitogenic response recover by 6 months after therapy completion (Alanko et al. 1992; Abrahamsson et al. 1995; Kantar et al. 2003; Ek et al. 2005; Kosmidis et al. 2008). Mackall et al. (1995) found that younger patients had greater recovery of CD4+ T-lymphocytes at 6 months compared to older patients who persisted with severe depletion. They theorized that thymic production is important in T-lymphocyte regeneration in the younger patients. Although Mustafa et al. (1998) did not show a statistical difference in immune recovery based on underlying malignancy, other studies have shown variable recovery between hematologic malignancies and solid tumors (Alanko et al. 1994, 1995).

In a complex statistical study using principal components analysis, Ek et al. (2011) found that increased treatment intensity led to poorer response to vaccination, even 6 months after therapy completion. Previously their group had shown that patients who received more intensive ALL therapy were significantly less likely to respond to tetanus toxoid after therapy completion (Ek et al. 2006). These results contrast to other studies such as Mustafa et al. (1998) and Ercan et al. (2005). Immune recovery after therapy completion is defined based on antibody seroresponse to vaccine-preventable disease although anamnestic response may occur even with low or absent antibody levels complicating measures of immunity and immune recovery (Banatvala and Van Damme 2003). Yetgin et al. (2007) studied 82 children with ALL who were vaccinated against HBV during maintenance therapy and 87 that were unvaccinated. Although the seroconversion rate was only 35.4 %, the HBV infection rate was significantly decreased as compared to the unvaccinated group (4.8 % vs. 28.7 %). This remained significant when comparing the vaccinated nonresponders with the unvaccinated (7.5 % vs. 28.7 %). On other hand, Ek et al. (2006) studied 31 pediatric patients with ALL and found that antibody avidity to tetanus toxoid and *Haemophilus influenzae* type b (Hib) correlated with antibody levels.

Among the multiple studies that have (re)vaccinated children after chemotherapeutic regimens, the timing of seroresponse is quite variable making generalizations about pace of immune recovery impossible. Some studies have shown a rapid response in all patients while others have shown persistence of immune dysfunction years after therapy completion. Smith et al. (1995), Nilsson et al. (2002) and Brodtman et al. (2005) all studied children with a history of ALL and found that even years after therapy completion some children failed to mount an appropriate postvaccination antibody response. In contrast, other studies have shown a uniform and rapid immune response after therapy completion. Ercan et al. (2005) immunized 21 patients 3–6 months after completion of ALL therapy and found no statistical difference compared with 14 healthy controls for tetanus, diphtheria,

pertussis, measles and mumps antibody response. Lehrnbecher et al. (2009) randomly assigned 24 patients who received non-high-risk treatment for ALL to receive booster vaccination for tetanus, diphtheria, polio and Hib 3, 6 or 9 months after the completion of therapy. Response at these different time points was not significantly different. Cheng et al. (2009) administered three doses of DTP booster vaccination 6, 8 and 10 months post-chemotherapy completion in patients with hematologic malignancies and solid tumors with a 100 % seroresponse rate which was maintained for at least 1 year (the end of the study period).

Most likely, antibody response is imperfect, and a subset of patients will not attain seroprotection even if immunized multiple times well after immune competence should be restored, especially to less immunogenic vaccines such as hepatitis B, measles and rubella. Reinhardt et al. (2003) studied 139 children with malignancies who showed a decline in antibody seropositivity to vaccine-preventable diseases through therapy. Patients were revaccinated 3–5 months after the completion of therapy to measles, mumps, rubella, diphtheria and tetanus. The majority of vaccinees recovered similar levels of seroprotection as was present prior to therapy; on the other hand, 6 of 83 children (7.2 %) did not respond to revaccination. Zignol et al. (2004) studied 192 pediatric oncology patients after the completion of chemotherapy. They found that a subset lost antibody protection to vaccine-preventable diseases. On reimmunization, 12 months after the completion of therapy, 93 % of those revaccinated had an appropriate seroresponse (three did not respond to hepatitis B, one did not respond to measles).

16.5 Defining the Risk from Vaccine-Preventable Diseases

In the setting of impaired immune competence both during therapy and for some time period after the completion of therapy, determining when and whom to (re)vaccinate should be based on population-based assessment to define when the potential benefit of (re)vaccination outweighs the cost, potential lack of seroresponse and risk of immunization (with live virus vaccines).

Many of the studies regarding disease prevalence in children with malignancy from the United States are before routine vaccination campaigns to Hib, *Streptococcus pneumoniae* and varicella. The data from such studies can now be generalized to resource-limited settings in which routine immunization practice to these diseases is not yet in place but more children are being treated for malignancy. Varicella is the best example of change in practice over time due to routine vaccination in the United States and the subsequent protection of the immunocompromised from herd immunity. Over time, the potential risks of live attenuated varicella vaccination during chemotherapy and delay in treatment have begun to outweigh the risk of varicella exposure and disease during chemotherapy. Yet, practice must be based on risk assessment in each particular community.

Risk versus benefit of varicella vaccination during maintenance chemotherapy must be considered with increasing rates of immunization, especially in North America. Caniza et al. (2012) found a 0.057 % mortality from VZV infection, with 70 % of those children dying during the first year of treatment and 1 dying after varicella vaccination. Based on the available data and the need to hold chemotherapy for VZV immunization, they conclude that the benefit of vaccination during maintenance does not outweigh the risks. Although the incidence of varicella in immunocompromised children in the United States has dropped precipitously since the studies by Gershon and Steinberg (1989), outbreaks are still reported. Adler et al. (2008) discuss the dissemination of disease between pediatric oncology patients after an index case in a hospital group housing facility. Interestingly, more than half the children had previously received varicella vaccination. Poulsen et al. (1993) studied Danish children from 1986 to 1991 and found that among 67 children with ALL, 25 were susceptible to VZV and the cumulative risk of varicella exposure was 90 % at 32 months with 5 patients developing varicella during this time period.

Encapsulated bacteremia from Hib and pneumococcus are also exposures that have changed significantly over time. Surveillance reporting for the years 1994–1995 in the United States shows near elimination of invasive Hib disease with routine vaccination; invasive disease among children aged 4 years or younger declined by 98 % since the introduction of Hib conjugate vaccines (Bisgard et al. 1998). Pneumococcal disease has also declined sharply after introduction of the 7-valent conjugate vaccine. Surveillance data from eight children's hospitals in the United States showed a 66 % decline in invasive disease in children ≤24 months of age in 2002 compared with the mean number of annual infections from 1994 to 2000 (Kaplan et al. 2004). How this affects immunocompromised children, especially with the emergence of non-vaccine serotypes and now routine immunization with the 13-valent conjugate vaccine, is unknown.

Over a 6-year study period in a setting without routine pneumococcal vaccination, Meisel et al. (2007) studied the relative risk of invasive pneumococcal disease in pediatric ALL patients as compared to the general population. Eleven of 3,200 patients had invasive pneumococcal disease, 2 at diagnosis, 4 in induction therapy and 5 during maintenance therapy. One patient died of pneumococcal sepsis. The relative risk of invasive pneumococcal disease was 11.4 times the general population, with the highest risk being in those patients 5–9 years of age. Siber (1980) looked at the incidence of infection with *S. pneumoniae* and *H. influenzae* from 1968 to 1977 and found that the majority of episodes of infection occurred during therapy although a small fraction also occurred after therapy completion. Feldman et al. (1990) found eight cases of Hib among 5,288 pediatric cancer patients, a significantly greater incidence than the general population. The majority of Hib infection was in children <4 years, but it was also seen in those >14 years of age. Nevin et al. (2013) recently reported a case of invasive *H. influenzae* in a 7-year-old who was fully immunized prior to ALL therapy but received no additional vaccine doses after chemotherapy completion.

Consensus guidelines from the American Academy of Pediatrics (2012a) still recommend considering vaccination in patients with Hodgkin lymphoma against encapsulated organisms prior to the initiation of chemotherapy, a risk based on studies when splenectomy was a routine part of Hodgkin staging. Donaldson et al. (1978) studied 181 pediatric patients with Hodgkin lymphoma and found that although the risk of any bacterial infection was not different in the splenectomized versus non-splenectomized group, all incidents of encapsulated bacteremia with vaccine-preventable disease (specifically *S. pneumoniae* and *H. influenzae*) occurred in the splenectomized group. Similarly, Chilcote et al. (1976) found that 60 % of infections in splenectomized children treated for Hodgkin lymphoma were due to encapsulated bacteria (pneumococcus in 50 %, hemophilus and meningococcus in 5 % each). The risk of encapsulated bacteremia and necessity of vaccination in Hodgkin lymphoma in the setting where routine splenectomy is no longer practiced are unclear but appear unnecessary. Additionally, it is impractical to delay chemotherapy initiation for vaccine delivery and response in such a context.

In areas of high prevalence, risk of HBV transmission is significant during chemotherapeutic regimens. Sevinir et al. (2003) studied 198 Turkish children with cancer and found 6.0 % became positive for HBsAg during therapy after failing HBV prophylaxis. One patient died of fulminant hepatitis B infection and most subsequently developed chronic disease. Yetgin et al. (2007) reported a similar transmission rate of 7.5 % in Turkish children that failed HBV prophylaxis and a 28.7 % rate in the unvaccinated cohort. Meral et al. (2000) described a 39 % infection rate in Turkish pediatric oncology patients that failed HBV prophylaxis. In an Indian study of pediatric ALL patients, Somjee et al. (1999) reported an HBV infection rate of 43 % even after an intensified HBV vaccination schedule. Finally, in Iraq, Al-Jadiry et al. (2013) recorded a 27.3 % seroconversion rate in children, with decreasing risk in those receiving multiple HBV vaccinations.

Increased risk from influenza is well documented in immunocompromised children. In a study of US associated deaths from influenza in 2003–2004, 5 of the 149 children (3.3 %) with

reportable health status who died were immunocompromised (4 from long-term corticosteroids, 1 from long-term rituximab) (Bhat et al. 2005). Moulik et al. (2013) recently reported on a measles outbreak in an Indian pediatric oncology unit in which 2 of 15 infected children died; those who were previously immunized to measles had milder disease. The risk of disseminated tuberculosis (miliary TB or TB meningitis) in high-prevalence settings and the potential benefit of BCG vaccination after chemotherapeutic regimens are unknown.

16.6 Immunization Practice Prior to Chemotherapy Initiation

Using a population-based risk stratification for vaccine-preventable disease, a more rational approach to vaccination can be employed. The potential benefit of vaccination in high-risk populations prior to the start of chemotherapy is unclear. In a Dutch study of ALL patients, van Tilburg et al. (2012) reported a cohort of patients who recently received booster immunization to tetanus, diphtheria and *B. pertussis*. This recent immunization, however, did not impact the decline in antibody levels with treatment which was not statistically different from those children without recent booster immunization. Thus, it is uncertain what protection, if any, would be afforded by pre-chemotherapy immunizations.

In his review of varicella vaccination practice in immunocompromised children, Levin (2008) discusses the potential to provide varicella vaccination prior to the delivery of chemotherapy in seronegative children in higher-risk populations. Considering that 70 % of the mortality from VZV occurred in the first year of treatment in the report by Caniza et al. (2012) (a window where varicella vaccination is contraindicated), this is a recommendation that deserves further study. Cristófani et al. (1991) administered live attenuated varicella vaccine to pediatric oncology patients on the first day of chemotherapy. Twenty-two children without clinical history of varicella (retrospectively, 13 that were seronegative and 9 that were seropositive) were immunized. No serious adverse events were noted although three patients developed a small number of vesiculopapular lesions. Three of the 13 seronegative children (23 %) failed to seroconvert. As seen by Heath et al. (1987), antibody protection was lost with time; 42 % lost seropositivity by 3 years. Eight of the immunized children (all seroconverters) were exposed to varicella and none developed disease. Of the seven control subjects that were exposed to VZV, four developed symptomatic disease. In their recommendation for pre-chemotherapy immunization for Hodgkin lymphoma patients, the AAP (2012a) mentions that efficacy is increased if vaccination is given 10–14 days prior to the start of chemotherapy; this delay is not always feasible with the urgency of commencing therapy, especially in leukemia patients. Additional randomized controlled trials are required to determine the safety and efficacy of this recommendation in at-risk populations which will be difficult from a feasibility standpoint.

Sinisalo et al. (2007) vaccinated adult patients with chronic lymphocytic leukemia (CLL) and controls to determine response to the 7-valent pneumococcal conjugate vaccine (PCV7) as pneumococcal disease is an important cause of morbidity in this patient population. Response to PCV7 was significantly decreased in the CLL group as compared to controls, although almost all patients that became seropositive were immunized prior to the onset of chemotherapy and subsequent development of hypogammaglobulinemia. In a separate report, Sinisalo et al. (2002) showed a moderate seroresponse rate in adult patients to immunization with Hib. They conclude, as with their study on PCV7, that immunization with Hib should occur prior to the onset of chemotherapy to have the highest seroresponsivity rate.

Many of the studies on HBV vaccination begin with immunization at the time of chemotherapy initiation with variable efficacy (Goyal et al. 1998; Somjee et al. 1999; Meral et al. 2000). Meral et al. (2000) had the highest seroconversion rate (78 %) when giving vaccination at diagnosis and then at months 1, 2 and 12 of therapy in addition to monthly passive immunization during the intensive parts of leukemia therapy. Using the same regimen without the passive immunization, Goyal et al. (1998) showed only a 10.5 % seroconversion rate in 162 pediatric ALL patients. To follow up

their previous study, the same group (Somjee et al. 1999) gave a more intensified regimen with five doses at monthly intervals followed by a booster at 1 year but only showed 19 % seroconversion.

16.7 Recommendations for Vaccination During Chemotherapy

Five of the six cited guidelines on immunization practice come to similar conclusions in regard to immunization with inactivated or killed vaccines during chemotherapy (Centers for Disease Control and Prevention 1993; Sung et al. 2001; Royal College of Paediatrics and Child Health 2002; Allen 2007; Esposito et al. 2010a). All agree that it is reasonable to continue with the primary immunization series during the less intensive parts of therapy (i.e., ALL maintenance) in addition to providing yearly inactivated influenza vaccination (Table 16.1). Among the group, only Esposito et al. (2010a) give consideration to providing varicella vaccination in settings of high exposure risk and lack of universal vaccination. Here we review the evidence for each particular vaccination.

16.7.1 Diphtheria, Tetanus, and Acellular Pertussis

Two studies were found in regard to response to diphtheria-tetanus-pertussis (DTP) during chemotherapy. Ercan et al. (2005) immunized 17 patients with ALL during maintenance chemotherapy and found no statistical difference compared with 14 healthy controls for tetanus and diphtheria antibody response, although pertussis titers were significantly lower. No adverse reactions were seen. Kung et al. (1984) administered DTP vaccination to 27 children during maintenance chemotherapy for various malignancies and found response to at least 1 of the 2 antigens in 26 of the children (only tetanus and diphtheria were measured for response). Based on their findings, they recommended continuing with the primary vaccination series for inactivated or killed vaccines during maintenance therapy.

16.7.2 Pneumococcal Conjugate Vaccine

In areas without routine pneumococcal vaccination, invasive pneumococcal disease remains a potential risk during and after chemotherapy (Meisel et al. 2007). Allen and Weiner (1981) reviewed 40 episodes of sepsis in 28 children with leukemia and lymphoma and found that 35 % of these episodes were secondary to *S. pneumoniae*, the most commonly isolated organism. Interestingly, *S. pneumoniae* was the only organism that caused infection during remission therapy; five of the 40 episodes (12.5 %) were during this time and due to *S. pneumoniae*. Lehrnbecher et al. (2009) studied 53 children treated for ALL and found persistent lack of protection to pneumococcal antigens which was significantly lower than age-matched, unvaccinated, healthy controls up to 9 months after the completion of therapy (the study period).

Protection during chemotherapy from vaccine strains in those with previous immunization is unknown. Patel et al. (2012) studied 42 children with a history of leukemia ≥6 months off of chemotherapy to assess for serotype-specific antibodies to *S. pneumoniae*. None of the subjects were noted to have protective antibody concentrations to pneumococcal conjugate vaccine serotypes. Cheng et al. (2012) administered two doses of PCV7 to 44 pediatric oncology patients, including 20 ALL patients in maintenance. Eighty-six to 100 % of patients obtained seropositivity depending on the pneumococcal serotype. No subgroup analysis was reported to determine if differences in seropositivity occurred with different underlying malignancies or based on timing of vaccination. Beyond patients that have received splenectomy as part of their therapy, there is no indication for immunization with the 23-valent pneumococcal polysaccharide vaccine.

16.7.3 Hemophilus Influenzae Type b

In settings with routine vaccination to Hib, invasive disease has plummeted (Bisgard et al. 1998). Risk still remains though in areas without routine

immunization (Siber 1980; Feldman et al. 1990). Multiple studies have described the effect of Hib conjugate immunization during chemotherapy (Feldman et al. 1990; Kaplan et al. 1992; Shenep et al. 1994; Cheng et al. 2012). Feldman et al. (1990) vaccinated 50 children with Hib; the overall response rate was 50 %. Shenep et al. (1994) studied 50 children with solid tumors who had not previously been vaccinated for Hib. Seroresponse was noted in 42 % after first vaccination and another 45 % responded to a second dose. Kaplan et al. (1992) studied 18 children with malignancy and found a 50 % seroresponse rate to Hib after 1 immunization. One-third of children responded to a second dose. Weisman et al. (1987) studied 27 children with malignancy, 6 of whom had completed therapy to measure response to Hib vaccination. Eighty-five percent of patients had an appropriate response. Solid tumor patients had a 100 % response; there was no difference in response for those off therapy. Of note, all of these studies were done at a time of significantly decreased chemotherapeutic intensity making it unclear as to their generalizability with modern therapeutic protocols.

16.7.4 Inactivated Poliovirus

The risk of polio is negligible due to the near worldwide eradication of the virus. Only one relevant study by Ogra et al. (1971) could be found, comparing antibody response in patients with leukemia, solid tumors and healthy controls. Response in healthy controls and solid tumor patients was similar while those with leukemia had a blunted response. Again, due to the age of this study, the generalizability to modern therapeutic protocols is unknown. Of note, oral poliovirus (OPV) is contraindicated.

16.7.5 Influenza

16.7.5.1 Inactivated Influenza Vaccine
Although in a Cochrane review Goossen et al. (2009) conclude that there is a paucity of well designed randomized controlled trials to define

whether influenza vaccination in children with malignancy during therapy is beneficial considering their blunted response to vaccination, no significant adverse effects were seen in the studies reviewed, and the general consensus is that the benefit of vaccination outweighs cost and any other potential risks, even if seroresponse is blunted (Centers for Disease Control and Prevention 1993; Sung et al. 2001; Royal College of Paediatrics and Child Health 2002; Allen 2007; Esposito et al. 2009, 2010a; Ruggiero et al. 2011; Kersun et al. 2013a).

Multiple small studies have analyzed response to influenza vaccination, mainly during maintenance of ALL therapy and reviewed by Esposito et al. (2009) and Kersun et al. (2013a) (Allison et al. 1977; Sumaya et al. 1977; Ganz et al. 1978; Gross et al. 1978; Smithson et al. 1978; Lange et al. 1979; Schafer et al. 1979; Steinherz et al. 1980; Brydak et al. 1996, 1998; Chisholm et al. 2001; Porter et al. 2004; Matsuzaki et al. 2005; Bektas et al. 2007; Shahgholi et al. 2010; Wong-Chew et al. 2012; Kersun et al. 2013a). In general, the vaccine was well tolerated with no serious adverse side effects. When comparing response for patients receiving chemotherapy versus patients off therapy and healthy controls, rate of seroconversion was lower in patients still receiving therapy. Additionally, response in patients with solid tumors was more similar to patients off therapy and healthy controls. Kersun et al. (2013b) showed that ALL patients vaccinated during induction had an improved response compared to patients receiving the vaccine post-induction or in maintenance. Timing of immunization during an ALL maintenance cycle has not been studied to determine if the rate of response is improved when the vaccine is given separated from a 5-day steroid pulse. Additionally, patients are recommended to receive a two-shot series their first year of immunization and subsequently one annual shot. It is unclear if there would be additional benefit by continuing with a yearly two-shot series or increased dose while immunocompromised.

16.7.5.2 2009 H1N1 Pandemic Vaccine

Seven studies have reported on efficacy of the 2009 H1N1 pandemic influenza vaccine (Bate et al. 2010b; Cheng et al. 2011; Yen et al. 2011; Hakim et al. 2012; Shahin et al. 2012; Leahy et al. 2013; Mavinkurve-Groothuis et al. 2013). In general, response rates were increased after two doses of vaccine in those patients with solid tumors and in those not receiving treatment. For a mixed pediatric oncology cohort, seroresponse ranged from 25.6–100 % (Bate et al. 2010b; Cheng et al. 2011; Yen et al. 2011; Hakim et al. 2012; Leahy et al. 2013; Mavinkurve-Groothuis et al. 2013). Absolute lymphocyte counts greater than the upper limit of normal for age (or ≥ 1.0–1.5×10^9/L depending on the study) were a significant factor in antibody response in three studies (Yen et al. 2011; Hakim et al. 2012; Mavinkurve-Groothuis et al. 2013). Leahy et al. (2013) showed significantly improved seropositivity in children who received the higher 0.5 mL dose on univariate but not multivariate analysis. No severe adverse reactions were noted in any of the studies. As with the annual trivalent influenza vaccine, clear data as to the most efficacious timing of immunization during ALL therapy, appropriate dose and the need for one versus two doses of vaccine are lacking although repeated, higher doses appear most effective.

16.7.5.3 Live Attenuated Influenza Vaccine

Two studies have been completed to measure seroresponse and safety of the live attenuated influenza vaccine (LAIV) in immunocompromised patients (Carr et al. 2011; Halasa et al. 2011). Halasa et al. (2011) conducted a small pilot study on the safety and immunogenicity of LAIV in mild to moderately immunocompromised children with cancer. Children with severe immunodeficiency as defined by an absolute neutrophil count (ANC) <0.5×10^9/L, concurrent high-dose steroid usage (≥ 2 mg/kg/day) or CD4+ T-lymphocyte percentage <15 % were excluded. The ten patients with hematologic malignancies and solid tumors who were immunized did not have any serious adverse events or an excessive period of viral shedding. Immunogenicity ranged from 33–44 % depending on the assay utilized. Carr et al. (2011) compared seroresponse in 52 children who were mild to moderately immunocompromised and randomly assigned to LAIV or inactivated vaccine. Seroprotection was found to be greater to influenza A strains with the inactivated vaccine. No difference was seen in seroprotection to influenza B. No serious adverse events were noted; specifically, viral shedding was not increased with the live attenuated vaccine. With limited safety data and no evidence of increased immunogenicity with LAIV, this form of the influenza vaccine remains relatively contraindicated in pediatric oncology patients.

16.7.6 Hepatitis B Virus Vaccine

In areas of high prevalence, especially East Asia and lower-income countries, the risk of HBV transmission during chemotherapeutic regimens is significant and therefore vaccination in these settings should be strongly considered (Somjee et al. 1999; Meral et al. 2000; Sevinir et al. 2003; Yetgin et al. 2007). Multiple studies using different vaccination schedules, a combination of passive and active immunization, and significant difference in transmission risk are present in the literature (Berberoğlu et al. 1995; Hovi et al. 1995; Kavakli et al. 1996; Goyal et al. 1998; Somjee et al. 1999; Meral et al. 2000; Yetgin et al. 2001; Somjee et al. 2002; Köksal et al. 2007; Yetgin et al. 2007; Baytan et al. 2008). The lowest rate of HBV transmission appears to be in those patients that receive a combination of passive and active immunization although the cost-effectiveness of this approach is questionable (Kavakli et al. 1996; Meral et al. 2000; Somjee et al. 2002). For seronegative patients with ALL in maintenance, seroconversion rates ranged from 35.1–62.5 % after a 2–5 shot HBV series (Yetgin et al. 2001, 2007; Baytan et al. 2008). Although HBV transmission still occurs in those that are immunized during therapy,

Yetgin et al. (2007) showed that infection was significantly decreased compared to unvaccinated patients, even if seroconversion did not occur. Additional studies among pediatric oncology patients with variable timing of immunization and vaccination schedules showed a seroconversion rate of 50–78 % (Berberoğlu et al. 1995; Hovi et al. 1995; Köksal et al. 2007). Hovi et al. (1995) studied 165 pediatric oncology patients; of the 51 on therapy, 67 % responded to a three-dose immunization schedule as compared to a 97 % seroresponse in the 114 off therapy. HBV immunization is important in settings outside of the United States and Western Europe where risk of transmission during therapy is high, although firm recommendations on the optimal timing and schedule of vaccination cannot be made based on the studies to date.

16.7.7 Meningococcal Conjugate Vaccine

The risk of meningococcus in immunocompromised pediatric oncology patients is unknown. Yu et al. (2007) studied vaccine response to protein-conjugated meningococcal C vaccine in 25 children with ALL and found improved response in those vaccinated 3 months after the completion of chemotherapy as compared to those in maintenance therapy (4 of 15 responders in maintenance versus 9 of 10 responders after chemotherapy completion).

16.7.8 Varicella Zoster Virus

Due to the herd immunity provided by routine varicella vaccination, especially in North America, guidelines for immunization during ALL maintenance have changed, and immunization is no longer recommended in these settings (Centers for Disease Control and Prevention 2007; American Academy of Pediatrics 2012c; Caniza et al. 2012). However, varicella immunization should still be a consideration in higher-risk populations, especially lower-income countries and, potentially, those higher income countries without universal varicella vaccination campaigns (Levin 2008; Esposito et al. 2010a).

Sartori (2004) provides an excellent review of varicella vaccination in immunocompromised patients. Early studies of the efficacy and safety of live attenuated varicella vaccine in children with acute leukemia were done in Japan with further safety data in the United States (Gershon et al. 1984; Takahashi et al. 1985; Gershon et al. 1986; Gershon and Steinberg 1989).

In their initial study, Gershon et al. (1984) showed the safety of live attenuated varicella vaccination when given to children with ALL that were in continuous clinical remission for 1 year, had a lymphocyte count $\geq 0.7 \times 10^9$/L, an IgG level ≥ 100 mg/dL, responded to at least one mitogen, and had all chemotherapy suspended for 1 week before and after vaccination. Seroresponse was 80 % after one dose of VZV. Rash was the only side effect which also increased seroconversion as well as the chance of transmission. Vaccination was quite protective, decreasing rate of infection after exposure to 18 % from an expected 90 % and also presenting as mild disease in those with clinical illness after exposure. A follow-up study by the same group with a larger cohort showed 88 % seroconversion after one dose of vaccination and 98 % seroconversion after two doses with no notable serious adverse events (Gershon and Steinberg 1989). Multiple other small studies have shown similar results with no serious adverse events (Heath and Malpas 1985; Ninane et al. 1985; Heath et al. 1987; Ecevit et al. 1996; Cakir et al. 2012).

A recent case report by Schrauder et al. (2007) on a child with ALL who developed fulminant varicella infection 32 days after varicella vaccination deserves mention. Vaccination was given with an interruption in chemotherapy, 1 week prior and 1 week after, but was given 5 months after complete remission had been achieved and prior to intensive reinduction chemotherapy, not in accordance with the stringent guidelines set forth by Takahashi et al. (1985) and Gershon et al. (1984, 1986; Gershon and Steinberg 1989). Based on their case, the authors recommend waiting at least 9 months after all therapy completion (including maintenance chemotherapy) prior to administering varicella vaccination. Their recommendation is not supported by the existing literature but does emphasize the care and attention that is necessary when administering this live attenuated vaccine to children that remain immunocompromised (Centers for Disease Control and Prevention 2007).

16.8 Recommendations for Vaccination After Chemotherapy Completion

Immune reconstitution is variable after the completion of chemotherapy leading to inconsistent guidelines for (re)vaccination. Among the published guidelines, four authors recommend commencing (re)vaccination 3 months after therapy completion (Centers for Disease Control and Prevention 1993; Sung et al. 2001; Allen 2007; Esposito et al. 2010a). For three of the four authors, this recommendation is inclusive of live viral vaccines (Centers for Disease Control and Prevention 2007). Esposito et al. (2010a) recommend waiting 6 months for live vaccines. The UK guidelines (Royal College of Paediatrics and Child Health 2002) recommend waiting 6 months for all vaccinations while Ruggiero et al. (2011) recommend waiting 6 months for inactivated/killed vaccines and measles but 12 months for VZV. Fioredda et al. (2005) also recommend waiting 6 months after therapy completion. Guidelines are unclear in regard to children that interrupted their primary immunization series (Esposito et al. 2010a; Ruggiero et al. 2011). Based on their review, van Tilburg et al. (2012) conclude that although revaccination is important, further study is still required to determine what the appropriate immunizations are, depending on the local herd immunity and risk for vaccine-preventable disease after chemotherapy. They do feel based on their review that 3 months after the completion of therapy is a good time point to begin the evaluatory process. Whether the evaluatory process should include pre- and/or post-immunization titers is also unclear; additionally there is a significant associated cost with such a strategy and seroprotection may not always equate with seropositivity by antibody level. The main factors that must be considered are minimizing the period of risk to the patient while balancing the risk for lack of seroconversion with premature immunization. Risk of vaccine-related infection from live viral vaccination seems less of a concern after therapy completion since patients can safely be immunized with varicella during ALL maintenance. For influenza, Esposito et al. (2010b) show that the biggest risk to pediatric patients with malignancy is during treatment and 6 months after the completion of therapy (including risk of infection and hospitalization). Beyond this point, risk becomes similar to the general pediatric population.

Based on the UK guidelines as outlined in the Royal College of Paediatrics and Child Health (RCPCH) best practice statement from 2002, Patel et al. (2007) enrolled 59 children with a history of leukemia ≥6 months after chemotherapy completion for revaccination. They found the large majority who were deficient achieved optimal antibody concentrations that persisted when rechecked 12 months after immunization. Based on their results they recommend following the RCPCH timing for booster vaccination. Of their studied vaccinations, inactivated poliovirus vaccine was the least immunogenic (HBV was not part of the study) but seroconversion rates were similar to published response in healthy individuals. Treatment intensity was not significantly associated with seroresponse. Similar rates of seroconversion are plausible with earlier vaccination as well; thus, 3 months post the completion of therapy is recommended by several authors based on their data (Lehrnbecher et al. 2009; Zengin and Sarper 2009). Large, randomized controlled trial data are lacking to make firm recommendations.

16.9 Active/Passive Immunization After Disease Exposure

16.9.1 Varicella

Live virus vaccination is contraindicated after varicella disease exposure (2 days prior to rash or before all lesions crusted over in contact) in immunocompromised individuals, although passive immunization and antivirals may be of utility. Multiple studies of variable quality have shown the potential benefit of varicella zoster immune globulin (VariZIG; VZIG) in immunocompromised children, nicely summarized by Fisher et al. (2011) (Brunell et al. 1972; Gershon et al. 1974; Judelsohn et al. 1974; Feldman et al. 1975; Evans et al. 1980; Orenstein et al. 1981; Hanngren et al. 1983; Zaia et al. 1983; Feldman and Lott 1987). VZIG often will not prevent disease in immunocompromised patients but has been shown to decrease disease severity (in most patients). Efficacy of VZIG has been shown to decline if given >72 h after exposure; therefore, previous US recommendations were to administer it within 96 h of exposure (Feldman and Lott 1988; American Academy of Pediatrics 2006). With the potential to attenuate disease even beyond this 72–96 h window, newer US guidelines as well as UK guidelines recommend VZIG up to 10 days after exposure (Royal College of Paediatrics and Child Health 2002; American Academy of Pediatrics 2012c). Due to the lack of quality studies, VariZIG remains an investigational agent in the United States and requires institutional review board approval and completion of an investigational new drug form. If VZIG is not available, intravenous immunoglobulin (IVIG) may be given.

Oral acyclovir antiviral prophylaxis has been claimed to show benefit in multiple studies, summarized by Fisher et al. (2011) (Ishida et al. 1996; Goldstein et al. 2000; Martin-Hernandez 2000; Shinjoh and Takahashi 2009). As with VZIG, these studies are case reports or nonrandomized uncontrolled studies. Studies in healthy children have specifically shown a decrease in disease when acyclovir is given as a 7-day course starting 1 week after exposure; efficacy was decreased when prophylaxis was started 3 or 11 days after exposure (Asano et al. 1993; Suga et al. 1993; Huang et al. 1995; Fisher et al. 2011). Current US guidelines recommend a 7-day course starting 7–10 days after exposure, while UK guidelines recommend a 14-day course starting 7 days after exposure (Royal College of Paediatrics and Child Health 2002; American Academy of Pediatrics 2012c). See Table 16.2 for VZIG, IVIG and acyclovir dosing recommendations. Fisher et al. (2011)

Table 16.2 Passive immunization after varicella or measles disease exposure[a]

Exposure to varicella 2 days prior to rash or before crusting of all lesions in contact:

If within 4–10 days of exposure:

VZIG 125 units/10 kg for the first 10–40 kg; >40 kg, 625 units IM (max 2.5 mL per injection site)

Or

IVIG 400 mg/kg IV

Or

If within 7–10 days of exposure and neither VZIG nor IVIG administered:

Acyclovir 80 mg/kg/day PO div QID (max dose 800 mg QID), for 7–14 days

Exposure to measles 5 days prior to or 4 days after onset of rash in contact:

If within 6–14 days of exposure:

Immunoglobulin 0.5 mL/kg IM (max dose 15 mL; max 3 mL per injection site in children)

Or

IVIG 400 mg/kg IV

VZIG varicella zoster immunoglobulin, *IVIG* intravenous immunoglobulin

Adapted from Royal College of Paediatrics and Child Health (2002), American Academy of Pediatrics (2012b, c)

[a]See text for details; level of evidence 1C per Guyatt et al. (2006); see Preface

comment in their review that a formal comparison between VZIG and acyclovir is lacking.

16.9.2 Measles

Measles immunization is contraindicated after measles exposure in immunocompromised patients. Passive immunization with immunoglobulin (Ig) should be utilized especially with virologic confirmation of exposure and exposure occurring 5 days prior to and up to 4 days after the onset of rash in the infectious contact. Ig may be given either intramuscularly or intravenously, especially if thrombocytopenic. Ideally passive prophylaxis should be given within 72 h of exposure; US guidelines recommend Ig up to 6 days after exposure, UK guidelines up to 14 days after contact (Royal College of Paediatrics and Child Health 2002; American Academy of Pediatrics 2012b). See Table 16.2 for dosing. Of note, a washout period after any immunoglobulin product (and blood products) is required prior to administration of measles vaccination. In the previously immunocompromised patient, MMR should be given a minimum of 6 months after Ig (American Academy of Pediatrics 2012b). In settings without Ig availability, early initiation of ribavirin for the treatment or postexposure prophylaxis of measles can be considered (Moulik et al. 2013).

16.10 Treatment of Hypogammaglobulinemia During Chemotherapy

The impact of low immunoglobulin levels on the risk of infectious sequelae during chemotherapy has not been well characterized. Although van Tilburg et al. (2012) showed that IgG levels were significantly lower in ALL patients receiving more intensive therapy and these patients also suffered more infectious complications, this fact could not be directly correlated to IgG levels. Kovacs et al. (2008) analyzed 88 children 1 year after the completion of chemotherapeutic regimens for malignancies. Leukemia patients suffered a statistically increased number of febrile episodes as compared to solid tumor patients, although this did not correlate with immunoglobulin levels. Similarly, solid tumor patients with low immunoglobulin levels suffered more febrile episodes than those with normal Ig levels, but not to the point of statistical significance. Multiple consensus statements on the use of IVIG do not include routine use in acquired hypogammaglobulinemia due to chemotherapy (Hemming 2001; Orange et al. 2006; Robinson et al. 2007). In a Canadian consensus statement, Robinson et al. (2007) note that IVIG is often a part of oncologic study protocols (though not evidence-based) and may also be considered in patients with a history of severe invasive infection or recurrent sinopulmonary infection in the setting of acquired hypogammaglobulinemia.

16.11 Vaccination of Household Contacts

Minimizing the risk of exposure in immunocompromised patients to vaccine-preventable diseases by immunization of household contacts is a vital

Table 16.3 Vaccination recommendations in household contacts of immunocompromised patients[a]

Vaccines that should be routinely given[b]

Yearly inactivated influenza vaccine

Live attenuated varicella vaccine in susceptible individuals

Rotavirus vaccine per routine schedule

All inactivated/killed vaccines and measles-mumps-rubella per routine schedule

Vaccines that are contraindicated

Live attenuated influenza vaccine

Oral poliovirus vaccine

Smallpox vaccine

Adapted from Centers for Disease Control and Prevention (1993), American Academy of Pediatrics (2012a)
[a]Level of evidence 1C per Guyatt et al. (2006); see Preface
[b]Live attenuated yellow fever vaccine may be given if necessary; unclear evidence for BCG and oral typhoid in high-risk settings

aspect of supportive care (Table 16.3). As discussed, immunogenicity to vaccine-preventable disease will be blunted during the period of highest risk; thus, minimizing any potential infectious contacts is more important than vaccine guidelines in those receiving therapy. Immunization of healthcare workers is therefore also important and summarized in Chap. 14. Live virus vaccines including measles-mumps-rubella, rotavirus and varicella have all been deemed safe due to the minimal risk of disease spread. Oral poliovirus vaccine is contraindicated and live attenuated influenza vaccine is relatively contraindicated (American Academy of Pediatrics 2012a). Household contacts should receive yearly inactivated influenza vaccine and young, susceptible contacts should be immunized against varicella. Vaccinees who develop a postvaccination rash should be separated from susceptible individuals due to the theoretical risk of infection transmission (Hughes et al. 1994; LaRussa et al. 1997; Chaves et al. 2008; Galea et al. 2008). However, no transmission of vaccine strain varicella has been reported to immunocompromised patients in the United States after 55 million doses of vaccine have been given (Chaves et al. 2008; Galea et al. 2008). Outside of the United States, in countries without national varicella vaccination programs, immunization of household contacts has been problematic due to concerns of safety as

well as a lack of identification by pediatric oncologists (Timitilli et al. 2008; Fisher et al. 2011).

16.12 Summary

Much is yet to be understood in regard to the pace of immune recovery after current chemotherapeutic regimens due to the lack of large, prospective studies. Likely, due to multifactorial reasons, the tempo will be variable when considering the array of ages, diagnoses and treatment regimens employed in pediatric oncology. In settings with expansive vaccine programs, immunocompromised children will be well protected from vaccine-preventable diseases due to herd immunity. In high-prevalence settings, vaccination during chemotherapy and periods of risk is more vital and further study is required as to the optimal timing and safety of such recommendations. (Re)vaccination after chemotherapy is important although the optimal timing and extent of (re)immunization is unclear. Large, randomized controlled trials are required to make firm decisions. Patients should be offered booster immunization 3–6 months after therapy completion by either the pediatric oncologist or in concert with the general pediatrician. Prevention of exposure by stringent vaccination of household contacts and treatment of exposure with passive immunization are also important aspects of supportive care in regard to vaccine-preventable disease.

References

Abrahamsson J, Marky I, Mellander L (1995) Immunoglobulin levels and lymphocyte response to mitogenic stimulation in children with malignant disease during treatment and follow-up. Acta Paediatr 84:177–182

Adler AL, Casper C, Boeckh M et al (2008) An outbreak of varicella with likely breakthrough disease in a population of pediatric cancer patients. Infect Control Hosp Epidemiol 29:866–870

Alanko S, Pelliniemi TT, Salmi TT (1992) Recovery of blood B-lymphocytes and serum immunoglobulins after chemotherapy for childhood acute lymphoblastic leukemia. Cancer 69:1481–1486

Alanko S, Pelliniemi TT, Salmi TT (1994) Recovery of blood lymphocytes and serum immunoglobulins after treatment of solid tumors in children. Pediatr Hematol Oncol 11:33–45

Alanko S, Salmi TT, Pelliniemi TT (1995) Recovery of natural killer cells after chemotherapy for childhood acute lymphoblastic leukemia and solid tumors. Med Pediatr Oncol 24:373–378

Alavi S, Rashidi A, Arzanian MT et al (2010) Humoral immunity against hepatitis B, tetanus, and diphtheria following chemotherapy for hematologic malignancies: a report and review of the literature. Pediatr Hematol Oncol 27:188–194

Al-Jadiry MF, Al-Khafagi M, Al-Darraji AF et al (2013) High incidence of hepatitis B infection after treatment for paediatric cancer at a teaching hospital in Baghdad. East Mediterr Health J 19:130–134

Allen UD (2007) Immunizations for children with cancer. Pediatr Blood Cancer 49:1102–1108

Allen JB, Weiner LB (1981) Pneumococcal sepsis in childhood leukemia and lymphoma. Pediatrics 67:292–295

Allison JE, Glezen WP, Taber LH et al (1977) Reactogenicity and immunogenicity of bivalent influenza A and monovalent influenza B virus vaccines in high-risk children. J Infect Dis 156:S672–S676

American Academy of Pediatrics (2012a) Active and passive immunization: immunization in special clinical circumstances—immunocompromised children. In: Pickering LK (ed) Red book: 2012 report of the committee on infectious diseases, 29th edn. American Academy of Pediatrics, Elk Grove Village

American Academy of Pediatrics (2012b) Summaries of infectious diseases: measles. In: Pickering LK (ed) Red book: 2012 report of the committee on infectious diseases varicella-zoster, 29th edn. American Academy of Pediatrics, Elk Grove Village

American Academy of Pediatrics (2012c) Summaries of infectious diseases: infections. In: Pickering LK (ed) Red book: 2012 report of the committee on infectious diseases, 29th edn. American Academy of Pediatrics, Elk Grove Village, IL

American Academy of Pediatrics (2006) Summaries of infectious diseases: infections. In: Pickering LK (ed) Red book: 2006 report of the committee on infectious diseases, 27th edn. American Academy of Pediatrics, Elk Grove Village, IL

Asano Y, Yoshikawa T, Suga S et al (1993) Postexposure prophylaxis of varicella in family contact by oral acyclovir. Pediatrics 92:219–222

Azuma E, Nagai M, Qi J et al (1998) CD4+ T-lymphocytopenia in long-term survivors following intensive chemotherapy in childhood cancers. Med Pediatr Oncol 30:40–45

Banatvala JE, Van Damme P (2003) Hepatitis B vaccine—do we need boosters? J Viral Hepat 10:1–6

Bate J, Patel SR, Chisholm J et al (2010a) Immunisation practices of paediatric oncology and shared care oncology consultants: a United Kingdom survey. Pediatr Blood Cancer 54:941–946

Bate J, Yung CF, Hoschler K et al (2010b) Immunogenecity of pandemic (H1N1) 2009 vaccine in children with cancer in the United Kingdom. Clin Infect Dis 51:e95–e104

Baytan B, Gunes AM, Gumay U (2008) Efficacy of primary hepatitis B immunization in children with acute lymphoblastic leukemia. Indian Pediatr 45:265–270

Bektas O, Karadeniz C, Oguz A et al (2007) Assessment of the immune response to trivalent split influenza vaccine in children with solid tumors. Pediatr Blood Cancer 49:914–917

Berberoğlu S, Büyükpamkcu M, Sarialioglu F et al (1995) Hepatitis B vaccination in children with cancer. Pediatr Hematol Oncol 12:171–178

Bhat N, Wright JG, Broder KR et al (2005) Influenza-associated deaths among children in the United States, 2003–2004. N Engl J Med 353:2559–2567

Biggar RJ, Christiansen M, Rostgaard K et al (2009) Immunoglobulin subclass levels in patients with non-Hodgkin lymphoma. Int J Cancer 124:2616–2620

Bisgard KM, Kao A, Leake J et al (1998) Haemophilus influenzae invasive disease in the United States, 1994–1995: near disappearance of a vaccine-preventable childhood disease. Emerg Infect Dis 4:229–237

Brodtman DH, Rosenthal DW, Redner A et al (2005) Immunodeficiency in children with acute lymphoblastic leukemia after completion of modern aggressive chemotherapeutic regimens. J Pediatr 146:654–661

Brunell PA, Gershon AA, Hughes WT et al (1972) Prevention of varicella in high risk children: a collaborative study. Pediatrics 50:718–722

Brydak LB, Rokicka-Milewska R, Jackowska T (1996) Kinetics of humoral response in children with acute lymphoblastic leukemia immunized with influenza vaccine in 1993 in Poland. Pediatr Hematol Oncol 13:231–238

Brydak L, Rokicka-Milewska R, Machala M et al (1998) Immunogenicity of subunit trivalent influenza vaccine in children with acute lymphoblastic leukemia. Pediatr Infect Dis J 17:125–129

Cakir FB, Timur C, Yoruk A et al (2012) Seroconversion status after single dose and double doses of varicella vaccination in children with leukemia. Pediatr Hematol Oncol 29:191–194

Caniza MA, Hunger SP, Schrauder A et al (2012) The controversy of varicella vaccination in children with acute lymphoblastic leukemia. Pediatr Blood Cancer 58:12–16

Carr S, Allison KJ, Van De Velde L et al (2011) Safety and immunogenicity of live attenuated and inactivated influenza vaccines in children with cancer. J Infect Dis 204:1475–1482

Caver TE, Slobod KS, Flynn PM et al (1998) Profound abnormality of the B/T lymphocyte ratio during chemotherapy for pediatric acute lymphoblastic leukemia. Leukemia 12:619–622

Centers for Disease Control and Prevention (1993) Recommendations of the Advisory Committee on Immunization Practices (ACIP): use of vaccines and immune globulins in persons with altered immunocompetence. MMWR Recomm Rep 42:1–24

Centers for Disease Control and Prevention (2007) Prevention of varicella: recommendations of the Advisory Committee on Immunization Practice (ACIP). MMWR Recomm Rep 56:25

Chaves SS, Haber P, Walton K et al (2008) Safety of varicella vaccination after licensure in the United States: experience from reports to the vaccine adverse event reporting system, 1995–2005. J Infect Dis 197:S170–S177

Cheng FW, Leung TF, Chan PK et al (2009) Humoral immune response after post-chemotherapy booster diphtheria-tetanus-pertussis vaccine in pediatric oncology patients. Pediatr Blood Cancer 52:248–253

Cheng FW, Leung TF, Chan PK et al (2010) Recovery of humoral and cellular immunities to vaccine-preventable infectious diseases in pediatric oncology patients. Pediatr Hematol Oncol 27:195–204

Cheng FW, Chan PK, Leung WK et al (2011) Pandemic (H1N1) 2009 vaccine in paediatric oncology patients: one dose or two doses? [letter]. Br J Haematol 154:408–409

Cheng FW, Ip M, Chu YY et al (2012) Humoral response to conjugate pneumococcal vaccine in paediatric patients. Arch Dis Child 97:358–360

Chilcote RR, Baehner RL, Hammond D (1976) Septicemia and meningitis in children splenectomized for Hodgkin's disease. N Engl J Med 295:798–800

Chisholm JC, Devine T, Charlett A et al (2001) Response to influenza immunization during treatment for cancer. Arch Dis Child 84:496–500

Crawford NW, Heath JA, Ashley D et al (2010) Survivors of childhood cancer: an Australian audit of vaccination status after treatment. Pediatr Blood Cancer 54:128–133

Cristófani LM, Weinberg A, Peixoto V et al (1991) Administration of live attenuated varicella vaccine in children with cancer before starting chemotherapy. Vaccine 9:873–876

De Vaan GA, van Munster PJ, Bakkeren JA (1982) Recovery of immune function after cessation of maintenance therapy in acute lymphoblastic leukemia (ALL) of childhood. Eur J Pediatr 139:113–117

Donaldson SS, Glatstein E, Vosti KL (1978) Bacterial infections in pediatric Hodgkin's disease. Cancer 41:1949–1958

Ecevit Z, Büyükpamukçu M, Kanra G et al (1996) Oka strain live varicella vaccine in children with cancer. Pediatr Infect Dis J 15:169–170

Ek T, Mellander L, Hahn-Zoric M et al (2004) Intensive treatment for childhood acute lymphoblastic leukemia reduces immune responses to diphtheria, tetanus, and Haemophilus influenzae type b. J Pediatr Hematol Oncol 26:727–734

Ek T, Mellander L, Andersson B et al (2005) Immune reconstitution after childhood acute lymphoblastic leukemia is most severely affected in the high risk group. Pediatr Blood Cancer 44:461–468

Ek T, Mellander L, Hahn-Zoric M et al (2006) Avidity of tetanus and Hib antibodies after childhood acute lymphoblastic leukaemia—implications for vaccination strategies. Acta Paediatr 95:701–706

Ek T, Josefson M, Abrahamsson J (2011) Multivariate analysis of the relation between immune dysfunction and treatment intensity in children with acute lymphoblastic leukemia. Pediatr Blood Cancer 56:1078–1087

El-Chennawi FA, Al-Tonbary YA, Mossad YM et al (2008) Immune reconstitution during maintenance therapy in children with acute lymphoblastic leukemia, relation to co-existing infection. Hematology 13:203–209

El-Din HM, Loutfy SA, Abdel-Rahman H et al (2012) Measles, mumps, varicella zoster, diphtheria and hepatitis B surface antibody status in pediatric acute leukemic patients. J Blood Disord Transfus S1:S1–S8

Ercan TE, Soycan LY, Apak H et al (2005) Antibody titers and immune response to diphtheria-tetanus-pertussis and measles-mumps-rubella vaccination in children treated for acute lymphoblastic leukemia. J Pediatr Hematol Oncol 27:273–277

Esposito S, Cecinati V, Russo FG et al (2009) Influenza vaccination in children with cancer receiving chemotherapy. Hum Vaccin 5:430–432

Esposito S, Cecinati V, Brescia L et al (2010a) Vaccinations in children with cancer. Vaccine 28:3278–3284

Esposito S, Cecinati V, Scicchitano B et al (2010b) Impact of influenza-like illness and effectiveness of influenza vaccination in oncohematological children who have completed cancer therapy. Vaccine 28:1558–1565

Evans EB, Pollock TM, Cradock-Watson JE et al (1980) Human anti-chickenpox immunoglobulin in the prevention of chickenpox. Lancet 1:354–356

Eyrich M, Wiegering V, Lim A et al (2009) Immune function in children under chemotherapy for standard risk acute lymphoblastic leukaemia—a prospective study of 20 paediatric patients. Br J Haematol 147:360–370

Feldman S, Hughes WT, Daniel C (1975) Varicella in children with cancer: 77 cases. Pediatrics 80:388–397

Feldman S, Lott L (1987) Varicella in children with cancer: impact of antiviral therapy and prophylaxis. Pediatrics 80:465–472

Feldman S, Lott L (1988) Passive immunization against varicella in children receiving chemotherapy. Pediatrics 82:954–955

Feldman S, Gigliotti F, Shenep JL et al (1990) Risk of haemophilus influenzae type b disease in children with cancer and response of immunocompromised leukemic children to a conjugate vaccine. J Infect Dis 161:926–931

Feldman S, Andrew M, Norris M et al (1998) Decline in rates of seropositivity for measles, mumps, and rubella antibodies among previously immunized children treated for acute leukemia. Clin Infect Dis 27:388–390

Fioredda F, Plebani A, Hanau G et al (2005) Re-immunisation schedule in leukaemic children after intensive chemotherapy: a possible strategy. Eur J Haematol 74:20–23

Fisher JP, Bate J, Hambleton S (2011) Preventing vari-cella in children with malignancies: what is the evi-dence? Curr Opin Infect Dis 24:203–211

Fuks Z, Strober S, Bobrove AM (1976) Long term effects of radiation on T and B lymphocytes in peripheral blood of patients with Hodgkin's disease. J Clin Invest 58:803–814

Galea SA, Sweet A, Beninger P et al (2008) The safety profile of varicella vaccine: a 10-year review. J Infect Dis 197:S165–S169

Ganz PA, Shanley JD, Cherry JD (1978) Responses of patients with neoplastic diseases to influenza virus vaccine. Cancer 42:2244–2247

Gershon AA, Steinberg SP (1989) Persistence of immu-nity to varicella in children with leukemia immunized with live attenuated varicella vaccine. N Engl J Med 320:8892–8897

Gershon AA, Steinberg SP, Brunell PA (1974) Zoster immune globulin. A further assessment. N Engl J Med 290:243–245

Gershon AA, Steinberg SP, Gelb L et al (1984) Live atten-uated varicella vaccine: efficacy for children with leu-kemia in remission. JAMA 252:355–362

Gershon AA, Steinberg SP, Gelb L (1986) Live attenuated varicella vaccine use in immunocompromised chil-dren and adults. Pediatrics 78:757–762

Goldstein SL, Somers MJ, Lande MB et al (2000) Acyclovir prophylaxis of varicella in children with renal disease receiving steroids. Pediatr Nephrol 14:305–308

Goossen GM, Kremer LC, van de Wetering MD (2009) Influenza vaccination in children being treated with chemotherapy for cancer. Cochrane Database Syst Rev (2):CD006484

Goyal S, Pai SK, Kelkar R et al (1998) Hepatitis B vacci-nation in acute lymphoblastic leukemia. Leuk Res 22:193–195

Gross PA, Lee H, Wolff J et al (1978) Influenza immuni-zation in immunosuppressed children. J Pediatr 92:30–35

Guyatt G, Gutterman D, Baumann MH et al (2006) Grading strength of recommendations and quality of evidence in clinical guidelines: report from an American College of Chest Physicians Task Force. Chest 129:174–181

Hakim H, Allison KJ, Van De Velde L et al (2012) Immunogenicity and safety of inactivated monovalent 2009 H1N1 influenza A vaccine in immunocompro-mised children and young adults. Vaccine 30:879–885

Halasa N, Englund JA, Nachman S et al (2011) Safety of live attenuated influenza vaccine in mild to moderately immunocompromised children with cancer. Vaccine 29:4110–4115

Hanngren K, Falksveden L, Grandien M et al (1983) Zoster immunoglobulin in varicella prophylaxis. A study among high-risk patients. Scand J Infect Dis 15:327–334

Heath RB, Malpas JS (1985) Experience with the live Oka-strain varicella vaccine in children with solid tumours. Postgrad Med J 61:107–111

Heath RB, Malpas JS, Kangro HO et al (1987) Efficacy of varicella vaccine in patients with solid tumours. Arch Dis Child 62:569–572

Hemming VG (2001) Use of intravenous immunoglobu-lins for prophylaxis or treatment of infectious dis-eases. Clin Diagn Lab Immunol 8:859–863

Hovi L, Valle M, Siimes M et al (1995) Impaired response to hepatitis B vaccine in children receiving anticancer chemotherapy. Pediatr Infect Dis J 14:931–934

Huang YC, Lin TY, Chiu CH (1995) Acyclovir prophy-laxis of varicella after household exposure. Pediatr Infect Dis J 14:152–154

Hughes P, LaRussa PS, Pearce JM et al (1994) Transmission of varicella-zoster virus from a vaccinee with underlying leukemia, demonstrated by poly-merase chain reaction. J Pediatr 124:932–935

Ishida Y, Tauchi H, Higaki A et al (1996) Postexposure prophylaxis of varicella in children with leukemia by oral acyclovir. Pediatrics 97:150–151

Judelsohn RG, Meyers JD, Ellis RJ et al (1974) Efficacy of zoster immune globulin. Pediatrics 53:476–480

Kantar M, Çetingül N, Kansoy S et al (2003) Immune deficiencies following cancer treatment in children. J Trop Pediatr 49:286–290

Kaplan SL, Duckett T, Mahoney DH et al (1992) Immunogenicity of Haemophilus influenzae type b polysaccharide-tetanus protein conjugate vaccine in children with sickle hemoglobinopathy or malignan-cies, and after systemic Haemophilus influenzae type b infection. J Pediatr 120:367–370

Kaplan SL, Mason EO, Wald ER et al (2004) Decrease of invasive pneumococcal infections in children among 8 children's hospitals in the United States after the intro-duction of the 7-valent pneumococcal conjugate vac-cine. Pediatrics 113:443–449

Kavakli K, Cetingul N, Oztop S (1996) Combined admin-istration of hepatitis B vaccine and hepatitis B immune globulin in children with cancer. Pediatr Hematol Oncol 13:295–298

Kersun LS, Reilly A, Coffin SE, Sullivan KE (2013a) Protecting pediatric oncology patients from influenza. Oncologist 18:204–211

Kersun LS, Reilly A, Coffin SE et al (2013b) A prospec-tive study of chemotherapy immunologic effects and predictors of humoral influenza vaccine responses in a pediatric oncology cohort. Influenza Other Respir Viruses 7:1158–1167

Köksal Y, Varan A, Aydin GB (2007) Comparison of accel-erated and rapid schedules for monovalent hepatitis B and combined hepatitis A/B vaccines in children with cancer. Pediatr Hematol Oncol 24:587–594

Kosmidis S, Baka M, Bouhoutsou D et al (2008) Longitudinal assessment of immunological status and rate of recovery following treatment in children with ALL. Pediatr Blood Cancer 50:528–532

Kostaridou S, Polychronopoulou S, Psarra K et al (2004) Decrease of CD4+ and B-lymphocyte populations is not associated with severe infectious complications in children with acute lymphoblastic leukemia during maintenance. Int J Hematol 80:354–360

Kovacs GT, Barany O, Schlick B et al (2008) Late immune recovery in children treated for malignant diseases. Pathol Oncol Res 14:391–397

Kung FH, Orgel HA, Wallace WW et al (1984) Antibody production following immunization with diphtheria and tetanus toxoids in children receiving chemotherapy during remission of malignant disease. Pediatrics 74:86–89

Kwon HJ, Lee JW, Chung NG et al (2012) Assessment of serologic immunity to diphtheria-tetanus-pertussis after treatment of Korean pediatric hematology and oncology patients. J Korean Med Sci 27:78–83

Lange B, Shapiro SA, Waldman MT et al (1979) Antibody responses to influenza immunization of children with acute lymphoblastic leukemia. J Infect Dis 140:402–406

LaRussa PS, Steinburg S, Meurice F et al (1997) Transmission of vaccine strain varicella-zoster from a healthy adult with vaccine-associated rash to susceptible household contacts. J Infect Dis 176:1072–1075

Leahy TR, Smith OP, Bacon CL et al (2013) Does vaccine dose predict response to the monovalent pandemic H1N1 influenza A vaccine in children with acute lymphoblastic leukemia? A single-centre study. Pediatr Blood Cancer 60:1656–1661

Lehrnbecher T, Schubert R, Behl M et al (2009) Impaired pneumococcal immunity in children after treatment for acute lymphoblastic leukaemia. Br J Haematol 147:700–705

Levin MJ (2008) Varicella vaccination of immunocompromised children. J Infect Dis 197:S200–S206

Luczynski W, Stasiak-Barmuta A, Krawczuk-Rybak M (2004) Immunologic monitoring of maintenance therapy for acute lymphoblastic leukaemia in children—preliminary report. Pediatr Blood Cancer 42:416–420

Mackall CL, Fleisher TA, Brown MR et al (1995) Age, thymopoiesis, and CD4+ T-lymphocyte regeneration after intensive chemotherapy. N Engl J Med 332:143–149

Martin-Hernandez E (2000) Acyclovir prophylaxis of varicella in children with nephritic syndrome. Pediatr Nephrol 15:326–327

Matsuzaki A, Suminoe A, Koga Y et al (2005) Immune response after influenza vaccination in children with cancer. Pediatr Blood Cancer 45:831–837

Mavinkurve-Groothuis AM, van der Flier M, Stelma F et al (2013) Absolute lymphocyte count predicts response to new influenza virus H1N1 vaccination in pediatric cancer patients. Clin Vaccine Immunol 20:118–121

Mazur B, Szczepański T, Karpe J et al (2006) Decreased numbers of CD4+ T lymphocytes in peripheral blood after treatment of childhood acute lymphoblastic leukemia. Leuk Res 30:33–36

Meisel R, Toschke AM, Heiligensetzer C et al (2007) Increased risk for invasive pneumococcal diseases in children with acute lymphoblastic leukaemia. Br J Haematol 137:457–460

Meral A, Sevinir B, Günay Ü (2000) Efficacy of immunization against hepatitis B virus infection in children with cancer. Med Pediatr Oncol 35:47–51

Moritz B, Eder J, Meister B et al (2001) Intact T-cell regenerative capacity in childhood acute lymphoblastic leukemia after remission induction therapy. Med Pediatr Oncol 36:283–289

Moulik NR, Kumar A, Jain A, Jain P (2013) Measles outbreak in a pediatric oncology unit and the role of ribavirin in prevention of complications and containment of the outbreak. Pediatr Blood Cancer 60:e122–e124

Mustafa MM, Buchanan GR, Winick NJ et al (1998) Immune recovery in children with malignancy after cessation of chemotherapy. J Pediatr Hematol Oncol 20:451–457

Nevin J, Washko JK, Arnold J (2013) Haemophilus influenzae type b in an immunocompetent, fully vaccinated ALL survivor. Pediatrics 131:e1639–e1642

Nilsson A, De Milito A, Engström P et al (2002) Current chemotherapy protocols for childhood acute leukemia induce loss of humoral immunity to viral vaccination antigens. Pediatrics 109:e91

Ninane J, Latinne D, Heremans-Bracke MT et al (1985) Live varicella vaccine in severely immunodepressed children. Postgrad Med J 61:97–102

Ogra PL, Sinks LF, Karzon DT (1971) Poliovirus antibody response in patients with acute leukemia. J Pediatr 79:444–449

Orange JS, Hossny EM, Weller CR et al (2006) Use of intravenous immunoglobulin in human disease: a review of evidence by members of the Primary Immunodeficiency Committee of the American Academy of Allergy, Asthma, and Immunology. J Allergy Clin Immunol 117:S525–S553

Orenstein W, Heymann D, Ellis R et al (1981) Prophylaxis of varicella in high risk children: response effect of zoster immune globulin. J Pediatr 98:368–373

Patel SR, Ortin M, Cohen BJ et al (2007) Revaccination of children after completion of standard chemotherapy for acute leukemia. Clin Infect Dis 44:635–642

Patel SR, Bate J, Borrow R et al (2012) Serotype-specific pneumococcal antibody concentrations in children treated for acute leukaemia. Arch Dis Child 97:46–48

Paulides M, Stöhr W, Laws H et al (2011) Antibody levels against tetanus and diphtheria after polychemothearpy for childhood sarcoma: a report from the Late Effects Surveillance System. Vaccine 29:1565–1568

Porter CC, Edwards KM, Zhu Y et al (2004) Immune responses to influenza immunization in children receiving maintenance chemotherapy for acute lymphoblastic leukemia. Pediatr Blood Cancer 42:36–40

Poulsen A, Schmiegelow K, Yssing M (1993) Varicella zoster infections in children with acute lymphoblastic leukemia. Leuk Lymphoma 9:177–192

Reinhardt D, Houliara K, Pekrun A et al (2003) Impact of conventional chemotherapy on levels of antibodies against vaccine-preventable diseases in children treated for cancer. Scand J Infect Dis 35:851–857

Robinson P, Anderson D, Brouwers M et al (2007) Evidence-based guidelines on the use of intravenous immune globulin for hematologic and neurologic conditions. Transfus Med Rev 21:S3–S8

Royal College of Paediatrics and Child Health (RCPCH) (2002) Immunisation of the immunocompromised child—best practice statement. London, RCPCH

Ruggiero A, Battista A, Coccia P et al (2011) How to manage vaccinations in children with cancer. Pediatr Blood Cancer 57:1104–1108

Sartori AM (2004) A review of the varicella vaccine in immunocompromised individuals. Int J Infect Dis 8:259–270

Schafer AI, Churchill H, Ames P et al (1979) The influence of chemotherapy on response of patients with hematologic malignancies to influenza vaccine. Cancer 43:25–30

Schrauder A, Henke-Gendo C, Seidemann K et al (2007) Varicella vaccination in a child with acute lymphoblastic leukaemia. Lancet 369:1232

Sevinir B, Meral A, Günay Ü et al (2003) Increased risk of chronic hepatitis in children with cancer. Med Pediatr Oncol 40:104–110

Shahgholi E, Ehsani MA, Salamati P et al (2010) Immunogenicity of trivalent influenza vaccine in children with acute lymphoblastic leukemia during maintenance therapy. Pediatr Blood Cancer 54: 716–720

Shahin K, Lina B, Billaud G et al (2012) Successful H1N1 influenza vaccination of children receiving chemotherapy for solid tumors. J Pediatr Hematol Oncol 34:e228–e231

Shenep JL, Peldman S, Gigliotti F (1994) Response of immunocompromised children with solid tumors to a conjugate vaccine for Haemophilus influenzae type b. J Pediatr 125:581–584

Shinjoh M, Takahashi T (2009) Varicella zoster exposure on paediatric wards between 2000 and 2007: safe and effective postexposure prophylaxis with oral acyclovir. J Hosp Infect 72:163–168

Siber GR (1980) Bacteremias due to Haemophilus influenzae and Streptococcus pneumoniae: their occurrence and course in children with cancer. Am J Dis Child 134:668–672

Sinisalo M, Aittoniemi J, Käyhty H et al (2002) Haemophilus influenzae type b antibody concentrations and vaccination responses in patients with chronic lymphocytic leukaemia: predicting factors for response. Leuk Lymphoma 43:1967–1969

Sinisalo M, Vipo J, Itälä M et al (2007) Antibody response to 7-valent conjugated pneumococcal vaccine in patients with chronic lymphocytic leukaemia. Vaccine 26:82–87

Smith S, Schiffman G, Karayalcin G et al (1995) Immunodeficiency in long-term survivors of acute lymphoblastic leukemia treated with Berlin-Frankfurt-Münster therapy. J Pediatr 127:68–75

Smithson WA, Siem RA, Ritts RE et al (1978) Response to influenza virus vaccine in children receiving chemotherapy for malignancy. J Pediatr 93:632–634

Somjee S, Pai S, Kelkar R et al (1999) Hepatitis B vaccination in children with acute lymphoblastic leukemia: results of an intensified immunization schedule. Leuk Res 23:365–367

Somjee S, Pai S, Parikh P et al (2002) Passive active prophylaxis against hepatitis B in children with acute lymphoblastic leukemia. Leuk Res 26:989–992

Steinherz PG, Brown AE, Gross PA et al (1980) Influenza immunization of children with neoplastic diseases. Cancer 45:750–756

Suga S, Yoshikawa T, Ozaki T et al (1993) Effect of oral acyclovir against primary and secondary viraemia in incubation period of varicella. Arch Dis Child 69: 639–642

Sumaya CV, Williams TE, Brunell PA (1977) Bivalent influenza vaccine in children with cancer. J Infect Dis 156:S656–S660

Sung L, Heurter H, Zokic KM et al (2001) Practical vaccination guidelines for children with cancer. Paediatr Child Health 6:379–383

Takahashi M, Kamiya H, Baba K et al (1985) Clinical experience with Oka live varicella vaccine in Japan. Postgrad Med J 61:61–67

Timitilli A, Bertoluzzo L, Micalizzi C et al (2008) Antivaricella-zoster vaccination in contacts of children receiving antineoplastic chemotherapy: a prospective pilot study. Infez Med 16:144–147

Van der Does-van den Berg A, Hermans J, Nagel J et al (1981) Immunity to diphtheria, pertussis, tetanus, and poliomyelitis in children with acute lymphocytic leukemia after cessation of chemotherapy. Pediatrics 67:222–229

Van Tilburg CM, Sanders EA, Rovers MM et al (2006) Loss of antibodies and response to (re-)vaccination in children after treatment for acute lymphocytic leukemia: a systematic review. Leukemia 20: 1717–1722

Van Tilburg CM, Bierings MB, Berbers GA et al (2012) Impact of treatment reduction for childhood acute lymphoblastic leukemia on serum immunoglobulins and antibodies against vaccine-preventable disease. Pediatr Blood Cancer 58:701–707

Von der Hardt K, Jüngert J, Beck JD et al (2000) Humoral immunity against diphtheria, tetanus and poliomyelitis after antineoplastic therapy in children and adolescents—a retrospective analysis. Vaccine 18: 2999–3004

Weisman SJ, Cates KL, Allegretta GJ et al (1987) Antibody response to immunization with Haemophilus influenzae type b polysaccharide vaccine in children with cancer. J Pediatr 111:727–729

Wong-Chew RM, Frías MN, García-León ML et al (2012) Humoral and cellular immune responses to influenza vaccination in children with cancer receiving chemotherapy. Oncol Lett 4:329–333

Yen TY, Jou ST, Yang YL et al (2011) Immune response to 2009 pandemic H1N1 influenza virus A monovalent vaccine in children with cancer. Pediatr Blood Cancer 57:1154–1158

Yetgin S, Tunç B, Koç A et al (2001) Two booster dose hepatitis B virus vaccination in patients with leukemia. Leuk Res 25:647–649

Yetgin S, Tavil B, Aytac S et al (2007) Unexpected protection from infection by two booster hepatitis B virus vaccination in children with acute lymphoblastic leukemia. Leuk Res 31:493–496

Yu JW, Borkowski A, Danzig L et al (2007) Immune response to conjugated meningococcal C vaccine in pediatric oncology patients. Pediatr Blood Cancer 49:918–923

Zaia J, Levin M, Preblud S et al (1983) Evaluation of varicella-zoster immune globulin: protection of immunosuppressed children after household exposure to varicella. J Infect Dis 147:737–743

Zengin E, Sarper N (2009) Humoral immunity to diphtheria, tetanus, measles, and hemophilus influenzae type b in children with acute lymphoblastic leukemia and response to re-vaccination. Pediatr Blood Cancer 53: 967–972

Zignol M, Peracchi M, Tredello G et al (2004) Assessment of humoral immunity to poliomyelitis, tetanus, hepatitis B, measles, rubella, and mumps in children after chemotherapy. Cancer 101:635–641

Central Venous Catheters: Care and Complications

17

Connie Goes

Contents

C. Goes, PNP
Department of Hematology/Oncology,
Children's Hospital and Research Center Oakland,
747 52nd Street, Oakland, CA 94609, USA
e-mail: cgoes@mail.cho.org

Abstract

Central venous catheters are an essential component of care in children and adolescents with cancer and allow for safe and compassionate administration of chemotherapy and supportive medications, infusions, and transfusions in an efficient and cost-effective manner. With these benefits also come a host of decisions and potential complications. Catheter choice includes implanted versus external catheter, those meant for short- versus longer-term usage, as well as catheters that may be utilized for hematopoietic stem cell harvesting. Complications are primarily infection and thrombosis. This chapter provides evidence-based graded recommendations from the medical literature regarding choice and care of catheters specific for each patient and provides techniques for prevention, recognition and treatment of the most common complications.

J. Feusner et al. (eds.), *Supportive Care in Pediatric Oncology:*
A Practical Evidence-Based Approach, Pediatric Oncology,
DOI 10.1007/978-3-662-44317-0_17, © Springer Berlin Heidelberg 2015

17.1 Introduction

Central venous catheters (CVCs) are an important component of the supportive care of pediatric oncology patients and allow for the utilization of increasingly intensive and complex therapeutic regimens which has contributed to the increased survival rate in high-income countries. CVCs allow for safe delivery of chemotherapy, antibiotics and other medications, parenteral nutrition, blood products, hematopoietic stem cell infusions, and fluids. Frequent blood sampling, required to monitor side effects of therapy and disease status, can be accomplished comfortably and efficiently through an external CVC. Despite these advantages, challenges exist with the use of CVCs, primarily infection and occlusion. Ongoing research to develop strategies to prevent and treat these problems is needed. Here we review the existing literature and provide graded recommendations based on the evidence as well as consensus and expert opinion when firm evidence is lacking (Table 17.1).

17.2 Types of Central Venous Catheters

CVCs are divided into two categories: non-tunneled and tunneled. Each catheter type has specific line care needs, advantages, disadvantages and complications (Table 17.2). Selection of the optimal type of CVC for use in a specific disease or treatment protocol is not standardized. Factors to consider in catheter selection include the age and weight of the child, the length and intensity of therapy, frequency of blood sampling, anticipated supportive care interventions including transfusions, infusions and nutrition, level of patient activity, body image, and family ability to understand teaching and properly care for the line.

17.2.1 Peripherally Inserted Central Catheter

A peripherally inserted central catheter (PICC) is the most frequently inserted non-tunneled CVC for short-term intravenous therapy and can remain in place for weeks to months. A PICC is the ideal central access device for oncology patients that present acutely ill and too unstable for anesthesia (e.g., mediastinal mass, airway compromise). Some institutions prefer a PICC during induction therapy for acute leukemia due to concern of an increased risk of catheter thrombosis associated with asparaginase therapy. The thin flexible silicone or polyurethane catheter is typically inserted into the basilic vein due to the ease of threading within this vessel. The catheter tip is placed into a large vessel, typically the distal superior vena cava (SVC), allowing for rapid dilution of medications and prevention of vessel damage from vesicants and hyperosmolar solutions (Pettit 2002; Burns 2005). Insertion complications include curling of the catheter, difficulty threading the catheter, multiple attempts to place the catheter, malposition or failure to insert the catheter and medial nerve damage (Pettit 2002; Burns 2005; Alomari and Falk 2006). Post-insertion imaging either with a chest radiograph or fluoroscopy should be obtained to document proper placement of the catheter tip.

Advantages of PICCs include the ability to insert at either the bedside or in interventional radiology, ability to remove at the bedside, decreased cost and decreased potential complications related to anesthesia or a surgical procedure. After insertion, the external portion of the catheter is measured and documented. Remeasurement with each dressing change ensures proper positioning. Smaller gauge (larger diameter) PICCs allow for blood sampling and red blood cell transfusions. The manufacturer's recommendations and established institutional guidelines should be strictly followed. Disadvantages of a PICC include the need for sterile dressing changes, frequent flushing and a risk of phlebitis. The catheter lacks a cuff for stabilization creating an increased risk of dislodgement. Securing a PICC line is especially important in young or unstable patients. A sutureless securement device, StatLock®, is a housing unit that clips the PICC line suture wings into place with an adhesive patch, improving stabilization over tape. A prospective,

Table 17.1 Summary of recommendations for prevention of infectious complications with central venous catheters (CVCs)

	Recommendation	Level of evidence[a]
Insertion	Hand hygiene with soap and water or waterless alcohol gel	1A
	Maximal sterile barrier precautions: cap, mask, sterile gown, sterile gloves, sterile full body drape	1A
	Skin antisepsis with 2 % chlorhexidine	1A
	Trained, competent provider to insert or oversee inexperienced personnel	1A
	No prophylactic antibiotic	1B
	Use of totally implanted device whenever possible due to decreased risk of infection	1B
	Use of ultrasound-guided assistance not recommended with subclavian line placement	2A
	Subclavian site is the preferred insertion site	2C
	CVC placement can occur with ALL induction or be delayed	2C
Site care	Hand hygiene with soap and water or waterless alcohol gel	1A
	Use either sterile transparent semipermeable dressing or sterile gauze and tape dressing (especially if diaphoretic or bleeding from site)	1A
	Change sterile transparent semipermeable dressing every 5 days or when loose, wet, or soiled	1C
	Change sterile gauze and tape dressing daily or if loose, wet, or soiled	1C
	Chlorhexidine gluconate for exit site antisepsis	1A
	Monitor site for evidence of infection	1C
	No topical antibiotic at exit site	1B
	Use of StatLock® for securement of PICC line	1B
	Antiseptic-impregnated catheters are not routinely recommended	2C
Hub care	Scrub hub for 15 s with either 70 % isopropyl alcohol or 2 % chlorhexidine in 70 % isopropyl alcohol prior to every access	1B
Assessment	Daily assessment of site for evidence of infection	1C
	Daily assessment of need for CVC	1A
Locking line	External catheters: daily (when not in use) and after intermittent use with heparinized saline (concentration/volume per institutional policy)	1C
	Totally implanted device: monthly and after intermittent use with heparinized saline (concentration/volume according to institutional policy)	1C
Education	Dedicated CVC team to evaluate current literature	1B
	Ongoing training for personnel of new policies, procedures, equipment	1B
Infection	Antibiotic ointment alone should not be used for exit site infections	1B
	Catheter removal is indicated for tunnel infection	2A
	Port catheter removal is indicated for pocket infection	1A
Occlusion[b]	Utilization of tPA dwell for CVC occlusion	2A
	Low-dose systemic tPA if tPA dwell unsuccessful	2C
	Imaging with compression US with Doppler and CT with venography if US nondiagnostic with a high level of suspicion	2A

ALL acute lymphoblastic leukemia, *PICC* peripherally inserted central catheter, *tPA* tissue plasminogen activator, *US* ultrasound, *CT* computed tomography
[a]Per Guyatt et al. (2006); see Preface
[b]See text for further detail

randomized trial to evaluate the use of StatLock® versus sutures found an overall reduction in complications and specifically with a significant decrease in bloodstream infections (Yamamoto et al. 2002).

17.2.2 External Tunneled Central Venous Catheter

A Broviac catheter is the most commonly inserted external tunneled CVC in pediatrics (other external

Table 17.2 Advantages and disadvantages of central venous catheters (CVCs)

Type of CVC	PICC	Broviac	Implanted port	Powerline
Advantages	Immediate access	Immediate access	No required daily care (when not accessed)	Immediate access
	Bedside insertion	Painless blood sampling	Blood sampling (when accessed)	Blood sampling
	Bedside removal	External portion repairable	Lower infection risk	Compatible with CT power injection
	Blood sampling with ≥2.8 F		No restriction of activities	Use for stem cell pheresis
	Transfusions with ≥4.0 F			
Disadvantages	Frequent flushing	Surgical placement	Needle required for access	Surgical placement
	Sterile dressing changes	Daily flushing		Daily flushing
	Phlebitis	Sterile dressing changes	Potential needle dislodgement	Sterile dressing changes
		Increased infection risk		Bathing limitations
		Bathing limitations		No swimming
		No swimming		Potential for self-removal
		Potential for self-removal		External portion not repairable
		Impact on body image		Impact on body image

PICC peripherally inserted central catheter, *F* French, *CT* computed tomography

tunneled CVCs include Hickman, Groshong, Leonard, Hemocath and Powerline) and is available in either a single- or double-lumen system. Tunneled catheters are placed into a vein in the chest or neck and tunneled under the skin to secure for long-term use. Made of silicone or polyurethane, Broviac catheters are surgically inserted into either the internal jugular vein or subclavian vein with the tip placed into the distal SVC. The line is tunneled under the skin and exits on the anterior or lateral chest. A Dacron cuff stimulates tissue growth stabilizing the line in place while inhibiting bacterial migration. The cuff may be felt under the skin approximately 2 cm above the exit site.

A Powerline is a newer less frequently used cuffed polyurethane tunneled CVC available in single-, dual- or triple-lumen systems. In addition to the advantages of an external CVC, a Powerline is compatible with power injection of CT contrast (as needed for imaging) with a maximum flow rate of 5 mL/s and can be utilized for stem cell harvesting (BARD website 2014). Routine daily line care is similar to a Broviac though Powerlines are made of a firmer material and breaks in the external portion are not repairable, thereby requiring removal.

Advantages of an external CVC include easy access for delivery of intravenous therapies and painless blood sampling. In the event of tears or blockages, the external portion of the catheter is repairable with kits available from the manufacturer. Repair kits for each CVC size should be kept in stock at the institution. Disadvantages of an external CVC are requirement of surgical placement with anesthesia, increased risk of infection and thrombosis compared to implanted catheters, requirement for sterile dressing changes, daily heparin flushes, risk of kinking and breaking particularly with larger gauge (smaller diameter) sizes, limitations on activity (swimming and bathing), impact on body image, and potential for self-removal, especially with infants and toddlers. External CVCs carry a greater risk of infection than implanted ports as a result of the external site of the hubs and possibly secondary to the frequency of access for infusion, line flushing and blood sampling (Adler et al. 2006; Maki et al. 2006; Perdikaris et al. 2008).

17.2.3 Implanted Port

A port is a totally implanted tunneled CVC consisting of two sections, a plastic or titanium reservoir with a self-sealing rubber septum and a silicone or polyurethane catheter. The reservoir is placed in a surgically created pocket in the subcutaneous tissue below the clavicle and sutured to the fascia to ensure stabilization. The reservoir should not be placed directly beneath the surgical incision as accessing through the incision may lead to infection or skin breakdown (Baggott et al. 2002). The catheter is tunneled and inserted into either the internal jugular or subclavian vein with the tip in the distal SVC. The use of a non-coring Huber needle prolongs the life of the septum to approximately 2,000 punctures with a 22 gauge needle and 1,000 punctures if using a 19 gauge needle (BARD website 2014). If the port is to be used immediately, the surgeon may access the device in the operating room prior to development of postoperative swelling thereby preventing patient discomfort.

Advantages of an implanted port include decreased risk of infection, ease of blood sampling when accessed for use, no restrictions on swimming or bathing and no required daily care when not accessed (O'Grady et al. 2002; Adler et al. 2006). A disadvantage, particularly in small children, is the requirement for needle access through the skin. A lidocaine-based topical anesthetic cream (or ethyl chloride "cold" spray) is frequently used prior to access to decrease the discomfort of needle insertion. While accessed, site assessment is necessary as dislodgment may occur due to the patient's activity or use of an inappropriate length Huber needle, potentially leading to infiltration or extravasation of infusions. Implanted ports may stay accessed for long periods of time, but it is recommended to reaccess with a fresh needle every 7 days. Mechanical complications, although quite rare, include damage to the port reservoir, separation of the catheter from the reservoir and erosion of the reservoir through the skin (Schulmeister 2010).

17.3 Catheter Insertion

Though rare, complications during insertion can arise and cause significant morbidity and include pneumothorax, hemothorax, chylothorax, malpositioning, arterial puncture and failure to place. Factors associated with complications include physician inexperience, multiple insertion attempts, prior catheterizations, patient anatomy, prior surgery or radiation in the area and a high body mass index (Mansfield et al. 1994; Lefrant et al. 2002; Kusminsky 2007). An insertion failure rate of up to 43 % and complication rate up to 24 % occurs with ≥3 insertion attempts leading to a recommendation of limiting each operator to a maximum of two unsuccessful attempts (Mansfield et al. 1994; Eisen et al. 2006). The definition of an "attempt" varies among studies ranging from one puncture to multiple punctures by one operator at one site making comparisons difficult (Eisen et al. 2006; Balls et al. 2010).

Several studies have been completed evaluating the advantage of using real-time ultrasound-guided assistance (UGA) rather than the anatomic landmark technique for placement of a CVC (Augoustides and Cheung 2009; Pittiruti et al. 2009; Balls et al. 2010). A meta-analysis by Randolph et al. (1996) concluded that this technique led to an improved insertion success rate and a decrease in complications in both internal jugular and subclavian vein insertions. McGee and Gould (2003) found that UGA is effective in catheterization of the internal jugular vein with a decreased incidence of mechanical complications and placement failure. However, they found no benefit using this technique with subclavian vein insertions as the clavicle lies directly over the vessel, impeding visualization. In their studies, Mansfield et al. (1994) and Troianos et al. (2011) reached a similar conclusion. A retrospective observational study by Balls et al. (2010) assessed 1,222 CVC placement attempts concluding that the use of UGA did not improve the success of placement on the first attempt but overall saw a reduced number of total attempts. Further study is required to determine whether the routine use of UGA is feasible due to the high cost of equipment, required personnel training and equipment maintenance (Randolph et al. 1996).

Catheter insertion in the subclavian vein carries a higher risk of pneumothorax, malpositioning and failure to place compared to internal jugular insertion, while internal jugular catheterization is associated with a higher incidence of arterial puncture and hematoma (McGee and Gould 2003; Eisen et al. 2006). Although the subclavian vein carries the greater risk of insertion complications, it remains the preferred approach due to a lower rate of infection noted in some studies (McGee and Gould 2003). A prospective, observational study by Deshpande et al. (2005) found no difference in CVC infection rates for subclavian, internal jugular or femoral vein insertion sites in adult patients. The 2011 Centers for Disease Control (CDC) Guidelines for the Prevention of Intravascular Catheter-Related Infections declined to make a recommendation for the preferred CVC insertion site leaving the issue unresolved (O'Grady et al. 2011).

Children with acute lymphoblastic leukemia (ALL) often present with neutropenia and thrombocytopenia theoretically putting them at increased risk for complications with CVC placement. However, two separate studies evaluating 172 and 98 children, respectively, found no increased rate of complication with early CVC placement in newly diagnosed ALL patients (Handrup et al. 2010; Gonzalez et al. 2012). Platelet thresholds for CVC placement are undefined (see Chap. 2). Handrup et al. (2010) also concluded that the nonelective removal rate was similar between early and later placed CVCs. A retrospective analysis of 362 patients with ALL assessed complication rates between timing of insertion (early, ≤day 15 of induction, vs. late, >day 15 of induction) and type of CVC (ports vs. external CVCs) and found that early placement was associated with an increased risk of a positive blood culture and external CVCs were associated with an increased risk of positive blood cultures, thrombotic complications, and early removal (McLean et al. 2005). Due to the conflicting evidence, institutions providing initial care of newly diagnosed oncology patients must decide on the benefit of CVC placement timing, with ongoing monitoring for early complications and of line care in this setting.

17.4 Infection

Infection remains the major complication of an indwelling CVC, with bloodstream infection causing the most significant risk of morbidity and mortality. Terms used to describe intravascular catheter-related infection are confusing with central line-associated bloodstream infection (CLABSI) and catheter-related bloodstream infection (CRBSI) often used interchangeably. CLABSI is defined as an infection occurring in the patient with a CVC and not related to an infection at another site and is the term used by the CDC National Healthcare Safety Network (NHSN). CRBSI is a clinical definition requiring specific laboratory testing, quantitative blood cultures, differential time to positivity or culture of a segment of the removed catheter (O'Grady et al. 2011). Common organisms causing CLABSI include *Staphylococcus epidermis*, *Staphylococcus aureus*, *Enterococcus faecalis*, *Klebsiella pneumoniae*, *Pseudomonas aeruginosa* and *Candida albicans*. See Chaps. 1 and 14 for prevention, recognition and treatment of suspected infection or sepsis.

Most CVC-related infections are thought to occur by one of two methods: colonization at the exit site with pathogen migration along the external catheter surface or hub contamination leading to intraluminal colonization with spread into the circulation (McGee and Gould 2003). Within hours of CVC placement, a protein-rich sheath begins developing, covering the external and internal surfaces of the catheter. The protein sheath allows adherence of microbes which then produce a slimy substance (biofilm) becoming embedded in the matrix (Raad et al. 1993). Pathogens within a biofilm behave differently with an increased rate of reproduction and a greater resistance to antimicrobial therapy (Raad et al. 1993; Donlan 2011).

Antiseptic-impregnated catheters (AIC) coated with either chlorhexidine and silver sulfadiazine (CSS) or minocycline-rifampin (MR) have been studied in an effort to determine their effectiveness in decreasing the rate of CLABSI. Randomized clinical trials have generally not shown these catheters to be beneficial (McGee and Gould 2003). In a randomized clinical trial evaluating 232 catheters inserted in 180 critically ill hospitalized adult patients in use <10 days, there was no significant difference in the rates of colonization between antiseptic-impregnated and non-impregnated catheters (Theaker et al. 2002). Separate meta-analyses reviewing randomized controlled trials comparing AICs and non-AICs with a median insertion duration of 7–12 days concluded the efficacy of CSS catheters to be <2 weeks with MR catheters being effective somewhat longer (Mermel 2000; Walder et al. 2002). The results of numerous studies are difficult to compare with no type of catheter showing a definitive advantage. The CDC recommends that institutions develop strategies to provide education of personnel who insert and maintain catheters, with use of maximal sterile barrier precautions (i.e., cap, mask, sterile gown, sterile gloves and a sterile full body drape for line insertion) and skin antisepsis with >0.5 % chlorhexidine with alcohol for insertion. The use of antimicrobial-coated catheters is recommended at institutions where implementation of these CDC strategies fails to decrease CLABSI rates (O'Grady et al. 2011). Maki et al. (2006) determined that institutions with a baseline CLABSI rate of >2 % would benefit from use of AICs as this was the threshold at which AICs would decrease overall costs.

17.4.1 Exit Site Infection

An exit site infection is characterized by the presence of erythema, tenderness, induration or drainage within 2 cm of the catheter exit site, without signs or symptoms of systemic infection (O'Grady et al. 2011). Culture of the site should be obtained. Though not evidence-based, gener-

ally Gram-positive infections may be treated with oral antibiotics, while broad-spectrum parenteral antibiotics are indicated for Gram-negative organisms and for children with neutropenia (Baggott et al. 2002). Once the organism is identified, antibiotic therapy should be tailored to sensitivities. An exit site infection due to water-borne organisms, such as *Pseudomonas* spp., or fungus generally requires catheter removal as these organisms are notoriously difficult to clear. Antibiotic ointment alone should not be used at the exit site as this significantly increases the risk of *Candida* spp. infection and promotes antibiotic resistance (Zakrzewska-Bode et al. 1995; O'Grady et al. 2011).

17.4.2 Tunnel Infection

A tunnel infection is defined as tenderness, erythema, drainage or site induration >2 cm from the catheter exit site along the subcutaneous tract in the absence of concomitant CLABSI (O'Grady et al. 2011). Blood cultures from the CVC and skin cultures should be obtained. Catheter removal is indicated and parenteral antibiotics tailored to sensitivities of the cultured organism are given for 7–10 days (Mermel et al. 2009). A PICC may be placed to complete the recommended course of antibiotics.

17.4.3 Pocket Infection

A pocket infection involves erythema, tenderness and swelling over the site of an implanted port with purulent fluid noted in the subcutaneous tissue. Drainage or necrosis of the overlying skin may be present (O'Grady et al. 2011). Drainage should be obtained and cultured. Removal of the port is indicated with debridement, if necessary. A course of parenteral antibiotics is essential with medication tailored to the sensitivity of the infecting organism (O'Grady et al. 2002). Prior to insertion of another CVC, the wound should be healed, the course of antibiotics completed and the child should have defervesced. Consideration may be given to placement of a PICC should a CVC be needed to complete therapy.

17.4.4 Prevention of Infection

A CVC bundle is a set of evidence-based care practices implemented to decrease the risk of infection due to the presence of a CVC. Components include hand hygiene, selection of the optimal insertion site, use of maximal barrier technique, chlorhexidine skin antisepsis and prompt removal of the catheter when it is no longer needed (O'Grady et al. 2011). Development of institutional guidelines and ongoing staff education are essential in decreasing infection rates (O'Grady et al. 2011). Each institution's infection control department is instrumental in tracking rates of CLABSI. Cooperation with the hematology/oncology service is imperative for ongoing evaluation with changes to institutional practices as indicated. A local expert on CVC care and management and infection control will enhance education, monitor adherence to policy, follow rates of infection and evaluate the current literature (Teichgraber et al. 2011). Placement of the institution's hand hygiene guidelines in patient care areas is a great reminder for practitioners, patients and family members. Further discussion of prevention of CVC line infection is detailed in Chap. 14.

17.5 Occlusions

A functioning CVC is a catheter that flushes easily, infuses without difficulty and has brisk blood return (Baskin et al. 2009). Occlusion is the most common noninfectious complication of CVCs with an occurrence rate of 25 % and resulting in delays in the administration of chemotherapy and supportive care (Stephens et al. 1995). Rapid assessment is needed to determine both the cause of the obstruction and the appropriate interventions. Causes of CVC occlusion include mechanical complications, drug precipitate or lipid residue and thrombosis. Each of these problems can result in either partial or complete obstruction of the catheter. A partial occlusion allows for fluid infusion but either a sluggish or complete inability to withdraw blood (ball-valve effect). A complete occlusion allows neither fluid infusion nor blood withdrawal. An unusual problem may occur with implanted ports allowing blood withdrawal but not fluid administration due to a thrombus inside the reservoir at the outlet port (a reverse ball-valve effect).

17.5.1 Mechanical Occlusion

The cause of a mechanical obstruction may be as simple as a closed clamp, a kink in the external portion of the line or an exit site suture that is too tight, all of which are easily corrected after careful inspection and manipulation. An improperly inserted Huber needle is corrected by re-accessing the implanted port. A "pinch-off" syndrome (Fig. 17.1) can occur with catheter compression between the clavicle and first rib at a reported 1 % incidence rate. This complication is associated with insertion into the subclavian vein via an infraclavicular approach (Fazeny-Dorner et al. 2003; Baskin et al. 2009).

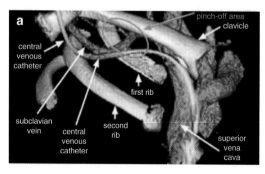
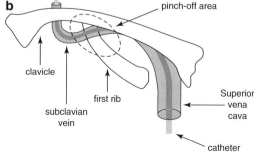

Fig. 17.1 Pinch-off syndrome (with permission from Baskin et al. [2009])

Rolling the shoulder forward or raising the arm on the opposite side may allow blood withdrawal. Over time, compression may lead to fracture of the catheter. A chest radiograph or fluoroscopic examination aids in diagnosis with immediate removal indicated if confirmed. A rare but life-threatening complication is fragmentation of a distal portion of the catheter with migration to the heart or pulmonary artery. Symptoms include shoulder and chest pain, palpitations and arrhythmias (Nace and Ingle 1993). Patients may be asymptomatic except for pain with attempted infusion (Dillon and Foglia 2006). Retrieval of the embolized catheter is generally accomplished by interventional radiology or cardiology using loop snares, baskets or guide wires (Sagar and Lederer 2004).

17.5.2 Drug Precipitate or Lipid Residue Occlusion

An intraluminal occlusion may result from precipitation of incompatible medications or lipid residue. Review of the patient's medications and parenteral nutrition formula may assist in evaluating the cause of occlusion. Precipitation resulting from calcium phosphate crystals or medications with a low pH may be cleared with 0.1 % hydrochloric acid (Baskin et al. 2009). However, many institutions refrain from this practice due to concern of catheter wall damage. Precipitations caused by high pH medications have been cleared by the use of sodium bicarbonate or sodium hydroxide (Baskin et al. 2009).

17.5.3 Thrombotic Occlusion

Fibrin begins forming on the external catheter wall within 24 h of insertion, starting at either the catheter entrance site into the vessel or where infused fluid comes into contact with the vessel wall. Blood cells adhere to the fibrin potentially interfering with blood flow and promoting bacterial growth. A variety of thrombotic occlusions are reported including fibrin sheath, mural thrombus and intraluminal thrombus (Fig. 17.2). Risk factors include prior catheterization of the same vessel, difficulty with insertion, poor tip placement, high catheter to vessel size ratio, suboptimal catheter care, underlying malignancy and type of chemotherapy (Kuter 2004). A fibrin sheath develops on the external catheter wall covering the catheter tip and resulting in withdrawal occlusion (Baskin et al. 2009). The sheath may extend up the entire length of the catheter with infused fluid traveling a path upward between the fibrin sheath and the catheter. Extravasation of medications and fluids is possible if the thrombus extends up to the site where the catheter enters the vessel (Mayo 1998). An intraluminal occlusion develops as a result of the buildup of fibrin and blood products with development of either a partial or complete occlusion. The incidence is decreased with strict adherence to institutional flush guidelines (Baskin et al. 2009). A mural thrombus forms as fibrin on the vessel wall attaches to fibrin covering the catheter. A withdrawal occlusion develops, but more significantly a mural thrombus may lead to venous thrombosis (Baskin et al. 2009).

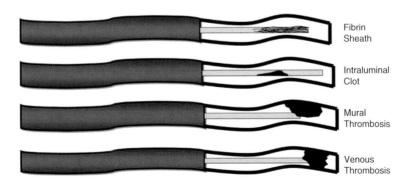

Fibrin Sheath

Intraluminal Clot

Mural Thrombosis

Venous Thrombosis

Fig. 17.2 Pictorial representation of central catheter occlusion and thrombosis (with permission from Baskin et al. [2009])

A suspected CVC-related thrombus may be evaluated by a radiographic study such as a dye study, computed tomography (CT) or ultrasound with Doppler flow (Fig. 17.3). However, common initial practice for treatment of a suspected thrombotic occlusion is instillation of a thrombolytic, most commonly tissue plasminogen activator (tPA) (Baskin et al. 2009). tPA converts plasminogen to plasmin resulting in local fibrinolysis (Fig. 17.4). tPA is simple and safe to use as well as being cost-effective. Our local institu-

tional protocol for administration of tPA for dwell and infusion is summarized in Table 17.3.

17.6 Central Venous Catheter-Related Deep Vein Thrombosis

A catheter-related thrombus (CRT) is generally the result of a mural thrombus that has enlarged, leading to complete occlusion of the vein. Kuter

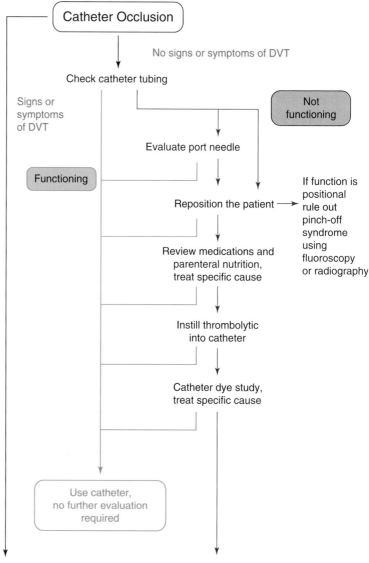

Fig. 17.3 Assessment of catheter occlusion (with permission from Baskin et al. [2009]). *DVT* deep venous thrombosis, *CT* computed tomography, *MRI* magnetic resonance imaging, *MRA* magnetic resonance arteriography

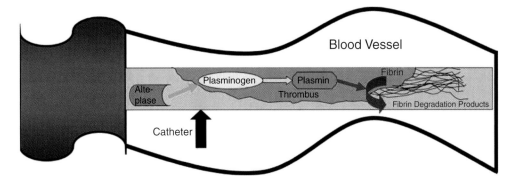

Fig. 17.4 Mechanism of action for tissue plasminogen activator (tPA) (with permission from Baskin et al. [2009])

(2004) reported an incidence of 5–41 % with differences related to a wide variety of catheter types, tip position, duration of insertion and underlying disease. Male et al. (2002) found a thrombosis rate of 29 % in a study of 66 children with ALL and a tunneled CVC. Clinical signs of a CRT include jaw, neck, chest, or shoulder pain, warmth, swelling, or development of visible collateral circulation. The majority of CRTs (up to 71 %) are asymptomatic, being diagnosed by imaging obtained to determine the cause of obstruction or with the occurrence of a pulmonary embolism (Kuter 2004).

17.6.1 Evaluation of Catheter-Related Thrombosis

Although the reference standard for the diagnosis of a CRT is contrast venography, compression ultrasound (CUS) with Doppler and color imaging is frequently used as CUS is noninvasive and does not require contrast medium (Rooden et al. 2005). In the patient with a negative CUS but a high clinical suspicion of a CRT, contrast venography is indicated (Rooden et al. 2005). Evaluation of the etiology of the CRT (in addition to the presence of a CVC) may guide treatment and prevention. A detailed family history of thrombosis will assist in determining the need for an evaluation for thrombophilia (see Chap. 8 for more detail). Other risk factors to consider are immobility, dehydration and administration of medications with thrombotic risk, particularly steroids and asparaginase (Table 17.4).

17.6.2 Treatment of Catheter-Related Thrombosis

Treatment of CRT is discussed in detail in Chap. 8 and is based on the 2012 American College of Chest Physicians (ACCP) guidelines with the following principles (Monagle et al. 2012):

- Anticoagulation therapy for 3 months following a first CRT.
- Continued anticoagulation with prophylactic dosing until removal of the CVC.
- For recurrent thrombosis during prophylaxis, increase to therapeutic dosing until line removal (but for a minimum of 3 months).
- A CVC that is no longer functional or required should be removed; a minimum of 3–5 days of anticoagulation at therapeutic dosing should be given prior to removal.

If a replacement CVC is medically indicated, consideration should be given to prophylactic anticoagulation to prevent recurrence of a thrombus. Low-molecular-weight heparin (LMWH) is an excellent anticoagulant for use in pediatrics due to predictable dosing (based on weight), limited need for blood level monitoring and short half-life. The updated 2012 ACCP guidelines recommend no routine monitoring of LMWH levels (Monagle et al. 2012). However, infants who are gaining weight and children with renal insufficiency do require monitoring to ensure appropriate levels. LMWH levels should be drawn 4 h after a dose (peak level) with a therapeutic target of 0.5–1 unit/mL. At least two to three doses should be given to reach steady state prior to obtaining a peak level.

Table 17.3 tPA dwell administration guidelines

General instructions
- Reconstitute tPA with 2.2 mL sterile water for injection (not bacteriostatic water) yielding a concentration of 1 mg/mL
- A 10 mL syringe is used for all dose administrations
- Instill one dose into each lumen of the catheter and allow to dwell for 30–120 min (optimal efficacy is achieved with a 120 min uninterrupted dwell time)
- A second dose is indicated if unable to obtain a brisk blood return after the initial treatment and dwell time

Broviac catheters
- Children <10 kg: dilute 0.5 mL tPA with 0.5 mL 0.9 % NaCl; instill 1 mL (0.5 mg) for each lumen
- Children ≥10 to <30 kg: 1 mL (1 mg) tPA for each lumen
- Children ≥30 kg: 2 mg (2 mL) tPA for each lumen

Implanted ports
- Children <10 kg: draw up 2.5 mL of 0.9 % NaCl into a 10 mL syringe and mix with 0.5 mL (0.5 mg) reconstituted tPA; total volume is 3 mL (0.5 mg) tPA
- Children ≥10 kg: draw up 1 mL 0.9 % NaCl into a 10 mL syringe and mix with 2 mL (2 mg) reconstituted tPA; total volume is 3 mL (2 mg) tPA

Completely occluded CVC
- Remove cap, cleanse hub per institutional policy and attach a 3-way stopcock to the catheter
- Attach tPA syringe to one of the stopcock ports
- Attach a 10 mL syringe to the remaining port
- Turn the stopcock off to the tPA syringe
- Gently pull back the plunger of the 10 mL syringe to the 3–5 mL mark and clamp the catheter to maintain negative pressure
- Turn the stopcock off to the 10 mL syringe
- Unclamp the catheter and allow tPA to be drawn into the line
- Clamp catheter, remove stopcock, apply positive pressure cap and allow tPA to dwell for 120 min
- May repeat a second dose of alteplase if needed

tPA (alteplase) infusion
If the CVC occlusion is not cleared after a second tPA dwell, a tPA infusion (6–24 h) may be indicated based on radiographic findings
Alteplase 0.03–0.06 mg/kg/h for 6–24 h
- Initial infusion 0.03 mg/kg/h for 6 h; if no clinical improvement (working line) may sequentially increase dose to 0.06 mg/kg/h (max 2 mg/h)
- Do not exceed 48–72 h of infusion
- Monitor patient for signs of sepsis as bacteria may be released into the bloodstream with dissolution of the thrombus
- Monitor labs including: PT, aPTT, fibrinogen, plasminogen, D-dimers, platelets; replete plasminogen with FFP for concentrations <50 %
- Repeat radiographic study to assess for improvement in dissolution of thrombus every 24 h
- Remove the catheter if the thrombus is not cleared after 48–72 h of tPA infusion (based on radiographic findings and functional improvement)

tPA tissue plasminogen activator, *PT* prothrombin time, *aPTT* activated partial thromboplastin time, *FFP* fresh frozen plasma

Table 17.4 Proposed risk factors for central venous catheter (CVC)-related thrombotic occlusions

Change in normal blood flow	Vascular endothelial damage	Hypercoagulable state
Immobility	Traumatic insertion	Malignancy
Large catheter to vessel ratio	Multiple insertion attempts	Sepsis
Dehydration	Catheter tip malposition	Chemotherapy
Compression of vessel by tumor	CVC placement time >14 days	Thrombophilia
Left-sided insertion		

17.6.3 Special Considerations During Anticoagulation Therapy

- LMWH should be held for 24 h prior to and 12 h after a lumbar puncture.
- LMWH should be held for 24 h prior to and 24 h after a minor surgical procedure.
- LMWH should be held during periods of thrombocytopenia (i.e., platelets <50×10⁹/L).

17.6.4 Contraindications of Anticoagulant Therapy

- Intracranial hemorrhage
- Ongoing hemorrhage
- Uncorrected coagulopathy
- Hypersensitivity to heparin or pork products
- Poor renal function (i.e., creatinine clearance < 30 mL/min)

17.7 Catheter Maintenance

Catheter maintenance refers to all activities undertaken to keep the line functioning properly while decreasing the risk of infection. CVC insertion bundles have dramatically reduced infectious complications related to surgical placement. Development of a maintenance bundle with institutional policies on hand hygiene, site cleansing, dressings, line flushing, hub care and line stabilization enhance catheter longevity and decrease morbidity (O'Grady et al. 2011). Hand hygiene, an inexpensive and easily implemented strategy, is the most effective measure in decreasing healthcare-associated infections (see Chap. 14) (Kline 2005).

17.7.1 Skin Antisepsis

Chlorhexidine has been shown to be a superior cleansing agent prior to CVC placement and for skin antisepsis with routine dressing changes. Chaiyakunapruk et al. (2002) reviewed 8 randomized controlled trials, totaling 4,143 catheters, comparing efficacy of chlorhexidine gluconate with povidone-iodine for skin disinfection. Results revealed a significant reduction in bloodstream infection with chlorhexidine.

17.7.2 Central Venous Catheter Dressings

CVC dressings serve a dual purpose: prevention of infection and stabilization of the line to decrease accidental removal. Semipermeable transparent and sterile gauze with tape are the two most commonly used types of dressings. The transparent dressing allows for evaporation of moisture and direct visualization of the site. Dressing changes are required every 5–7 days or more frequently as needed if the dressing becomes loose, wet, or soiled, which may decrease skin irritation and breakdown. A sterile gauze and tape dressing is recommended when there is bleeding or drainage at the site and for patients who are diaphoretic, requiring changes every 1–2 days. The literature has shown no difference in CLABSI rates between semipermeable transparent and sterile gauze and tape dressings (Mermel 2000; Gillies et al. 2003; O'Grady et al. 2011). The choice of dressing may be left to institutional guidelines or patient preference. Chlorhexidine has been shown to be the superior choice for skin antisepsis prior to CVC insertion (O'Grady et al. 2011). In the past decade several studies were undertaken to determine the effectiveness of a chlorhexidine-impregnated dressing (BIOPATCH, Johnson & Johnson, Somerville, NJ) in reducing rates of CLABSI. Findings revealed that although colonization was decreased there was no difference in the rate of CLABSI between semipermeable transparent dressings and BIOPATCH (Levy et al. 2005; Hatler et al. 2009).

17.7.3 Hub Care

Needleless connectors were introduced 20 years ago in an effort to decrease the incidence of needlestick injuries among healthcare workers.

Since then, emphasis has been placed on developing connectors that lessen the risk of CLABSI. Currently, several types of connectors are available, each with unique recommendations for flushing, locking and clamping the catheter. Strategies to decrease occlusion and CLABSI related to the use of needleless connectors include use of a single product within the institution, education on proper use including disinfection prior to access, and adherence to institutional policy for flushing and clamping.

Catheter hub colonization and contamination is a significant cause of CLABSI (Sannoh et al. 2010). In an observational study by Soothill et al. (2009), a change in catheter hub cleansing agent to 2 % chlorhexidine in 70 % isopropyl alcohol significantly decreased the rate of bloodstream infections in pediatric patients undergoing hematopoietic stem cell transplant. CDC guidelines recommend scrubbing the hub with friction for 15 s using 70 % isopropyl alcohol or 2 % chlorhexidine in 70 % isopropyl alcohol (O'Grady et al. 2011).

17.7.4 Central Venous Catheter Flushing and Locking

CVC flushing with normal saline is instrumental in assessing catheter patency and clearing the catheter after medication administration (preventing precipitation from incompatible drugs), blood sampling and blood transfusions. Locking a catheter, typically with heparinized saline, prevents reflux of blood into the catheter. However, wide variation exits in the frequency, concentration and volume of heparin utilized, with the majority of data from adult patients (Stephens et al. 1997; Hadaway 2006; Cesaro et al. 2009). Following institutional guidelines with ongoing assessment of efficacy and intermittent review of the literature will aid in decisions to change clinical practice. Examples of guidelines are in Tables 17.5 and 17.6.

Healthcare providers need to be cognizant of rare but potentially significant complications related to heparin locking solutions, specifically heparin-induced thrombocytopenia, heparin-induced thrombosis and bleeding. The cost and risk of replacing an occluded catheter outweigh the potential risks of heparin locks. A safe practice is strict adherence to institutional policy, awareness of potential complications and development of local expert resources.

17.7.5 New Strategies to Prevent Central Line-Associated Blood Stream Infection (CLABSI)

17.7.5.1 Chlorhexidine Bathing

Chlorhexidine has been shown to be effective in decreasing cutaneous colonization and is the recommended skin antiseptic prior to CVC insertion (O'Grady et al. 2002). Researchers are now investigating the effect of daily chlorhexidine bathing of pediatric oncology patients. Initial studies have demonstrated a significant decrease in CLABSI rates (Munoz-Price et al. 2009; Popovich et al. 2009; Montecalvo et al. 2012). A meta-analysis by O'Horo et al. (2012) concluded that the CLABSI rate is decreased in medical intensive care units with daily chlorhexidine bathing, whether 2 % chlorhexidine-impregnated cloths (Sage® products) or a 1:2 dilution of 4 % chlorhexidine was used. A current two-armed, randomized, double-blind study through the Children's Oncology Group is assessing the efficacy of 2 % chlorhexidine gluconate bathing in prevention of CLABSI in children with cancer and in those undergoing hematopoietic stem cell transplantation.

Table 17.5 Heparin lock guidelines

Device	Heparin strength, volume and frequency
PICC	2 F: 1 mL heparinized saline (10 U/mL) every 6 h
	2.6 F and larger: 2–3 mL heparinized saline (10 U/mL) every 12 h
Tunneled catheter	2 mL heparinized saline (10 U/mL) every 24 h
Implanted port	If locked >1 time daily: 5 mL heparinized saline (10 U/mL)
	Daily to monthly flush: 5 mL heparinized saline (100 U/mL)

PICC peripherally inserted central catheter, *F* French

Table 17.6 Example of central venous catheter (CVC) maintenance bundle

Care practice	Bundle recommendations
Hand hygiene	Hand hygiene performed before and after CVC insertion, care, and catheter entry or after contact with any inanimate object; use clean gloves for all CVC access as needed; glove use does not preclude use of hand hygiene
Surface disinfection	Clean work surfaces with germicidal wipe prior to CVC care
Use of maintenance kits/CVC cart	Procedure kits/carts containing supplies help to ensure all required supplies are available at the time of the procedure, including those required for insertion, dressing change and CVC removal
Insertion	*Bundle recommendations*
Hand hygiene	Hand hygiene is followed by waterless surgical scrub application
Maximal sterile barrier precautions	Patient is covered from head to toe with sterile drapes; mask, cap, sterile gown and sterile gloves during insertion procedure; all staff (including the assistant and family members) to wear regular face mask and cap when within 3 ft of sterile field
Skin antisepsis	Skin disinfected with chlorhexidine gluconate; apply back and forth friction scrub for 30 s and allow to dry completely for 30 s (2 min scrub for wet sites, such as the groin); site must be dry before skin puncture
Universal protocol utilized	Staff observers are skilled in monitoring elements of sterile technique; staff empowered to stop non-emergent procedure if sterile technique not followed
Assessment	*Bundle recommendations*
Ongoing assessment of catheter site	Inspect catheter site for cleanliness and dressing integrity; assess CVC site for complications hourly when infusing solutions and every 4 h when locked
Daily assessment of need for CVC	Discuss ongoing need for CVCs daily with medical team during rounds; assess patient for appropriateness of their vascular access device based on infusates/length of therapy and available vessels; promptly remove unnecessary CVCs
Catheter site care/management	*Bundle recommendations*
Skin antisepsis	Use clean gloves for all CVC access; maintain clean disposable towel or 4×4 gauze under CVC access port before accessing; skin disinfected with chlorhexidine gluconate; apply back and forth friction scrub for 30 s and allow to dry for 30 s (2 min scrub for wet sites, such as the groin)
CVC dressing assessment and change	Routine dressing changes performed by clinicians with demonstrated competency; use of catheter securement device with PICC dressing changes; mask and sterile gloves for dressing changes; dressing change frequency: transparent dressing, every 7 days and as needed for soiled dressing or loss of integrity; gauze and non-occlusive dressing, every 48 h and as needed
Antisepsis of needleless connectors, IV junctions and catheter hub	Vigorously scrub needleless connectors, IV junctions and hub (diaphragm and sides) prior to accessing with an alcohol swab using friction for a minimum of 15 s
CRBSI criteria	*Bundle recommendations*
Blood culture sampling	Consider DTP protocol when drawing blood cultures with significant time differential of CVC culture versus peripheral culture positivity of >2 h; generally peripheral blood cultures are not drawn on oncology patients who have central lines (see Chap. 1)
Administrative	*Bundle recommendations*
Education	Education of clinicians responsible for managing CVCs to include: care and maintenance strategies, identification and management of complications
Routine surveillance of CVCs	Collect and benchmark outcome data with the National Healthcare Safety Network

PICC peripherally inserted central catheter, *IV* intravenous, *CRBSI* catheter-related bloodstream infection, *DTP* differential time to positivity
Adapted from Mermel (2000), Marschall et al. (2008), Horan et al. (2011)

17.7.5.2 Antiseptic Needleless Connectors and Antiseptic Port Barrier Caps

Contamination of the CVC hub is the main source of CLABSI 10 days after insertion. Novel products are now available to decrease the incidence of this complication. Three such devices are currently marketed. *V-link with VitaShield* protective coating (Baxter) is a needleless connector with an antimicrobial coating (silver) on the interior and exterior surface. *Curos®* port protector is a barrier cap with a sponge saturated with 70 % isopropyl alcohol (IPA). Disinfection occurs 3 min after being threaded onto the connector. The cap may be left in place up to 7 days protecting the connector from airborne and contact contamination. Caps should be placed on all needleless injection sites and changed after each access. *Saralex-CL* (Menyhay) is an antimicrobial barrier cap that threads onto the needless connector bathing the connector in 2 % chlorhexidine gluconate in 70 % IPA. Disinfection occurs in 5 min and may be left in place up to 96 h. The cap protects the connector from airborne and contact contamination. A new cap is applied after each access.

A prospective simulation study by Menyhay and Maki (2006) evaluated the efficacy of cleansing a CVC hub with 70 % alcohol compared to the use of a Saralex barrier cap. One hundred five needleless connectors from three manufacturers were tested. The septum of each device was contaminated with *Enterococcus faecalis* and allowed to dry for 24 h. A control group of 15 connectors were not disinfected, 30 were cleansed with a 70 % alcohol swab and 60 had a Saralex barrier cap applied and removed after 10 min. Nutrient broth was injected through each connector, collected and cultured. Cultures from all control connectors were positive. Twenty connectors (67 %) with conventional disinfection with 70 % alcohol were culture positive, whereas only 1 (1.6 %) of the connectors disinfected with use of the Saralex cap was culture positive. Further study through randomized trials is needed to determine if practice changes are indicated.

17.8 Summary

CVCs are a central component in the care of pediatric oncology patients and allow for safe and effective administration of chemotherapeutic agents in addition to antibiotics, blood products, parenteral nutrition and multiple additional medications. Blood can be easily drawn from externally tunneled CVCs and in accessed implanted ports. Infection and thrombosis are the most common risk factors with CVC placement, and practitioners must be aware of the clinical signs and symptoms associated with these complications, methods to prevent these side effects, and treatment of these problems. Generally, practice and management are based on consensus guidelines and expert opinion as robust evidence is lacking, especially in pediatric patients.

References

Adler A, Yaniv I, Steinberg R et al (2006) Infectious complications of implantable ports and Hickman catheters in paediatric haematology-oncology patients. J Hosp Infect 62:358–365

Alomari A, Falk A (2006) Median nerve bisection: a morbid complication of a peripherally inserted central catheter. J Vasc Access 7:129–131

Augoustides JG, Cheung AT (2009) Pro: ultrasound should be the standard of care for central catheter insertion. J Cardiothorac Vasc Anesth 23:720–724

Baggott CR, Kelly KP, Fochtman D, Foley GV (eds.) (2002) Nursing care of children and adolescents with cancer, 3rd edn. Elsevier Saunders, Philadelphia

Balls A, LoVecchio F, Kroeger A et al (2010) Ultrasound guidance for central venous catheter placement: results from the Central Line Emergency Access Registry Database. Am J Emerg Med 28:561–567

Bard Access Systems. https://www.bardaccess.com. Accessed 21 Apr 2014

Baskin JL, Pui CH, Reiss U et al (2009) Management of occlusion and thrombosis associated with long-term indwelling central venous catheters. Lancet 374:159–169

Burns D (2005) The Vanderbilt PICC service: program, procedural, and patient outcomes successes. J Assoc Vasc Access 10:183–192

Cesaro S, Tridello G, Cavaliere M et al (2009) Prospective, randomized trial of two different modalities of flushing central venous catheters in pediatric patients with cancer. J Clin Oncol 27:2059–2065

Chaiyakunapruk N, Veenstra DL, Lipsky BA, Saint S (2002) Chlorhexidine compared with povidone-iodine solution for vascular catheter-site care: a meta-analysis. Ann Intern Med 136:792–801

Deshpande KS, Hatem C, Ulrich HL et al (2005) The incidence of infectious complications of central venous catheters at the subclavian, internal jugular, and femoral sites in an intensive care unit population. Crit Care Med 33:13–20

Dillon PA, Foglia RP (2006) Complications associated with an implantable vascular access device. J Pediatr Surg 41:1582–1587

Donlan RM (2011) Biofilm elimination on intravascular catheters: important considerations for the infectious disease practitioner. Clin Infect Dis 52:1038–1045

Eisen LA, Narasimhan M, Berger JS et al (2006) Mechanical complications of central venous catheters. J Intensive Care Med 21:40–46

Fazeny-Dorner B, Wenzel C, Berzlanovich A et al (2003) Central venous catheter pinch-off and fracture: recognition, prevention and management. Bone Marrow Transplant 31:927–930

Gillies D, O'Riordan E, Carr D et al (2003) Central venous catheter dressings: a systematic review. J Adv Nurs 44:623–632

Gonzalez G, Davidoff AM, Howard SC et al (2012) Safety of central venous catheter placement at diagnosis of acute lymphoblastic leukemia in children. Pediatr Blood Cancer 58:498–502

Hadaway L (2006) Heparin locking for central venous catheters. J Assoc Vasc Access 11:224–231

Handrup MM, Moller JK, Frydenberg M, Schroder H (2010) Placing of tunneled central venous catheters prior to induction chemotherapy in children with acute lymphoblastic leukemia. Pediatr Blood Cancer 55:309–313

Hatler C, Buckwald L, Salas-Allison Z, Murphy-Taylor C (2009) Evaluating central venous catheter care in a pediatric intensive care unit. Am J Crit Care 18:514–520

Horan TC, Arnold KE, Rebmann CA, Fridkin SK (2011) Network approach for prevention of healthcare-associated infections. Infect Control Hosp Epidemiol 32:1143–1144

Kline AM (2005) Pediatric catheter-related bloodstream infections: latest strategies to decrease risk. AACN Clin Issues 16:185–198

Kusminsky RE (2007) Complications of central venous catheterization. J Am Coll Surg 204:681–696

Kuter DJ (2004) Thrombotic complications of central venous catheters in cancer patients. Oncologist 9:207–216

Lefrant JY, Muller L, De La Coussaye JE et al (2002) Risk factors of failure and immediate complication of subclavian vein catheterization in critically ill patients. Intensive Care Med 28:1036–1041

Levy I, Katz J, Solter E et al (2005) Chlorhexidine-impregnated dressing for prevention of colonization of central venous catheters in infants and children: a randomized controlled study. Pediatr Infect Dis J 24:676–679

Maki DG, Kluger DM, Crnich CJ (2006) The risk of bloodstream infection in adults with different intravascular devices: a systematic review of 200 published prospective studies. Mayo Clin Proc 81:1159–1171

Male C, Chait P, Ginsberg JS et al (2002) Comparison of venography and ultrasound for the diagnosis of asymptomatic deep vein thrombosis in the upper body in children: results of the PARKAA study. Prophylactic Antithrombin Replacement in Kids with ALL treated with Asparaginase. Thromb Haemost 87:593–598

Mansfield PF, Hohn DC, Fornage BD et al (1994) Complications and failures of subclavian-vein catheterization. N Engl J Med 331:1735–1738

Marschall J, Mermel LA, Classen D et al (2008) Strategies to prevent central line-associated bloodstream infections in acute care hospitals. Infect Control Hosp Epidemiol 29:S22–S30

Mayo DJ (1998) Fibrin sheath formation and chemotherapy extravasation: a case report. Support Care Cancer 6:51–56

McGee DC, Gould MK (2003) Preventing complications of central venous catheterization. N Engl J Med 348:1123–1133

McLean TW, Fisher CJ, Snively BM, Chauvenet AR (2005) Central venous lines in children with lesser risk acute lymphoblastic leukemia: optimal type and timing of placement. J Clin Oncol 23:3024–3029

Menyhay SZ, Maki DG (2006) Disinfection of needleless catheter connectors and access ports with alcohol may not prevent microbial entry: the promise of a novel antiseptic-barrier cap. Infect Control Hosp Epidemiol 27:23–27

Mermel LA (2000) Prevention of intravascular catheter-related infections. Ann Intern Med 132:391–402

Mermel LA, Allon M, Bouza E et al (2009) Clinical practice guidelines for the diagnosis and management of intravascular catheter-related infection: 2009 update by the Infectious Diseases Society of America. Clin Infect Dis 49:1–45

Monagle P, Chan AK, Goldenberg NA et al (2012) Antithrombotic therapy in neonates and children: antithrombotic therapy and prevention of thrombosis, 9th ed: American College of chest physicians evidence-based clinical practice guidelines. Chest 141:e737S–e801S

Montecalvo MA, McKenna D, Yarrish R et al (2012) Chlorhexidine bathing to reduce central venous catheter-associated bloodstream infection: impact and sustainability. Am J Med 125:505–511

Munoz-Price LS, Hota B, Stemer A, Weinstein RA (2009) Prevention of bloodstream infections by use of daily chlorhexidine baths for patients at a long-term acute care hospital. Infect Control Hosp Epidemiol 30:1031–1035

Nace CS, Ingle RJ (1993) Central venous catheter "pinch-off" and fracture: a review of two under-recognized complications. Oncol Nurs Forum 20:1227–1236

O'Grady NP, Alexander M, Dellinger EP et al (2002) Guidelines for the prevention of intravascular catheter-related infections. Centers for Disease Control and Prevention. MMWR Recomm Rep 51:1–29

O'Grady NP, Alexander M, Burns LA et al (2011) Guidelines for the prevention of intravascular catheter-related infections. Clin Infect Dis 52:e162–e193

O'Horo JC, Silva GL, Munoz-Price LS, Safdar N (2012) The efficacy of daily bathing with chlorhexidine for reducing healthcare-associated bloodstream infections: a meta-analysis. Infect Control Hosp Epidemiol 33:257–267

Perdikaris P, Petsios K, Vasilatou-Kosmidis H, Matziou V (2008) Complications of Hickman-Broviac catheters in children with malignancies. Pediatr Hematol Oncol 25:375–384

Pettit J (2002) Assessment of infants with peripherally inserted central catheters: part 1. Detecting the most frequently occurring complications. Adv Neonatal Care 2:304–315

Pittiruti M, Hamilton H, Biffi R et al (2009) ESPEN guidelines on parenteral nutrition: central venous catheters (access, care, diagnosis and therapy of complications). Clin Nutr 28:365–377

Popovich KJ, Hota B, Hayes R et al (2009) Effectiveness of routine patient cleansing with chlorhexidine gluconate for infection prevention in the medical intensive care unit. Infect Control Hosp Epidemiol 30:959–963

Raad I, Costerton W, Sabharwal U et al (1993) Ultrastructural analysis of indwelling vascular catheters: a quantitative relationship between luminal colonization and duration of placement. J Infect Dis 168:400–407

Randolph AG, Cook DJ, Gonzales CA, Pribble CG (1996) Ultrasound guidance for placement of central venous catheters: a meta-analysis of the literature. Crit Care Med 24:2053–2058

Rooden CJ, Tesselaar ME, Osanto S et al (2005) Deep vein thrombosis associated with central venous catheters–a review. J Thromb Haemost 3:2409–2419

Sagar V, Lederer E (2004) Pulmonary embolism due to catheter fracture from a tunneled dialysis catheter. Am J Kidney Dis 43:e13–e14

Sannoh S, Clones B, Munoz J et al (2010) A multimodal approach to central venous catheter hub care can decrease catheter-related bloodstream infection. Am J Infect Control 38:424–429

Schulmeister L (2010) Management of non-infectious central venous access device complications. Semin Oncol Nurs 26:132–141

Soothill JS, Bravery K, Ho A et al (2009) A fall in bloodstream infections followed a change to 2 % chlorhexidine in 70 % isopropanol for catheter connection antisepsis: a pediatric single center before/after study on a hematopoietic stem cell transplant ward. Am J Infect Control 37:626–630

Stephens LC, Haire WD, Kotulak GD (1995) Are clinical signs accurate indicators of the cause of central venous catheter occlusion? JPEN J Parenter Enteral Nutr 19:75–79

Stephens LC, Haire WD, Tarantolo S et al (1997) Normal saline versus heparin flush for maintaining central venous catheter patency during apheresis collection of peripheral blood stem cells (PBSC). Transfus Sci 18:187–193

Teichgraber UK, Pfitzmann R, Hofmann HA (2011) Central venous port systems as an integral part of chemotherapy. Dtsch Arztebl Int 108:147–153

Theaker C, Juste R, Lucas N (2002) Comparison of bacterial colonization rates of antiseptic impregnated and pure polymer central venous catheters in the critically ill. J Hosp Infect 52:310–312

Troianos CA, Hartman GS, Glas KE et al (2011) Guidelines for performing ultrasound guided vascular cannulation: recommendations of the American Society of Echocardiography and the Society of Cardiovascular Anesthesiologists. J Am Soc Echocardiogr 24:1291–1318

Walder B, Pittet D, Tramer MR (2002) Prevention of bloodstream infections with central venous catheters treated with anti-infective agents depends on catheter type and insertion time: evidence from a meta-analysis. Infect Control Hosp Epidemiol 23:748–756

Yamamoto AJ, Solomon JA, Soulen MC et al (2002) Sutureless securement device reduces complications of peripherally inserted central venous catheters. J Vasc Interv Radiol 13:77–81

Zakrzewska-Bode A, Muytjens HL, Liem KD, Hoogkamp-Korstanje JA (1995) Mupirocin resistance in coagulase-negative staphylococci, after topical prophylaxis for the reduction of colonization of central venous catheters. J Hosp Infect 31:189–193

Knowledge Gaps and Opportunities for Research

18

Anurag K. Agrawal, Caroline A. Hastings, and James H. Feusner

Abstract

Through the process of researching, writing and editing this book, many knowledge gaps within supportive care for pediatric oncology patients are quite evident, leading to a multitude of possible avenues for research in the supportive care field. Although the majority of research dollars go toward projects whose goal is to improve patient survival through treatment of the underlying malignancy, improvement in supportive care practices has been a vital aspect of the survival gains made to date. Continued assessment and advancement in this field will continue to yield results in improvement in patient quality of life and potentially treatment-related morbidity and mortality. Here we outline some of the areas that necessitate further work.

Through the process of researching, writing and editing this book, many knowledge gaps within supportive care for pediatric oncology patients are quite evident, leading to a multitude of possible avenues for research in the supportive care field. Although the majority of research dollars go toward projects whose goal is to improve patient survival through treatment of the underlying malignancy, improvement in supportive care practices has been a vital aspect of the survival gains made to date. Continued assessment and advancement in this field will continue to yield results in improvement in patient quality of life and potentially treatment-related morbidity and mortality. Here we outline some of the areas that necessitate further work.

As a general practice, pediatric oncology patients with febrile neutropenia continue to be monitored in the inpatient setting. Although multiple groups have devised risk stratification models, none of these have been validated across populations—further research is required to validate one risk stratification model. As a corollary to this question is the development of standard criteria for outpatient management of febrile neutropenia as well as early discharge criteria for low-risk patients. Although many institutions have developed local protocols to define low-risk populations that can be managed as outpatients

A.K. Agrawal (✉) • C.A. Hastings • J.H. Feusner
Department of Hematology/Oncology,
Children's Hospital and Research Center Oakland,
747 52nd Street, Oakland, CA 94609, USA
e-mail: aagrawal@mail.cho.org

J. Feusner et al. (eds.), *Supportive Care in Pediatric Oncology:*
A Practical Evidence-Based Approach, Pediatric Oncology,
DOI 10.1007/978-3-662-44317-0_18, © Springer Berlin Heidelberg 2015

after an initial inpatient stay, work remains to determine more universal criteria that can be used across institutions which will both improve patient and family quality of life as well as decrease healthcare costs. Duration of antimicrobial therapy both in patients with febrile neutropenia without a source as well as in those with a proven infection in the face of continued neutropenia is undefined. Many practitioners will continue antibiotics until count recovery even if the patient has no known source of infection and has defervesced. It is unclear if this is necessary and potentially can lead to side effects such as antibiotic-associated diarrhea and development of *C. difficile* as well as development of resistant bacterial strains. Similarly, for the patient with a known source who has cleared the infection with negative cultures and a sufficient time on antibiotics, it is unclear whether antibiotics can be discontinued or should be continued through some period of count recovery.

Prevention of infection continues to have many questions. The role of bacterial prophylaxis is still unclear and is generally not utilized although may be beneficial in high-risk populations; this question is currently being researched by the Children's Oncology Group in a study of levofloxacin prophylaxis in high-risk patients. Similarly, it remains unclear if central venous catheter lock therapy, either with ethanol or antibiotics, has universal benefit in the prevention of infection in pediatric oncology patients. Although lock therapy is not standard at our institution, it likely is used in other institutional protocols; whether such a protocol should be universal is unanswered. The benefit of chlorhexidine bathing as a method to prevent central venous catheter infection is also currently being studied by the Children's Oncology Group. The management of fungal prophylaxis also remains an area with many unanswered questions. Additional biomarkers of invasive fungal infection such as polymerase chain reaction (PCR) and $(1,3)$-β-D glucan require further testing and validation in the pediatric oncology population. Similarly, underlying genetic markers which may impact the development of invasive fungal infection are unknown. The utility of empiric antifungal therapy in febrile neutropenia beyond patients with acute myelogenous leukemia and those undergoing hematopoietic stem cell transplantation remains undefined as to which additional pediatric oncology cohorts may benefit; in addition, appropriate choice of antifungal as well as dose required (prophylactic versus treatment dosing) remains unclear. Additional questions include the optimal fluconazole prophylaxis dose and when anti-mold coverage is important as prophylaxis. Finally, pediatric data are lacking in regard to a preemptive or prophylactic approach with viral infection.

Although utilization of packed red blood cells and platelets for anemia and thrombocytopenia is generally standard for pediatric oncology patients, little research has investigated the iron burden associated with frequent red blood cell transfusion in high-risk patients such as those with acute myelogenous leukemia, relapsed leukemia, or high-risk acute lymphoblastic leukemia and those patients undergoing hematopoietic stem cell transplantation. How this transfusional iron burden impacts the development of late effects such as notably long-term left ventricular dysfunction with concomitant anthracyclines and potentially metabolic syndrome with liver and pancreatic iron burden is unstudied. Similarly, appropriate hemoglobin thresholds for anesthesia and hemoglobin and platelet thresholds for different types of surgical procedures are unknown in pediatric oncology patients. The current thresholds utilized may lead to increased transfusions than what is safely necessary, posing both short- and long-term risks. Secondarily, utilization of higher red blood cell thresholds as a radiosensitizer is often utilized and advocated by radiation oncologists, although data describing the utility of this approach in impacting response and survival are unknown; again, patients may be unnecessarily receiving additional blood products with the perception that such a strategy is low-risk when in fact such a mentality may be increasing long-term risks for survivors. Pediatric oncology patients receive frequent red blood cell transfusion over the historic standard of 4 hours, although more rapid rate of transfusion in the patient with normal underlying cardiopulmonary status would likely be safe, decrease time in the hospital and infusion centers, and improve quality of life parameters but has not been investigated. Finally, utility of granulocyte transfusion in patients that are severely ill with profound neutropenia requires further evidence to determine whether this is a useful and cost-effective strategy.

As with many supportive care practices, utilization of newer, more expensive therapies often becomes the "standard" without proper, systematic study. Recommendations for rasburicase are a prime example of such a practice, and further evidence is required to determine the appropriate dose and proper utilization of this expensive agent as the majority of patients can be managed safely and effectively without rasburicase. One argument for the use of rasburicase is the effect of xanthine precursors on the development of acute kidney injury in patients with hyperuricemia on allopurinol. This theory remains unproven and is not a satisfactory reason to use rasburicase at this time without further study. Finally, settings exist where urine alkalinization may still be valuable, such as in the patient with hyperuricemia but without hyperphosphatemia or evidence of need for rasburicase. What the appropriate parameters are for the use of alkalinization with the availability of rasburicase is also unknown.

Multiple new pharmacologic agents are being tested and utilized in adult oncology patients but are as yet to make it downstream to pediatric oncology patients. These agents all require further pediatric study to determine their potential benefit and cost-effectiveness. For example, newer 5-HT$_3$ receptor antagonists such as palonosetron may be more effective both from a therapeutic and cost standpoint in pediatric cancer patients due to frequency of dosing required (i.e., one versus multiple doses), but further evidence is required on appropriate dosing and efficacy. Palonosetron has shown benefit in delayed chemotherapy-induced nausea and vomiting and likely with be useful in the pediatric population. Neurokinin-1 (NK$_1$) receptor antagonists (aprepitant; substance P antagonists) have been shown to be beneficial in chemotherapy-induced nausea and vomiting in adult oncology patients, and aprepitant has begun being utilized in pediatric

patients although further study is required to determine the appropriate weight-based dosing as well as to delineate whether the drug is effective from a therapeutic and cost standpoint in this cohort. Interaction between aprepitant and chemotherapy remains a concern and requires more investigation before routine use of this new antiemetic. Palifermin, a keratinocyte growth factor, has potential benefit in the prevention and treatment of severe oral mucositis in high-risk pediatric oncologic and transplant populations; further evidence is required as to which pediatric populations may benefit from this expensive medication. Many institutions are still utilizing filgrastim as opposed to pegfilgrastim with potential decrement in quality of life with the necessity of daily subcutaneous doses as compared to one single dose of pegfilgrastim. The therapeutic and cost-efficacy of pegfilgrastim in pediatric oncology patients needs further study although this agent could likely be used more universally in our population. Oral anti-Xa inhibitors (e.g., rivaroxaban) are being utilized in adult patients for treatment and prophylaxis of thrombosis; early-phase studies are being conducted in pediatric patients with thrombosis and can likely be generalized to the pediatric oncology cohort with benefit in quality of life with an oral as compared to subcutaneous (i.e., low-molecular-weight heparin) medication. With the advent of oral anti-Xa inhibitors, it will become more crucial to delineate pediatric oncology risk factors for development of venous thromboembolism and secondarily determine a population that would benefit from anticoagulation prophylaxis as is utilized in the adult setting. Finally, subcutaneous methylnaltrexone has shown benefit in opioid-induced constipation without reduction in pain control and should be further studied in the pediatric oncology population, especially those receiving palliative therapy.

Many other supportive care interventions have shown promise in the adult literature but require more rigorous study in the pediatric oncology cohort. Low-level laser therapy in the prevention and treatment of oral mucositis, especially in the transplant population, has been shown beneficial in adult patients but needs more systematic study in the pediatric population. Glutamine, previously studied by the Children's Oncology Group, may have benefit in the prevention and treatment of oral mucositis but more evidence is required. Similarly, utilization of multiple complementary and alternative therapies for pain management as well as prevention and treatment of mucositis and chemotherapy-induced nausea and vomiting require further study. Finally, systematic review of medications for appetite stimulation, especially cannabinoids, is necessary to make evidence-based recommendations.

Genetic risk factors that may impact treatment and side effects of cancer therapy are generally unknown in oncology patients but are likely to significantly affect our approach to cancer therapy in the future. Currently it has been shown that over- and undernutrition impacts both therapeutic efficacy and development of side effects. Whether there are underlying genetic factors which regulate this effect is unknown; appropriate dosing in these populations also needs to be further delineated. Similarly, genetic factors which may modulate the development of invasive fungal infection, chemotherapy-induced nausea and vomiting, pain, mucositis, and acute radiation side effects are undefined. The effect of such genetic factors on the development of long-term complications of cancer therapy such as left ventricular dysfunction is also unknown but likely significant.

Other areas for consideration include the appropriate utilization of blood draws and imaging, both during and after the completion of therapy. Currently blood draws are done with frequency even after the completion of leukemia therapy; whether this is necessary and cost-effective is unknown. Similarly, imaging is done quite frequently during and after completion of therapy for solid tumors. Evidence is mounting that frequency of computed tomography (CT) should be curtailed both due to the long-term risks of radiation and the ability to diagnosis occult relapse. Magnetic resonance imaging (MRI) can likely replace CT for acute abdominal pathology as well as for surveillance, although again, the necessity of frequent scanning as surveillance after therapy completion is in question.

Finally, appropriate supportive care in unique populations, specifically those with Down syndrome and adolescent and young adult (AYA) patients, is yet to be defined but has special features which must be considered such as increased toxicity in both patient cohorts. Though not specifically discussed in this book, evidence-based guidelines for long-term follow-up are lacking and will become increasingly important as more survivors reach adulthood and need to be transitioned to competent adult care. Important components such as nutritional and cardiac health must be addressed so that practitioners can make effective interventions that impact longer-term health.

Paralleling gains in overall survival, supportive care in pediatric oncology has made great strides in the last 50 years and has been a vital component in the effective treatment of these patients. Lower resource settings which are developing pediatric oncology programs must be cognizant of the importance of building a supportive care infrastructure concomitant with the development of pediatric treatment protocols and chemotherapy drug pipelines. Without these elements in concert, treatment of these patients will not be effective. As shown here, a multitude of areas of research remain to optimize the supportive care of pediatric oncology patients which, at the minimum, will improve quality of life and may ultimately impact morbidity and mortality.